S0-BTZ-867

Pathology
OF THE Fetus
& THE Infant

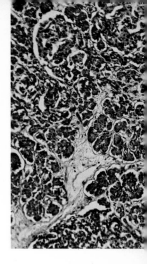

EDITH LOUISE POTTER, M.D., PH.D.

Doutor Honoris Causa (Brasil)
Doctor of Medical Sciences, Women's Medical College of Pennsylvania
Professor Emeritus of Pathology, Department of Obstetrics
and Gynecology, University of Chicago
Former Pathologist, Chicago Lying-in Hospital

JOHN M. CRAIG, M.D.

Pathologist-in-Chief, Boston Hospital for Women
Professor of Pathology, Harvard Medical School
Consultant in Pathology, Children's Hospital Medical Center
Boston, Massachusetts

YEAR BOOK MEDICAL PUBLISHERS · INC.
35 EAST WACKER DRIVE · CHICAGO

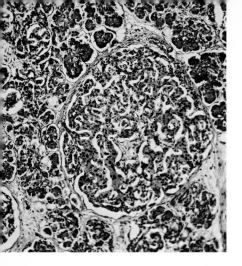

PATHOLOGY

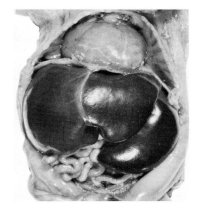

OF The Fetus

AND The Infant

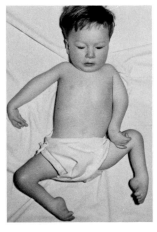

THIRD EDITION

Reprinted, 1953

Reprinted, 1957

Second Edition, 1961

Reprinted, 1962

Third Edition, 1975

Library of Congress Catalog Card Number: 75-16021
International Standard Book Number: 0-8151-6760-1

Preface to Third Edition

MORE THAN a quarter of a century now has passed since preparation of the material included in this book first was commenced, and in that time the scope of our knowledge related to the fetus and young infant has increased immeasurably. Thirty years ago publications were few and widely scattered and interest in this age period was very limited. Because of this it seemed possible that by bringing together information derived from wide reading and an extensive personal experience, help might be provided for those engaged in disciplines concerned with this age period and that enough interest might be stimulated in the problems of the physiology and pathology of the newborn to initiate research into these areas. What part this book may have played in the gradual growth of interest is impossible to know, but now the condition of the unborn and newly born infant and the processes responsible for its development and state of health are major subjects of investigation and clinical interest. The fetus has become recognized as an individual whose welfare can be modified and who can be treated before birth. Improvement in care of the pregnant and parturient woman as well as improved delivery room care of the newborn have increased the chances of survival of the infant and its growth into a healthy child. Fetology and neonatology have become recognized branches of pediatrics and are constantly assuming increasingly important roles.

The present edition of this book was prepared in order to add new and important information to the basic material contained in the earlier editions. The pathologic lesions resulting from specific causes do not change, but the relative frequency with which they are observed may be greatly modified and their significance more completely understood. Some abnormalities, such as the intracranial hemorrhage that results from birth injury and which was such a frequent cause of death earlier in this century, have now largely disappeared. On the other hand, the then little-known viruses, inborn errors of metabolism, chromosomal abnormalities, fetal-maternal incompatibility and so on now have become widely recognized as causes of disease and death. We have learned a great deal about the illnesses for which they are responsible and the pathologic lesions they produce.

Inasmuch as the senior author has retired from the active practice of pathology, it was thought desirable to enlist the aid of a younger pathologist still intimately concerned with the problems of fetuses and young infants and who is associated with another large maternity hospital. Consequently, Dr. John Craig of the Boston Hospital for Women has helped with this revision and is responsible for most of the new material included in the text. He is indebted to Dr. Gordon Vawter for allowing access to material from the Children's Hospital Medical Center. Both authors are indebted also to other collaborators and to the staff of the Year Book Medical Publishers for unfailing assistance and encouragement. It is hoped that the book will find a place in the working library of all pathologists, pediatricians and obstetricians.

—E. L. P.

Preface to First Edition

For the past 18 years I have been intensely interested in the fetus as it develops in the uterus and in the infant as it adapts, after birth, to a new environment and a new type of existence. This interest has included the normal variations in growth and development, the physiologic adjustments necessitated by birth, and the behavior of the newborn infant as well as the more extreme variations that are generally considered pathologic.

The pathologist is too often considered as living in a world apart from clinical medicine, but nothing is farther from the truth. The aim of the pathologist is to promote the well-being of the living by any means at his disposal; and one of the avenues of approach is a study of the dead. The death of a fetus or infant is even yet often taken as "an act of God," regrettable but unexplainable, and dismissed as unavoidable. Every time a sperm cell and ovum unite a new being is created which is alive and which will continue to live unless its death is brought about by some specific condition. What the lethal factors are is to some extent still unknown, especially in the very young fetus, but our knowledge is being increased constantly and this is being reflected in the decreasing stillbirth and infant mortality rates.

The description of the body of a dead infant is of no value as an isolated piece of information, but if it is integrated with the various aspects of heredity, conception, development, intrauterine and extrauterine environment and behavior it becomes part of an important chronicle. Only by correlating all the facts of one case with all those of many cases can we hope to elicit the etiologic factors responsible for clinical and pathologic observations. Needless to say, studies in the associated disciplines of embryology, anatomy, physiology and chemistry are necessitated in the attempt to answer the questions constantly being posed by the abnormalities under observation.

In addition to the ultimate aim of the pathologist, of immediate practical importance is the demonstration to the attending physician of the pathologic changes found in any fetus or infant who fails to survive and the correlation of these findings with the symptoms observed during life. When symptoms can be recognized as associated with specific pathologic processes a great stride has been made toward their prevention and cure.

The pathology of the fetus and young infant has until recently been greatly neglected. The pathologic changes that occur during the infant's brief life are often meager and overlooked by the inexperienced investigator. He becomes discouraged and loses interest because he sees little and does not know how to interpret even the little that he may discover. This volume has been prepared to help those who are attempting to discover the reasons for nonsurvival and to stimulate those who have the opportunity and the material with which to work. It is also hoped that it will be of practical value to the pediatrician and the obstetrician as well as to the pathologist. An attempt has been made to present a brief but complete picture of the infant and to correlate its embryologic development, intrauterine environment and postnatal physiologic adaptations with specific conditions responsible for morbidity and mortality. Only if this work ultimately helps save the lives of infants who otherwise might die will it have been worth the effort expended in its production.

During the time that material for this book has been collected, over 6,000 autopsies have been performed at the Chicago Lying-in Hospital on infants and fetuses dying in that hospital and those received from other sources, and tissues have been examined from over 3,000 additional autopsies performed elsewhere by pathologists from the Chicago Department of Health. During this period more than 50,000 infants have been delivered in the Chicago Lying-in Hospital. In addition, it has been possible to review over 10,000 protocols of autopsies on liveborn infants dying under 1 year of age from other hospitals in Chicago.

Our material has rarely included children over 1 year of age and much of it is limited to the fetus and newborn. As a result, the greatest emphasis is placed on the latter groups, but since a few important conditions may not be manifested until slightly beyond the newborn period, other lesions that may be found during the first three months of extrauterine life have been included. This takes the infant through the first year of life, dating from conception, and by this time most of the conditions that are found during any part of infancy are at least occasionally observed.

This first year is unique in the life of any individual. During three fourths of it, existence is parasitic and the environment is very limited. The last one fourth is a period of transition and a time of adaptation to extrauterine conditions and an independent existence. Pathologic disturbances are much less varied than later and are largely a result of abnormal development, of trauma incurred in passage through the birth canal and of interference with oxygenation as a result either of disturbance in circulation through the cord or placenta before birth or of inadequate functioning of the lungs after birth. Infections are responsible for a fairly large number of deaths; in fact, for many more deaths in the newborn period than in later infancy even though during the latter part of the first year after birth they are the cause of a much greater proportion of the total deaths.

I am extremely grateful to the many people who have contributed directly or indirectly to this project. These are, of course, especially the members of the Department of Obstetrics and Gynecology of the Chicago Lying-in Hospital, the pediatric staff of the Bobs Roberts Memorial Hospital, the staff of the Department of Pathology of the Albert Merritt Billings Hospital and the Photographic Department, all of The University of Chicago Clinics. The Chicago Department of Health has contributed immeasurably. The Department of Puericultura of the University of Brazil made it possible to compare at first hand the conditions affecting infants in Rio de Janeiro with those in Chicago. Individuals in Australia, Turkey, Czechoslovakia, England, Scotland, Canada, Mexico, Argentina, Brazil and many parts of the United States have supplied specimens or photographs of unusual conditions.

One always expects publishers to do a good job, but the staff of the Year Book Publishers have exerted themselves so far beyond what is ordinarily expected that words become an inadequate expression of appreciation. To them and to the many others who have contributed so much, I am immeasurably indebted.

—E.L.P.

Table of Contents

1

Early Development of the Fetus and Placenta

Ovulation

OVULATION NORMALLY TAKES PLACE near the middle of the intermenstrual period, most often between the 12th and 16th days counting from the 1st day of menstruation. It is convenient to use the 1st day of the last menstruation before the beginning of pregnancy to calculate the expected date of delivery, and most often pregnancy ends in approximately 40 weeks. The fetus, however, at this time is only 38 weeks old.

It is customary for embryologists to calculate age from a known or assumed date of ovulation but it is common clinical practice to estimate age from the last menstrual period, and many of the discrepancies in measurement of fetuses at stated ages are due to the use by some investigators of actual age and by others of so-called menstrual age.

Endometrial Changes Incident to Pregnancy

At the time of ovulation, the endometrium, under the influence of estrogen from the developing follicle, is composed of long, slightly undulating glands lined by tall columnar cells that show little secretory activity. They are separated by loose connective tissue stroma. After ovulation, under the influence of progesterone from the newly formed corpus luteum, the glands increase in length and tortuosity, and their constituent cells enlarge as they become actively secretory. The cells of the stroma increase in size and prominence. If pregnancy is established, either in the uterus or in an abnormal location, the enlargement of the stromal cells and the secretory changes in the glands become still more pro-

nounced and the endometrium is known as decidua. With these changes the endometrial lining of the uterus greatly thickens, a condition that has been called gestational hyperplasia (Hertig). The parts of the glands running through the superficial decidua are less tortuous than those in the deeper portions, and the stromal cells are proportionately more numerous. This superficial one third is known as the decidua compacta because of the close approximation of the large stromal cells. The term decidual cells is often applied to these cells although they have no more right to this name than do the cells lining the glands. The deeper two thirds of the decidua is called the decidua spongiosa because of the spongy appearance produced by the great tortuosity of the actively secreting glands and the relative lack of stromal cells (Fig. 1–1).

Fertilization

Fertilization is ordinarily accomplished in the outer third of the fallopian tube. Sperm cells do not appear to survive more than 24 hours in the vagina, and Hertig concluded from his own observations that the normal life of the ovum after expulsion from the ovary is limited to 8 hours. After that time degenerative changes begin to take place, and even if the egg is fertilized, abortion or malformation is the usual outcome. Consequently the introduction of sperm cells into the vagina must coincide closely with ovulation in order to permit normal fertilization.

The ovum, when liberated from the ovary, has already completed the first meiotic division and begun the preliminary stages of the second. If it is

1

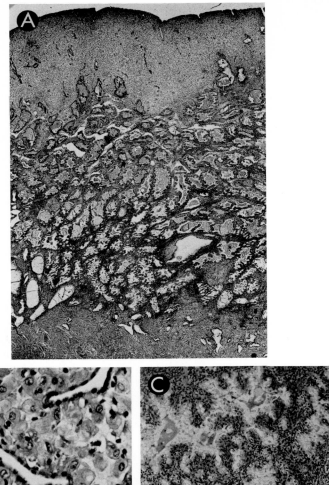

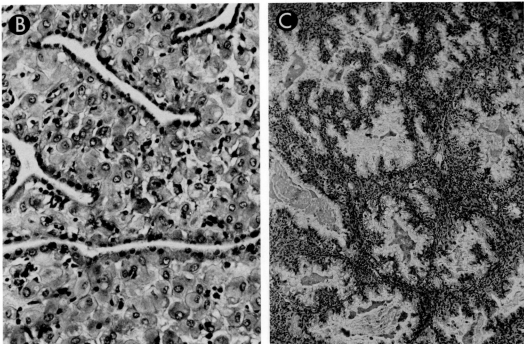

Fig. 1—1.—Decidual lining of the uterus at 8th week of gestation. **A,** entire thickness, showing superficial decidua compacta and basal decidua spongiosa. **B,** decidua compacta, showing isolated, ovoid stromal cells found only in pregnancy or after prolonged exposure to high levels of progestational agents. **C,** decidua spongiosa with saw-toothed glands filled with mucus.

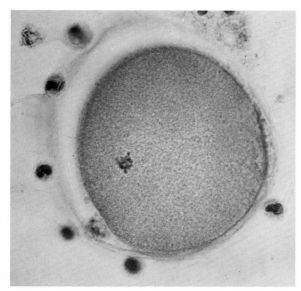

Fig. 1–2.—Unfertilized human ovum showing chromosomes in the second meiotic division; the first polar body lies adjacent to the cytoplasmic membrane. (Courtesy Drs. W. J. Hamilton, Josephine Barnes and Gladys H. Dodds.)

appear, each containing 23 pairs of chromosomes, one member of each pair derived from the sperm and the other from the ovum.

Implantation

Division continues as the fertilized ovum moves down through the fallopian tube and out onto the uterine lining. Six or seven days after its expulsion from the ovary, the ovum normally comes to rest high in the uterus, most often on the posterior wall. By this time it has developed into a blastocyst and is a hollow sphere composed of trophoblast cells arranged in a single layer everywhere except at one point where the small group of cells known as the inner cell mass remains (Fig. 1–3). As the blastocyst penetrates the decidual lining of the uterus, the superficial part of the decidua comes together over it and hides it from view. The decidua over the blastocyst is called decidua capsularis, that between the blastocyst and the uterine musculature the decidua basalis and the part lining the remainder of the uterus the decidua vera (Figs. 1–4 and 1–5).

successfully penetrated by a sperm, the second meiotic division is completed and the second polar body is formed (Fig. 1–2). The chromosomes of the sperm enlarge and mingle with those remaining in the ovum. All divide by mitosis and two new cells

Development of the Chorionic Vesicle

As soon as the blastocyst is embedded in the decidua, the trophoblast cells grow rapidly to form a thick outer coat, and the cells of the inner cell mass differentiate into the ectodermal and entodermal

Figs. 1–3.—Human blastocysts. **A,** two-celled stage, approximately 36 hours' postcoital age, recovered from the fallopian tube. **B,** morula of about 96 hours' gestational age found in the uterine cavity. **C,** morula of about 108 hours' gestational age; the inner cell mass can be distinguished. (Courtesy Dr. A. T. Hertig and Carnegie Institute of Embryology.)

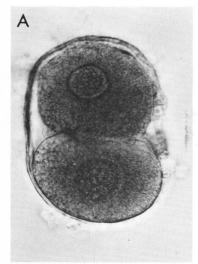
A

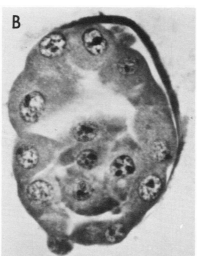
B

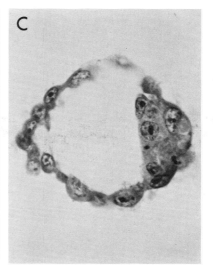
C

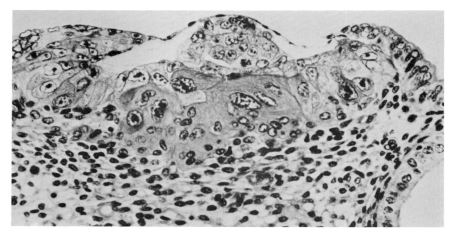

Fig. 1–4.—An implanting human blastocyst of 7½ days' gestational age.

Fig. 1–5.—**A,** implanted blastocyst, age 11½ days, with layer of decidua covering the outer surface. The blastocyst wall has begun to differentiate into cytotrophoblast and syncytial trophoblast. The embryonic disk is composed of ectoderm and entoderm; yolk sac and amniotic sac are present, and mesoderm is visible on the inner surface of the blastocyst wall. (Courtesy Drs. John Rock and A. T. Hertig.) **B,** opened uterus showing chorionic vesicle of 8 weeks covered by decidua capsularis. The rest of the uterus is lined by decidua vera. Opened vesicle shown in Figure 1–10, B.

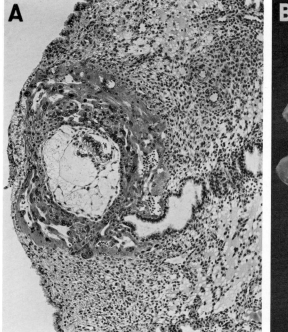

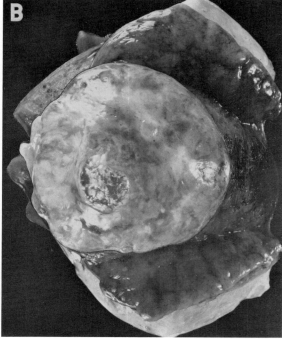

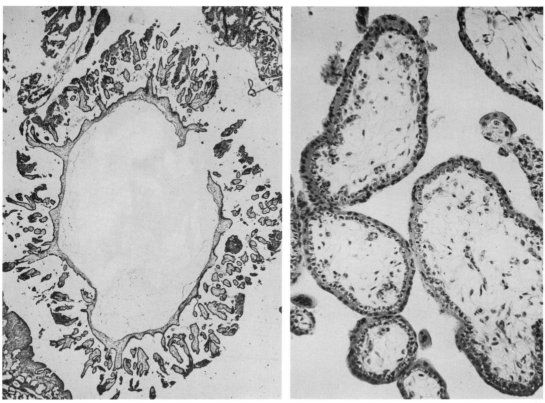

Fig. 1–6 (left).—Wall of chorionic vesicle with attached villi; age 21 days.

Fig. 1–7 (right).—Villi (from a chorionic vesicle age 28 days) covered by inner cytotrophoblast and outer plasmoditrophoblast.

layers of the germinal disk and the cavities associated with them. The amniotic cavity is visible as a dome above the ectodermal layer and is lined by cells that are continuous with those of the ectoderm. The yolk sac lies beneath the entoderm and is lined by a layer of cells continuous with it. Mesodermal cells appear at the margins of the germinal disk at about the time of implantation and invade the space between the ectoderm and the entoderm to form a third part of a three-layered disk. At the same time they spread peripherally to form the inner lining of the blastocyst and project outward into the proliferating trophoblast in fingerlike processes (Fig. 1–6). As the trophoblast spreads over the mesodermal projections, it differentiates into two layers, the inner cytotrophoblast or Langhans' layer and the outer plasmoditrophoblast or syncytial layer (Fig 1–7). The cells of the Langhans' layer have definite boundaries which are lacking in the syncytial layer. The latter is covered superficially with microvilli visible only by electron microscopy (Fig. 1–8). The mesodermal projections with their trophoblastic covering are the chorionic villi. They branch repeatedly and soon assume complicated treelike patterns. At this stage the blastocyst is called a chorionic vesicle.

In the first months of pregnancy the chorionic villi have abundant cytotrophoblast. As pregnancy proceeds, the cytotrophoblast becomes a thinner layer and more sparsely cellular, but electron microscopy shows that, although much attenuated, it persists as a continuous layer throughout pregnancy.

The local destruction of decidua at the site of implantation permits the blastocyst to sink below the surface, and the necrotic decidual cells provide the blastocyst with nourishment during the early stages of implantation. Subsequent destruction of portions of the walls of the decidual blood vessels permits maternal blood to flow out into the spaces between the villi, establishing a more efficient source of nutrition.

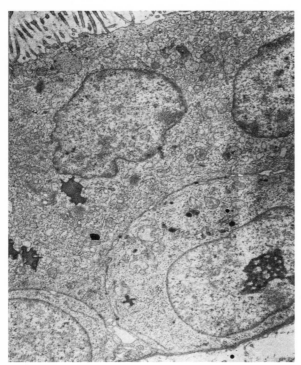

Fig. 1–8. — Electron photomicrograph of a portion of the covering of a placental villus; 21 days' gestational age. Above are syncytial cells with well-developed microvilli, no indication of cell boundaries and numerous organelles; below are Langhans' cells with distinct boundaries and fewer organelles. (Courtesy Dr. M. Knoth.)

The elaboration and release of specific chemical substances give the trophoblast the ability to induce vascular growth and differentiation in the decidua, thus increasing vascularity in the region occupied by the placenta.

Delineation of Placenta

While the chorionic vesicle is small, maternal blood surrounds all villi equally, and all grow at approximately the same rate (Fig. 1–9). As it becomes larger, the most superficial villi, which are farthest from the source of maternal blood, become less well nourished and fail to develop as luxuriantly as those on the side adjacent to the uterine wall (Fig. 1–10, A). Gradually they cease to grow, soon degenerate and at term are found only as hyalinized acellular "ghost villi" on the nonplacental portions of the chorionic membrane. This portion of the early chorion is known as the chorion laeve, in contrast to the chorion frondosum, from which the placenta arises. At the end of the first trimester the placenta occupies almost one half of the surface area of the chorionic vesicle, at the end of pregnancy only about one fifth. This is because the extraplacental portion of the sac enlarges to accommodate the growing fetus more rapidly than does the part covered by villi.

Elaboration of Membranes

The amniotic sac, which originally forms a small dome over the ectodermal layer of the germinal disk, enlarges as pregnancy proceeds. When the ectoderm spreads to enclose the embryo and form the epidermis, the amnion, which is attached to the margins of the ectodermal plate, is carried along. It forms a sac that surrounds the embryo but is attached to it only at the umbilicus. Fluid is present both within the amniotic sac and between it and the wall of the chorionic vesicle. As a result the embryo lies in a sac within a sac (Fig. 1–10, B). The amnion enlarges more rapidly than the chorion, and by the middle of pregnancy the fluid between the layers has disappeared and the amnion is in contact with the chorion. The fetus thenceforth lies in a single sac composed of an inner layer of amnion and an outer layer of chorion. The amnion fuses with the umbilical cord but not with the chorion, and amnion and chorion can still be easily separated at the end of pregnancy.

Fetal Blood Supply

Before the end of the 3d week after fertilization, groups of cells making up blood islands can be distinguished in the mesoderm of the embryonic disk, the yolk sac and the chorionic villi. They differen-

Fig. 1–9. — External surface of chorionic vesicle completely covered by villi; age 21 days.

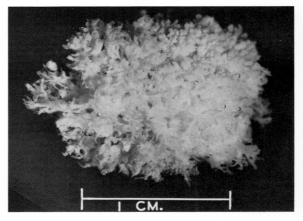

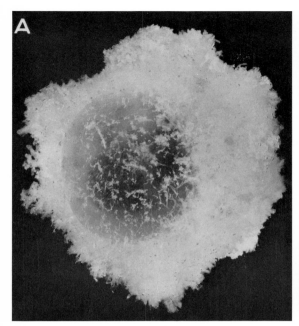

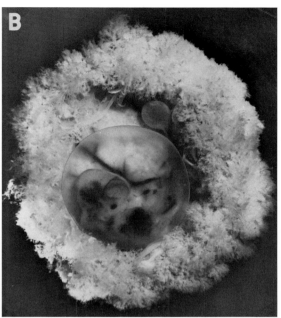

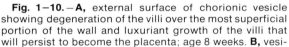

Fig. 1–10.—A, external surface of chorionic vesicle showing degeneration of the villi over the most superficial portion of the wall and luxuriant growth of the villi that will persist to become the placenta; age 8 weeks. B, vesi-cle of the same age with chorionic membrane incised to show space between walls of amnion and chorion. Yolk sac and embryo are also visible.

tiate rapidly into vascular channels, and those in the yolk sac also produce circulating blood cells; the ends of the channels come in contact with each other and fuse, and by the 28th day a circulation is established between the embryo and the yolk sac and chorionic vesicle. Blood of the embryo circulates in these vessels; maternal blood circulates in the spaces between the villi. Normally there is no communication between the two, and exchange of foodstuffs, minerals, oxygen and fetal waste products is accomplished by diffusion, pinocytosis and active transfer across the layers of cells that separate maternal and fetal blood. The four layers across which foodstuffs must pass are endothelial cells of the fetal blood vessels, the mesoderm and the Langhans' and syncytial cells covering the outer surface of the villi.

Differentiation of Embryonic Disk

ECTODERM.—While the accessory embryonic structures are differentiating, the embryo itself begins to emerge from the germinal disk. The neural groove appears, forms a closed tube and becomes detached from the layer of ectoderm in which it originates. The neural tube gives rise to the brain; spinal cord; cranial, spinal and sympathetic nerves; chromaffin tissue; retina; and a few other structures. The remaining ectoderm forms the epidermal layer of the skin.

ENTODERM.—The entodermal tube is formed by evagination of the portions of the yolk sac that are in close contact with the elongating neural tube. For a time much of the entodermal tube is confluent with the yolk sac, but gradually the open area diminishes and eventually the tube is completely closed. The ends come in contact with the surface covering of the embryo and break through to form the oral and anal orifices. The tube differentiates into the lining of the pharynx, esophagus, stomach and intestines. A diverticulum arising from the anterior portion branches repeatedly and develops into the lungs. The organs intimately associated with digestion such as the liver, pancreas and salivary glands arise as buds from the entodermal tube.

MESODERM.—Part of the early mesoderm that lies near the sides of the neural and entodermal tubes condenses into masses of cells called somites. From these come the vertebrae and from closely adjacent

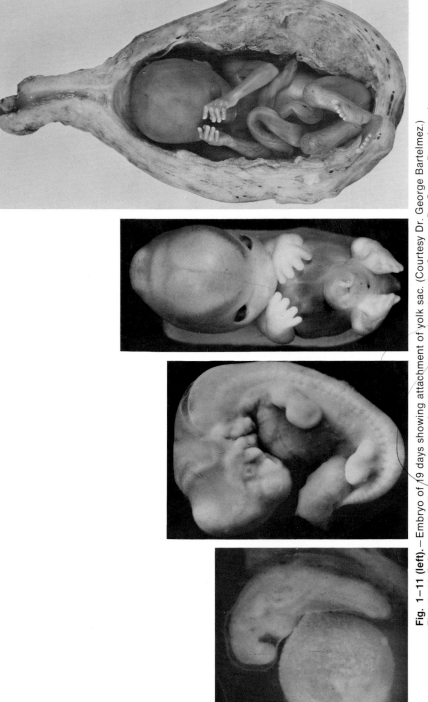

Fig. 1–11 (left).—Embryo of 19 days showing attachment of yolk sac. (Courtesy Dr. George Bartelmez.)
Fig. 1–12 (left center).—Embryo of 22 days; 10.2 mm in greatest length. (Courtesy Dr. George Bartelmez.)
Fig. 1–13 (right center).—Embryo of 8 weeks; 20 mm in greatest length.
Fig. 1–14 (right).—Fetus of 14 weeks showing position in uterus and attachment to placenta. Fetus 11 cm long and weighs 34 gm.

cells come the remainder of the skeleton and the muscles. Also from mesoderm come the heart, blood vessels and blood cells, genitourinary organs and spleen.

Periods of Intrauterine Growth

The rate of growth in the early part of pregnancy is proportionately much more rapid than that in the latter part. Organogenesis is largely completed by the end of the 2d month, and development thereafter consists principally of an increase in size and elaboration of cellular patterns.

For the first 2 weeks after fertilization, or until it is well implanted in the uterine wall, the growing organism is known as a zygote or fertilized ovum; for the next 6 weeks, while major differentiation of organs and tissues is being accomplished, it is an embryo (Figs. 1–11 to 1–13), and during the rest of intrauterine life, after it has acquired recognizable human form, it is a fetus (Fig. 1–14). A fetus becomes an infant when it is completely outside the body of the mother, even before the cord is cut.

Keibel and Mall suggested that the word conceptus be used for products of conception at any stage of development from fertilization to birth. This is a convenient term since it includes the accessory structures of cord, amnion, chorionic membrane and villi and could well be used more often than it is.

The size of the uterus increases greatly during

Fig. 1–15. – Sagittal sections of normal nonpregnant uterus and uterus containing a mature fetus.

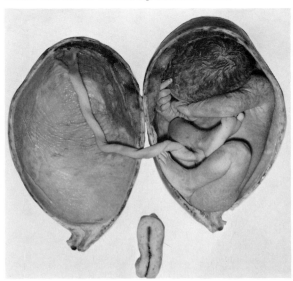

the 38 weeks of pregnancy (Fig. 1–15) and gains about tenfold in weight. Muscle cells are increased in size and number, interstitial fluid is increased, and blood vessels, especially those of the placental site, are increased in number, length and caliber.

The Structure of the Mature Placenta

The placenta at maturity is usually an oval or circular mass measuring 12–14 cm in diameter and 2–3 cm in thickness. Without cord or membranes it weighs about one seventh as much as the infant. The in situ placenta is spread out over the surface of the uterine wall, but when seen outside the uterus following delivery, is considerably thicker and has a smaller surface area than before separation. The fetal surface is covered by easily separable amnion and the maternal surface by a thin irregular layer of adherent decidua (Fig. 1–16). Beneath the amnion lies the chorionic plate, derived from the inner portion of the chorion frondosum. The chorionic cells in the region of the chorionic plate are largely replaced by relatively acellular tissue studded with small nodules of hyaline. The major fetal vessels course over the surface of the chorionic plate, the narrower, thicker-walled arteries lying superficial to the wider, thinner-walled veins. The two umbilical arteries anastomose near their entrance into the placenta, making it possible for either vessel to supply the entire arterial bed. The surface vessels give off branches that are directed down into the substance, the last branch usually being located about 1 cm from the margin so that beyond this point major vessels are not visible on the surface. The branches of the arteries and veins lie adjacent to each other within the villi. They are held together by a small amount of connective tissue and are covered by the cyto- and syncytiotrophoblast layers (Fig. 1–17). Recent work of Freese, who filled the fetal vessels with plastic material and subsequently removed surrounding tissues by corrosion, shows that the major vessels, as they leave the surface of the placenta, give off many branches that divide repeatedly and are distributed around a central cavity (Figs. 1–18 and 1–19). Each of these major vessels and its branches forms a hummock on the maternal surface known as a cotyledon. The blood pressure is believed to be highest in the center of the cotyledons and lowest in the region of the maternal veins.

Freese *et al.* showed by cineradiography and plastic injection that maternal blood flow through the placenta follows a definite pattern: an artery from the uterine wall empties into a space in the center

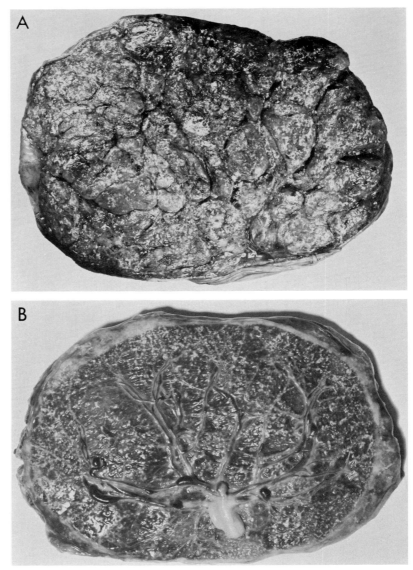

Fig. 1–16.—Mature placenta. **A,** maternal surface with calcification of the decidual layer. Cotyledons vary in size. **B,** fetal surface with a narrow marginate ring. The major vessels normally disappear from the surface 1–2 cm from the margin of the chorionic plate.

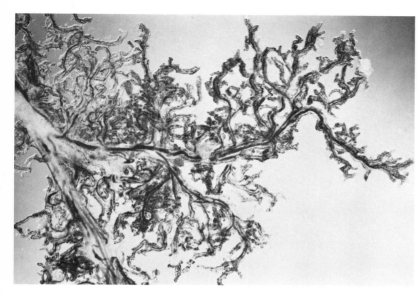

Fig. 1–17.—Terminal villi of a minute fragment of placenta teased out in saline. Blood-filled vessels appear as black lines.

Fig. 1–18.—Side view of mature placenta showing external appearance of cotyledons after plastic injection of fetal blood vessels followed by corrosion. (Courtesy Drs. U. E. Freese and B. J. Maciolek.)

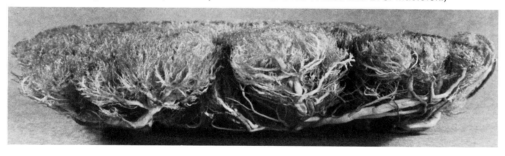

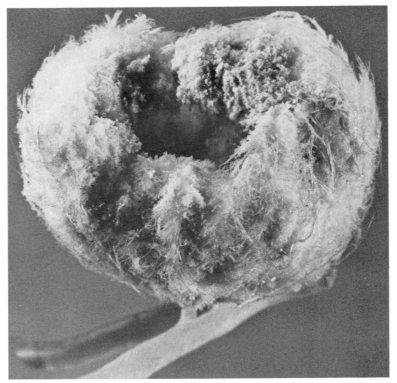

Fig. 1–19.—Single cotyledon following plastic injection and corrosion. Divisions of artery and vein produce the villus mass which surrounds a central cavity. (Courtesy Drs. U. E. Freese and B. J. Maciolek.)

Fig. 1–20.—Cineradiograph of pregnant rhesus monkey showing peripheral dispersion of material entering the centers of the cotyledons. (Courtesy Dr. U. E. Freese.)

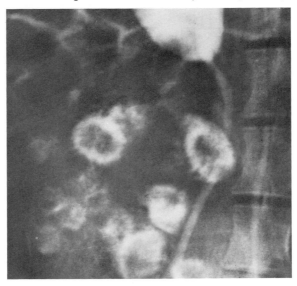

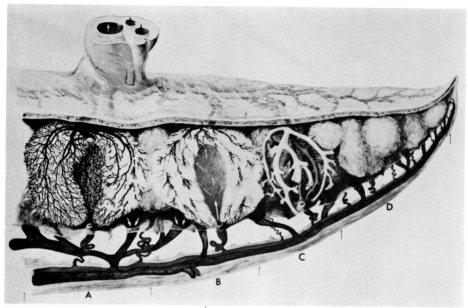

Fig. 1–21.—Diagram of maternal and fetal circulation showing how fetal blood from umbilical artery enters vessels within villi *(A);* maternal blood from a spiral artery enters the center of a cotyledon and disperses peripheral- ly *(B);* oxygenated fetal blood leaves the placenta from the outer circumference of the cotyledons *(C)* and maternal blood leaves placenta from randomly distributed maternal veins *(D).*

of each cotyledon; the blood flows laterally and seeps slowly through the peripheral portion of the cotyledon, from which it returns to the maternal surface of the placenta and enters randomly distributed maternal veins in the placental site (Fig. 1–20). This work and that of Ramsey offer no support for the concept, long and widely held, of a flow of blood to the periphery of the placenta where it leaves by entering a circumferential marginal sinus.

REFERENCES

Arey, L. B.: *Developmental Anatomy* (7th ed.; Philadelphia: W. B. Saunders Co., 1965).

Brewer, J. I.: A human embryo in the bilaminar blastocyst stage, Contrib. Embryol. 27:85, 1938.

Brewer, J. I., and Fitzgerald, J. E.: Six normal and complete presomite human ova, Am. J. Obstet. Gynecol. 34:210, 1937.

Freese, U. E.: The fetal-maternal circulation, J. Reprod. Med. 1:161, 1968.

Freese, U. E., and Maciolek, B. J.: Plastoid injection studies of the uteroplacental vascular relationship in the human, Obstet. Gynecol. 33:160, 1969.

Freese, U. E., Ranninger, K., and Kaplan, H.: The fetal-maternal circulation of the placenta, Am. J. Obstet. Gynecol. 94:361, 1966.

Harris, J. W. S., and Ramsey, E. M.: The morphology of the human placental vasculature, Contrib. Embryol. 38:45, 1966.

Hertig, A. T.: Involution of tissues in fetal life; a review, J. Gerontol. 1:96, 1946.

Hertig, A. T.: Gestational hyperplasia of early pregnancy. A morphologic correlation of ova endometrium and corpora lutea of pregnancy, Lab. Invest. 13:1153, 1964.

Hertig, A. T.: *Human Trophoblast* (Springfield, Ill.: Charles C Thomas, 1968).

Hertig, A. T., and Rock, J.: On the development of the early human ovum, with special reference to the trophoblast of the previllous stage: Description of 7 normal and 5 pathologic human ova, Am. J. Obstet. Gynecol. 47:149, 1944.

Hertig, A. T., and Rock, J.: Two human ova of the previllous stage, having a developmental age of about 7 and 9 days respectively, Contrib. Embryol. 31:65, 1945.

Hertig, A. T., Rock, J., Adams, E. C., and Mulligan, W. J.: On the preimplantation stages of the human ovum. Description of four normal and four abnormal specimens from the second to the fifth day of development, Contrib. Embryol. 35:199, 1954.

Heuser, C., Hertig, A. T., and Rock, J.: Two human embryos showing early stages of the definitive yolk sac, Contrib. Embryol. 31:85, 1945.

Keibel, F., and Mall, F. M. (eds.): *Manual of Human Embryology* (Philadelphia: J. B. Lippincott Co., 1910).

Potter, E. L.: *Fundamentals of Human Reproduction* (New York: McGraw-Hill Book Co., 1948).

Rock, J., and Hertig, A. T.: Information regarding the time of human ovulation derived from a study of 3 unfertilized and 11 fertilized human ova, Am. J. Obstet. Gynecol. 47:343, 1944.

Lanman, J. T.: Delays during reproduction and their effects on the embryo and fetus, N. Engl. J. Med. 278:1077, 1092, 1968.

Mitchell, F. F.: Steroid metabolism in the fetal placental unit and in early childhood, Vitam. Horm. 25:191, 1967.

Patten, B. M.: *Human Embryology* (New York: McGraw-Hill Book Co., 1968).

Ramsey, E. M.: Circulation in the maternal placenta of the rhesus monkey and man, with observations on marginal lakes, Ann. Anat. 98:159, 1956.

Rhodin, J. A. G., and Terzakis, J. A.: The ultrastructure of the human full term placenta, J. Ultrastruct. Res. 6:88, 1962.

Terzakis, J. A.: The ultrastructure of the normal human first trimester placenta, J. Ultrastruct. Res. 9:268, 1963.

Wislocki, G. W., and Padykula, H. A.: Histochemistry and Electron Microscopy of the Placenta, in Young, W. C. (ed.): *Sex and Internal Secretions* (Baltimore: Williams & Wilkins Co., 1961).

Wolstenholme, E., and O'Connor, M.: *Symposium on Pre-Implantation Stages of Pregnancy* (Ciba Foundation Symposia) (Boston: Little, Brown and Co., 1965).

2

Rate of Antenatal Growth

THE RATE OF BODY GROWTH, even in the absence of pathologic states, varies considerably from one individual to another before as well as after birth. Variation in length of gestation too is to some extent responsible for weight differences, although in any given week weight may vary by several hundred grams. In lay circles pregnancy is expected to last 9 months, and the general obstetric practice of calculating the due date by counting back 3 months and adding 7 days from the 1st day of the last menstrual period gives 280–282 days or about 40 weeks. This is sometimes called menstrual age in recognition of the fact that pregnancy begins in the middle of the menstrual cycle and is actually about 2 weeks shorter than generally calculated. The baby is expected to weigh about 7½ lb (3,400 gm) and to be about 20 in. (50 cm) long.

In order to test the validity of these established assumptions and to determine the range in length of pregnancy and its relation to the size of the infant, several studies have been made. The outcome of all has been much the same. All have shown a considerable variation within any given parameter, but mean weight and length of gestation have not varied greatly from Gruenwald's figures of a mean weight of 3,270 gm at 40 weeks and those of Lubchenko et al. of 3,226 at 40 weeks. A study carried out at the Chicago Lying-in Hospital showed a mean weight for 4,418 single white infants over 1,000 gm of 3,320 gm and a mean gestation of 282 days, yet only 22% were in the weight category of 3,250–3,500 gm and only 25% were born during the 41st week; only 6.2% fulfilled both criteria (Table 2–1).

As shown in Table 2–1 and the model constructed from these data (Figs. 2–1 and 2–2), births are distributed fairly symmetrically around the peak of 3,320 gm and 282 days. There is a group of infants with short gestation and low birth weight that keeps the model from having the symmetric form of a Bell curve. Clinical data suggest that the slight preponderance of such births results from complications of pregnancy and if such cases were excluded, distribution would be entirely symmetric.

When an attempt is made to estimate fetal weight from the length of gestation or the length of gestation from fetal weight, considerable inaccuracy is inevitable. Table 2–2, in which mean length of gestation is calculated for infants over 1,000 gm divided according to weight, and mean weight is calculated for infants arranged according to length of gestation, shows that although 1,113 infants born at the Chicago Lying-in Hospital during the 41st week had a mean weight of 3,290 gm, 1,518 infants had birth weights ranging from 3,500 to 5,000 gm, all whose mean length of gestation was 41 weeks. The same relation of weight and length of gestation for infants under 500 gm is shown in Tables 2–3 and 2–4.

Twins

Twins grow more slowly in utero than do single infants. Potter and Fuller, who compared the weight of 249 twin pairs with 1,000 single infants delivered concurrently, found that the mean weight of twin infants born during the 40th week was 2,753 gm, while that for single infants was 3,325 gm. The latter figure is higher than that found in a later study from the same institution (see Table 2–2), but the twin study shows a weight approximately 600 gm less for twins than for single infants. Mean difference in weight of the two members of a twin pair during the 40th week was 521 gm.

Naeye et al., in a similar study, separated twins according to type of placenta, and found that at 40

TABLE 2–1.—GESTATION IN WEEKS AND BIRTH WEIGHT IN GRAMS FOR 4,418 CONSECUTIVELY BORN SINGLE WHITE INFANTS (Chicago Lying-in Hospital).*

GRAMS	29†	30	31	32	33	34	35	36	37	38	39	40	41	42	43	44	45	46	47+	%
5,000												1	2	1		1				0.1
4,750									1		1	1	2	4	3	1	1			0.3
4,500								1				4	6	6	7	4	1			0.7
4,250						1				2	5	17	27	30	13	10	2	2		2.5
4,000						1	2	2	1	1	15	27	53	44	35	10	6	2		4.4
3,750							2		3	7	23	76	137	108	41	22	3	1	5	9.5
3,500					1		2	5	11	12	70	166	224	146	57	24	10	4	8	17.0
3,250			1	2		2	4	3	19	38	113	229	276	157	70	20	12	5	6	21.6
3,000				1		2	3	9	22	52	142	244	215	96	46	27	6	1	4	20.0
2,750		1	2		4	5	5	10	24	42	112	124	117	49	14	9	4		8	12.0
2,500		1				4	8	15	24	33	69	64	39	17	8	4		1	1	6.4
2,250		1		2	1	9	16	11	17	20	15	14	9	4	2	1		1	1	2.7
2,000		1	1	2	5	9	9	7	6	2	6			4		1				1.2
1,750				3	2	2	2	3	1	2	2	1	1							0.4
1,500			2	5	3		2	3	2		2	1	1		2	2				0.6
1,250	3	7		3		2	1	1		1										0.4
1,000‡	1	2				3	2		1											0.2
%	0.1	0.3	0.2	0.4	0.4	0.8	1.2	1.7	3.0	4.3	13.0	22.2	25.3	15.3	6.9	3.0	1.0	0.4	0.8	100

*Based on 5,000 consecutive births, with twins, nonwhite infants and infants under 1,000 gm excluded. No pregnancies artificially terminated because of gestational duration. Gestational data calculated from 1st day of last menstrual period as given by patient.

†Data are given for 29th week (days 197–203 inclusive), 30th week (days 204–210 inclusive), etc.

‡Includes infants 1,000–1,249 gm.

TABLE 2–2.—BIRTH WEIGHT BY GESTATION, AND GESTATION BY BIRTH WEIGHT FOR 4,418 CONSECUTIVELY BORN SINGLE WHITE INFANTS OVER 1,000 GM*

GESTATION LENGTH (WEEK)	$\bar{X}$	BIRTH WEIGHT SD	N
29th†	1,187	125	4
30th	1,431	548	11
31st	2,321	672	7
32d	1,900	772	15
33d	2,178	540	14
34th	2,348	837	28
35th	2,475	705	51
36th	2,555	599	77
37th	2,809	533	127
38th	2,879	450	213
39th	3,032	433	577
40th	3,174	425	975
41st	3,290	428	1,113
42d	3,386	475	674
43d	3,439	508	301
44th	3,425	525	134
45th	3,445	516	46
46th	3,426	543	18
47th	3,210	381	33

Mean weight 3,320 gm

BIRTH WEIGHT	$\bar{X}$ (WEEK)	GESTATION LENGTH SD	N
1,000–1,249	31st	2.7	9
1,250	33d	2.6	18
1,500	34th	4.0	25
1,750	35th	2.8	19
2,000	36th	2.7	53
2,250	38th	2.6	124
2,500	39th	2.0	288
2,750	39th	2.1	530
3,000	40th	1.7	870
3,250	40th	1.7	957
3,500	41st	1.7	740
3,750	41st	1.5	428
4,000	41st	1.8	199
4,250	41st	1.7	109
4,500	41st	1.7	29
4,750	41st	1.9	13
5,000	42d	1.5	6

Mean gestation 282 days

*Summation of data given in Table 2–1.
†Day 197–203, etc.

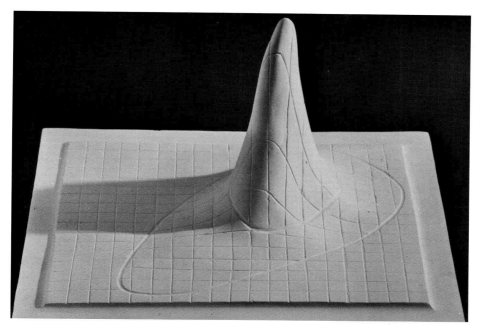

Fig. 2–1. — Model constructed from data given in Table 2–1 showing distribution according to weight and length of gestation of 4,418 consecutive single white births at the Chicago Lying-in Hospital. The two *oval lines* include 75% and 95% of births.

Fig. 2–2. — Same model shown in Figure 2–1 viewed from above.

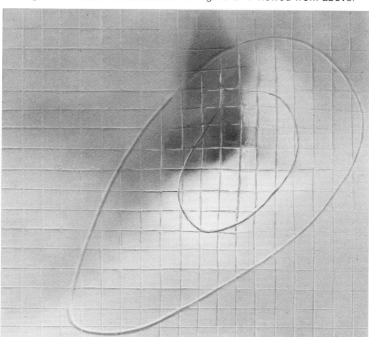

TABLE 2–3. – DURATION OF PREGNANCY FROM LAST MENSTRUAL PERIOD, FETAL LENGTH IN CENTIMETERS AND ORGAN WEIGHT IN GRAMS GROUPED BY BODY WEIGHT OF FETUSES OF 0–500 GM (Chicago Lying-in Hospital)*

Body Weight	Duration of Pregnancy (Days)	Body Length Crown-Heel	Crown-Rump	Brain	Heart	Lungs (Both)	Liver	Adrenals (Both)	Kidneys (Both)	Spleen	Pancreas	Thymus	Thyroid	No. of Cases
0–4	63	3	3	0.8	0.1	0.1	0.2	0.1	0.1					23
5–9	80	6	5	1.2	0.1	0.1	0.2		0.1					30
10	81	8	6	1.5	0.2	0.3	0.7	0.1	0.1					27
15	85	9	6	2.6	0.2	0.4	0.8	0.1	0.1					15
20	87	10	7	4.3	0.3	0.4	1.1	0.1	0.2					21
25	90	10	7	4.8	0.4	0.7	1.1		0.2					14
30	93	11	8	5.4	0.4	1.0	1.3	0.2	0.2					15
35	98	12	9	6.2	0.5	1.4	2.0	0.2	0.3					14
40	102	12	9											14
45	103	13	9	7.4	0.5	1.9	2.5	0.4	0.4					22
50	104	14	10	8.5	0.5	1.9	3.0	0.5	0.5	0.1		0.1		23
60	105	14	10	10	0.5	2.5	3.4	0.6	0.6	0.1		0.2		21
70	106	15	11	11	0.6	3.0	3.6	0.6	0.8	0.1	0.1	0.2		24
80	110	16	11	12	0.7	3.0	4.3	0.6	0.8	0.2	0.1	0.2		7
90	114	16	12	14	0.9	3.0	4.7	0.7	0.9	0.2	0.2	0.2		15
100	119	18	12	17	1.1	3.9	5.6	0.7	1.4	0.2	0.2	0.3	0.2	28
125	123	19	13	23	1.3	4.1	7.4	0.7	1.4	0.2	0.2	0.3	0.2	21
150	129	20	14	23	1.4	5.3	9.2	0.8	1.4	0.3	0.2	0.3	0.2	20
175	131	21	14	23	1.4	5.6	11	0.8	1.8	0.4	0.4	0.3	0.2	27
200	132	22	15	33	1.7	7.2	12	1.1	2.2	0.4	0.4	0.4	0.2	39
250	138	24	16	39	2.2	9.1	15	1.2	2.7	0.5	0.4	0.4	0.2	37
300	144	25	17	46	2.4	10	17	1.5	3.1	0.6	0.5	0.7	0.3	43
350	147	26	18	54	2.9	11	21	2.0	3.8	0.7	0.5	0.8	0.3	31
400	157	27	18	61	3.4	11	23	2.2	4.2	0.8	0.6	1.0	0.3	32
450+	163	28	19	70	3.4	12	23	2.3	4.7	0.8	0.6	1.0	0.3	29
No. of cases	592	592	592	152	183	187	187	184	180	149	113	139	78	592

*Figures include only normal nonmacerated fetuses. Most of those under 200 gm were obtained by hysterotomy or hysterectomy. Category 450+ includes 450 – 499 gm.

TABLE 2–4.—FETAL WEIGHT AND LENGTH FROM 8 TO 26 WEEKS' GESTATION (Chicago Lying-in Hospital)

| GESTATION (Week) | WEIGHT (GM) | | | LENGTH (CM) | | | | | |
| | | | | CROWN-HEEL | | | CROWN-RUMP | | |
	X̄	SD	N	X̄	SD	N	X̄	SD	N
8th*	10	2	2		1	2	2	2	9
9th	11	11	4		1	3	3	3	16
10th	14	20	14		3	8	4	3	22
11th	14	16	23	6	3	35	5	2	20
12th	25	20	29	7	3	38	6	2	30
13th	27	24	36	9	3	41	7	2	38
14th	38	17	33	10	3	41	8	2	35
15th	53	22	36	13	3	38	9	2	37
16th	73	46	35	14	4	37	10	2	36
17th	122	59	35	17	3	35	12	2	34
18th	161	91	31	19	4	32	13	3	32
19th	188	87	41	20	4	43	14	3	43
20th	227	99	39	21	4	40	15	3	40
21st	303	75	34	24	2	34	16	2	33
22d	348	112	36	25	4	35	17	3	35
23d	384	111	38	26	3	38	18	2	35
24th	361	121	13	25	3	13	18	3	12
25th	379	142	8	27	3	8	19	2	8
26th	394	140	6	27	6	7	18	4	7

*Day 49–55.

weeks the mean weight of twins with monochorionic placentas was 2,698 gm, while for those with dichorionic placentas it was 2,806 gm. Since all of the first group are monozygous and the majority of the second group are dizygous, they concluded that twins emanating from one egg grow slightly more slowly than those from two eggs. At 29 weeks their mean weight for twins of 1,202 and 1,190 gm respectively were similar to the figures of Lubchenko *et al.* for single infants. On this basis Naeye *et al.* concluded that a decrease in rate of growth occurred only in the last trimester. In the study made by Potter and Fuller the mean weight of twins born during the 29th week was 951 gm, while that of single infants was 1,187 gm. This suggests that the rate of growth for these twins was slightly slower even before the last trimester.

Prematurity

Prematurity is the factor considered responsible for more neonatal deaths than any other, and consequently prevention of prematurity and the need for specialized care of infants born prematurely are important areas of investigation if mortality is to be reduced.

There has been much discussion as to which infants should be considered premature—whether this designation should be based on length of gestation or fetal length or weight. In the first third of this century it was customary to use length of gestation, and in some studies normal infants of 3,500 gm and more were considered premature because the stated length of gestation was less than 37 weeks. With the realization that length of gestation is dependent on memory, which is often faulty, birth weight gradually came to be substituted as a more accurate measurement. On the basis of autopsy material, Scammon urged the use of fetal length, particularly the crown-rump measurement, as the most accurate of all; but this never became popular, largely because of the difficulty encountered in obtaining accurate measurements of living infants. Attempts were also made to combine two or three criteria, and from the opening of the Chicago Lying-in Hospital in 1931, body length, weight and duration of gestation were all taken into consideration in assessing the maturity of an infant.

In recent years it has become popular to disparage the use of weight to estimate degree of maturity or to classify infants for any reason and to revert to the supposed gestational age. The data in Table 2–1 show that neither method is perfect and that of 248 infants weighing less than 2,500 gm at birth, 118 (47%) had gestational lengths in excess of 37 weeks, and of 334 born before the end of the 37th week, 204 (61%) weighed more than 2,500 gm.

Several studies based on large numbers of cases have shown that for infants of low birth weight the mortality rate is lower among those with a longer than those with a shorter length of gestation. Yerushalmy believed that much could be gained by dividing infants into 5 groups: group 1 consisting of all under 1,500 gm regardless of length of gestation; groups 2 and 3 consisting of those weighing 1,500-2,500 gm, divided into those of less than and those of more than 37 completed weeks of gestation; and groups 4 and 5 consisting of those weighing over 2,500 gm divided into those of less than and those of more than 37 completed weeks. He found mortality rates higher (104.7) in infants under 2,500 gm whose gestational periods were shorter than among those whose gestation was longer (32). In infants weighing less than 2,500 gm, malformations were proportionately more frequent among those with longer than those with shorter gestations.

The difficulty in arriving at a weight that is "normal" for a given length of gestation is compounded by the definitions used by different investigators. For instance, 40 weeks for Lubchenko *et al.* meant 40 completed weeks (280–286 days); Gruenwald used the day nearest to 40 weeks (277–284 days); and Potter and Fuller spoke of the 40th week

(274–280 days). In spite of this the variation among the three was less than 100 gm (Gruenwald 3,270; Lubchenko *et al.* 3,226; Potter and Fuller 3,174).

Realizing the inadequacy of using either weight or presumed length of gestation as a basis for assessing the relative maturity of an infant, Graziani *et al.* recommended the use of neurologic maturation as an indicator, and Usher *et al.* recommended certain external characteristics including creases on the sole of the foot, size of the mass of breast tissue, cartilaginous development of the ear lobe and character of the hair. Such data are of value in determining proportionate maturity of a given infant but cannot be used as a basis for comparison of groups of infants. If infants must be categorized as being mature or premature on the basis of a single criterion, weight seems the least objectionable. Its use, combined with length of gestation as recommended by Yerushalmy, will give better results.

In a study published in 1972 by the National Center of Health Statistics, which was made to determine change in frequency of premature birth, it was concluded that on a national level weight gave a more accurate measurement of prematurity than stated length of gestation. The former can be measured accurately, while the latter is subject to patient recall and differences in recording.

Growth Retardation

The terms intrauterine growth retardation and small-for-date have come to be used in recent years to indicate infants who are believed to be abnormally small for the stated length of gestation. Warkany has been particularly instrumental in popularizing these terms and has pointed out that such infants fall into several groups based on those who are small because of some fetal abnormality and those who appear normal except for small size. The latter fall into two groups, one consisting of those who do well after birth, grow at a normal rate and soon attain a normal size, and another consisting of infants who fail to thrive and, if they survive, remain unusually small.

The total frequency with which infants are born weighing appreciably less than expected is difficult to determine. Warkany quoted several studies that appeared to give an incidence of between 0.1% and 0.2% for infants who weighed less than 2,000 gm at more than 37 weeks' gestation. In the study of 4,418 consecutively born white single infants at the Chicago Lying-in Hospital 15 (0.34%) fell into this category.

Warkany found a great variety in the clinical disease pictures sometimes associated with intrauterine growth retardation, although he concluded that almost no known condition is invariably associated with such retardation and that a large proportion of these small infants demonstrate no abnormality. He stressed that many microcephalic dwarfs, including the "bird-headed" dwarfs of Seckel and some infants with microcephaly resulting from prenatal rubella, toxoplasmosis or exposure to x-ray, are abnormally small at birth. This is true also for the de Lange, Silver and Russell syndromes, leprechaunism, progeria and for many infants with malformations affecting individual organs. Infants with complete renal agenesis are usually small. Although most infants with cardiac malformations have a normal birth weight, Yerushalmy found that among 14 infants with major malformations who weighed less than 2,500 gm and had a gestation of more than 37 weeks, half of the abnormalities were cardiac.

Warkany, in discussing the etiology of intrauterine growth retardation, stressed the undesirability of considering such infants as a single group and pointed out that the retardation might be of genetic or chromosomal origin or a result of maternal malnutrition, vitamin deficiency, chronic hypoxia, exposure to x-ray and so on. Whether placental insufficiency per se is responsible for retarded growth is a subject of debate, but in favor of the possibility that it may play a role is the fact that when major weight differences are found in twins, organ maturation in the small twin is usually commensurate with that of the larger twin. Also, in occasional twin pregnancies in which one fetus is malformed, that fetus usually is small and supplied by a smaller portion of the placenta than is its normal mate.

Fetal Length

Until after 2 months' gestation, because the back of the fetus is curved and the legs are short, only a single measurement for length can be obtained. After about 3 months the legs are proportionately longer, and from then until the end of pregnancy the crown-rump (sitting height) measurement is approximately two thirds of the crown-heel (standing height) measurement. When abnormalities of the head or legs exist, this known relationship may be helpful in calculating what the normal measurement of the abnormal part would have been. Interrelationships of length of gestation and birth weight and length of the fetus are shown in Tables 2–2–2–5.

TABLE 2–5.—ORGAN WEIGHT IN GRAMS, BODY LENGTH AND FETAL AGE IN RELATION TO BODY WEIGHT (Chicago Lying-in Hospital)*

ORGAN		BODY WEIGHT								
		500–999	1,000–1,499	1,500–1,999	2,000–2,499	2,500–2,999	3,000–3,499	3,500–3,999	4,000–4,499	4,500+
Brain	$\overline{X}$	109	180	250	308	359	403	421	424	406
	SD	45	53	55	76	67	60	72	55	56
	N	267	181	148	149	127	138	76	41	28
Lungs	$\overline{X}$	18	27	38	44	49	55	58	66	74
	SD	6	7	10	10	11	13	12	15	16
	N	256	130	108	83	69	88	51	20	21
Heart	$\overline{X}$	6	9	13	15	19	21	23	28	36
	SD	2	5	5	5	5	4	5	5	10
	N	368	257	226	198	186	213	127	58	41
Liver	$\overline{X}$	39	60	76	98	127	155	178	215	275
	SD	11	16	17	25	31	33	38	36	54
	N	376	269	232	207	188	226	135	59	43
Spleen	$\overline{X}$	2	3	5	7	9	10	12	14	17
	SD	3	3	3	5	4	4	5	5	7
	N	367	267	228	211	187	220	134	61	43
Kidneys	$\overline{X}$	7	12	16	20	23	25	28	31	33
	SD	3	4	4	4	5	5	7	7	8
	N	340	220	219	186	171	204	121	54	37
Adrenals	$\overline{X}$	3	4	5	6	8	10	11	12	15
	SD	1	1	2	2	3	3	3	4	4
	N	356	262	227	205	184	216	128	60	36
Thymus	$\overline{X}$	2	4	7	8	9	11	13	14	17
	SD	1	2	3	4	4	4	5	5	6
	N	366	262	228	208	188	223	125	59	42
Thyroid	$\overline{X}$	0.8	0.8	0.9	1.0	1.3	1.6	1.7	1.9	2.3
	SD	0.7	0.8	0.6	0.7	0.9	0.9	0.8	0.9	1.1
	N	255	177	153	141	128	148	84	45	34
Pancreas	$\overline{X}$	1.0	1.4	2.0	2.3	3.0	3.5	4.0	4.6	6.0
	SD	1.3	1.0	1.3	1.1	1.2	1.2	1.5	2.1	6.2
	N	245	170	127	143	125	131	85	45	34
		LENGTH (CM)								
Crown-heel	$\overline{X}$	33	39	43	47	50	52	53	54	56
	SD	3	2	3	2	2	2	2	2	2
	N	386	276	241	217	191	230	136	63	43
Crown-rump	$\overline{X}$	22	26	29	32	34	36	37	38	40
	SD	2	2	2	2	2	2	2	2	2
	N	386	275	241	217	187	230	134	63	42
		FETAL AGE (1ST DAY LMP TO BIRTH)								
Day	$\overline{X}$	180	208	230	250	270	276	281	281	283
	SD	23	23	24	28	22	20	16	12	12
	N	220	181	153	124	111	126	56	28	25

*Based on 1,878 autopsies of fetuses and infants less than 2 hours of age who were not macerated, malformed, erythroblastotic or one of twins. Also excluded were lungs with pneumonia, hyaline membranes and large amounts of amniotic fluid.
$\overline{X}$ = mean weight; SD = standard deviation; N = number; LMP = last menstrual period.

TABLE 2–6.—TIME OF FIRST APPEARANCE OF CENTERS OF OSSIFICATION (White House Conference on Child Health and Protection)

	Week
Head	
Mandible	7
Occipital bone (squamous portion)	8
Occipital bone (lateral and basilar portion)	9–10
Superior maxilla	8
Temporal bone (petrous portion, mastoid and zygoma)	9
Sphenoid (inner lamella of pterygoid process)	9
Sphenoid (great wings)	10
Sphenoid (lesser wings)	13
Sphenoid (anterior body)	13–14
Nasal bone	10
Frontal bone	9–10
Bony labyrinth	17–20
Milk teeth (rudiments)	17–28
Hyoid bone (greater cornua)	28–32
Body	
Clavicle (diaphysis)	7
Scapula	8–9
Ribs	
5th, 6th, 7th	8–9
2d, 3d, 4th, 8th, 9th, 10th, 11th	9
1st	10
12th (very irregular)	10
Sternum	21–24
Upper extremity	
Humerus (diaphysis)	8
Radius (diaphysis)	8
Ulna (diaphysis)	8
Phalanges	
Terminal	9
Basal 3d and 2d	9
Basal 4th and 1st	10
Basal 5th	11–12
Middle 3d, 4th, 2d	12
Middle 5th	13–16
Metacarpals	
2d and 3d	9
4th, 5th, 1st	10–12
Vertebrae	
Arches	
All cervical and upper 1st or 2d dorsal	9
All dorsal and 1st or 2d lumbar	10
Lower lumbar	11
Upper sacral	12
4th sacral	19–25
Bodies	
From 2d dorsal to last lumbar	10
From lower cervical to upper sacral	11
From upper cervical to lower sacral	12
5th sacral	13–28
1st coccygeal	37–40
Structural arrangement	13–16
Odontoid process of axis	17–20
Costal process	
6th and 7th cervical	21–32
5th cervical	32–36
4th, 3d and 2d cervical	37–40
Transverse processes	
Cervical and dorsal	21–24
Lumbar	25–28
Pelvic girdle	
Ilium	9
Ischium (descending ramus)	16–17
Os pubis (horizontal ramus)	21–28
Lower extremity	
Femur (diaphysis)	8–9
Femur (distal epiphysis)	35–40
Tibia (diaphysis)	8–9
Tibia (proximal epiphysis)	40
Fibula	9
Os calcis	21–29
Astragalus	24–32
Cuboid	40
Metatarsals	
2d and 3d	9
4th, 5th and 1st	10–12
Phalanges	
Terminal 1st	9
Terminal 2d, 3d, 4th	10–12
Terminal 5th	13–14
Basal 1st, 2d, 3d, 4th, 5th	13–14
Middle 2d	20–25
Middle 3d	21–26
Middle 4th	29–32
Middle 5th	33–36

Initial Appearance of Centers of Ossification

In an attempt to determine accurately the age of infants at the time of birth, Cruikshank, Miller and Browne compared ossification, age, weight and length. Correlation was better between length and centers of ossification (78%) than between any other two sets of measurements; weight and ossification centers (66%), length and menstrual age (65%) and weight and menstrual age varied considerably more. Centers of ossification visible on roentgen examination before birth may give valuable information as to the stage of fetal development. Average time of initial ossification is shown in Table 2–6.

Individual Bone Growth

Individual bones normally grow in constant relation to total body growth. Consequently it is possible to calculate the approximate gestational age of a fetus from the length of a single bone or part of the body (Table 2–7). Measurements of the head at different months of gestation are given in Table 2–8. Diameters may be measured fairly well by appropriate roentgen technics while the fetus is still in the uterus.

TABLE 2–7.–CALCULATED VALUES OF LENGTH OF THE EXTREMITIES AT CLOSE OF EACH FETAL MONTH (IN MM) (Scammon and Calkins)

PORTION OF EXTREMITY MEASURED	3 Mo	4 Mo	5 Mo	6 Mo	7 Mo	8 Mo	9 Mo	10 Mo
Length of lower extremity	23.4	59.8	91.0	118.6	143.7	166.8	188.5	208.9
Thigh length (trochanter to knee)	11.5	27.5	41.3	53.5	64.6	74.8	84.4	93.4
Leg length (knee to lateral malleolus)	9.7	26.6	41.1	53.9	65.6	76.4	86.4	95.9
Foot length	4.8	18.4	30.0	40.2	49.6	58.2	66.3	73.8
Length of upper extremity	24.3	58.2	87.2	112.8	136.2	157.7	177.9	196.8
Arm length (acromion to elbow)	10.2	23.6	34.8	44.8	53.8	62.2	70.0	77.3
Forearm length	7.7	18.7	28.1	36.5	44.1	51.1	57.6	63.8
Hand length	3.5	15.6	24.3	32.0	39.1	45.5	51.6	57.2

TABLE 2–8.–CALCULATED VALUES OF EXTERNAL DIMENSIONS OF THE HEAD AT CLOSE OF EACH FETAL MONTH (IN MM) (Scammon and Calkins)

DIMENSIONS OF HEAD	3 Mo	4 Mo	5 Mo	6 Mo	7 Mo	8 Mo	9 Mo	10 Mo
Occipitofrontal circumference	60.8	117.9	166.8	210.1	249.6	285.9	319.9	351.9
Occipitofrontal diameter	20.6	40.5	57.6	72.6	86.4	99.0	110.9	122.0
Suboccipitobregmatic circumference	60.3	113.1	158.4	198.5	235.1	268.7	300.2	329.8
Suboccipitobregmatic diameter	20.2	37.1	51.6	64.4	76.1	86.9	96.9	106.4
Suboccipitofrontal circumference	61.0	116.0	163.1	204.8	242.8	277.8	310.6	341.3
Suboccipitofrontal diameter	22.2	40.4	56.0	69.8	82.4	93.9	104.8	114.9
Occipitomental circumference	53.6	106.9	152.6	193.0	229.8	263.7	295.5	325.3
Occipitomental diameter	18.6	38.5	55.6	70.6	84.4	97.0	108.9	120.0
Biparietal diameter	15.5	31.5	45.3	57.5	68.6	78.8	88.4	97.4

Organ Weights

Organ weight in general is closely related to total body weight. Occasionally there are independent variations in weight even though organs appear normal, but usually any appreciable divergence from the average is due to pathologic lesions. This must be remembered when a "normal" weight is given for an organ belonging to a fetus or newborn infant. The average weight of the liver, for instance, of a newborn weighing 2,500 gm is 127 gm, but of an infant weighing 4,500 gm it is 245 gm, or over twice the weight normal for the smaller infant. The term macrosomia should be applied only when organ weight is disproportionately great in relation to body weight. Figures for average organ weights are given in Tables 2–3 and 2–5.

Differences in body size are dramatically shown in Figure 2–3. These two stillborn fetuses weighed 6,750 and 2,095 gm. The age as derived from menstrual data was stated to have been 40 weeks for both, although it seems quite probable that it was correct for neither. The organ weights of both were normal in relation to individual body size but, compared with those of an average fetus of 3,400 gm, all would have been considered abnormal.

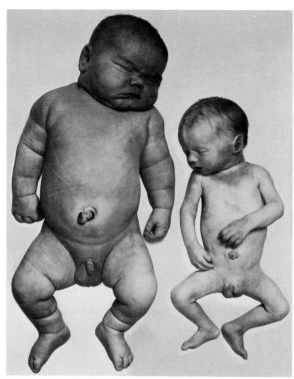

Fig. 2–3. — Stillborn fetuses weighing 6,750 and 2,095 gm demonstrating the great differences in size that may exist at time of delivery of infants at same estimated stage of gestation (40 weeks). Organ weights normal for one would be entirely abnormal for the other.

REFERENCES

Arey, L. B.: Correlation of fetal age and size, Am. J. Obstet. Gynecol. 54:872, 1947.

Bakwin, H., and Bakwin, R. M.: External dimensions of newborn, Am. J. Dis. Child. 48:1234, 1934.

Baumgartner, L., *et al.:* Weight in relation to fetal and newborn mortality: Influence of sex and color, Pediatrics 6:329, 1950.

Cruikshank, J. N., Miller, M. J., and Browne, F. J.: *The Estimation of Foetal Age, the Weight and Length of Normal Foetuses, and the Weights of Foetal Organs,* Medical Research Council Spec. Rep. Series No. 86 (London: His Majesty's Stationery Office, 1924).

Frazier, T. M.: Errors in reported date of last menstrual period, Am. J. Obstet. Gynecol. 77:95, 1959.

Graziani, L. J., Weitzman, E. D., and Velasco, M. S. A.: Neurologic maturation and auditory evoked responses in low birth weight infants, Pediatrics 41:483, 1968.

Gruenwald, P.: Growth of the human fetus, Am. J. Obstet. Gynecol. 94:1112, 1966.

Lubchenko, L. O., *et al.:* Intrauterine growth as estimated from liveborn birth-weight data 24 to 42 weeks of gestation, Pediatrics 32:793, 1963.

Mall, F. P.: On measuring the human embryo, Anat. Rec. 1:129, 1907.

Naeye, R. L., *et al.:* Intrauterine growth of twins as estimated from liveborn birth-weight data, Pediatrics 37:409, 1966.

Potter, E. L., and Fuller, H.: Multiple pregnancies at the Chicago Lying-in Hospital 1941 to 1947, Am. J. Obstet. Gynecol. 58:139, 1949.

Scammon, R. E.: Summary of the Anatomy of the Infant and Child, in *Abt's Pediatrics* (Philadelphia: W. B. Saunders Co., 1925), Vol. 1, p. 318.

Scammon, R. E., and Calkins, L. A.: Simple empirical formulae for expressing the lineal growth of the human fetus, Proc. Soc. Exp. Biol. Med. 20:353, 1923.

Scammon, R. E., and Calkins, L. A.: *Growth in the Fetal Period* (Minneapolis: University of Minnesota Press, 1929).

Schulz, D. M., Giordano, D. A., and Schulz, D. H.: Weights of organs of fetuses and infants, Arch. Pathol. 74:244, 1962.

Schuyler, W. B. J.: Fetal gigantism, Obstet. Gynecol. 6:538, 1956.

Scott, R. B., Jenkins, M. E., and Crawford, R. P.: Growth and development of Negro infants, Pediatrics 6:425, 1950.

Streeter, G. L.: Weight, sitting height, head size, foot length, and menstrual age of the human embryo, Embryology 11:143, 1920.

Usher, R., McLean, F., and Scott, K. E.: Judgment of fetal age. II. Clinical significance of gestational age and objective method for its assessment, Pediatr. Clin. North Am. 13:835, 1966.

Vital and Health Statistics: *Trends in "Prematurity," United States: 1950–1967.* Analytical Study Series #18 (Washington, D. C.: National Center of Health Statistics, 1972).

Warkany, J.: *Congenital Malformations: Notes and Comments* (Chicago: Year Book Medical Publishers, Inc., 1971).

White House Conference on Child Health and Protection: *Growth and Development of the Child* (New York: Century Company, 1933).

Yerushalmy, J., *et al.:* Birth weight and gestation as indices of "immaturity," Am. J. Dis. Child. 109:43, 1965.

Yerushalmy, J.: Relation of birth weight, gestational age, and the rate of intrauterine growth to perinatal mortality, Clin. Obstet. Gynecol. 13:107, 1970.

$\underline{3}$

Placenta and Umbilical Cord

Site of Implantation

THE FERTILIZATION OF the ovum by a sperm cell normally occurs in the distal portion of the fallopian tube, and cell division begins immediately. The growing structure passes down the fallopian tube over part of the uterine lining and comes to rest at about the 8th day on the endometrial surface of the uterus, most frequently high on the posterior wall.

PLACENTA PREVIA.—In about 0.5% of all pregnancies the blastocyst travels too far down in the uterus and implants in the lower uterine wall. As pregnancy progresses, a constantly increasing share of the uterine wall is covered by the placenta. When implantation is sufficiently low the placenta grows into the vicinity of, or spreads over, the internal cervical os. This condition is known as marginal, partial or central placenta previa, depending on the proportionate amount of the cervical opening that is covered by placental tissue (Fig. 3–1). The lower part of the uterus generally provides an adequate blood supply and pregnancy progresses normally.

Symptoms related to low implantation are ordinarily absent until late in pregnancy when the

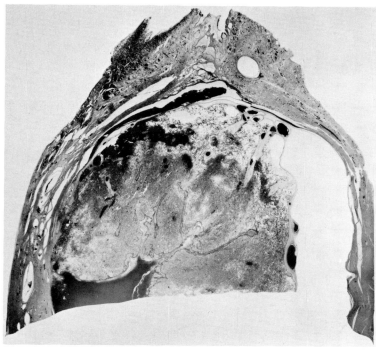

Fig. 3–1.—Placenta previa. Section through lower part of uterus showing placenta covering inner surface of cervix.

uterus begins to undergo changes preparatory to expulsion of the fetus. The amount of separation and the time of its occurrence depend largely on the relation of the placental site to the internal cervical os. If the placenta covers the os, even slight effacement may cause some placental detachment. If the placenta is adjacent to the os but does not cover it, effacement and dilatation may be almost complete before separation takes place.

Separation is characterized by painless vaginal bleeding. If the placenta is so attached that the dilated cervix is completely covered by placental tissue (central or complete placenta previa), delivery of the fetus through the vaginal canal is impossible except by manual separation or incision of the placenta. To detach the placenta exposes the mother to the risk of fatal hemorrhage. To make a hole in it subjects the fetus to the probability of death from exsanguination.

Anoxia resulting from premature separation of the placenta is the most common cause of fetal death in association with placenta previa. Exsanguination resulting from laceration of fetal vessels is less frequent and does not occur without manual intervention. When it is deemed necessary to deliver the fetus through an incompletely dilated cervix because of maternal hemorrhage, traumatic intracranial hemorrhage may result. When the undilated cervix is covered by placental tissue, the treatment of choice to prevent serious maternal hemorrhage and fetal damage is delivery by cesarean section.

CERVICAL PREGNANCY.—Because it is usually not recognized as a pregnancy, implantation of the embryo in the cervix often leads to massive hemorrhage following attempts at biopsy or removal of what is believed to be a cervical tumor. The absence of underlying decidua and the fibrous nature of the cervical stroma make a placenta located on the cervix difficult to remove, and the absence of muscle in the cervix prevents the blood vessels from being closed in a normal manner by muscular contraction.

DOUBLE UTERUS.—Implantation in one side of a double uterus usually leads to normal development. Implantation in different sides may occur in different pregnancies when both sides are well developed. One specimen observed at the Chicago Lying-in Hospital consisted of two equally developed uteri with a single vagina removed from a woman who had had 12 normal pregnancies with 12 living children. Rarely, implantation of two fertilized zygotes occurs simultaneously in the two parts of a double uterus. When a gestational sac is present in only one side, the endometrium of the other becomes converted into decidua in the same manner as that of the side in which the pregnancy is located. If a double uterus is asymmetrical and one part is rudimentary, implantation in that portion may be associated with uterine rupture because of muscular hypoplasia. Implantation on the uterine septa often results in abortion because of inadequate blood supply.

FALLOPIAN TUBE.—Tubal pregnancies account for 98% of all ectopic pregnancies. Infection may cause adhesions between tubal folds and produce pockets and distorted channels that interfere with normal movement. Abnormalities in peristaltic or ciliary action may also interfere with normal passage.

Downward movement may be arrested in any part of the tube; thus the vesicle may continue its development in the ampulla, isthmus or interstitial portion. The middle and distal parts of the isthmus are the most common sites of arrest, and a characteristic ovoid swelling is usually produced (Fig. 3–2). The lining of the tube makes a poorer implantation site than does the lining of the uterus. A few decidual cells may be found in the stroma of the tubal folds or in the muscular wall, but a complete layer of decidua never develops. The blood supply is inadequate and, as a result, the differentiation of the proliferating trophoblast into villi is retarded. Masses of cells resembling cytotrophoblast, often

Fig. 3–2.—Bisected fallopian tube and ovary. Fetus and chorionic vesicle are in the distal part of the tube and the rest is filled with blood. Corpus luteum and large follicle are present in the ovary. Pregnancy of about 7 weeks.

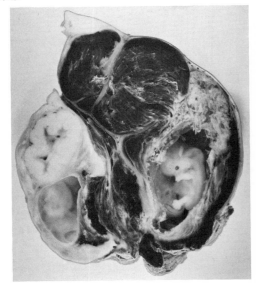

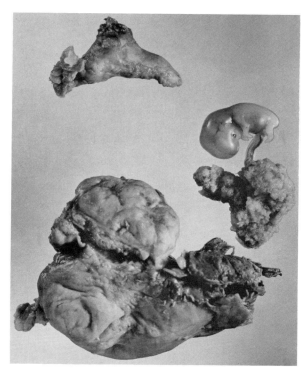

Fig. 3–3.—Two tubal pregnancies. The upper tube ruptured 32 days after the last menstrual period. The lower tube with attached ovary ruptured about 10 weeks after the last menstrual period; operation revealed the fetus and ruptured vesicle in the abdominal cavity.

several centimenters before the tube ruptures or the embryo is expelled through the ampulla into the abdominal cavity (Fig. 3–3). If this occurs in the early stages of development, the fact that pregnancy existed may remain unrecognized. More often it is associated with intra-abdominal hemorrhage. The tubal lumen is capable of great enlargement if the increase is gradual, and excessive distention is almost never a cause of rupture. The site of blastocyst implantation largely determines the time of rupture; when it is on the wall of the tube, erosion and subsequent perforation occur earlier than when it is on the surface of a tubal fold.

In many tubal pregnancies separation of the chorionic vesicle from the tubal wall is responsible for hemorrhage and embryonic death before perforation or operative intervention. Such separation from the tubal wall is generally designated tubal abortion.

INTERSTITIAL PORTION OF FALLOPIAN TUBE.—Interstitial implantation occurs when the zygote is arrested in the portion of the fallopian tube that traverses the uterine wall. As growth proceeds, the vesicle usually extends into the uterine cavity and either is aborted or continues to grow in the uterine cornu. When the vesicle remains interstitial, it produces a local swelling (Fig. 3–4) that may be

Fig. 3–4.—Interstitial pregnancy with chorionic vesicle and degenerated embryo. Ovary and fallopian tube are visible beneath implantation site.

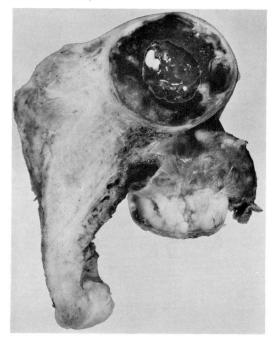

found in tubal pregnancies, are not seen in intrauterine pregnancies.

The ability of the trophoblast to destroy tissues with which it comes in contact is often responsible for erosion of the wall of the fallopian tube and its blood vessels. In an intrauterine pregnancy syncytial cells grow for short distances along the inner surface of the blood vessels that are opened by this erosive process, and blood loss is thus controlled and excessive bleeding prevented. When the trophoblast penetrates blood vessels in the fallopian tube, such control of hemorrhage does not occur. When the involved vessels are small, the bleeding is often confined to the lumen of the tube or the tissues immediately surrounding it. If such blood becomes organized, it may be responsible for numerous adhesions between the tube and adjacent structures. Bleeding from larger vessels causes massive intra-abdominal hemorrhage and is accompanied by symptoms of shock.

The tube may be perforated by trophoblastic erosion while the vesicle is still only a few millimeters in diameter, or the vesicle may reach a diameter of

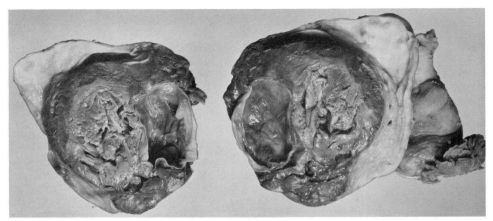

Fig. 3–5.—Ovarian pregnancy with chorionic vesicle embedded in blood clot and contained entirely within the ovary. The adjacent fallopian tube is normal.

mistaken for a leiomyoma. Penetration of the uterine wall by villi may be followed by local rupture and expulsion of the fetus into the abdominal cavity. Interstitial pregnancy, like implantation in other parts of the tube, never proceeds to term if the vesicle remains in its original location.

OVARY.—Fertilization and development of a chorionic vesicle in the ovary is rare, occurring in only about 0.4% of all ectopic pregnancies. In earlier years many investigators contended that ovarian pregnancies could not take place, but there are now over 200 authentic cases in the literature and one was observed at the Chicago Lying-in Hospital (Fig. 3–5).

ABDOMINAL CAVITY.—A vesicle growing in the fallopian tube may escape by rupturing the tubal wall, growing out through the ampulla or, less often, by being expelled into the abdominal cavity. If

Fig. 3–6.—Abdominal pregnancy. **A,** fetus weighing 2,900 gm partially surrounded by amniotic membrane and attached by umbilical cord to placenta. **B,** lipiodol in uterine cavity and both fallopian tubes. Fetus is visible in abdominal cavity.

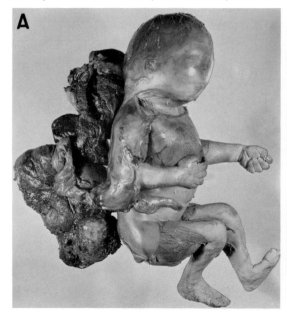

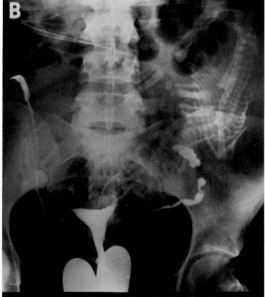

alive it may implant on adjacent structures such as the ovary, broad ligament, intestine or omentum. It seems possible also, in rare instances, that fertilization may occur in the abdominal cavity and that development may be intra-abdominal from the beginning. Abdominal pregnancy may continue to or near term (Fig. 3–6,A), and the first indication that the fetus is not in the uterus may be the absence of labor pains at the expected time. Most often the fetus is dead before the diagnosis is made, but if it is alive, delivery by laparotomy may save its life. In a thin patient the diagnosis can usually be made from the ease with which fetal parts can be palpated. The diagnosis can be confirmed by the injection of a radiopaque substance into the uterus. If the cavity can be visualized, no doubt as to the diagnosis remains (Fig. 3–6,B). The placenta in an abdominal pregnancy may be fairly normal except that it is often somewhat thinner and covers a greater surface area than in an intrauterine pregnancy. Villi, which are usually attached to the omentum, are often spread out over the surface of the intestines and occasionally over the pelvic organs. As long as the fetus is alive, growth proceeds fairly normally and the villi are so firmly adherent that they cannot be separated without injury to the tissues from

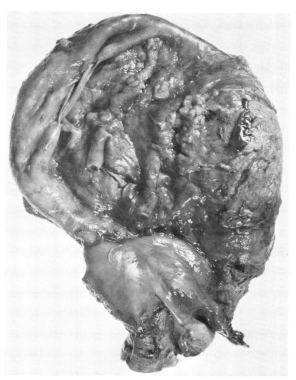

Fig. 3–8.—Uterus with placenta and membranes extruded through rupture at the site of a previous cesarean section. Fetal development continued following escape from the uterus, with fetus attaining a weight of 2,430 gm. View shows external, unattached surface of placenta.

Fig. 3–7.—Lithopedion resulting from retention of fetus in abdominal cavity for several years after death. (Courtesy Dr. Henry W. Edmonds.)

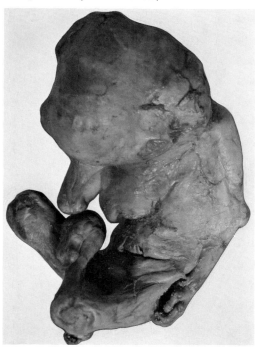

which they are deriving their blood supply. When the fetus dies or is surgically removed and the villi no longer contain circulating blood, they gradually degenerate and separate spontaneously from the abdominal organs.

If the fetus of an abdominal pregnancy is not removed surgically, it may remain in the abdomen for many years, seldom producing symptoms other than those of a local tumor. Such fetuses become calcified and are called lithopedions (Fig. 3–7). Formation of a fistulous tract with the discharge of fetal skeletal parts through the abdominal wall, vagina or rectum has been known to occur when a fetus has remained in the abdomen for a long period.

One case was observed at the Chicago Lying-in Hospital in which fetus and placenta were expelled in early pregnancy through a dehiscence of the site of a previous cesarean section and continued to grow in the abdomen until the fetus weighed 2,430 gm (Fig. 3–8). No symptoms were produced and the patient presented herself for the first time at 42 weeks because she failed to go into labor.

RELATION OF ABNORMAL SITE OF IMPLANTATION TO FETAL MALFORMATIONS. — The fact that the incidence of fetal malformations has been reported as increased when associated with abnormal sites of implantation has been cited as direct proof that abnormalities of environment are responsible for many malformations. Mall reported that 96% of the embryos he found in tubal pregnancies were pathologic, and Greenhill reported a 2.5% incidence of fetal malformations in 4,466 cases of placenta previa, in contrast to 0.94% for all obstetric cases. The incidence of malformations has varied among the abdominal pregnancies described by various authors; in seven abdominal pregnancies observed at the Chicago Lying-in Hospital only one of the fetuses was malformed. Embryos were seldom found in tubal pregnancies in that hospital, but among the few that were discovered almost none had demonstrable malformations. However, if hydropic changes in villi are considered evidence of malformation, the incidence would be higher than in intrauterine pregnancies. If malformations are more commonly associated with abnormal than with normal implantation sites, it is possible either that a disturbance already exists in the blastocyst, which is responsible for both conditions, or that the embryo receives a poorer blood supply because of its abnormal location and that the relative anoxia thus produced is the cause of the maldevelopment.

Placental Configuration

Degeneration of part of the villi that originally cover the entire outer surface of the chorionic vesicle leads to localization of the placenta in the wall of the vesicle and determines its size and shape. During the middle part of the first trimester of pregnancy the villi on that portion of the vesicle most elevated above the surface of the uterine wall and most poorly oxygenated because of the distance from the maternal blood supply begin to atrophy and gradually disappear. By midpregnancy the placenta is delineated and at term it ordinarily occupies only about one fifth of the surface of the chorionic sac. The portion in which functioning villi persist is known as the chorion frondosum. The inner (fetal) surface, which usually becomes somewhat hyalinized, is known as the chorionic plate; the major placental vessels are contained in its substance. The part from which villi disappear is known as the chorion laeve. This becomes the chorionic membrane and at term is composed of a thin fibrinous layer in which a few ghosts of degenerated villi are still discernible. It forms an outer covering for the amniotic sac.

The shape of the placenta is most frequently round or oval because the villi ordinarily degenerate in an evenly progressive manner. If, for unknown reasons, degeneration proceeds irregularly, the shape of the mature placenta may be bizarre. If it is divided into two or three lobes of fairly similar size that are attached to one another in the region in which the umbilical cord originates, it is designated a bipartite (Fig. 3–9) or tripartite placenta. If one or more groups of villi persist at a little distance from the main portion of the placenta, they form accessory or succenturiate lobes (Fig. 3–10). Rarely, groups of villi persist over much of the surface of the chorionic vesicle and are separated by irregular areas from which they have disappeared. This gives rise to a succenturiate or membranous placenta (Fig. 3–11). The area in which villi persist may rarely assume an elongate or horseshoe shape. One horseshoe-shaped placenta observed at the Chicago Lying-in Hospital almost completely encircled the lower uterine segment. Had it been delivered with

Fig. 3–9. — Bipartite placenta with velamentous insertion of vessels. Transilluminated.

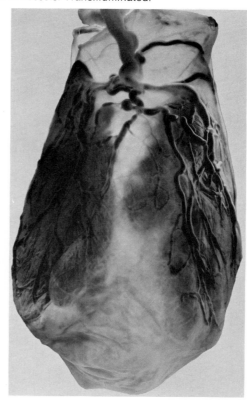

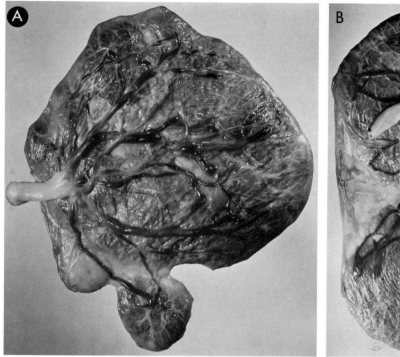
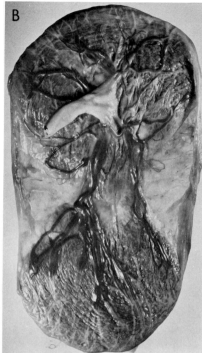

Fig. 3—10.—Placentas with succenturiate lobes. **A**, small lobe. **B**, large lobe.

the infant's body, it would have formed a cape covering the back and both shoulders. Only once in over 100,000 deliveries at the Chicago Lying-in Hospital did the placenta completely encircle the uterus (Fig. 3–12).

PLACENTA EXTRACHORIALIS (PLACENTA MARGINATA AND CIRCUMVALLATA).—The fetal surface of the placenta occasionally has a sharply demarcated circumferential zone of hyaline that varies from a narrow, thin, flat, somewhat irregular ring closely adherent to the surface of the placenta to a complete wide, thick ring elevated above the surface of the placenta. This has been designated extrachorial placenta (Scott) because of the belief that the extension of the placenta peripheral to the zone of hyaline is a secondary growth of villi beyond the original chorionic plate; those with a thin superficial ring have been designated placenta marginata (see Fig. 1–16,B), those with a thick elevated ring, placenta circumvallata (Fig. 3–13). In attempts to explain why these abnormalities occur the two conditions have usually been considered together and the following reasons have been given:

1. The size of the original placenta is inadequate and subsequent growth produces the extrachorial part of the placenta.

2. Because the implantation of the blastocyst is too deep in the decidua, part of the fetal surface is covered by decidua.

3. Early in placental development the outer edge of the chorion splits so that the amnion and superficial chorion come to lie above the decidua while the lateral major cotyledons lie below and lateral to the inner decidual border. Further growth of the exposed fetal surface of the placenta causes hemorrhage, focal thrombosis, villous infarction and fibrin deposition, which give rise to the in-rolled cufflike appearance of the circumvallate placenta.

4. The lesion follows partial early separation of the placenta with consequent infarction, thrombosis and necrosis resulting in the heaped-up area, while the placenta continues to grow more distally in a deeper plane.

There is such a marked difference in form and structure of the two varieties of placentas that the adequacy of any single explanation seems somewhat questionable, and the term extrachorialis may be misleading. In placenta marginata the superficial zone of hyaline is without clinical significance, villi beneath and beyond this zone are similar to those in the rest of the placenta and there is no conclusive evidence that their formation differs in time or manner from those in the remainder of the placenta. In placenta circumvallata the inner edge of the hyaline ring is the area that was originally at the margin of the placenta. Detachment of the periphery causes degeneration and hyalinization of villi, and the separation from the uterine wall permits the margin to roll inward, producing the characteristic cuffing. The chorionic membrane and its adherent amnion are attached to the inner edge of the ring (Fig. 3–13,B) and while the fetus remains in the uterus, hydrostatic pressure forces them backward against the in-rolled portion of the placenta. Such separation prevents further growth of the original margin, which shrinks as it becomes hyalinized. The portion still attached continues to grow and the cotyledonary pattern gives a scalloped edge. The total placenta is thicker and has a smaller diameter than normal. Many patients with such placentas have a history of midpregnancy bleeding and threatened miscarriage. In an extensive study carried out at the Chicago Lying-in Hospital the frequency of premature delivery was

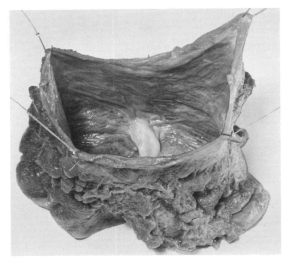

Fig. 3–12.—Placenta completely encircling the uterus in a continuous wide band 9 cm wide.

slightly increased but the percentage of malformations was no higher than in total pregnancies.

Attachment of the Umbilical Cord to the Placenta

The relation of the attachment of the umbilical cord to the surface of the placenta is determined at the time of implantation by the position that the inner cell mass assumes in relation to the uterine wall. The blastocyst ordinarily implants in such a way that the inner cell mass is on the side of the blastocyst that first penetrates the decidua and comes to lie nearest the uterine musculature. The inner cell mass is the region in which the embryo develops, and when the body stalk forms, it connects the embryo with this same section of the vesicle wall. It thus normally attaches to the part where the villi persist and the placenta develops. As a result, the umbilical cord, which is the mature body stalk, is connected with the placenta near its central portion.

If implantation is such that the inner cell mass, and consequently the body stalk, is not in the deepest-lying portion of the blastocyst but on the upper or lateral surface, the umbilical cord will be attached to the wall of the chorionic vesicle some distance from the placenta. The relation of the body stalk to the part of the chorionic vesicle that lies closest to the uterine wall and becomes the placenta determines whether the attachment of the umbilical cord to the placenta is central, eccentric, marginal or velamentous.

The major blood vessels of the placenta usually consist of about five pairs that are branches of the

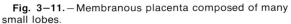

Fig. 3–11.—Membranous placenta composed of many small lobes.

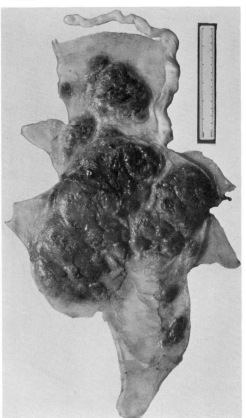

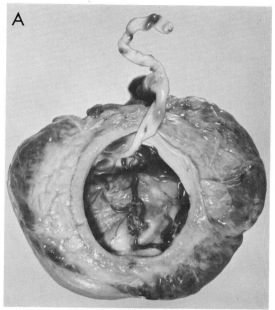

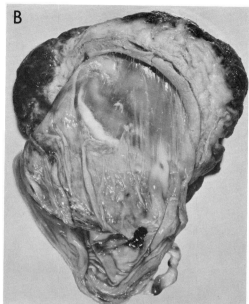

Fig. 3–13.—Circumvallate placenta. **A,** amniotic and chorionic membranes turned back and under to show surface of placenta. **B,** membranes drawn to one side to show in-rolled hyalinized edge of placenta and attachment of membranes.

Fig. 3–14.—**A,** placenta with velamentous origin of umbilical cord. **B,** vasa previa in which one vessel crossed the cervical os. Umbilical cord originated in the chorionic membrane on the side opposite the placenta.

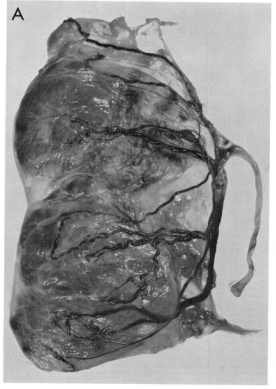

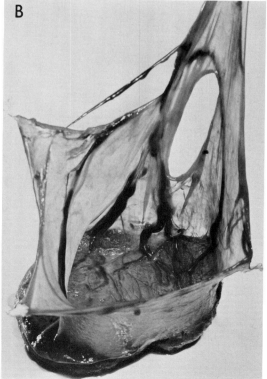

veins and arteries of the umbilical cord. They run over the fetal surface, disappearing into the fetal substance about 1 cm from the outer margin of the chorionic plate. If the cord arises eccentrically, two pairs are usually found on the narrow portion and three on the wider portion of the placenta. If the cord is attached at the margin, all vessels run in the same direction toward the opposite edge of the placenta, and if it is velamentous they leave the placenta and extend through part of the chorionic membrane before they meet to form the cord (Fig. 3–14,A). The distance between the edge of the placenta and the origin of the umbilical cord is usually short, but occasionally some of the blood vessels form an arc and traverse a much greater distance than would be necessary if they took the shortest possible course to the cord.

If implantation is such that the inner cell mass is in the wall of the blastocyst opposite that attached to the uterine wall and in a position the reverse of that usually assumed, the superficial blood vessels will extend peripherally from the surface of the placenta and encircle the chorionic sac to unite as the umbilical cord on the portion of the chorionic

membrane directly opposite the placenta (Fig. 3–14,B). If velamentous blood vessels cross the opening formed by the cervix as it dilates during labor, the condition in designated vasa previa. Unsupported blood vessels are somewhat more susceptible to rupture than are those within the umbilical cord, but even those crossing the cervical opening often remain uninjured. The membranes usually rupture between the blood vessels, and they are simply pushed aside as the fetus passes between them. Any vessels, however, may be ruptured, even those on the surface of the placenta, and it must be remembered that any vaginal bleeding may be fetal in origin. If the vessels on the surface of the placenta are involved, bleeding is between amnion and chorion (Fig. 3–15).

Placental Separation

Normally the placenta separates as soon as the uterus contracts after delivery of the infant. The plane of separation passes through the spongy layer of the decidua where large, cystically dilated glands and sinusoidal spaces are common. Conse-

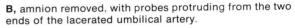

Fig. 3—15.—Ruptured placental blood vessel. **A,** surface of placenta with blood between amnion and chorion.   **B,** amnion removed, with probes protruding from the two ends of the lacerated umbilical artery.

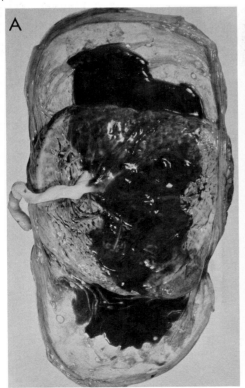
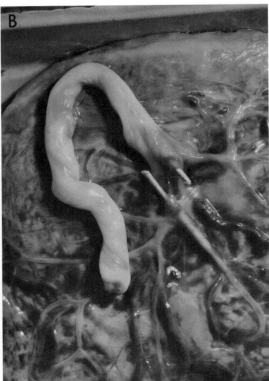

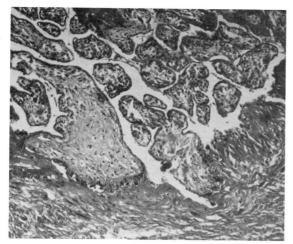

Fig. 3—16.—Placenta accreta. Anchoring villi are attached to the underlying uterine muscle with no intervening decidua.

quently part of the decidua adheres to the placenta while part remains attached to the myometrium where separation occurs.

PLACENTA ACCRETA.—On the rare occasions when the placenta does not separate spontaneously, manual examination often fails to reveal a plane of cleavage. It may be impossible to separate all or part of the placenta from the uterine wall mechanically, and hysterectomy may be necessary to prevent exsanguinating hemorrhage. Microscopic examination usually shows villi attached directly to the uterine muscle separated only by a layer of fibrin with no intervening decidua (Fig. 3—16), or the villi may actually penetrate the uterine muscle. Both are usually called placenta accreta, although some authors have substituted the term increta for growth of villi into uterine muscle, reserving the term accreta for a placenta that is abnormally adherent but not actually invasive. Rarely, as occurred in one patient at the Chicago Lying-in Hospital, the villi penetrate the entire thickness of the uterine wall (placenta percreta).

ABRUPTIO PLACENTAE.—The placenta occasionally becomes partially or completely detached before the birth of the infant (Fig. 3—17). This is known as abruptio placentae, ablatio placentae or premature detachment of the normally implanted placenta. The detachment is associated with rupture and bleeding from decidual vessels. If the separation extends to the margin of the placenta, blood escapes into the vagina. If the separation involves only the central portion, a hematoma is formed between the placenta and the uterine wall, and the villi in this area may be compressed into a solid mass resembling an infarct. This is sometimes

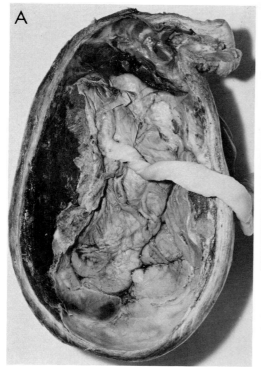

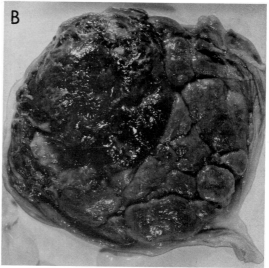

Fig. 3—17.—Abruptio placentae. **A,** bisected uterus showing a large retroplacental hematoma that completely detached the placenta. **B,** placenta with a localized hematoma caused by an area of premature separation.

called placental apoplexy. If the area of separation is extensive, the fetus usually dies of anoxia. In a condition designated as a Couvelaire uterus, which is occasionally associated with premature placental detachment, the wall of the uterus, especially the lateral portions, becomes infiltrated by blood. Hemorrhage is present in muscle bundles, perivascular connective tissue and the subserosa, where it gives the uterus a deep purple color.

Abruptio placentae is sometimes accompanied by a severe disturbance in the clotting mechanism. The fibrinogen level may be low, presumably due to precipitation of fibrin in the retroplacental clot, and bleeding may become generalized. The cause of the placental detachment and its sequelae is not known for certain. Although Hibbard and colleagues showed a relationship between low levels of folic acid and abruptio placentae, this has not been substantiated by other investigators. The simultaneous occurrence of abruptio and preeclampsia or eclampsia has often been reported, but Hibbard's observations suggest that albuminuria and hematuria may occur as a direct result of abruptio placentae and may lead to a false diagnosis of toxemia of pregnancy.

Placental Size

The size of the placenta increases throughout pregnancy because of continuous growth of the vil-li. Early in pregnancy the weight of the vesicle wall and villi exceeds that of the fetus. At about the 4th month the weights are equal, and thereafter the weight of the fetus becomes increasingly greater than that of the placenta. At term the weight of the placenta without cord or membranes normally averages about one seventh—with cord and membranes, about one sixth—that of the fetus. Weights ranging from one fifth to one tenth that of the fetus are usually considered within a normal range.

Little studied the placentas of 956 mature infants (37–41 weeks) and concluded that a placental coefficient of less than 0.10 and greater than 0.18 should be considered indicative of a relatively small or large placenta and that less than 0.08 and more than 0.2 should be considered definitely abnormal. Dodds calculated from data obtained by light microscopy that at term the chorionic villi have a surface covering of 7 m². If the microvilli seen by electron microscopy are taken into account, this figure will be increased severalfold.

If the fetus dies, the placenta ordinarily stops growing, becomes detached from the uterine wall and is expelled from the uterus with the fetus. Delivery may not occur for weeks or even months after death of the fetus, and most of the villi then show complete loss of nuclear structure and are embedded in a solid mass of acellular fibrinoid material. Occasionally, trophoblast cells covering part of the villi remain alive and may show small

Fig. 3–18.—Placental hyperplasia. Diffuse cystic hyperplasia with continued growth of the placenta following fetal death. Fetus was normal except for advanced maceration. Single pregnancy.

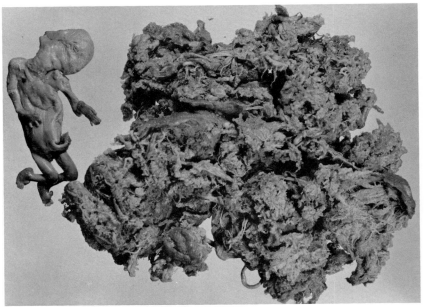

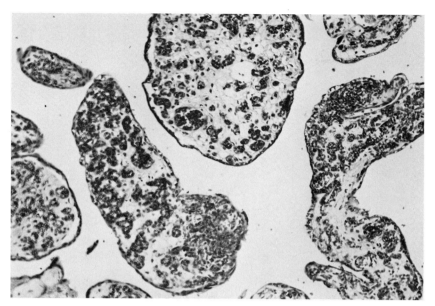

Fig. 3—19.—Excessive number of blood vessels in villi causing diffuse placental hypertrophy (chorioangiosis). Fetus was not macerated but was abnormally small for the size of the placenta.

areas of excessive growth. As long as trophoblast cells are alive, pregnancy tests remain positive regardless of the condition of the fetus.

PLACENTAL HYPERTROPHY.—Excessive size may be found in several conditions. In some instances the placenta appears to continue to grow after fetal death. In such cases the villi often become mildly cystic, and this contributes to the disproportionately large size of the placenta (Fig. 3 – 18). Diffuse enlargement may be associated with an increase in size of individual villi resulting from an abnormal proliferation of blood vessels. The vessels are similar to those of normal villi, but instead of the usual four to six in a cross-section of a villus, 25 – 50 or more may be found (Fig. 3 – 19). In the cases seen at the Chicago Lying-in Hospital the placenta and fetus had been delivered before the period of viability. This abnormality, which has been called chorioangiosis, may be related to the chorioangiomas described later in this chapter.

Excessive size most often results from erythroblastosis, although in former years it was usually attributed to syphilis. These conditions are also described later in this chapter.

PLACENTAL HYPOPLASIA.—Except with twins there is little evidence that fetal death is ever a result of insufficient placental size. If some disturbance causes cessation of placental growth, fetal growth is interrupted because of an inadequate source of food materials and oxygen. The fetus probably never outgrows the placenta for it can increase in size only in relation to the size of the capillary bed in the villi and, once formed, this continues to be adequate unless the area of circulation is reduced by some pathologic change.

Degenerative Changes in the Placenta

INFARCTION.—Infarcts of the placenta are the result of disturbances in the maternal blood supply. Many kinds have been described, but almost all are a result of variation in size, shape, location and age of only two principal varieties. They are rarely of clinical significance and almost never cause fetal death.

The most common variety is composed of groups of degenerated villi that are held together in a firm, compact mass by the intervillous deposit of a homogeneous acellular material composed of coagulated fibrin, often without enmeshed red blood cells (Fig. 3 – 20). The age of the infarcts determines their color. They are red in the early stages but gradually become pink and finally yellow-white as a result of disintegration of whatever blood cells are contained in and between the villi. The most frequent location is the margin of the placenta in the area where maternal circulation is the least adequate. However, they may be found on any portion of the maternal surface. They are often roughly cone-shaped, with the base directed toward the surface in

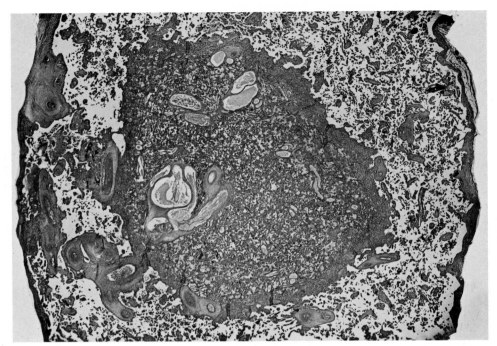

Fig. 3–20.—Photomicrograph of portion of placental infarct composed of degenerated villi embedded in fibrin. Central part of infarct extended to decidual surface.

contact with the uterine wall. In such a location they ordinarily result from local interference with maternal blood supply, and their cone shape is due to the deeper portions of the placental substance receiving blood from adjacent areas. Such infarcts are most often superficial and only 0.5–1 cm thick. Sometimes they extend through the entire thickness of the placenta (Fig. 3–21) and may involve several cotyledons. They are somewhat more common with preeclamptic toxemia or chronic renal disease than with normal pregnancies, and some investigators believe that they precede the toxemia and are responsible for its development. The latter view is not generally accepted.

The infarcts just described are sharply circumscribed and have a uniform structure. Occasionally the placenta contains irregular areas of degeneration scattered throughout much of its substance, and the entire placenta may be composed of an intermixture of hyaline, degenerated villi and normally functioning placental tissue. Surprisingly large amounts of the placenta may appear degenerated without producing discernible fetal hypoxia (Fig. 3–22).

Little thought that one third of the placenta must be infarcted to be a significant cause of placental insufficiency. The only reliable method of estimating the degree of infarction is to excise the infarcted areas and ascertain their weight in relation to the whole placenta.

The second type of lesion often considered an infarct is more accurately designated a thrombus. It is usually cuboidal, less than 2 cm in diameter and ordinarily located in the center of a cotyledon. Such areas are almost never visible from the surface and are discovered only when the placenta is incised. When sectioned they are smooth and glistening and are composed of red and white blood cells and platelets, giving a gross appearance similar to the layering found in a thrombus (Fig. 3–23). Although villi are not present within the thrombus, they may be compressed around the margin, producing a peripheral zone similar in structure to the type of infarction described above. These thrombi are in the central cotyledonary space described by Freese and result from the stasis of maternal blood. That they consist of maternal blood was shown earlier by Potter. One or many such thrombi may be present.

CHANGES WITH AGE.—The villi show considerable variability in relation to maturation and aging. The early villus is short and thick with only a few small vessels situated at some distance from the surface. The connective tissue is abundant and loosely arranged with much fluid between the cells.

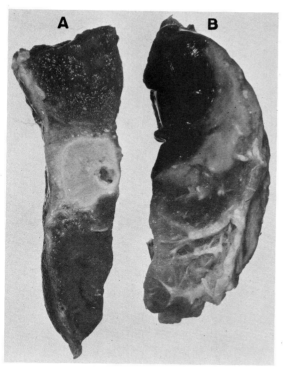

Fig. 3–21.—Placental infarcts in cross-section. **A,** infarct composed of degenerated villi embedded in fibrin extending through entire thickness of placenta. **B,** retroplacental hematoma with secondary infarct caused by compression of villi.

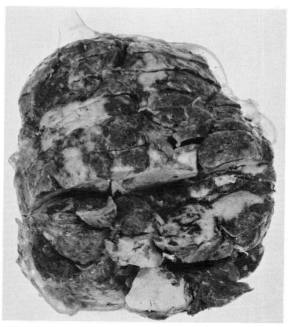

Fig. 3–22.—Term placenta with normal infant and no pregnancy complications. Multiple large old white infarcts throughout the placenta.

Fig. 3–23.—Thrombotic type of infarct composed of grossly visible layers of leukocytes, platelets and fibrin in the mass of erythrocytes.

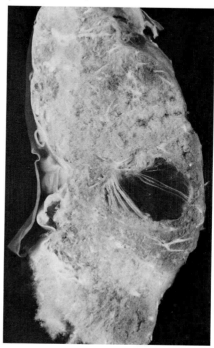

The outer syncytial layer and the inner Langhans' layer are easily identifiable (see Fig. 1–7). Even with the light microscope, in well-prepared sections one can see microvilli on the outer surface. As aging progresses, the syncytial cells become thinner, the microvilli less prominent and the nuclei smaller and more pyknotic. The Langhans' layer appears discontinuous by light microscopy, although with the electron microscope it can be seen to surround the entire villus. The stromal core of the villus at term is less voluminous and is nearly filled with small blood vessels. The connective tissue becomes hyalinized and more prominent. Hofbauer cells, the macrophages of the villi, which are common in the immature villus, are rarely recognized in the full-term placenta. Changes accompanying villus aging that are demonstrable by electron microscopy include gradual reduction in size and number of microvilli, reduction of pinocytotic vacuoles and tubules in the syncytial cells and reduction of endoplasmic reticulum in Langhans' cells. It is now generally agreed that the syncytial cells are incapable of dividing but are formed from the cells of the proliferating cytotrophoblast, which subsequently undergo fusion, to form multinucleated cells on the surface of the villi. While "syncytial knots" (clumps of syncytial cell nuclei) are increased in frequency in all older placentas (Fig. 3–24), an excessive increase in knotting was described by Tenney in cases of toxemia. In an experimental study, using in vitro technics, he showed that villi exposed to anoxic conditions developed more syncytial knots than those kept in a medium with more oxygen. This was considered an adaptive phenomenon to reduce the diffusion distance from the intervillous space to the fetal capillaries in the presence of reduced oxygen tension, since the movement of the cells into clumps reduces the number of cells covering the remainder of the surface and hence the thickness of this cellular layer. However, in a study of 500 placentas examined without knowledge of clinical data, Potter found no correlation between clumping of syncytial nuclei and the presence of toxemia (unpublished).

Calcium and iron are present in varying amounts in almost all placentas at term. They appear earliest in the decidua, the connective tissue of the fetal surface and the major trunks of the villi. They appear last in the stroma of the terminal villi and are found there only when the placenta contains unusually excessive amounts. Calcium is ordinarily present in the form of sheets and crystals, and the tissues may be so densely infiltrated that they require decalcification before sections can be prepared for microscopic examination. No correlation has been demonstrated between the amount of calcium in the placenta and any condition in the mother or infant.

Hyalinelike material, largely fibrin, is always present on the fetal surface of the placenta near term. It may be scattered over the entire surface in small nodules 2–4 mm in diameter that can be palpated even more readily than they can be seen. Such nodules afford an approximate means of determining the age of the fetus since they increase in size and number with increasing maturity. At other times similar material is arranged in irregularly circumscribed plaques that may attain a thickness of several millimeters. Occasionally, cystic cavities several centimeters in diameter are present in the superficial portions of such hyalinized areas (Fig. 3–25). They, too, have no known significance.

PLACENTAL DYSFUNCTION SYNDROME.—This phrase has become popular among some clinicians as a means of designating certain newborn infants who are of less than average weight for the estimated length of gestation, who have a disproportionately small amount of subcutaneous fat and seemingly increased desquamation and who may have expelled meconium before birth. It has been said, by way of explanation, that the placenta does not function normally and that chronic oxygen lack may be responsible for fetal malnutrition and expulsion of meconium. This is the same description and explanation used earlier by some observers to justify the phrase "postmaturity syndrome," since

Fig. 3–24 (left).—Villi from a term placenta showing increase in syncytial knots.
Fig. 3–25 (right).—Chorionic cyst on surface of placenta.

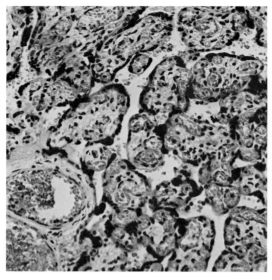
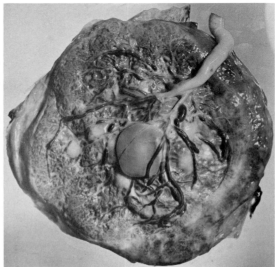

it was thought that certain infants were retained in the uterus longer than the placenta could adequately supply their nutritional needs. When it was shown that infants of normal gestational age might resemble those thought to be postmature, the less limiting designation of placental dysfunction was substituted.

Doubtless, placental function may vary, and transfer of metabolites may be more satisfactory in some instances than in others. Since rabbit and rat fetuses invariably die when pregnancy is artificially prolonged more than about 20% of normal time, it is reasonable to assume that this may be true also for the human, although it has not yet been conclusively demonstrated.

Many authors have described an increase in perinatal mortality in association with an estimated duration of pregnancy beyond 42 or 43 weeks and have recommended artificial termination to prevent fetal death. This increased mortality appears to be associated only with fetal and not with infant death; once a postmature infant is born alive, the mortality is no greater than that of an infant of a normal length gestation—yet such an infant rarely may have other difficulties such as hypoglycemia in the neonatal period. Twelve per cent of all births were found to occur after the end of the 42d week of pregnancy in the study described in Chapter 1 conducted at the Chicago Lying-in Hospital. Fetal and neonatal mortality were not increased in this group.

It is impossible to correlate any gross or histologic changes in the placenta with supposed abnormal prolongation of pregnancy or with any characteristic change in the infant. Placental dysfunction syndrome is an entirely clinical diagnosis and one that cannot be substantiated pathologically.

Diseases of the Placenta

ERYTHROBLASTOSIS FETALIS.—The changes produced in the placenta by erythroblastosis fetalis are of varying degree. If the infant is not edematous at birth, the size and gross appearance of the placenta are often normal. If immature erythrocytes are present in the fetal circulation they will be visible in the capillaries of the villi and in the larger blood vessels; but, in general, the placenta is not abnormally large unless the fetus is edematous and then the more edematous the fetus the larger is the placenta. Rarely, however, even in the absence of fetal edema the placenta is very large and microscopically resembles that of a hydropic fetus.

If the infant is edematous, the placenta may weigh one half or more as much as the infant. Both surface area and thickness are greatly increased. The cotyledons are enlarged and unusually well demarcated (Fig. 3–26). The color is light gray-pink instead of the usual dark red. Fragments of placenta teased out in water show individual villi thicker and the terminal portions larger than normal. Much fluid exudes from the placenta if it is permitted to stand. Microscopic examination reveals large edematous villi with numerous bulbous projections (Fig. 3–27). The stroma of the villi resembles loose connective tissue and often contains Hofbauer cells. The capillaries are most numerous at the periphery of the villi and ordinarily contain many normoblasts and erythroblasts (Fig. 3–28). Some investigators have observed erythropoiesis in the stroma of villi, but none of the large number of erythroblastotic placentas examined at the Chicago Lying-in Hospital have shown unequivocal evidence of local formation of blood cells. The cellular covering of the villi is often detached from the underlying stroma as a result of the fluid loss that occurs when the placenta is permitted to stand or of the shrinkage that occurs during preparation for microscopic examination.

On rare occasions the villi are covered by two complete layers of cells that closely resemble those normally present in the 1st trimester of pregnancy. Normally, the Langhans' layer becomes inconspicuous before the middle of pregnancy, leaving only the syncytial layer, but in some cases of erythroblastosis the Langhans' layer persists and is as

Fig. 3—26.—Placenta with large, thick, sharply demarcated cotyledons characteristic of erythroblastosis.

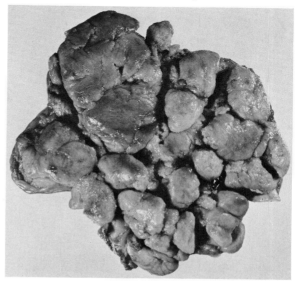

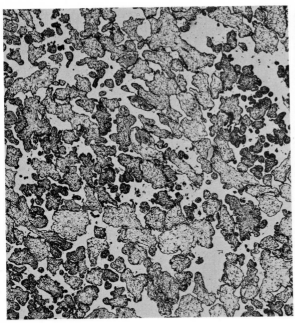

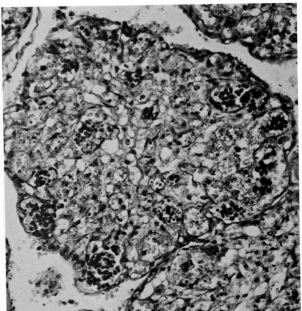

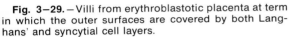

Fig. 3—27 (left).—Erythroblastotic placenta showing increased size of villi.

Fig. 3—28 (right).—Villi from erythroblastotic placenta showing margination and increase in number of blood vessels. Vessels are filled with nucleated red blood cells.

Fig. 3—29.—Villi from erythroblastotic placenta at term in which the outer surfaces are covered by both Langhans' and syncytial cell layers.

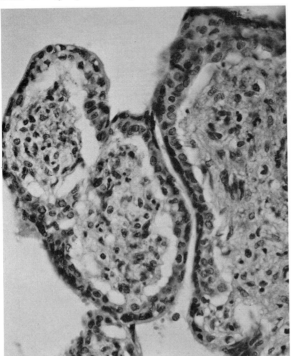

prominent at term as it is normally at 8 or 10 weeks (Fig. 3–29). In other cases fewer cells remain, and in some placentas almost none are visible with the light microscope.

VIRAL INFECTIONS.—When the fetus is anemic at birth, the placenta is usually enlarged. This is especially true in erythroblastosis but it is also found in cytomegalic inclusion disease caused by the salivary gland virus. These two conditions ordinarily destroy more fetal erythrocytes and incite a greater erythropoietic response than any other conditions. Occasionally, similar changes may be found in other placentally transmitted infections or in the absence of known cause. Cytomegalic inclusion disease has been recognized in the placenta by the presence in scattered villi of large cells containing characteristic inclusions accompanied by a focal inflammatory reaction, but most often no such cells are visible and the only change is a diffuse villous hypertrophy (Fig. 3–30). Rubella and variola may also cause inflammation in placental villi, the former a mild mononuclear response, the latter a granulomatous reaction with thickening of the villi. Fetal herpes simplex infection, with hepato-adrenal necrosis, may produce a more severe placentitis characterized by mononuclear infiltration of the villi.

TOXOPLASMA GONDII.—In most cases of congenital

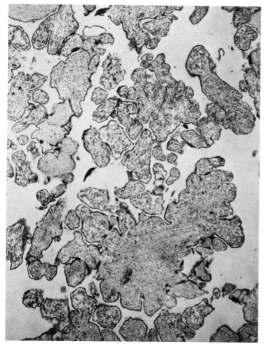

Fig. 3–30.—Placenta in cytomegalic inclusion disease (salivary gland virus infection) showing hypertrophy and branching of villi identical to changes produced by severe erythroblastosis.

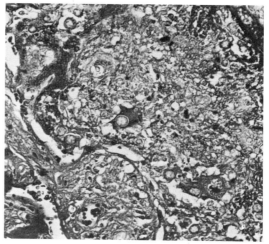

Fig. 3–31.—Coccidioidomycosis infection of the placenta. Large spore forms about 40 μ in diameter with double contours are present in masses of fibrin in the intervillous space.

toxoplasmosis placental membranes, cord or maternal decidua contain identifiable pseudocysts. These are sharply defined, often within identifiable cells, are between 20 and 50 μ in diameter and contain many nucleated organisms 1–2 μ in diameter. They have been seen most often in the connective tissue of the umbilical cord, the chorionic plate, the chorion laeve and the maternal decidua. In the placenta they are often unaccompanied by local inflammatory response although there may be infiltration of mononuclear cells in the villi or lymphocytes in the maternal decidua.

LISTERIA MONCYTOGENES.—Alone among the nontuberculous bacterial infections Listeria gives a characteristic distribution of lesions in the placenta. In this infection individual villi are enlarged and are the site of focal granulomas. Similar granulomas may appear in the chorionic plate.

CANDIDA ALBICANS.—Infection may reach the amniotic sac by ascent from the vagina and may involve the surface of the amnion or umbilical cord or, less often, the substance of the placenta. The organisms grow as spores or pseudohyphae on the surface and invade the underlying chorion where they cause an acute localized polymorphonuclear

reaction with focal necrosis. The infection is usually confined to these structures, but the presence of organisms in the amniotic fluid may lead to infections of the esophagus, stomach or lungs as a consequence of deglutition or inhalation.

COCCIDIOIDOMYCOSIS.—Several cases of coccidioidomycosis have been described in pregnant women

Fig. 3–32.—Villi from a syphilitic placenta in which blood vessels are surrounded by an increased amount of connective tissue.

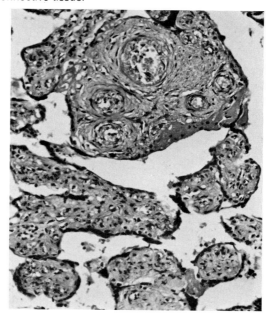

but the generative tract is usually spared and no involvement of the fetus has been recorded (Baker). In spite of this the placenta is occasionally involved (Fig. 3–31). A few cases have been described in older infants (see Chapter 9).

SYPHILIS. — Syphilis may produce striking changes in the placenta, although in mild cases the appearance is usually not abnormal. When the fetus is severely affected and the viscera show the generalized fibrosis characteristic of severe congenital syphilis, the placenta is ordinarily enlarged and paler than normal. The pale color is caused by the greater size of the villi in relation to the number of capillaries — the same condition responsible for the pallor in the erythroblastotic placenta except that in erythroblastosis anemia is often more extreme and is responsible for an even lighter color. Microscopic examination reveals enlarged villi with bulbous projections similar to those found in erythroblastosis. The stroma is made up of dense connective tissue. The capillaries are often surrounded by a considerable local increase in connective tissue (Fig. 3–32) and are distributed through-

out the substance of the villi instead of being concentrated at the periphery as they are in erythroblastosis. Hofbauer cells are numerous and zones of necrosis and leukocyte infiltration common. *Treponema pallidum* can sometimes be demonstrated in the tissues but their absence does not exclude the diagnosis. McCord pointed out the difficulty of making a histologic diagnosis of syphilis from the appearance of the placenta even when the organism has been identified in the fetal tissues. This difficulty is heightened by prematurity and intrauterine death.

TUBERCULOSIS. — The placenta is infrequently affected by tuberculosis because tubercle bacilli ordinarily are not found in the circulation except with miliary or fulminating pulmonary infections. If bacilli are present in the circulation, the placenta is as susceptible to infection as any other organ. Lesions have been described and tubercle bacilli are reported to have been obtained from the placenta by animal inoculation in a few instances of minimal or nondemonstrable maternal infections. Such lesions, if they occur, must be extremely rare. One

Fig. 3–33. — Nonspecific placentitis. Leukocytes are present in amnion, chorion and walls of superficial blood vessels. **A,** low power view. **B,** high power view showing leukocytes in zone between amnion and chorion.

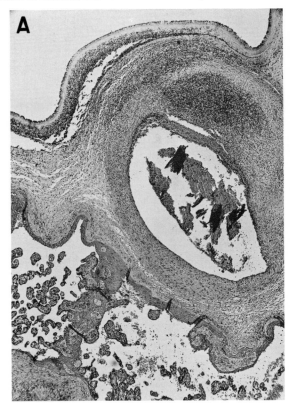
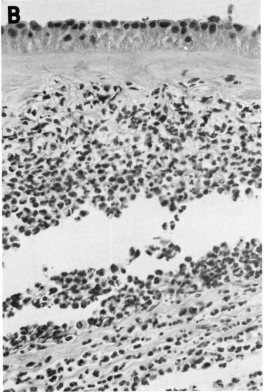

of the most complete descriptions of placental tuberculosis was given by Warthin, who studied the placenta of a 7-month-old fetus born dead 12 hours before the mother died of miliary tuberculosis. He described generalized involvement of all parts of the placenta. Changes in the decidua began with the formation of hyaline or agglutination thrombi in blood vessels at the point of endothelial injury. They progressed to the point of caseation with peripheral lymphocytic infiltration but without epithelioid or giant cell reaction. Intervillous involvement began as lesions of the syncytium with superficial hyaline or agglutination thrombi caused by tubercle bacilli on the syncytial surfaces. Caseation followed and some of the stromal cells in the villi were converted into epithelioid cells. Intravillous tubercles with epithelioid and giant cells were found both with and without involvement of the syncytium. The location of these tubercles was thought to prove that tubercle bacilli might pass through the intact chorionic epithelium, leaving it undamaged. Tubercles and tuberculous thrombi were rarely observed in the vessels of the chorion. The amnion was occasionally secondarily involved by large caseating or epithelioid tubercles primary in the chorion, and portions of amnion lying in the neighborhood of chorionic tubercles were thickened, infiltrated by lymphocytes and partially caseous.

Lesions indistinguishable from tubercles have been found in rare instances in the placentas of normal women with normal babies. The cause is unknown.

MALARIA.—Malaria parasites do not produce changes in the structure of the placenta, but in the presence of a maternal infection they are often found in great numbers in the maternal blood in the intervillous spaces of the placenta. In spite of this they have been observed in the blood vessels of the villi only rarely. Although some investigators have disclaimed the possibility that the fetus may acquire malaria, the evidence seems fairly conclusive that, although rare, it does occur. Most cases thought to have been transmitted through the placenta have been of the estivo-autumnal type.

NONSPECIFIC INFECTIONS.—After early rupture of the membranes, a long and complicated delivery or, occasionally, even when membranes are unruptured, bacteria may enter the amniotic cavity and produce inflammation of the membranes and the chorionic plate (Fig. 3–33). The inflammation, a polymorphonuclear infiltrate, appears first in the fibrin layer between the chorion and intervillous space. The inflammatory cells are considered to be

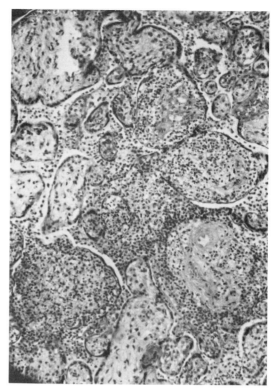

Fig. 3–34.—Placentitis. Polymorphonuclear cells in the intervillous space and in the substance of the villi in a case of septic abortion.

of maternal origin. The process extends toward the amnion, and the vessels of the chorionic plate are frequently involved.

Inflammation of the umbilical cord is most common near its connection to the fetal abdominal wall but may occur irregularly at any point throughout its length. The most common site of inflammation is the inner part of the wall of the umbilical vein. The inflammation is always an acute reaction consisting largely of polymorphonuclear cells. More extensive inflammation involves the entire thickness of the vein as well as the arteries and connective tissue. The inflammatory cells appear to congregate within the vessels and pass outward into the walls. Tissue destruction is rarely seen except with monilial infections, in which the organisms probably invade the cord structures from the amniotic sac, not from the vessels. Such inflammatory lesions are more frequent in smaller premature infants and may affect as many as 25% of those below 800 gm. These infiltrates seldom show evidence of chronicity and for the most part are of unknown etiology. They do not necessarily indicate the presence of bacterial infection, for in 50% of premature infants with such inflammation careful bacteriologic examination reveals no evidence of organisms. Though frozen sections of the cord have been recommended as a guide to prophylactic antimicrobial therapy, for the above reasons, and because of the occasional occurrence of fatal aspiration pneumonia without evidence of cord inflammation, this laboratory guide by itself is unreliable.

In early placentas the presence of intervillous collections of polymorphonuclear cells as well as acute inflammation of the maternal decidua are often associated with induced abortion (Fig. 3–34).

Tumors of the Placenta

CHORIOANGIOMAS.—Tumors of the placenta are largely limited to chorioangiomas, so called because they are composed of an abnormal overgrowth of blood vessels and chorionic tissue. They usually consist of a single, dark red-purple, sharply demarcated mass, varying in size from a few millimeters to several centimeters and located within the substance of the placenta (Fig. 3–35). The mass is sometimes composed of separate, closely packed lobules but is more often single and of a uniform consistency. Rarely, the tumor is entirely separate from the placenta and attached to it only by blood vessels (Fig. 3–36,A).

Microscopically, the tumors usually consist of small lobules composed of capillarylike blood vessels embedded in a small amount of myxomatous

tissue. The lobules are separated by varying amounts of connective tissue often containing calcium (Fig. 3–37). Less often the vascular spaces are not as well defined and endothelial cells have a greater tendency to form solid areas (Fig. 3–38). Benirschke and Driscoll reported that such tumors may be associated with hydramnios, which is responsible for premature labor and fetal death. They found cardiac enlargement in some such fetuses and postulated that the chorioangioma acts as an arteriovenous fistula responsible for cardiac hypertrophy because of the required increase in cardiac output, and that this in turn leads to heart failure and hydramnios.

Diffuse placental hypertrophy is sometimes caused by proliferation of blood vessels and myxomatous tissue within villi, a condition that has been designated chorionomatosis or chorioangiosis (see Fig. 3–19).

ANGIOMYXOMAS.—Angiomyxomas, like chorioangiomas, are composed of numerous capillarylike blood vessels similar to those in normal villi. These tumors, which often extend from the placenta into the umbilical cord (Fig. 3–36,B), contain varying amounts of myxomatous tissue resembling that in the normal cord. There is no sharp demarcation between chorioangiomas and angiomyxomas, and many intermediate forms have been observed.

HYDATIDIFORM MOLES.—An hydatidiform mole is a product of conception in which the embryo fails to develop or dies very early in pregnancy and the villi of the chorionic vesicle become cystic. In most cases the cause of fetal death and molar formation

Fig. 3–35.—Placenta with chorioangioma. **A,** chorionic surface showing tumor adjacent to umbilical cord. **B,** cross-section of placenta and tumor.

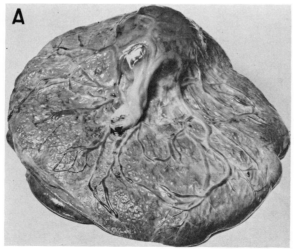
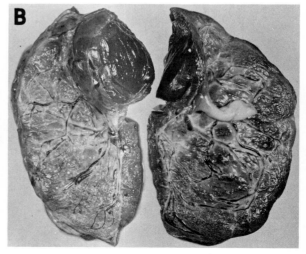

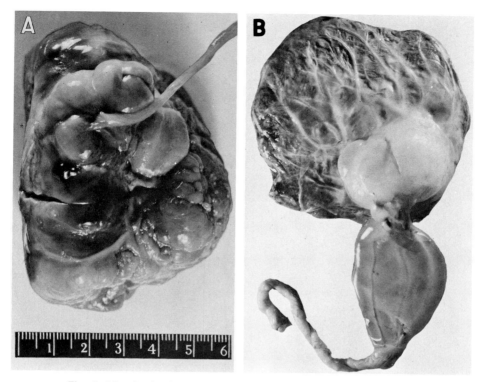

Fig. 3−36.−**A,** chorioangioma that was attached to placenta only by blood vessels. **B,** angiomyxoma involving both placenta and umbilical cord.

Fig. 3−37.−Chorioangioma of the placenta. Grossly this was a single compact mass. Microscopically it was divided into small segments by connective tissue containing calcium. Endothelial-lined spaces were separated by myxomatous and connective tissues.

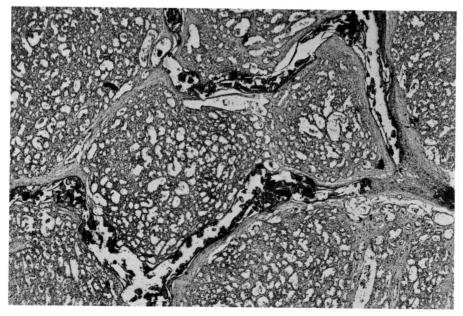

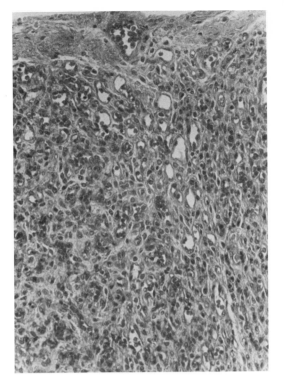

Fig. 3—38.—Chorioangioma of the placenta in which the vascular spaces are poorly defined and the endothelial cells tend to form solid masses.

is unknown, although Carr identified triploid chromosomal patterns (69 chromosomes) in 17% of the hydatidiform moles he studied. Curiously, in abortions with extensive hydatid changes, the incidence of a triploid constitution is 70%.

Mild cystic changes in villi are found fairly often in early abortions even though a fetus is present (Fig. 3—39). In later pregnancy the placenta may be excessively large because of the presence of many small cysts, sometimes so small that they are discovered only on microscopic examination. A severely macerated fetus smaller than would be expected for the duration of pregnancy is usually delivered with such a placenta. The cause of cystic changes is unknown but those of early and late pregnancy are probably related.

Typical hydatidiform moles occur about once in every 2,000 pregnancies in urban America, but in Singapore, the Philippines and Hong Kong an incidence as high as 1 in 150 pregnancies has been reported. They consist of masses of cystic villi often having a total weight of 200–300 gm. The villi are attached to the chorionic membrane and may be 5–

10 cm long with many cysts scattered along their course (Fig. 3–40). Many branches, also containing cysts, arise at irregular points along the main villi, as do the branches of normal villi. The villi are distended to a diameter of 2–10 mm and are divided into round or oval globules by interspersed points of constriction. They are usually colorless or light gray after being washed free of maternal blood.

The cavities of the cysts contain no blood vessels and are filled with filmy anuclear material and fluid rich in estrogen. The outer surfaces are covered by irregularly proliferating trophoblast, and both Langhans' and syncytial cells can be identified (Fig. 3–41). They are benign growths, although about 5% are generally considered to result in chorionepitheliomas. However, at the Chicago Lying-in Hospital about 60 well-developed hydatidiform moles occurred among approximately 100,000 deliveries and none were followed by chorionepitheliomas.

In the presence of a mole the uterus enlarges with excessive rapidity in early pregnancy and often seems unusually small in mid or late pregnancy. Gonadotropic hormone is present in abnormally high concentration. Roentgen examination fails to reveal a fetus. An angiogram may reveal a grossly disturbed pattern in the maternal circulation in the uterus. The ovaries are often enlarged by numerous follicles with excessively thick walls composed of luteinized theca cells. Early in pregnancy a diagnosis may be difficult to establish clinically unless some of the cysts are expelled.

CYSTIC PLACENTAS WITH A FETUS.—On three occa-

Fig. 3—39.—Hydatid degeneration of villi in abortus of 13 weeks' gestational age.

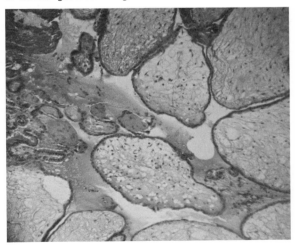

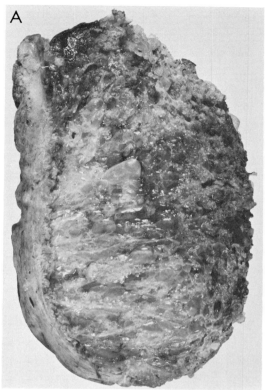

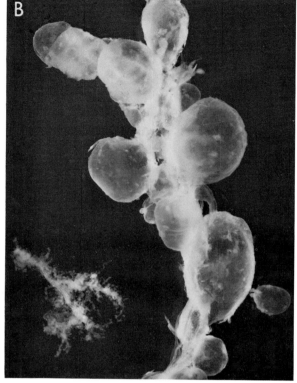

Fig. 3–40.—Hydatidiform mole. **A,** bisected uterus with attached mole. **B,** comparison of size of normal villi with cysts of hydatidiform mole. Characteristic arrangement of cysts is well shown.

sions scattered cysts of varying size, the largest measuring about 3 cm in diameter, were intermingled with normal villi in placentas observed at the Chicago Lying-in Hospital. One fetus was hydrocephalic; the other two were normal. All were delivered prematurely. In each instance the cystic villi were filled with fluid, but the peripheral villous connective tissue contained blood vessels (Fig. 3–42). Such placentas have been called transitional moles.

CHORIOADENOMA DESTRUENS.—A great difference appears in rate of growth of hydatidiform moles, manifested histologically by different degrees of thickening of the Langhans' and syncytial layers of the villi. Their biologic behavior also varies, particularly in their propensity for invading the myometrium. When invasion is active and the wall of the uterus deeply penetrated, fragments of the mole remaining after evacuation may be the cause of serious hemorrhage, infection or perforation of the uterus followed by peritonitis. Such moles are regarded as locally malignant.

CHORIONEPITHELIOMAS.—These are malignant tumors arising from chorionic tissue. They are found most commonly in the uterus (Fig. 3–43,A), although they may arise as part of a teratoma in the testis, mediastinum or other part of the body. In the uterus about half follow hydatidiform moles, one fourth follow abortions and one fourth follow pregnancies with viable fetuses. They are characterized by irregularly proliferating masses of trophoblast which show varying degrees of differentiation into Langhans' and syncytial cells (Fig. 3–43,B) without villous formation. They form extremely hemorrhagic tumors because their cells, like normal trophoblast, encourage increased vascularity and destroy tissues with which they come in contact. Such tumors are highly malignant and until recently the prognosis has been poor. Now, with prompt treatment with chemotherapeutic agents such as methotrexate and vincaleukoblastine, nearly 90% of all patients, including more than 50% of those with pulmonary metastases, can be cured.

A mild downgrowth of syncytiotrophoblast into the superficial portions of the uterine musculature

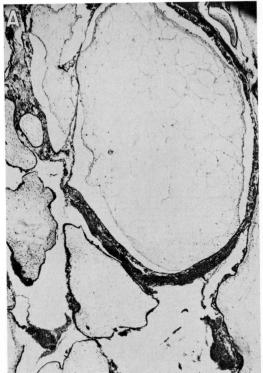
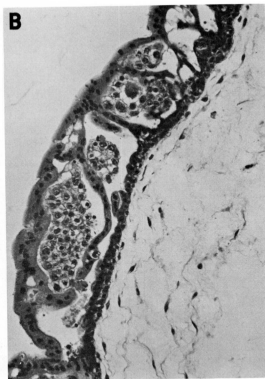

Fig. 3–41.—Hydatidiform mole. **A,** photomicrograph showing absence of blood vessels in interior of cysts. **B,** wall of a cyst showing irregular proliferation of Langhans' cells but fairly prompt transformation into syncytial cells.

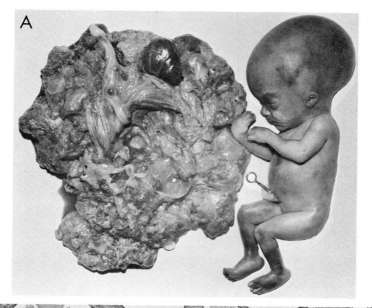

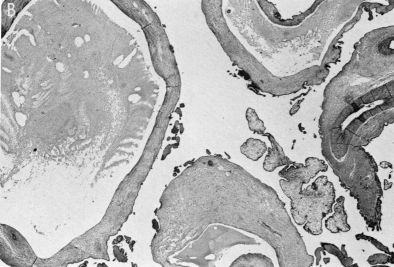

Fig. 3–42.—Cystic placenta. **A,** placenta with many cysts and hydrocephalic premature infant. **B,** photomicrograph of placenta showing multiple cysts and a few villi of normal size.

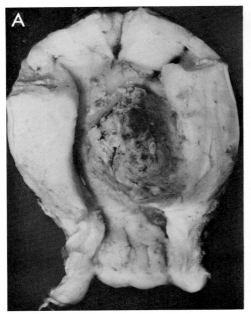

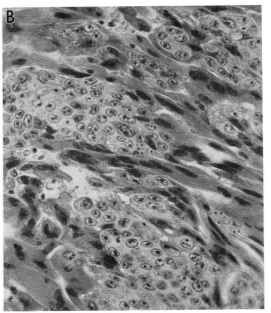

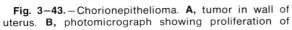

Fig. 3—43.—Chorionepithelioma. A, tumor in wall of uterus. B, photomicrograph showing proliferation of cytotrophoblast with some differentiation into syncytiotrophoblast.

Fig. 3—44.—Muscle adjacent to decidual surface of the uterus showing numerous multinucleate cells characteristic of syncytial "placental site giant cells." They disappear soon after termination of pregnancy.

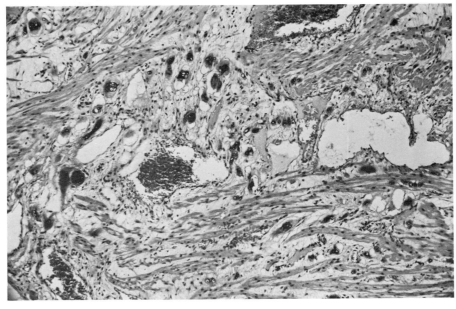

occurs in almost all uteri during pregnancy. The cells resemble multinucleated giant cells and may be widely scattered for a considerable distance below the surface (Fig. 3–44). At times, when the amount of downgrowth is pronounced, the presence of such cells has been designated syncytial metritis or syncytioma. Such invasion is of no consequence and disappears promptly after pregnancy ends. Unless there is an actual invasion by trophoblast with continued differentiation into both Langhans' and syncytial cells in the uterine wall after termination of the pregnancy, a diagnosis of malignant neoplastic growth is not warranted.

Umbilical Cord

LENGTH.—The umbilical cord averages 50 cm in length at fetal maturity, although it may be considerably longer or shorter. An excessively long cord is somewhat more subject to entanglement, knotting or prolapse than one of normal length. The cord may be absent or rudimentary and the placenta may be attached directly to the abdominal wall of the fetus and associated with visceral eventration as a result of maldevelopment of the body stalk (see Figs. 19–10 to 19–12), or it may be attached to the scalp and associated with a defect in the skull (see Fig. 25–44,B). In such cases the fetus is grossly malformed.

DIAMETER.—The diameter of the cord averages 1–2 cm at term, although it is variable, and the thickness is largely dependent on the amount of Wharton's jelly (Fig. 3–45). After pulsations through the cord have ceased following birth, the umbilical arteries are completely constricted and the umbilical vein frequently shows multiple zones of constriction throughout its entire length. Such cords give an inadequate impression of the usual size of the vessels in their functioning state, when blood is coursing through them (Fig. 3–46). In the hydropic form of erythroblastosis, or in fetal hy-

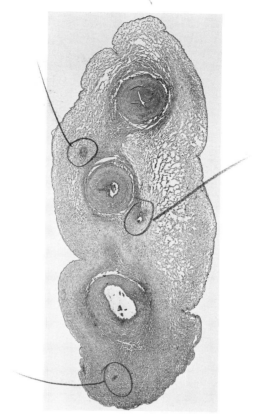

Fig. 3–45.—Microscopic section of umbilical cord showing two arteries and one vein embedded in an average amount of Wharton's jelly.

drops from other causes, the thickness is increased by extension of the edema into the cord. The maceration of the fetus following intrauterine death is generally accompanied by mild edema and discoloration of the cord. When a knot in the cord is drawn tight enough to occlude circulation, the diameter of the portion between the knot and the placenta increases, while that between the fetus and the knot

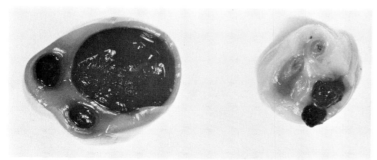

Fig. 3–46.—Two sections of umbilical cord, one with all vessels filled with blood, as they are while the fetus is in the uterus, and the other with arteries constricted as they are following birth.

shrinks. If the two portions of cord are of equal thickness, there is little likelihood that circulation through it was interrupted before delivery.

CONSTITUENTS.—Wharton's jelly is composed of myxomatous connective tissue and is normally colorless and translucent. In erythroblastosis fetalis the surface of the cord is often stained yellow if excessive amounts of bilirubin have been excreted into the amniotic fluid. Following fetal death the cord becomes pink-violet from hemolysis of blood cells.

Normally the cord contains two arteries, and one vein, which are embedded in Wharton's jelly. A single umbilical artery occurs in about 0.45–1.2% of placentas (Benirschke), and about 50% of the infants with this cord anomaly have an accompanying visceral anomaly. The cord always appears twisted because the greater length of the umbilical vein permits it to twist around the arteries. One or more vessels may show a local increase in length, and irregular loops and coils may be present. Actual varicosities are found occasionally (Fig. 3–47) and in rare instances they rupture. The blood is ordinarily retained in the substance of the cord and

the amount of bleeding is usually small. A few cases of ruptured varicosities causing exsanguinating hemorrhage have been reported.

The urachus continues into the proximal portion of the cord as a narrow tubular structure with a very small lumen. Rarely, this dilates to form a cyst that may reach several centimeters in diameter. Such a cyst is filled with clear fluid and lined by flattened cuboidal epithelium. It communicates with the remnant of urachus in the abdomen. (See also p. 473.)

Portions of a patent omphalomesenteric duct may on rare occasions extend for a short distance into the umbilical cord, and even less often a portion of the intestine that was not retracted into the abdominal cavity in embryonic life may be present in the cord several centimeters from the umbilicus with the intervening cord seemingly of normal caliber. Much more often the unretracted intestine lies immediately adjacent to the abdomen.

ABNORMALITIES.—Syphilis may cause a leukocytic infiltration of all layers of the walls of the umbilical vessels (Fig. 3–48), and organisms can sometimes be demonstrated. Scrapings from the

Fig. 3–47 (left).—Varicosities producing false knots in umbilical cord.

Fig. 3–48 (right).—Umbilical cord from an infant with

syphilis. *Treponema pallidum* identified in scrapings from the intima of the umbilical vein.

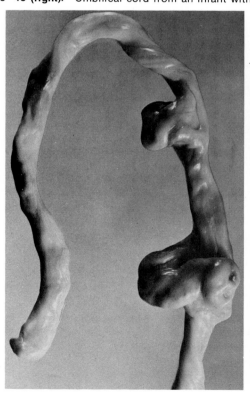
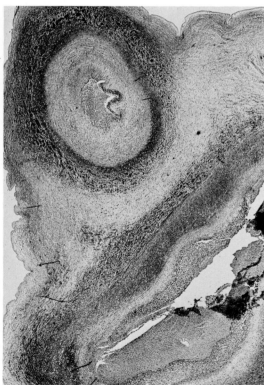

intima of the vessels may yield fluid in which *Treponema pallidum* can be demonstrated on dark-field examination. Pseudocysts of *Toxoplasma gondii* have been found in the connective tissues of the cord in generalized congenital toxoplasmosis. Nonspecific infections of the amnion and chorion may spread to the vessels of the cord and produce a leukocytic infiltration similar to that seen in syphilis.

Tumors of the umbilical cord are almost entirely limited to the angiomyxomas described for the placenta.

Any condition that reduces the amount of blood passing through the umbilical vessels will cause fetal anoxia. Prolapse of the cord with compression between the presenting part of the fetus and the maternal pelvis is the abnormality most often recognized. If the obstruction is partial or intermittent, little or no harm may be done the fetus, but if blood flow is completely interrupted, death soon follows. It is more frequent in breech than in cephalic deliveries because the breech is less often fixed in the pelvis when membranes rupture than is the head, and the rush of escaping fluid carries the cord down and out of the uterus through the space between the breech and the maternal pelvis.

Excessive tension that interferes with circulation through the cord is more difficult to diagnose than cord prolapse. The cord may be wrapped several times around the neck or an extremity without producing evidence of circulatory embarrassment, but if the portion of the cord between the placenta and the point of entanglement is short, this segment may be placed under excessive tension and the lumens of the blood vessels may be greatly reduced as the fetus moves downward in the birth canal during labor. It is also possible that some unexplained intrauterine deaths are due to tension exerted on the cord by movements of the fetus if a portion of the cord is wrapped around the neck or an extremity. At times, however, even excessive tension seems to be compatible with an adequate flow of blood. This is especially true in early stages of gestation, for fetuses are occasionally observed in which part of the body seems to have stopped growing because circulation to the part was at least partially cut off as a result of encirclement and constriction by the cord (Fig. 3–49). In such instances circulation must have been carried on for a time at least or death would have occurred before changes resulting from differences in rate of growth became visible.

Knots in the umbilical cord are fairly common, but fortunately they are rarely drawn tight enough to cut off circulation. It is probable that the pulsation of the cord and the forceful flow of blood

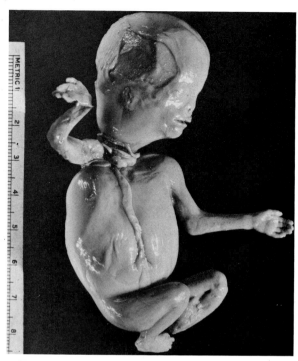

Fig. 3–49.—Hypoplasia of right arm due to constriction by umbilical cord. Subsequent obstruction to flow through the cord caused death and maceration.

through the vessels is sufficient to keep the knot loose. This is probably also the reason that circulation to a part of the fetus may be cut off by an encircling loop of cord without interfering with the circulation in the cord itself.

When twins are present in the same amniotic sac, there is great danger of circulatory obstruction. Movement of the fetuses causes intertwining of the cords, and if any part is drawn tight, circulation between the fetuses and the placenta is interrupted. Occasionally an amazing intertwining of the cords is produced without interference with the circulation (see Fig. 13–4).

Amniotic Sac

NORMAL STRUCTURE.—The amnion at term is composed normally of a single layer of columnar cells surrounded by a thin layer of connective tissue. It forms the inner lining of the chorionic membrane and placenta, from which it can be easily separated, and the outer covering of the umbilical cord with which it is fused. The amnion together with the chorionic membrane, by which it is surrounded, make up the extraplacental bag of waters.

The cells of the amnion are generally tall columnar cells that have a moderate amount of cytoplasm. They may contain large clear vacuoles, the presence of which has contributed to the belief that amniotic fluid is a secretory product of the amnion. Although the cells of the amnion cannot be excluded as contributing fluid to the total volume in the amniotic sac, especially early in pregnancy, they cannot be the sole source.

In the first few weeks the embryo almost completely fills the amniotic sac (Fig. 3–50,A), but by 9 or 10 weeks the sac is proportionately larger and the fetus is allowed greater freedom of movement (Fig. 3–50,B). Early in pregnancy the amniotic sac has a smaller diameter than the chorionic vesicle,

and fluid is present between the wall of the amnion and the chorion as well as in the amniotic sac (see Fig. 1–10). As pregnancy progresses, the amniotic sac enlarges proportionately faster than the chorion, and before the middle of pregnancy the two layers are in apposition.

ABNORMALITIES.—The amnion ordinarily is a transparent membrane, although opaque areas of varying size are occasionally scattered over part or all of the surface. They consist most often of several layers of cells that are generally a little larger and somewhat more irregular in shape than the normal cells and resemble zones of squamous metaplasia (Fig. 3–51). The occurrence of epithelial cells in

Fig. 3–50 (top).—**A,** gestation of 5 weeks showing close apposition of amniotic sac and body of embryo. **B,** gestation of 8 weeks showing relative increase in size of amniotic sac.

Fig. 3–51 (bottom).—Area of squamous epithelium in amniotic membrane (metaplasia).

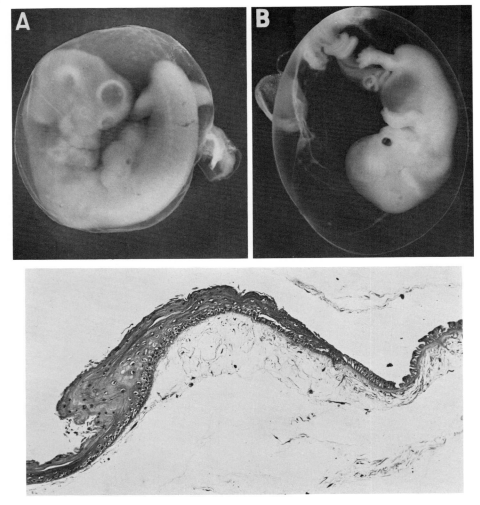

this location is not surprising in view of the close association of amnion and ectoderm in the young embryo.

Opaque nodules may also be found in association with the oligohydramnios that accompanies renal agenesis or severe bilateral cystic or noncystic renal dysplasia (Fig. 3–52). They may be present over the entire surface of the amnion but ordinarily are most readily observed in the portion of the amnion adherent to the placenta. The surface layer of amniotic cells is lost and masses composed of degenerated squamous epithelial cells (1–3 mm in diameter) adhere to the surface. Somewhat similar masses can be seen in the placentas of stillborn macerated infants that have remained in the uterus for a considerable time after fetal death (Fig. 3–53).

Inflammation of the amnion is most often associated with early rupture of membranes or a long and complicated labor. Mononuclear and polymorphonuclear leukocytes infiltrate the connective tissue, making up the deeper layer of the amniotic membrane, and often extend into the adjacent connective tissue of the chorion (see Fig. 3–33).

On rare occasions the amnion is incomplete and does not cover all of the chorionic surface. Instances have been reported in which the entire fetus was extra-amniotic, and in one infant observed at the Chicago Lying-in Hospital the amnion surrounded only half of the fetus. The free margin was attached in three places to the infant's body by pedunculated outgrowths of skin 3 cm long arising near the waistline (see Fig. 27–41). The umbilical cord, placenta and fetus were also abnormal in this case.

Amniotic adhesions connecting parts of the fetus to the amnion were formerly believed to be due to local inflammatory changes in the amnion that caused it to adhere to the parts of the fetus with which it came in contact. Such bands occasionally attach the head (Fig. 3–54) or a portion of the body to the amnion but are more often found extending between the ends of the fingers or toes and the amnion (see Fig. 27–39). The etiology is unknown, although there is no histologic evidence that they are inflammatory in nature.

Amniotic Fluid

Source.—While there is strong evidence that the source of amniotic fluid varies at different periods of development and is modified by abnormal states of the mother or fetus, a major source has not yet

Fig. 3–52 (left).—Amnion nodosum. Collection of keratinized squamous cells attached to the surface of the amnion. There is also a chorioamnionitis. (From an infant with renal agenesis.)

Fig. 3–53 (right).—Multiple nodules composed largely of hyaline on surface of placenta of macerated fetus.

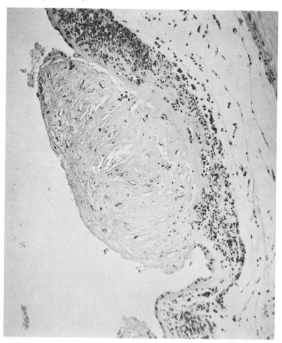
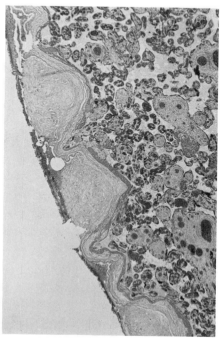

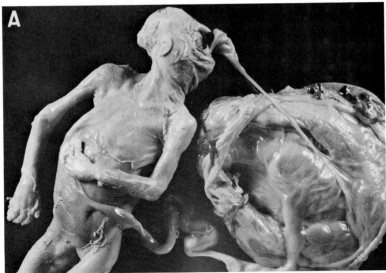

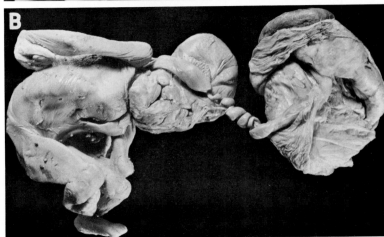

Fig. 3–54.—Amniotic bands. **A,** fetus without calvarium. Skin of upper part of head has a tubular connection with the amnion. **B,** malformed fetus with tubular communication between forehead and amnion. Cord was twisted around the amniotic band seven times.

been positively identified. Contributions to amniotic fluid could possibly be derived from (1) the amnion, by secretion from cells forming its lining; (2) maternal blood, by transudation through the amnion and chorion; (3) the umbilical cord, by secretion from Wharton's jelly or transudation from umbilical vessels; or (4) fetal skin, lungs, gastrointestinal tract or kidneys.

In the first few weeks of pregnancy the embryo and young fetus are snugly encased in the amniotic sac, which is contained within the larger chorionic sac. Fluid increase in both sacs is proportionately greater than increase in fetal size, with that in the amniotic sac increasing more rapidly than that between the walls of the two sacs. By about 14 weeks of pregnancy the walls of the two sacs are

juxtaposed, and for the next few weeks the amount of fluid within the sac is proportionately greater than at any other time. At 12–13 weeks the amount of fluid averages about 75 ml; the fetus weighs 25–30 gm and the placenta and membranes about twice as much. The lungs at this time have no alveoli and are composed of tubular structures as yet nonvascularized although capable of inspiring and absorbing amniotic fluid or of inspiring air if the fetus is alive outside the uterus. A few generations of glomeruli are present in the kidney, and urine is present in the bladder.

With maldevelopment of the conceptus so extreme that the embryo is absent or consists only of a nodular mass, fluid may nevertheless accumulate within both amniotic and chorionic sacs or within a single sac. In early weeks the amount of fluid under such circumstances may be about normal but it fails to continue to increase. Pregnancy without an embryo seldom endures more than 14–16 weeks, and the sac seldom contains more than 40–60 ml of fluid. Histologic structure of membranes in such pregnancies has not been studied, but since formation of the amnion is closely related to development of the embryo, it is probable that the amnion as well as the embryo is often lacking and that fluid within the sac is derived from the mother as a transudate through the chorion.

Pyloric or duodenal atresia is accompanied by distention of the tract proximal to the obstruction, narrowing and lack of development distal to the obstruction and an increased amount of amniotic fluid. This is interpreted as definite evidence that fluid is removed from the amniotic sac by fetal swallowing, is absorbed through the intestinal wall into the fetal bloodstream and is absorbed into the maternal circulation in the placenta and/or excreted back into the sac by the fetal kidneys.

After the middle of pregnancy the accumulation of amniotic fluid is proportionately less rapid than growth of the fetus, and although the fetus continues to be able to move, it is not "free-swimming" as it was earlier. From 500–1,500 ml of fluid is ordinarily considered normal at term, the amount most often being in the vicinity of 1,000 ml.

Attempts to determine the source of amniotic fluid experimentally have been responsible for numerous experiments, often giving seemingly contradictory evidence, and nature's experiments, in the form of malformations, are often ignored or dismissed as of no significance. The malformation most constantly associated with abnormal amniotic fluid volume is bilateral renal agenesis. Several hundred cases of renal agenesis have now been reported, all of which, with the exception of two anencephalic fetuses, have had little or no amniotic fluid. Bowing of the legs and varying degrees of pulmonary hypoplasia are always associated. These findings have been interpreted as showing that kidney secretion is responsible for the production of amniotic fluid and that the presence of amniotic fluid is necessary for normal pulmonary development.

Under experimental conditions in animals some investigators have been unable to confirm the kidney as the source of certain constituents of amniotic fluid. Certain materials injected into fetal vessels in the placentas of monkeys have appeared in the amniotic fluid in normal and nephrectomized fetuses in equal amounts. Amniotic fluid, however, has been conserved when nephrectomy has been performed, and studies have not shown whether amniotic fluid is replaced in the absence of fetal kidneys or whether transfer of these substances into amniotic fluid requires the initial presence of the fluid. Under normal circumstances in human beings, fluid is rapidly replaced following withdrawal.

Adams and co-workers are convinced that the lungs normally provide most of the fluid and assume that the pulmonary hypoplasia constantly associated with renal agenesis is responsible for lack of fluid when kidneys are absent. However, if pulmonary hypoplasia is an accompaniment and not a result of renal agenesis, it is a unique example of such a constant association. Other investigators, most notably Goodlin and Rudolph, have found the lungs making little or no contribution to the volume of fluid.

In over half of all cases of hydramnios no cause can be discovered, and it seems probable that the fluid is a transudate through the chorion. At times several liters of fluid may accumulate and be removed artificially within such a short time that it seems impossible for such large amounts to be secreted by the fetal kidney. Malformations of the fetus, especially anencephaly, are present in about one third of cases, and it has generally been assumed in such instances that the fluid was secreted by the choroid plexus, which is frequently hyperplastic. Benirschke and McKay believed fetal renal secretion to be normally controlled by an antidiuretic hormone derived from the hypophysis and that in anencephaly absence of the hypophysis leads to excessive urinary secretion. However, one case has been reported in which hydramnios accompanied anencephaly even though the kidneys were absent. The hydramnios accompanying anencephaly is generally greatest in cases of severe craniospinorachischisis and in such fetuses the lungs are always hypoplastic. This constitutes further evidence against the lungs being a source of amniotic fluid, and it might be argued that the hydramnios accompanying anencephaly results from inability of the hypoplastic lungs to absorb fluid normally.

The natural and experimental evidence provided thus far seems to warrant the conclusion that the source of amniotic fluid varies with period of gestation and pathologic states: under normal conditions it is a transudate from maternal tissues in early pregnancy and largely a secretion of the fetal kidney in late pregnancy; under pathologic conditions it may come as a transudate from maternal tissues at any time of pregnancy and possibly as a secretion from the hypertrophied choroid plexus in severe anencephaly. The fetus swallows and inhales fluid throughout the second and third trimesters (Davis and Potter), and anything that interferes with these functions permits excessive accumulation of fluid provided the kidneys are functioning. Any contribution made by the fetal skin and umbilical cord must be minimal.

COMPONENTS OF AMNIOTIC FLUID AS AN INDICATION OF FETAL MATURITY. — Attempts have been made to determine the maturity of the fetus by examination of the amniotic fluid. Creatinine, bilirubin and cellular constituents have received the most attention. Most authors agree that after 36 weeks, in comparison to the period prior to that time, the creatinine level is often higher, the bilirubin usually lower and the number of anuclear squames, often with attached lipid globules, considerably increased. The reverse of any of these findings does not necessarily mean prematurity; positive findings are more probably indicative of maturity than are negative findings indicative of prematurity (Droegemueller *et al.*, White *et al.*).

REFERENCES

Adair, F. L., and Thelander, H.: Study of the weight and dimensions of the human placenta in its relation to the weight of the newborn infant, Am. J. Obstet. Gynecol. 10:172, 1925.

Adams, E. H., Desilets, D. T., and Towers, B.: Control of flow of fetal lung fluid at the laryngeal outlet, Respir. Physiol. 2:302, 1967.

Baker, R. L.: Pregnancy complicated by coccidioidomycosis, Am. J. Obstet. Gynecol. 70:1033, 1955.

Benirschke, K.: Routes and types of infection in the fetus and newborn, Am. J. Dis. Child. 99:714, 1960.

Benirschke, K.: The incidence and prognostic implication of congenital absence of one umbilical artery, Am. J. Obstet. Gynecol. 79:251, 1960.

Benirschke, K., and Driscoll, S.: *Pathology of the Placenta* (Berlin: Springer Verlag, 1967).

Benirschke, K., and McKay, D. G.: The antidiuretic hormone in fetus and infant: Histochemical observations with special reference to amniotic fluid formation, Obstet. Gynecol. 1:638, 1953.

Blanc. W. A.: Amniotic infection syndrome: Pathogenesis, morphology and significance in circumnatal mortality, Clin. Obstet. Gynecol. 2:705, 1959.

Boronow, R. C., McElen, T. W., West, R. H., and Buckingham, J. C.: Ovarian pregnancy, Am. J. Obstet. Gynecol. 91:1095, 1965.

Bourne, G.: *The Human Amnion and Chorion* (London: Lloyd-Luke, 1962).

Cantarow, A., Stuckert, H., and Davis, R. C.: Chemical composition of amniotic fluid: Comparative study of human amniotic fluid and maternal blood, Surg. Gynecol. Obstet. 57:63, 1933.

Carr, D. H.: Chromosomal anomalies in human reproduction, Res. Reprod. 4:3, 1972.

Chacko, A. W., and Reynolds, S. R. M.: Architecture of distended and nondistended human umbilical cord tissues, with special reference to arteries and veins, Contrib. Embryol. 35:135, 1954.

Davis, M. E., and Potter, E. L.: Intrauterine respiration of the human fetus, J.A.M.A. 131:1194, 1946.

Deglon, P., and Blanc, W. A.: Fetal and placental lesions in 100 cases of oligohydramnios, Am. J. Dis. Child. 6:408, 1972.

Dippel, A. L.: Hematomas of the umbilical cord, Surg. Gynecol. Obstet. 70:51, 1940.

Dodds, G. S.: The area of the chorionic villi in the full term placenta, Anat. Rec. 24:287, 1923.

Droegemueller, W., *et al.*: Amniotic fluid examination as an aid in the assessment of gestational age, Am. J. Obstet. Gynecol. 104:424, 1969.

Fox, H.: Vascular tumors of the placenta, Obstet. Gynecol. Surv. 22:697, 1967.

Freese, U. E.: The fetal-maternal circulation, J. Reprod. Med. 1:161, 1968.

Goodlin, R. C., and Rudolph, A. M.: Tracheal fluid flow and function in fetuses in utero, Am. J. Obstet. Gynecol. 106:597, 1970.

Greenhill, J. P.: The increased incidence of fetal anomalies in cases of placenta praevia, Am. J. Obstet. Gynecol. 37:624, 1939.

Hellman, L. M., and Hertig, A. T.: Pathologic changes in the placenta associated with erythroblastosis of the fetus, Am. J. Pathol. 14:111, 1938.

Hertig, A. T., and Edmunds, H. W.: The genesis of hydatidiform mole, Arch. Pathol. 30:326, 1940.

Hertig, A. T., and Mansell, H.: *Tumors of the Female Sex Organs: Hydatidiform Moles and Choriocarcinoma* (Washington, D.C.: Armed Forces Institute of Pathology, 1956).

Hertz, R., Ross, G. T., and Lipsett, M. S.: Chemotherapy in women with trophoblastic disease; choriocarcinoma, chorioadenoma destruens and complicated hydatidiform mole, Ann. N. Y. Acad. Sci. 144:884, 1964.

Hibbard, B. M., Hibbard, E. P., and Jeffcoate, T. N. A.: Folic acid and reproduction, Acta Obstet. Gynecol. Scand. 44:375, 1965.

Hirsch, A., and Waltman, R.: Primary ovarian pregnancy, Am. J. Surg. 79:341, 1950.

Hobbs, J. E., and Price, C. N.: Placenta circumvallata, Am. J. Obstet. Gynecol. 39:39, 1940.

Irving, F. C., and Hertig, A. T.: Study of placenta accreta, Surg. Gynecol. Obstet. 64:178, 1937.

Kobak, A. J.: Fetal bacteremia: A contribution to the mechanism of intrauterine infection and to the pathogenesis of placentitis, Am. J. Obstet. Gynecol. 19:299, 1930.

Laufer, A., Sadovsky, A., and Sadovsky, E.: Histologic appearance of placenta in ectopic pregnancy, Obstet. Gynecol. 20:350, 1960.

Lennon, C. G.: Some aspects of fetal pathology, with special reference to the role of placental bands, J. Obstet. Gynaecol. Br. Emp. 54:830, 1948.

LePage, F., and Schramm, B.: Aspects histologiques du placenta et des membranes dans la maladie des inclusions cytomegaliques, Gynecol. Obstet. 57:273, 1958.

Little, W. A.: Placental infarction, Obstet. Gynecol. 15:109, 1960.

Little, W. A.: Significance of placental-fetal weight ratios, Am. J. Obstet. Gynecol. 79:134, 1960.

Lopez, E., and Ackerman, K.: Intra-uterine infection by Candida, Am. J. Dis. Child. 115:663, 1968.

Mall, F. P.: *On the Fate of the Human Embryo in Tubal Pregnancy* (Washington, D. C.: Carnegie Institute, 1915), publication no. 221, p. 104.

McCord, J. R.: Syphilis of the placenta, Am. J. Obstet. Gynecol. 28:743, 1934.

Paalman, R. J., and McElen, T. W.: Cervical pregnancy, Am. J. Obstet. Gynecol. 77:1261, 1959.

Patterson, T. J. S.: Amniotic bands, in Bourne, G. (ed.): *The Human Amnion and Chorion* (London: Lloyd-Luke, 1962).

Potter, E. L.: Intervillous thrombi in the placenta and their possible relation to erythroblastosis fetalis, Am. J. Obstet. Gynecol. 56:959, 1948.

Scott, J. S.: Placenta extrachorialis (placenta marginata and placenta circumvallata), J. Obstet. Gynaecol. Br. Emp. 67:904, 1960.

Seeliger, H. P. R.: *Listeriosis* (New York: Hafner, 1961).

Sexton, L. I., *et al.:* Premature separation of the normally implanted placenta, Am. J. Obstet. Gynecol. 59:13, 1950.

Siddall, R. S.: Extramembranous pregnancy, Am. J. Obstet. Gynecol. 51:897, 1946.

Smalbraak, J.: *Trophoblastic Growths. Hydatidiform Mole and Chorionepithelioma* (Amsterdam: Elsevier, 1957).

Szulman, A. E.: Chromosomal aberrations in spontaneous human abortions, N. Engl. J. Med. 272:811, 1965.

Taylor, H. G.: Pregnancy and the double uterus, Am. J. Obstet. Gynecol. 46:388, 1943.

Tenney, B.: Syncytial degeneration in normal and pathologic placentas, Am. J. Obstet. Gynecol. 31:1024, 1936.

Thiede, H. A., and Sam, S. B.: Chromosome studies of human spontaneous abortions, Am. J. Obstet. Gynecol. 90:205, 1964.

Villee, C. (ed.): Symposium on the physiology of the placenta, Fed. Proc. 23:773, 1964.

Warthin, A. S.: Tuberculosis of the placenta, J. Infect. Dis. 4:347, 1907.

White, C. A., Doorenbos, D. E., and Bradbury, J. T.: Role of chemical and cytologic analysis of amniotic fluid in determination of fetal maturity, Am. J. Obstet. Gynecol. 104:664, 1969.

Yahia, C., and Montgomery, G., Jr.: Advanced extrauterine pregnancy, Obstet. Gynecol. 6:68, 1956.

4

Abortion

Definition

ABORTION IS GENERALLY DEFINED as the expulsion of the fetus from the uterus prior to the period of viability. This definition is inadequate, however, because of the different interpretations of the word viability and because of differences of opinion as to whether or not both living and dead fetuses should be included. In most states the law intimates, although it rarely states specifically, that all products of conception born alive should be registered as live births and that an appropriate certificate to this fact should be filed with the local health department. In many instances the law reads "when there is any sign of life . . . after the child is altogether outside the body of the mother . . .," but few hospitals or physicians consider a 50 or 100 gm fetus a child even though the heart is beating at delivery.

In all states there is a clearer ruling for stillborn fetuses. Those under 5, 7 or some other specified number of months need not be reported as births and consequently can be considered abortions. In many communities the same criteria are applied unofficially to liveborn fetuses, and all those born before the number of months specified for reporting stillbirths are considered abortions. In some hospitals an arbitrary limit is set for reporting fetal and neonatal mortality, and all products of conception whether born alive or dead under 400, 1,000 or 1,500 gm, as the case may be, are excluded and considered abortions. The eighth revision of the *International Classification of Diseases* (1965), adopted for use in the United States, includes under abortion "any interruption of pregnancy before 28 weeks of gestation with a dead fetus." This is somewhat ambiguous since with this definition the sec-

tion titled "Certain Causes of Perinatal Mortality and Morbidity" would include all infants born alive regardless of gestation but only those over 28 weeks if born dead. The World Health Organization has recommended that use of the word abortion be discontinued and that the term fetal death be applied to all fetuses dying in utero, with classification into four groups: group 1, less than 20 weeks; group 2, 20–28 weeks; group 3, over 28 weeks; group 4, unknown age. It has been the practice at the Chicago Lying-in Hospital to insist that at least two of the following criteria be present for a diagnosis of abortion: weight less than 400 gm, length less than 28 cm and gestational age less than 22 weeks. The term previable has been used for the group with a weight of 400–1,000 gm, length of 28–35 cm and gestational age of 22–28 weeks; such fetuses and infants have been included in fetal and neonatal mortality figures because in Illinois all births of over 22 weeks' gestation must be reported to the health department.

At the Boston Hospital for Women all fetuses born before 20 completed weeks of gestation, whether alive or dead, are regarded as abortions. All fetuses surviving in utero beyond 20 weeks' gestation must be reported to the health department whether live or stillborn.

The principal reason a uniform definition of abortion is needed is to allow comparison of the loss of life among different institutions or communities and thus evaluate accurately the importance of various complications and different forms of therapy. Few published discussions of abortion indicate the period to which the pregnancies were advanced in a particular study, and until this is done close comparison will be impossible. For statistical purposes many investigators use a fetal weight of 1,000 gm as a dividing line between an abortion and a birth or stillbirth. Although a few infants weighing less than 1,000 gm survive, the incidence is so low that it does not invalidate the fact that this is the approximate weight at which organ maturation is sufficient to permit independent existence. Ylppö maintained that 1,250 gm is a better point of division, and it is true that survival rates of infants weighing 1,250–1,500 gm are considerably higher than those of infants weighing 1,000–1,250 gm. It would not make a big difference which figures were used as long as they were uniform. Until we can have international, or at least national, agreement on a definition, every report dealing with pregnancy should state the weight or gestational age of the offspring of the patients under discussion. In the present discussion the general term abortion is used to indicate the termination of pregnancy before the fetus is capable of an independent existence regardless of whether it is born alive or dead.

Frequency

In a study of abortions at the Chicago Lying-in Hospital for an 8-year period ending in 1965, Sentrakul and Potter found that 12.3% of all pregnancies ended in abortion before 20 weeks of gestation, while only 1.4% terminated in fetal death after 20 weeks. The majority of early terminations were thought to have been spontaneous because the mothers had registered for prenatal care and in very few was there evidence of bacterial infection. The World Health Organization has recommended that all fetal deaths be made reportable in order to obtain information on total fetal loss. However, Sentrakul and Potter found the term fetal death unacceptable because, in their study, if the reporting had been limited to instances in which an embryo or fetus was found 1,696 (61%) of 2,451 intrauterine pregnancies terminating spontaneously would not have been reported (Table 4–1).

Among 1,000 specimens, Mikamo in Switzerland

TABLE 4–1.—PRODUCTS OF CONCEPTION OBSERVED IN 2,681 PREGNANCIES TERMINATING UNDER 20 WEEKS*

Intrauterine pregnancy with spontaneous termination				2,451
Embryo or fetus absent			1,696	
Decidua only		509		
Chorionic vesicle, ruptured		1,109		
Incomplete chorionic vesicle or placenta	544			
Complete chorionic vesicle or placenta	565			
Chorionic vesicle, intact		78		
Embryo or fetus present (part or all)			755	
Normal gross development		555		
Fresh	186			
Macerated	369			
Abnormal gross development		76		
Embryo with extreme abnormality: nodular, cylindrical, rudimentary, etc.	53			
Embryo or fetus with individually identifiable malformations	23			
Fragmented (probably but not definitely normal except for maceration)		124		
Other termination				230
Intrauterine pregnancy, therapeutic termination (all with fetus)			70	
Extrauterine pregnancy			145	
Embryo or fetus present		49		
Embryo or fetus not observed		96		
Hydatidiform mole			15	
TOTAL PREGNANCIES				2,681
TOTAL WITH FETUS				874

*From Sentrakul, P., and Potter, E. L., Am. J. Public Health 56:2083, 1966.

studied material from 318 spontaneous human abortions in which conceptuses were intact, or nearly so; 212 fetuses were normal. This comprised 21% of all abortions, a figure almost identical to the 22% found in the Chicago Lying-in Hospital material. However, Mikamo found definitely defective development in 33% of those in which a sac or embryo was complete, in contrast to only 20% in similar material at the Chicago Lying-in Hospital. Chromosome studies of 67 cases from his material yielded a 25% abnormality rate, with the frequency highest in the earliest weeks of pregnancy.

In eight states where health department regulations call for all products of conception to be reported, the frequency of fetal deaths under 20 weeks actually reported in 1963 varied from 0.3% of live births in Maine to 4.9% in Virginia and rose to 7.4% in New York City. This figure was 12.3% at the Chicago Lying-in Hospital for total pregnancies under 20 weeks, or 4% for those with a fetus or embryo.

The proportionate number of fertilized eggs that are delivered as liveborn infants is known only approximately. Data from rats, wild rabbits and pigs suggest that as many as 40% of fertilized eggs fail to come to delivery. In these species about 10% of the losses are thought to occur in the fallopian tube, nearly 85% at or near the time of implantation and the remainder from the postimplantation stage until delivery (Brambell, Perry). Although data are meager, they suggest that the total losses are equally high in human beings. It is certain that the losses are numerically greatest before a missed menstrual period would give clinical evidence of pregnancy. Hertig and Livingston found that among eight preimplantation blastocysts removed from the fallopian tubes or uterine cavities of normally fertile women, four were abnormal. Among 34 implanted blastocysts of less than 16 days' gestational age, Hertig *et al.* described abnormalities in 11 so severe that they would not have been expected to survive. The loss for clinically apparent abortions, i.e., those occurring after implantation has taken place and after the first missed period, is usually given as about 10–15%. This is obviously too low a figure for total pregnancy wastage according to Hertig's data and those derived from lower animals. One could speculate that this figure would be more than 30% of the eggs fertilized.

Etiology

The factors contributing to the occurrence of any given abortion are generally unknown, and even when an etiologic agent is suspected, it is usually impossible to prove that it was actually responsible. All causes are genetic, environmental or a combination of both and may produce such similar changes that no differentiation can be made.

Abortions are most frequent in the first 3 months of pregnancy, during which time a normal live fetus is rarely delivered. Some fetuses are malformed, but even of those that appear to be normally developed almost all have been dead for some time before expulsion from the uterus. Any proposed theory for the prevention of early abortion must be directed toward the maintenance of life and prevention of abnormality rather than expulsion from the uterus.

At different gestational ages different agents are effective in causing abortion or fetal loss, although many have only a restricted period of effectiveness. It is known from animal work and from the recognized clinical effectiveness of administration of high doses of estrogen soon after midcycle coitus for the prevention of pregnancy that the acceleration of the passage of the fertilized zygote through the fallopian tube will cause degeneration and loss of the blastocyst. Similarly, steroids given shortly after the first missed period can destroy the implanting embryo.

Chromosomal abnormalities, as identified by cultivation and karyotyping of the embryo or amnion, are now recognized as an important cause of abortion in the first 15 weeks of pregnancy. The incidence is greatest in young embryos. Carr thought the incidence of chromosomal anomalies to be about 20–25% in spontaneous abortions occurring between 60 and 150 days. According to Szulman, in studies of material obtained from spontaneous abortions a frequency as high as 65% has been reported in some series in which attention was focused on younger and more anomalous-appearing abortuses. Most series indicate that trisomy—the presence of an extra chromosome—is the most common form of abnormality. In Carr's own series, 27 of 50 abnormal karyotypes were trisomies. The smaller chromosomes were chiefly involved, but occasionally even a group B chromosome was duplicated. The latter is an abnormality not recognized in material obtained from full-term infants or adults. The loss of one sex chromosome, giving an XO karyotype, was present in 12 of the 50 cases. Curiously, Carr found germ cells in all of the identifiable gonads in this group despite the fact that adults with this anomaly usually have gonads devoid of such cells. The third major group of anomalies consisted of cells with triploid or tetraploid numbers, giving 69 or 96 chromosomes. Though mosaic triploids have been found in liveborn infants, tetraploids are known only in abortions. As might be expected, the incidence of chromosomal anomaly is higher in grossly deformed or anomalous abortuses than in those anatomically normal (Thiede and Sam).

Analysis of chromosomal data shows that abnormal chromosomal configurations are present in a higher proportion of female than male embryos even after exclusion of the XO cases which originally might have been either male or female genotype. In spite of this there are more male than female abortuses, indicating that other causes must be proportionately higher in males.

Evidence of an *immunologic etiology* for abortions in human beings hinges entirely on an inferred relationship based on statistical data. A relative deficiency of group A or B offspring has been noted in group O women with group A or B husbands (McNeil). This is presumed to be due to embryonic loss resulting from fetal-maternal incompatibility. There is no good evidence that abortion results from Rh incompatibility although late fetal deaths are common.

Teratogenic agents, experimentally effective in animals, frequently induce abortion in the litter mates of those with congenital anomalies. These two effects occur at the same dose levels and appear inextricably bound together. Methotrexate and 6-azoguanine are among the chemical antagonists, and x-rays are among the physical agents that have been proved to be effective abortifacients in human beings. It is highly probable that since, in experimental animals, an abortifacient drug is most effective soon after blastocyst implantation (8th–10th day in the rat), in human beings it would be most active before clinical pregnancy was apparent.

Infections have been thought to cause abortions, but few acceptable data are available to support this belief. Toxoplasmosis has been identified histologically in the endometrium or recovered following serial passage in mice of material removed from the uterine cavity of habitual and repeating aborters. These data need confirmation. Mycoplasma has also been recovered from the cervix and endometrium of repeated aborters, but since this organism is found in over 50% of random genital cultures, assessment of its role is difficult. There is a little evidence that rubella and measles virus present very early in pregnancy may cause abortion (Siegel *et al.*).

Increasing maternal age is correlated with an increasing frequency of abortion, congenital anomalies and the disjunctional chromosomal characteristics of classical Down's syndrome. "Tired eggs" as well as "tired mothers" give a high proportion of anomalies and abortuses in guinea pigs, the incidence of both rising with delayed fertilization of the egg. The values run from 12% when guinea pigs are inseminated 8 hours after ovulation to 90% when inseminated at 26 hours (Young). Some authors have suggested that the increased frequency of abnormal pregnancy in older mothers may be attributed to a decreased frequency of intercourse, with resulting delay in the fertilization of the egg. Mikamo felt that chromosomal abnormalities were often a result of overripeness of the egg and that this might be a result of chronologic age or delayed liberation from the follicle as well as delayed fertilization in the fallopian tube.

Local environmental disturbances have been suggested as causes of human abortions. Among these are submucous myomas with thinning of the overlying decidua, a septate uterus in which implantation on the septum may cause abortion due to lack of an adequate blood supply, and an incompetent cervix. It must be remembered, however, that in a broad sense the environment of the fetus is not limited to the uterus but includes the total milieu provided by the mother; anything affecting her in any way can have a possible effect on the development of the conceptus.

Habitual Abortion

Any woman may have one or several abortions. Some women seem unable to carry a fetus in the uterus for a normal length of time, and several successive pregnancies may terminate prematurely at about the same period of gestation. Any woman who has had three successive abortions is often called an habitual aborter. The data of Hertig and Livingston on the pathology of abortuses from habitual aborters suggest that the same ovular factors are present in successive abortions and that the greater the number of successive abortions, the more likely it is that a single factor is operating. Yet even with three successive abortions, the incidence of full-term pregnancy in the next gestation runs as high as 80%. The causes of repeated abortions usually cannot be identified, and there is probably as great a variety as in single abortions. Incompetence of the internal cervical os, most often a result of trauma, has received much attention as a cause of repeated midpregnancy abortions, and various operations have been devised to overcome this condition. There is no evidence that Rh incompatibility is responsible for habitual abortion, although an abortion may be responsible for maternal sensitization if an Rh negative woman is carrying an Rh positive fetus.

Pathologic States

When decidua only is observed, one cannot be certain that pregnancy was responsible for its production since many progestins given together with estrogens for prolonged periods can mimic the changes of pregnancy. In addition, uterine decidua may be cast off in an ectopic pregnancy. However, when tissues derived from the ovum are present, the various forms of "pathologic ova" described by Mall and Meyer can often be identified. Their group 1 included conceptuses with villi only and no embryonic sac; group 2, villi and an intact empty chorionic sac; group 3, villi, chorion and intact empty amniotic sac; group 4, the same as 3 but with an indication of an umbilical cord or body stalk; group 5, the same as 4 but with a nodular (nonaxial) embryo (Fig. 4–1); group 6, the same as 4 but with a cylindrical embryo without limb buds; and group 7, the same as 4 but with an embryo with a local malformation (Fig. 4–2). While Mall and Meyer

included macerated embryos with normal morphology as a last group of pathologic ova, maceration or sterile autolysis in itself is not evidence of intrinsic abnormality. Chromosomal studies of the amnions of the last group show a reduced incidence of abnormal karyotypes in comparison to those of groups 2–6.

Malformations found in young embryos are often so severe that they cannot be compared to those in older fetuses. They often appear to result from severe and lethal chromosomal anomalies since such chromosomal anomalies are not found in liveborn infants except as part of a mosaic karyotype. Once pregnancy has progressed beyond the first few weeks, malformations resemble those of infants delivered at or near term. Malformations most often observed at the Chicago Lying-in Hospital in the first half of pregnancy have involved the brain and spinal cord—hydrocephalus, anencephalus and spina bifida—and eventration of the abdominal viscera (Figs. 4–3 to 4–5). Abnormal twin fetuses were found occasionally and one chorionic vesicle contained three amniotic sacs and three malformed embryos, each less than 2 cm long (Fig. 4–6).

For the first few weeks the amniotic sac closely envelops the embryo, and only as it enlarges to

Fig. 4–1 (left).—Opened chorionic vesicle with intact amniotic sac. The embryo has failed to develop and is a small white mass 2 mm in diameter visible within the amniotic sac.

Fig. 4–2 (right).—Hydrocephalic embryo 1.5 cm long.

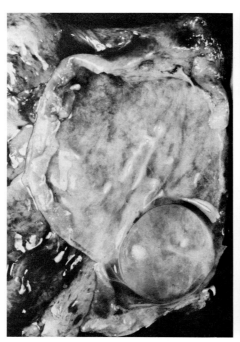
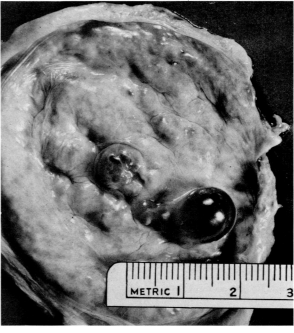

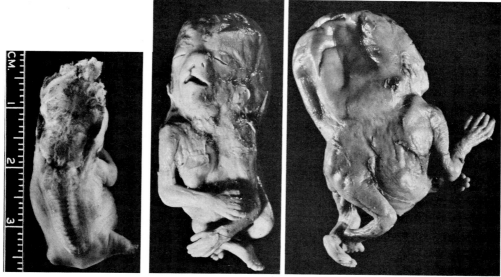

Fig. 4–3 (left). — Embryo 3 cm long with complete spina bifida and degeneration of the brain.

Fig. 4–4 (right). — Iniencephalic fetus with unilateral harelip. (Courtesy Dr. James Blair.)

Fig. 4–5 (left). — Fetus with anencephalus, spina bifida, clubfoot and omphalocele. (Courtesy Dr. Eleanor P. Cheydleur.)

Fig. 4–6 (right). — Monochorionic triplet pregnancy with three malformed embryos in individual amniotic sacs.

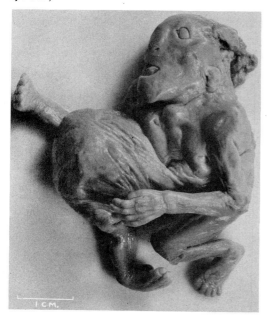

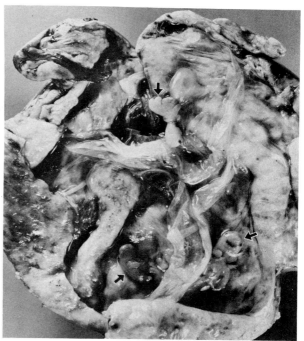

form the inner lining of the chorionic vesicle does it normally provide much free space around the embryo. Occasionally it grows at an excessive rate and becomes disproportionately large, or it may continue to grow after the death of the embryo (Fig. 4–7). Even in the absence of an embryo, the amnion and chorion seem able to develop fairly normally during the 1st trimester, but after this they begin to degenerate and are sooner or later expelled from the uterus.

For the first 2 months the normal chorionic vesicle is completely covered by luxuriantly growing villi, but in many abortuses the villi are abnormally short, sparsely distributed over the surface or otherwise abnormal (Fig. 4–8). Occasionally some or all of the villi are cystic (Fig. 4–9); in such villi blood vessels are often reduced in number or lacking altogether (Fig. 4–10). Abnormal growth of vil-

li is as much an abnormality as is failure of growth or differentiation of the embryo itself. About 70% of abortuses with true hydatidiform degeneration have a triploid karyotype (69 chromosomes) (Carr).

It has been suggested that placental abnormalities are responsible for a large share of abortions but, with the exception of hydatidiform moles, intrinsic abnormalities of trophoblast or associated mesoderm have never been proved to cause failure of normal fetal growth. In common with other investigators (Eckman and Carrow), Sentrakul and Potter, in a review of material from 317 abortuses at the Chicago Lying-in Hospital, found the most common changes to be edema, central condensation of stroma (Fig. 4–11) with eventual hyalinization (Fig. 4–12) or seemingly poor vascularization of villi, paucity and pyknosis of syncytiotrophoblastic nuclei and, in early pregnancy, decrease in cyto-

Fig. 4–7 (top).—Degenerated embryo in excessively large amniotic sac. The latter has become separated from the inverted chorionic vesicle.

Fig. 4–9 (bottom).—Cystic enlargement and sparse development of villi in chorionic vesicle 2.8 cm in diameter.
Fig. 4–8. (right).—Chorionic vesicle 1 cm in diameter showing inadequate development of villi.

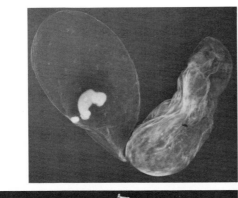

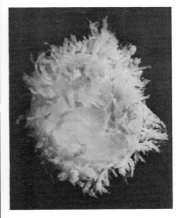

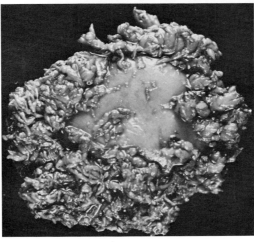

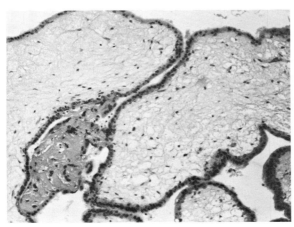

Fig. 4—10.—Hydatid degeneration of villi retained for a short period of time after early fetal death. The villi are enlarged and the stroma is edematous.

trophoblast. Deposits of anuclear, homogeneous, acidophilic material between all or part of the villi were present in all degenerated placentas and chorionic vesicles.

Varying degrees of decidual inflammation and degeneration accompany these changes. The early decidua of normal pregnancy often shows small foci of inflammation, necrosis and hemorrhage (McCombs and Craig). Such changes are almost universally present in spontaneous abortions but they seem probably to be caused by stromal breakdown resulting from lack of progesterone support of the decidua and probably do not indicate an inflammatory cause of abortion.

With the institution of more liberal abortion policies the appearance of the abortuses in artificially terminated pregnancies is of increasing interest. In gestational products obtained by curettage or suction the villi are well preserved with intact blood vessels containing nucleated red blood cells. When criminal abortion or an incomplete therapeutic abortion is followed by a delay of several days before it is completed by a subsequent curettage, two features not ordinarily seen in spontaneous abortions are found. First, the villi appear normal except for evidence of fetal death; they may be partially necrotic but there is no fibrin deposition or hydatid change. Second, severe acute intervillous and villous inflammation is almost invariably present.

When death of the fetus has been brought about by intra-amniotic injection of a hypertonic solution (glucose, saline, urea), the fetus is always macerated. The placenta shows characteristic changes, in-

Fig. 4—11 (left).—Villi from an abortion with collapse of the blood vessels and partial condensation of the edematous stroma.

Fig. 4—12 (right).—Material from a spontaneous abortion showing hyalinization of villi, clumping of syncytiotrophoblast nuclei and collapse of the maternal vascular space.

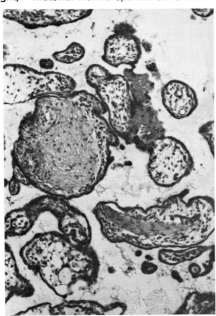

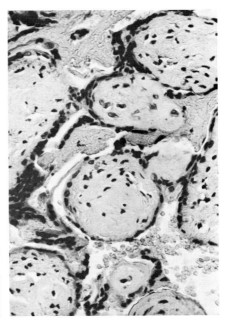

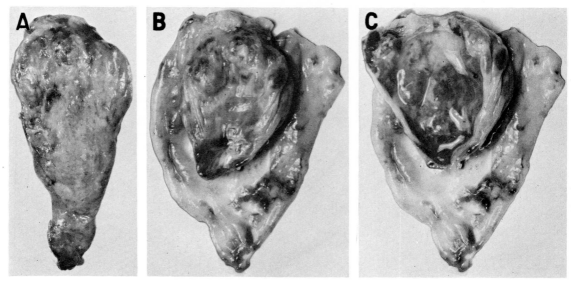

Fig. 4–13.—**A,** complete decidual cast of the uterus. **B,** decidual cast opened showing attached ruptured chorionic vesicle. **C,** chorionic vesicle opened. The embryo was expelled several days prior to passage of decidua and chorionic sac.

cluding necrosis of the amniotic and chorionic membranes and a zone of subchorionic thrombosis. The villi beneath the chorionic plate are often infarcted and inflamed. Near the maternal surface the villi show only the changes of recent fetal death, with collapse and necrosis of intravillous vessels and shrinkage of the villi.

Hydatid alteration that may follow death of the embryo in early pregnancy but is uncommon after the 16th week of gestation.

Mechanism

Abortion may follow one of several patterns. The decidual lining may separate from the uterus and, with the enclosed chorionic vesicle, be passed as a single unit (Fig. 4–13); the chorionic vesicle may become loosened from the decidua and be expelled intact, leaving the decidua behind; or the chorionic vesicle and amniotic sac may rupture and the fetus escape, temporarily leaving the other structures

Fig. 4–14.—Breus mole. **A,** degenerated chorionic vesicle with multiple subchorionic hematomas. **B,** higher magnification showing especially the small cylindroid mass that comprises the entire embryo. (Courtesy Dr. H. B. W. Benaron.)

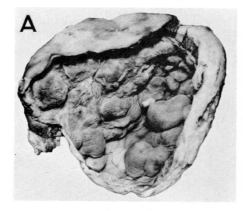
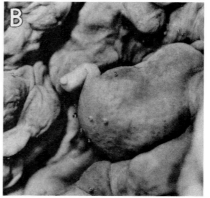

attached to the uterine wall. Before an abortion is complete, the fetus, chorionic vesicle and decidua must all be expelled or therapeutically removed. In most abortions the sac ruptures, the umbilical cord breaks and the fetus is passed first. However, the earlier in pregnancy that abortion takes place, the more often is the embryo or fetus expelled in an intact chorionic vesicle.

Missed abortion is the term applied when a chorionic vesicle is retained in the uterus for several weeks or months after death of the fetus. Breus' mole indicates a retained chorionic vesicle in which there are numerous small protuberant hematomas under the chorionic membrane (Fig. 4–14). The fetus is usually rudimentary. The condition is unrelated to hydatidiform moles.

REFERENCES

Brambell, F. W. R.: Prenatal mortality in mammals, Biol. Rev. 23:370, 1948.

Carr, D. H.: Cytogenetics of Abortion, in Benirschke, K. (ed.): *Comparative Aspects of Reproductive Failure* (New York: Springer-Verlag New York, Inc., 1967), p. 96.

Carr, D. H.: Chromosomal anomalies in human fetuses, Res. Reprod. 4:3, 1972.

Corner, G. W.: The problem of embryonic pathology in mammals with observations upon intrauterine mortality in pigs, Am. J. Anat. 31:523, 1922–23.

Eckman, T. R., and Carrow, L. A.: Placental lesions in spontaneous abortion, Am. J. Obstet. Gynecol. 84:222, 1962.

Fox, H.: Morphological changes in the human placenta following fetal death, J. Obstet. Gynaec. Br. Commonw. 75:839, 1968.

Hertig, A. T., and Livingston, R. G.: Spontaneous, threatened and habitual abortion: Their pathogenesis and treatment, N. Engl. J. Med. 230:797, 1944.

Hertig, A. T., Rock, J., and Adams, E.: A description of 34 human ova within the first 17 days of development, Am. J. Anat. 98:435, 1956.

MacMahon, B., Hertig, A. T., and Ingalls, A.: Association between maternal age and pathologic diagnosis in abortion, Obstet. Gynecol. 4:477, 1954.

Mall, F. P., and Meyer, A. W.: Studies on abortuses: A survey of pathologic ova in the Carnegie Embryological Collection, Contrib. Embryol. publication no. 275, 1923.

McCombs, H. L., and Craig, J. M.: Decidual necrosis in normal pregnancy, Obstet. Gynecol. 24:436, 1964.

McNeil, C.: The significance of blood group conflicts and aberrant salivary secretion in spontaneous abortion, Am. J. Clin. Pathol. 28:469, 1957.

Mikamo, K.: Anatomic and chromosomal anomalies in spontaneous abortion: Possible correlation with overripeness of the egg, Am. J. Obstet. Gynecol. 106:243, 1970.

Perry, J. S.: Fecundity and embryonic mortality in pigs, J. Embryol. Exp. Morphol. 3:308, 1954.

Pierce, G. B., and Midgely, A. R., Jr.: The origin and function of human syncytiotrophoblastic giant cells, Am. J. Pathol. 43:153, 1963.

Potter, E. L.: The abortion problem, G. P. 19:105, 1959.

Sentrakul, P., and Potter, E. L.: Pathologic diagnosis on 2,681 abortions at the Chicago Lying-in Hospital, 1957-65, Am. J. Public Health 56:2083, 1966.

Siegel, M., Fuerst, H. T., and Peress, W. S.: Comparative fetal mortality in maternal virus disease: A prospective study on rubella, measles, mumps, chicken pox and hepatitis, N. Engl. J. Med. 274:768, 1966.

Speert, H.: Pregnancy prognosis following repeated abortion, Am. J. Obstet. Gynecol. 68:665, 1954.

Szulman, A. E.: Chromosomal aberrations in spontaneous human abortions, N. Engl. J. Med. 272:84, 1965.

Thiede, H. A., and Sam, S. B.: Chromosomal studies of human spontaneous abortions, Am. J. Obstet. Gynecol. 90:205, 1964.

World Health Organization (Geneva): *Manual of the International Statistical Classification of Diseases, Injuries and Causes of Death* (8th rev., 1965).

Ylppö, A.: New classification and nomenclature for newborn infants including prematures and abortions, Acta Paediat. 35 (suppl. 1): 161, 1948.

5

Causes of Fetal and Infant Death

THE PRIMARY REASON for studying the dead is to save the living—to correlate the events that have transpired during life with the state of the body after death and to come to some conclusion as to cause and effect. To examine a dead body, to record the pathologic changes and to make no attempt to reconstruct events leading to those changes or to try to arrive at a conclusion as to why death occurred is to leave the job half done. The growing awareness that stillbirth and infant mortality rates are too high and are amenable to reduction has led to a widespread desire for more information regarding the causes of these deaths. Many studies have been instituted to learn more about this problem, and too often an obstacle has been met in the inadequacy of the autopsy report. The pathologist frequently lists gross and microscopic findings and leaves someone else, usually a clinician unaware of the significance of these findings, to make a diagnosis.

When any general study of stillbirths and infant deaths is undertaken, it is highly desirable that these deaths be classified as to cause: we should know what we are going to prevent if we are to expend our energy purposefully. The way in which data are arranged in a classification will depend to some extent on the purpose for which they are being used, but in general the causes of death are relatively few, and the following summary based on the time that they might occur during pregnancy or after birth is a logical basis for categorizing them.

1. *Malformations:* If the egg or the sperm carries abnormal genes or chromosomes or if they become abnormal because of environmental circumstances, or if the environment adversely affects the early constitution, the embryo can manifest this disturb-

ance only by an alteration in manner of development.

2. *Blood disturbances: Erythroblastosis fetalis and some instances of thrombocytopenic purpura:* If a fetus is developing normally but is incompatible with its mother, i.e., the fetus possesses antigens specific for antibodies reaching it from the maternal circulation, it will be injured by these antibodies. The only conditions now recognized are certain blood dyscrasias, especially erythroblastosis.

Hemorrhagic disease. A diminution of prothrombin resulting from lack of vitamin K reaching the fetus from the mother is thought to be the cause of some nontraumatic postnatal hemorrhage.

3. *Anoxia:* A fetus is completely dependent on oxygen obtained from maternal blood surrounding the villi in the placenta and transported to it through the vessels of the umbilical cord. Oxygen may not reach the fetus because of failure of blood to become oxygenated in the placenta (abruptio placentae, placenta previa, ruptured uterus, maternal shock) or because of obstruction to circulation through the cord (cord prolapse, entanglement or other compression). Death from any of these causes may follow quickly or may not occur until after birth even though the oxygen lack was sustained earlier.

4. *Infection:* Normally the fetus is surrounded by sterile amniotic fluid during intrauterine life. Following rupture of membranes or onset of labor, bacteria from the vagina enter the amniotic cavity and may be inspired into the lungs (intrauterine pneumonia). Bacteria or viruses in the maternal blood may penetrate fetal vessels in placental villi and infect the fetus (syphilis, cytomegalic inclusion body disease, toxoplasmosis, etc.). Bacteria may enter the cut umbilical stump (omphalitis, septi-

cemia) or the lungs, gastrointestinal tract, etc., after birth (postnatal pneumonia, gastroenteritis, etc.).

5. *Birth injury:* The fetus must make its exit from the uterus through the bony pelvis; abnormal tensions or pressures within the head resulting from cephalopelvic disproportion, abnormal presentations or other causes may lead to rupture of blood vessels and be responsible for hemorrhage into the cranial cavity. Less often, the viscera and spinal cord are involved.

6. *Prematurity, liveborn infants under 1,000 gm. only:* Fifty percent of infants are delivered between the beginning of the 39th and the end of the 40th week after the 1st day of the last menstrual period. Far more serious consequences are encountered when delivery occurs before this time than when it occurs later, and the earlier a child is born, the poorer its chances of survival. However, if the viscera have developed sufficiently to support extrauterine life, the child can be expected to survive unless it has been injured by trauma, anoxia or some other condition. Although it may contribute to a fatal outcome, prematurity should not ordinarily be considered a primary cause of death in a viable infant, i.e., one who has reached a degree of maturity compatible with extrauterine existence, generally associated with a weight of about 1,000 gm and a gestational length of about 28 weeks. Prematurity can never be considered to be a cause of stillbirth.

7. *Abnormal pulmonary function:* After birth the lungs must function immediately and adequately if the infant is to survive, and if the child is normal they invariably do so. Failure to breathe properly may be a result of anoxia, intracranial hemorrhage, malformations, intrauterine pneumonia and so on. The lungs may not become completely expanded or subsequently may become atelectatic. Atelactasis per se probably can never be considered a cause of death as it is only a manifestation of some underlying disturbance.

In a particular group of infants who exhibit marked dyspnea almost immediately after birth, die within a few hours or a few days and at autopsy show extreme atelactasis with characteristic hyalinelike deposits in the lung, a definite etiologic agent has not yet been established. The condition has been designated pulmonary hyaline membrane disease or respiratory distress syndrome. Without an autopsy the cause of respiratory disturbances can seldom be identified, and such infants cannot be more specifically classified than as suffering from "abnormal pulmonary function."

8. *Inborn errors of metabolism:* Such disturbances are ordinarily caused by the homozygous state of specific recessive genes. The genes are responsible for the absence of specific enzymes that normally control certain metabolic processes; the usual result is accumulation and/or excretion of abnormal substances. The absence of an enzyme is seldom manifested in the fetus and may not be apparent until food containing materials that cannot be properly metabolized is included in the infant's diet.

9. *Other specific diseases:* Other demonstrable causes of death are rare in the newborn period. A few cases of thrombosis of renal or other vessels have been described. Fetal hydrops, with or without pleural and peritoneal effusions, may occur in the absence of erythroblastosis or recognized infection. The liver may be the site of necrosis or other cellular abnormalities. None of these has a known etiology.

10. *Maternal disease without evidence in the fetus:* In some instances careful autopsy examination fails to disclose pathologic lesions. This is especially true in deaths occurring before the onset of labor and those involving small premature infants dying in the neonatal period (no pathologic lesions). In some, maternal complications exist that it is wise to mention because an associated increase in fetal or neonatal mortality is recognized even though the precise mechanism producing death in such conditions has not been demonstrated. These include maternal nephritis, toxemia, diabetes, heart disease and so on.

11. *Sudden infant death syndrome:* This syndrome is the major cause of death in infants over the age of 1 month and is responsible for more than 10,000 deaths a year in the United States (La Veck). Such infants are found dead in bed without a preceding recognized illness or a cause of death demonstrable at autopsy. Speculations as to possible etiology, none of which has been proved, include viral and bacterial infections, especially those involving the larynx, lungs or intestine, laryngospasm, breath holding, suffocation, hypothermia, ventricular fibrillation, metabolic acidosis, reduced gamma globulin, status thymicolymphaticus, hypoparathyroidism, abnormal karyotype, milk allergy, rickets and scurvy.

Classification of Causes of Death

The reason for any classification is to arrange data so they may be useful for whatever purpose they are gathered. The reason for classifying causes of fetal and neonatal deaths is to allow discovery of the factors that may be associated and to determine the areas in which the greatest effort must be concentrated to decrease the number of such deaths.

The problem of ascribing an exact cause of death in the age period with which we are dealing is somewhat more difficult than at most ages for several reasons. First, there are two persons involved and, except for malformations caused by inherited genes, all disturbances in the fetus are secondary to abnormal states in the mother or in its own accessory structures—the placenta, membranes and umbilical cord. It may even be possible that a third level of involvement exists: the mother may affect the accessory structures, which in turn may affect the fetus. Ideally, multiple tables showing such interrelationships would be made, and in a particular investigation they are often necessary. But if a single classification is to be made, a decision must be reached as to whether death should be attributed to the end-state in the fetus or to the underlying cause in the mother. One must choose, for instance, between intracranial hemorrhage and cephalopelvic disproportion or between anoxia and cord prolapse.

Second, the pathologist encounters difficulty in interpreting his observations. One of the main difficulties arises from the fact that there are no specific changes invariably produced in the fetus or newborn by anoxia even when reduction of oxygen supply is severe enough to cause death. The anoxia resulting from premature placental detachment is responsible for characteristic subpleural, subepicardial and thymic petechiae, but in most fetuses and infants dying of anoxia from other causes, hemorrhages are few or absent and other pathologic changes generally lacking. On the other hand, scattered ecchymoses and occasional petechiae may be found after death from any cause. Consequently the diagnosis of anoxia must often rest on the absence of any other demonstrable cause of death with a definite cause of anoxia apparent from the clinical history. In any autopsy it is as important to establish the absence as the presence of pathologic findings.

Other difficulties are encountered, especially in the lungs and the placenta. Almost all newborn infants exhibit some degree of atelectasis at autopsy, much of which may be terminal and in no way responsible for death. How extensive must the atelectasis be before it can be considered a cause of sufficient anoxia to lead to death and not simply an agonal state? Or is atelectasis never to be considered a primary cause of death? The most severely hyalinized and infarcted placentas we have observed were associated with normal infants. How much of the placental substance must be involved before placental insufficiency can be indicted as a cause of death? Is there ever a time when infarcts or other degenerative changes in the placenta can be shown positively to have caused death?

Maternal toxemia is associated with no recognizable state in the fetus, and most pathologists hesitate to ascribe a death to toxemia per se. The situation is quite different from anoxia in which the way death is produced is well recognized even though visible pathologic changes do not necessarily occur. No one has been able to demonstrate toxic substances or specific reasons why toxemia should cause death, and since most toxic women deliver normal children, there rarely seems justification for indicting toxemia as a definite cause of nonsurvival.

A classification of causes of fetal and neonatal deaths that has been found satisfactory at the Chicago Lying-in Hospital follows. It is arranged and numbered so that it may be used on a code sheet requiring only two columns on IBM punch cards.

CODE FOR CLASSIFICATION OF CAUSES OF FETAL AND NEONATAL DEATHS

Living

00__ Living (not included in study)

Malformations

10__ Brain and spinal cord
11__ Heart and blood vessels
12__ Lungs and trachea
13__ Stomach, intestine, including tracheo-esophageal fistulas
14__ Kidneys, bladder and organs of reproduction
15__ Skeleton
16__ Skin and muscle
17__ Tumors
18__ Inborn errors of metabolism
19__ More than one potentially lethal malformation
1x__ Other

Trauma

20__ No autopsy: symptoms interpreted as trauma
21__ Cranial cavity: hemorrhage from laceration of tentorium cerebelli or vein of Galen
22__ Cranial cavity: subdural hematoma
23__ Cranial cavity: other
24__ Spinal cord: hemorrhage or laceration
25__ Adrenal: gross hemorrhage
26__ Liver: gross hemorrhage
27__ Other

Anoxia

30__ Abruptio placentae
31__ Placenta previa
32__ Cord prolapse
33__ Cord knots and entanglement
34__ Maternal hypotension

35__ Anesthesia
36__ Shoulder dystocia
37__ Delayed delivery of aftercoming head
38__ Prolonged labor
39__ Other cause
3x__ Unknown cause

Infections

40__ Lungs, probably intrauterine
41__ Lungs, probably extrauterine
42__ Intestine, stomach or esophagus
43__ Heart or blood vessels
44__ Kidneys or bladder
45__ Brain or meninges
46__ Bone, muscle or skin
47__ Umbilicus
48__ Generalized, bacterial
49__ Generalized, viral
4x__ Syphilis
4y__ Other

Blood Dyscrasias

50__ ABO erythroblastosis
51__ Rh erythroblastosis with fetal hydrops
52__ Rh erythroblastosis with kernicterus
53__ Rh erythroblastosis without hydrops or kernicterus
54__ Hemorrhagic disease
55__ Leukemia
56__ Anemia from other than above causes

Abnormal Pulmonary Function

60__ Generalized atelectasis with hyaline membrane
61__ Generalized atelectasis without hyaline membrane
62__ Mild hyaline membrane without other recognizable cause of death

Inborn Errors of Metabolism

70__ Carbohydrate
71__ Amino acid
72__ Lipid
73__ Other

Other

80__ Kernicterus not due to erythroblastosis
81__ Hydrops without erythroblastosis
82__ Liver necrosis, cirrhosis, etc., without known cause
83__ Diffuse pulmonary hemorrhage without known cause
84__ Sudden infant death syndrome
85__ Other

Iatrogenic Causes

90__ Craniotomy or other destructive operation on living fetus
91__ Delivery for maternal cause prior to viability

No Pathologic State at Autopsy with or without Possible Maternal Factors and Not Elsewhere Classifiable

x0__ No known maternal factor
x1__ Toxemia of pregnancy
x2__ Glomerulonephritis
x3__ Pyelocystitis
x4__ Diabetes mellitus
x5__ Heart disease, symptomatic
x6__ Preceding accident
x7__ Preceding operation
x8__ Over 301 days' gestation without other complications
x9__ Other

Conceptuses Not Included as Fetal or Neonatal Deaths*

y0__ Fetus, with or without chorionic vesicle, normal, nonmacerated
y1__ Fetus, with or without chorionic vesicle, normal, macerated
y2__ Fetus, with or without chorionic vesicle, malformed (regardless of state of preservation)
y3__ Chorionic vesicle, intact, with absent or rudimentary embryo
y4__ Chorionic vesicle, ruptured, without embryo or fetus
y5__ Villi, with or without decidua
y6__ Decidua only
y7__ Hydatidiform mole
y8__ Ectopic pregnancy

Mortality rates have decreased everywhere and at all ages during the past 40 years. The greatest change has occurred in infants aged from 1 month to 1 year; this has been brought about especially as a result of the more universal availability of noninfected milk and improved control of communicable diseases. In the younger age group the most outstanding decreases have been in deaths from anoxia and birth injury, as a result of better management of labor and delivery, and in deaths from prematurity, as a result of improved nursery care. The experience of the Chicago Lying-in Hospital has been similar to that of many other hospitals. The total mortality for fetuses and infants weighing over 1,000 gm at the Chicago Lying-in Hospital fell from 42/1,000 in 1931, the year the hospital was opened, to 19 in 1966. Throughout all the years until the last year this has been almost equally divided between stillbirths and infant deaths (Fig. 5–1). At the Boston Hospital for Women, where fetal and neonatal deaths include those occurring after 20 weeks' gestation, the ratio of stillbirth and neonatal death has been undergoing a change, with the proportion of stillbirths increasing. These figures are distorted, however, by the large number of mothers who were referred to that hospital because they were sensitized to Rh or had diabetes mellitus. In some years this excess of stillbirths reached 50%.

The mortality rate for premature infants at the Chicago Lying-in Hospital fell from 28% in 1935 to 12% in 1966, which is still about 20 times as high as the mortality rate for infants over 2,500 gm, the

*Necessary only when classification of all unsuccessful pregnancies is required. Division is at 400 gm at the Chicago Lying-in Hospital.

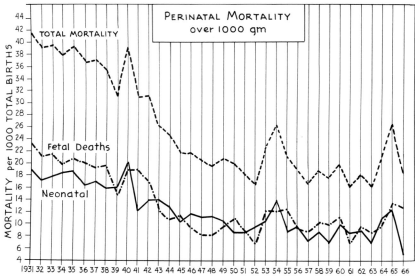

Fig. 5–1.—Perinatal mortality (over 1,000 gm) at the Chicago Lying-in Hospital, July 1, 1931 to July 1, 1966.

latter having fallen from about 1% to 0.25% (Fig. 5–2). The frequency of premature births has remained fairly constant, but in the last 5-year period, the percentage of premature infants delivered has shown a trend upward, which probably reflects the changing nature of the population serviced, with an increasing proportion of black poor (Potter and Davis), among whom premature delivery and small infants are more common. The areas in which these changes have been brought about in

Fig. 5–2.—Mortality among liveborn infants (over 1,000 gm) at the Chicago Lying-in Hospital, 1935–1966.

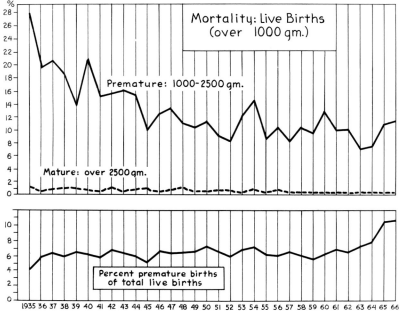

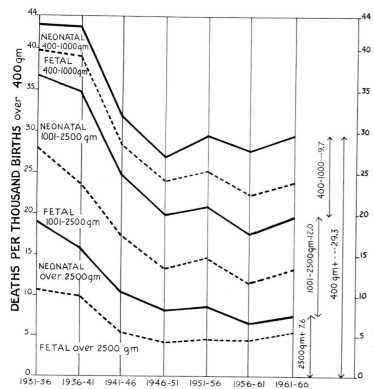

Fig. 5—3.—Total mortality per thousand live births (over 400 gm) at the Chicago Lying-in Hospital, 1931–1966.

antepartum, intrapartum and neonatal deaths are shown in Figures 5–3 to 5–6. Figures are based on a 95% autopsy rate.

Causes of death as determined by autopsy on all dead fetuses and infants born after 20 weeks' gestation at the Boston Hospital for Women from 1957–

1970 are shown in Table 5–1. Although the frequency of deaths among total births is not available for the Boston Hospital for Women, the relative frequency of causes of death was much the same as at the Chicago Lying-in Hospital. The majority of deaths (71% Chicago Lying-in Hospital

Fig. 5—4.—Fetal deaths (over 1,000 gm) in antepartum period at the Chicago Lying-in Hospital, July 1, 1931, to July 1, 1966.

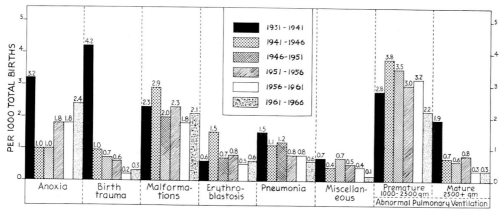

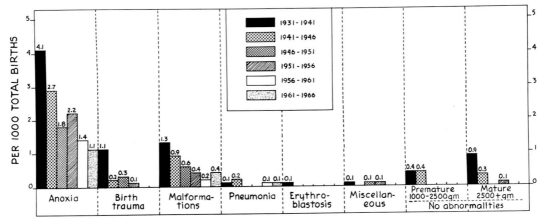

Fig. 5—5.—Fetal deaths (over 1,000 gm) in the intrapartum period at the Chicago Lying-in Hospital, July 1, 1931, to July 1, 1966.

1961–66, 65% Boston Hospital for Women 1957–70) were in fetuses and infants who showed no pathologic changes except for evidence of abnormally functioning lungs. They include the groups thought to have died of anoxia or hyaline membranes as well as those with no demonstrable pathologic changes. There is much overlap among these groups, and except for the small proportion of infants with specific evidence of anoxia from premature placental detachment or with massive hyaline membranes, whether death should be attributed to one cause or another is often subject to variable opinion. In both hospitals malformations ranked second, erythroblastosis third, and other conditions including birth trauma were far behind.

Definition of Live Births and Fetal Death

A uniform distinction between what constitutes a live birth and a stillbirth is important if figures for causes of stillbirth and death after birth are to be meaningful. At one time a distinction was made between deadbirth and stillbirth, the former being applied to a child with no signs of life at birth, the latter to one who either did not breathe at all or who never established a satisfactory extrauterine existence but whose heart was beating at the time of delivery.

The World Health Organization has recommended that the term fetal death be substituted for stillbirth, and its definition of fetal death, which is in

Fig. 5—6.—Neonatal deaths (over 1,000 gm) at the Chicago Lying-in Hospital, July 1, 1931, to July 1, 1966.

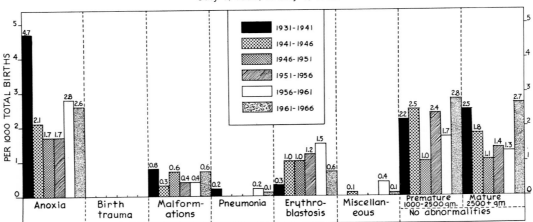

TABLE 5–1.—CAUSES OF DEATH AS DETERMINED BY AUTOPSY:
FETAL AND NEONATAL DEATHS OVER 20 WEEKS' GESTATION AT THE
BOSTON HOSPITAL FOR WOMEN 1957–1970

	FETAL DEATHS		NEONATAL DEATHS		TOTAL	
	No.	%	No.	%	No.	%
Anoxia	524	50.2	183	19.0	707	35.3
Hyaline membrane (under 2,500 gm)			359	37.4	359	18.0
Hyaline membrane (over 2,500 gm)			31	3.2	31	1.5
Birth trauma			24	2.5	24	1.2
Malformation	114	10.9	139	14.5	253	12.6
Pneumonia	30	2.8	90	9.3	120	6.0
Erythroblastosis	154	14.7	67	6.9	221	11.5
Miscellaneous	36	3.4	67	6.9	103	5.1
No abnormality (under 2,500 gm)	150	14.3			150	7.5
No abnormality (under 2,500 gm)	39	3.7			39	2.0
Totals	1,047	100%	960	100%	2,007	100%

use in the United States, has had wide acceptance. Fetal death is defined as death prior to the complete expulsion or extraction from its mother of a product of conception, irrespective of the duration of pregnancy; the death is indicated by the fact that after such separation the fetus does not breathe or show any other evidence of life such as heartbeat, pulsation of the umbilical cord or definite movement of voluntary muscles.*

Any child not fitting the description of fetal death is considered liveborn, for in live birth the heart is beating at the time of birth even though the fetus does not breathe.

Recommendations for Studies on Perinatal Mortality and Morbidity

Because of the increasing realization that mortality and morbidity among fetuses and newborn infants should be amenable to reduction, many hospitals and community groups have undertaken investigations of conditions pertaining to the health of the mother, of conditions existing at the time of labor and delivery and of the state of the infant at birth in relation to the ultimate health of the child. To provide a guide for the conduct of such studies the American Medical Association through its Committee on Maternal and Child Care held a

*From *Recommendations on Definitions of Live Birth and Fetal Death,* PHS publication no. 39 (Washington, D.C.: National Office of Vital Statistics, October, 1950).

series of conferences in different parts of the United States at which this subject was discussed by leading pediatricians, obstetricians, pathologists, statisticians, public health workers and others. The deliberations and recommendations of these groups were summarized and published in a special report by the American Medical Association in 1959. The section dealing with definitions is especially valuable and is reproduced here in the hope that the recommendations will be generally adopted.

Guide for Study of Perinatal Mortality and Morbidity*

TERMS, DEFINITIONS, AND RATES

I. PERINATAL MORTALITY is defined as those deaths of fetuses and newborn infants occurring before, during, and soon after birth.
   A. The Perinatal Period
      1. *Perinatal Period I* as a minimum basis for achieving nationwide, as well as international, comparability will begin with deaths of fetuses weighing 1,001 Gm. (28 weeks gestation) and include deaths of infants occurring in the first seven days of life (hebdomadal period). See chart.
      2. *Perinatal Period II* for more inclusive study, and recommended whenever and wherever possible, will begin with deaths of fetuses weighing 501 Gm. or more (20 weeks gestation) and include deaths of infants occurring in the first 28 days of life (full neonatal period). See chart.

*American Medical Association, Council on Medical Services, Committee on Maternal and Child Care (Chicago, 1959).

THE PERINATAL PERIOD CHART

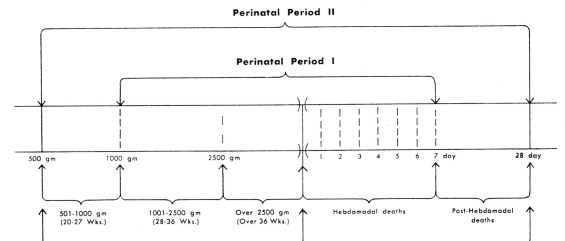

Perinatal Period I is the basic core on which perinatal mortality rates should be calculated in order to assure comparability of statistics. When Perinatal Period II or other combinations of end points are used in perinatal mortality studies, data should be collected and tabulated in such a manner that this basic core is always obtainable.

The commonly known "Intermediate" (20 completed weeks of gestation but less than 28) and "Late" (28 completed weeks of gestation and over) fetal deaths, known as Group II and Group III[1] respectively are both included in Perinatal Period II, whereas the "Late" only are included in Perinatal Period I. However, the weeks of gestation as shown in parentheses in the chart, and as indicated in the text, are not to be used as the basis of classification. Rather, the weight of the fetus is to be used in all possible cases and in minimum birth weight groupings similar to those recommended for grouping deaths of live born infants. The birth weight classification for fetal deaths as used in the text and as shown on the chart are consistent with the established definition by weight of an immature (premature) infant: *a liveborn infant with a birth weight of 2500 grams (5½ pounds) or less.*[2]

The chart further makes obvious the exact period of days involved in the hebdomadal, post-hebdomadal, and neonatal periods. The first 23 hours and 59 minutes after birth is under one day: an infant has lived 7 full days the moment it becomes 7 days of age; therefore, the correct designation of the hebdomadal period is "under 7 days". Similarly an infant has lived 4 full weeks or 28 full days the moment it becomes 28 days of age; therefore, the correct designation of the neonatal period is "under 28 days".

---

[1]*International Recommendations on Definitions of Live Birth and Fetal Death*, PHS Publication No. 39, National Office of Vital Statistics, October, 1950.

[2]*Manual of the International Statistical Classification of Diseases, Injuries, and Causes of Death,* Seventh (1955) Revision, World Health Organization, 1957. Volume I, p. 225.

Many hospitals and communities may wish to include other and additional combinations of endpoints in their study of perinatal mortality and morbidity (i.e., 501 Gm. to 7 days or 1,001 Gm. to 28 days). This is to be encouraged, but in order to have statistical results that have comparability on a nationwide (and international) basis it is essential that all study committees compile data and calculate rates based on Perinatal Period I and, whenever possible, the more inclusive Perinatal Period II also.

B. Fetal deaths (stillbirths) included in perinatal mortality and morbidity studies will be recorded by weight; in cases when the date of the last menstrual period is known, the estimated gestational age should be recorded for additional information but *not* as a basis for classification. These fetal deaths will be subclassified into *antepartum* (fetuses dying before delivery) and *intrapartum* (fetuses dying during delivery). These two subclassifications are further divided into the following minimum birth weight groupings:

1. *Perinatal Period I*
   a. 1,001 through 2,500 Gm.
   b. Over 2,500 Gm.
2. *Perinatal Period II*
   a. 501 through 1,000 Gm.
   b. 1,001 through 2,500 Gm.

Further subdivisions into 500 (or 250) Gm. birth weight groupings are desirable. (See table of equivalent weights below.)

C. Neonatal deaths (first 4 weeks—under 28 days)

1. *Hebdomadal (first week – under 7 days)* deaths are the only deaths of liveborn infants to be included in the study if Perinatal Period I is used. These are divided into the following minimum birth weight groupings:
   a. 501 through 1,000 Gm.
   b. 1,001 through 2,500 Gm.
   c. Over 2,500 Gm.
2. *Post-hebdomadal (second, third, and fourth week – 7 days and over to under 28 days)* deaths to be included in addition to hebdomadal deaths in studies using Perinatal Period II. This component of the neonatal deaths is similarly divided into minimum birth weight groupings as follows:
   a. 501 through 1,000 Gm.
   b. 1,001 through 2,500 Gm.
   c. Over 2,500 Gm.

In all instances birth weight will be recorded and used as a basis for classification. However, when the date of the last menstrual period is known, the estimated gestational age* should also be recorded for additional information but *not* as a basis for classification. As with the fetal death component of perinatal deaths, it is desirable to further subdivide all neonatal deaths of the above weight groupings at 500 (or 250) Gm. intervals:

Metric		English
500 Gm. or less	=	1 lb. 1 oz. or less
501 – 1,000 Gm.	=	1 lb. 2 oz. – 2 lb. 3 oz.
1,001 – 1,250 Gm.	=	2 lb. 4 oz. – 2 lb. 12 oz.
1,251 – 1,500 Gm.	=	2 lb. 13 oz. – 3 lb. 4 oz.
1,501 – 1,750 Gm.	=	3 lb. 5 oz. – 3 lb. 13 oz.
1,751 – 2,000 Gm.	=	3 lb. 14 oz. – 4 lb. 6 oz.
2,001 – 2,250 Gm.	=	4 lb. 7 oz. – 4 lb. 15 oz.
2,251 – 2,500 Gm.	=	5 lb. 0 oz. – 5 lb. 8 oz.
2,501 – 2,750 Gm.	=	5 lb. 9 oz. – 6 lb. 1 oz.
2,751 – 3,000 Gm.	=	6 lb. 2 oz. – 6 lb. 9 oz.
3,001 – 3,500 Gm.	=	6 lb. 10 oz. – 7 lb. 11 oz.
3,501 – 4,000 Gm.	=	7 lb. 12 oz. – 8 lb. 13 oz.
4,001 – 4,500 Gm.	=	8 lb. 14 oz. – 9 lb. 14 oz.
4,501 – 5,000 Gm.	=	9 lb. 15 oz. – 11 lb. 0 oz.
5,001 Gm. or more	=	11 lb. 1 oz. or more

D. The Perinatal Mortality Rate is to be calculated on the basis of total births in the perinatal period chosen for study. However, for those using Perinatal Period II, it is necessary to calculate and report both Perinatal Period I and Perinatal Period II rates. This is to insure that the Perinatal Period II rate of one study will not be confused and wrongly compared with the Perinatal Period I rate of another study, and in order that all studies reported in the United States may be compared on a common basis with each other, and in turn with the rates of other countries, many of which use Perinatal Period I in calculating their perinatal mortality rates.

1. *Perinatal Period I* rate is calculated by the following formula:

$$\frac{\text{Hebdomadal deaths and Fetal deaths 1,001 Gm. and over}}{\text{Live births and Fetal deaths 1,001 Gm. and over}} \times 1,000$$

*Based on the formula that the estimated gestational age is that period from the first day of the last menstrual period to the day of delivery.

2. *Perinatal Period II* rate is calculated by the following formula:

$$\frac{\text{Neonatal deaths and Fetal deaths 501 Gm. and over}}{\text{Live births and Fetal deaths 501 Gm. and over}} \times 1,000$$

3. *The proportion of deaths* of the various component parts and sub-parts of the perinatal period (such as hebdomadal and post-hebdomadal in the neonatal, and antepartum and intrapartum in the fetal) should be calculated on the basis of *total births* in question as used in calculating the particular total perinatal mortality rate that is under consideration.

   These component proportions are to be compiled in addition to — and the *neonatal proportion* is not to be considered a substitute for — the well-established *neonatal death rate* which traditionally and accurately has been calculated on the basis of live births only. The purpose for calculating component proportions of the total perinatal mortality rate for either Perinatal Period I or Perinatal Period II as outlined above is to provide more accurate statistical data to better delineate the problem of the perinatal period.

II. PERINATAL MORBIDITY is defined as a pathologic condition (or conditions) observed in the fetus or infant during the perinatal period. This condition may follow one of several courses:
A. It may terminate in death;
B. It may result in an obvious continuum requiring treatment, rehabilitation, or continuous care during the life span;
C. The infant may seem to recover from such a condition but in subsequent life show signs or symptoms probably due in full or in part to the perinatal morbidity; or
D. There may be complete recovery with no detectable sequelae.

   Effective perinatal study programs with resultant reduction in mortality will favorably influence the reduction of morbidity in the perinatal period as well. Currently, many hospitals do specifically include morbidity in their perinatal studies. The Committee recognizes that new committees may wish to become firmly established with an effective mortality study program before enlarging their scope to include morbidity. However, all committees studying perinatal mortality should look to this extension of their work at the earliest possible date.

REFERENCES

Bound, J. P., Butler, N. R., and Spector, W. E.: Classification and causes of perinatal mortality, Br. Med. J. 2: 1191, 1956.

Butler, N. R., and Bonham, D. G.: *Perinatal Mortality* (Edinburgh: E. & S. Livingstone, Ltd., 1960).

Clifford, S. H.: Diseases of the newborn, N. Engl. J. Med. 232:42, 1945.

Dickinson, F. G., and Welker, E. L.: Infant deaths and stillbirths in leading nations, J.A.M.A. 142:1014, 1950.

Engle, E. T. (ed.): *Pregnancy Wastage* (Springfield, Ill.: Charles C Thomas, 1953).

La Veck, G. D.: in *Sudden Infant Death Syndrome: Selected Annotated Bibliography, 1960–1971* (Washington, D. C.: U. S. Department of Health, Education and Welfare), publication no. (NIH) 73-237, 1972.

MacGregor, A. R.: *Pathology of Infancy and Childhood* (Edinburgh: E. & S. Livingstone, Ltd., 1960).

Mitchell, J. R., Hogg, G., DePape, A. J., Briggs, E. J. N., and Medovy, H.: Analysis of causes of perinatal death, Can. Med. Assoc. J. 80:796, 1959.

Morison, J. E.: *Fetal and Neonatal Pathology* (3d ed.; London: Butterworth & Co., Ltd., 1970).

Niswander, K. R., and Gordon, M.: *Collaborative Study of the National Institute of Neurological Diseases and Stroke: The Women and Their Pregnancies* (Philadelphia: W. B. Saunders Co., 1972).

Potter, E. L.: Fetal and neonatal deaths: Statistical analysis of 2,000 autopsies, J.A.M.A. 115:996, 1940.

Potter, E. L.: Abnormalities of intrauterine environment associated with 2,000 fetal and neonatal deaths, Ill. Med. J. 61:189, 1942.

Potter, E. L.: Trend of changes in causes of perinatal mortality, J.A.M.A. 158:1471, 1954.

Potter, E. L.: Planning perinatal mortality studies, Obstet. Gynecol. 13:243, 1959.

Potter, E. L., and Adair, F. L.: *Fetal and Neonatal Death* (2d ed.; Chicago: University of Chicago Press, 1949).

Potter, E. L., and Davis, M. E.: Perinatal mortality, The Chicago Lying-in Hospital, 1931–1966, Am. J. Obstet. Gynecol. 105:335, 1969.

Potter, E. L., and Jack, W.: Responsibility of the physician in perinatal mortality, Surg. Clin. North Am. 33: 141, 1953.

Shapiro, S., Schlesinger, E. J., and Nesbitt, R. E. L.: *Infant, Perinatal, Maternal and Childhood Mortality in the United States* (Cambridge, Mass.: Harvard University Press, 1968).

Silverman, W. E. (ed.): *Dunham's Premature Infants* (3d ed.; New York: Paul B. Hoeber, Inc., 1961).

Smith, C. A.: *The Physiology of the Newborn Infant* (3d ed.; Springfield, Ill.: Charles C Thomas, 1959).

Stowens, D.: *Pediatric Pathology* (2d ed.; Baltimore: Williams & Wilkins Co., 1966).

Wallace, H. M., Gold, E. M., Baumgartner, L., and Losty, M. A.: Trends in maternal and perinatal mortality in New York City, J.A.M.A. 155:716, 1954.

Wegman, M. E.: Annual summary of vital statistics—1969, Pediatrics 47:461, 1969.

6

Postmortem Examination

General Requirements

THE POSTMORTEM EXAMINATION of the fetus and newborn does not differ appreciably from that of the child and adult. Anyone familiar with adult pathology can easily make an examination of the newborn that technically is entirely satisfactory. Interpretation of the changes disclosed by the examination, however, requires interest and experience in the clinical fields of obstetrics and pediatrics.

The infant at best has had only a short life—9 months in the uterus and a few days or weeks of extrauterine existence. During this interval few pathologic changes have had time to develop and none are of the degenerative variety that make up a large share of the lesions found in older age groups. The findings at autopsy are much less spectacular than those in older individuals and consequently are frequently overlooked. It is only when the pathologist is aware of the fundamental obstetric and pediatric problems that he can observe adequately and correlate accurately the observations he makes at autopsy with clinical states that existed before death.

A complete record of every postmortem examination should become part of the permanent files of the institution in which death occurred. It should include a complete history of the mother's general health, previous pregnancies and health during the current pregnancy; a complete description of labor and delivery; and immediate and subsequent postnatal course of the infant. This should be available to the pathologist at autopsy. The body of the infant should be thoroughly examined and completely described, and the placenta should be included in this examination. Representative tissues should be examined microscopically and appropriate bacteriologic, serologic or chemical studies made as indicated. When the investigations are completed, the data should be assembled and a final summary made that takes into account the maternal and infant clinical history as well as the laboratory investigations. Only after this final correlation and evaluation of all the material collected should the autopsy be considered complete. With such an investigation it is almost always possible to give a probable cause of death.

A postmortem examination is made to obtain as much information as possible both for immediate use in determining the causes of the specific death and for wider use in studying the causes of fetal and infant deaths in general. Any procedure that will give information is of value. Blood cultures, which are frequently desirable, can be made during the examination by searing the surface of the heart and withdrawing blood by pipet. Blood can also be obtained by inserting a needle into the posterior fontanel and directing it posteriorly, keeping it close to the skull. It will enter the confluence of sinuses in the posterior part of the head and a large amount of blood can be withdrawn easily. This method may be used for obtaining blood for chemical or serologic study or in the event that permission for autopsy is refused.

Technic

WEIGHTS AND MEASUREMENTS

Estimation of weight of the body or the organs varies so greatly among examiners that the figures obtained are useless and should never be allowed. All organs should be freed of extraneous tissues and weighed on an accurate scale. (See Chapter 2 for normal organ weights.)

The postmortem examination begins with weighing the body and measuring both the standing (crown-heel) and sitting (crown-rump) height. The latter is approximately two thirds of the former. If malformations cause an abnormal shortening or lengthening of the sitting height, as in anencephalus or hydrocephalus, the length that the individual could have been expected to attain in the absence of such an anomaly may be calculated by multiplying by 3 the figure obtained by subtracting sitting height from standing height. In calculating total expected length in the presence of abnormalities of the legs, the sitting height may be considered two thirds of the total length.

External Examination

The external surface of the body is carefully inspected for evidence of maceration, cyanosis, injury and skin lesions. The orifices are examined for patency, exudations or other abnormalities. The state of the umbilicus is investigated. All abnormalities of development that are visible on external examination are described.

MACERATION — When death occurs before delivery, degenerative changes begin immediately and all tissues lose tone and soften. If membranes are intact and labor has not started, the amniotic cavity contains no bacteria, and tissue changes are nonputrefactive. Early changes are most pronounced in the skin, and within a few hours oblique pressure on the skin will cause separation of the epidermis from the dermis—a condition known as skin-slipping. Fluid may accumulate beneath the epidermis and produce large bullae (see Fig. 27–1). Bullae usually rupture during delivery and this, or the simple manipulation of the body incident to delivery, is responsible for separation of large areas of skin from the body surface. Hemolysis causes reddish discoloration, and muscles, connective tissue

Fig. 6–1.—Normal newborn skull. **A,** superior surface. **B,** anterior surface. **C,** lateral surface.

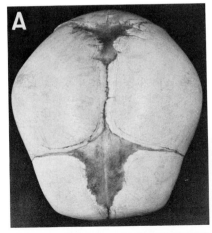
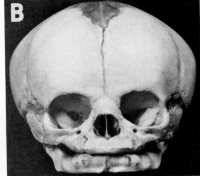
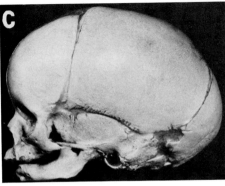

and viscera become a fairly uniform red-purple color. Hemolyzed blood and fluid diffuse into the pleural and peritoneal cavities.

If the fetus is retained for more than a week or 10 days after death, the color gradually begins to fade and changes to a light olive-brown. The younger the fetus, the more rapid the change because of the fewer red cells per milliliter of blood.

Within a few days of death the brain becomes semiliquid. The abdominal viscera degenerate more rapidly than those in the chest. The intestinal wall gradually disintegrates, freeing meconium into the abdominal cavity. The total body weight and the weight of individual organs progressively decrease after death, a fact that must be taken into account in attempts to determine whether or not they are of normal size.

Rigor mortis is almost never observed in a fetus at delivery regardless of when death occurs. Occasionally it has been reported as responsible for difficulty in delivery but we have been unable to find anyone who has observed it during or after delivery of a stillborn fetus.

HEAD. — The general appearance of the face is examined for possible resemblance to any of the conditions that have facial characteristics such as mongolism, renal agenesis and so on. The position and shape of the eyes and eyeballs, the presence of conjunctival hemorrhage, the appearance of the nose and its patency, the character of the buccal cavity, the state of the tongue, gums and palate and the size, shape and general appearance of the ears are all noted. The shape and symmetry of the bones of the face and skull may give evidence of abnormal forces that were active during labor or delivery. The tissues beneath the scalp, the skull bones, the sutures and fontanels are all inspected before the skull is opened. The bones, fontanels and sutures of the normal newborn skull are shown in Figure 6–1.

The method of opening the head is one of the principal differences between the technic of autopsy performed on the newborn and that on older individuals. If the skull of the newborn is removed in the manner accepted for adults, no important information can be obtained. In the method of choice a large window is cut in each parietal bone in such a way that the tentorium cerebelli and falx cerebri remain intact. One blade of a pair of scissors is inserted in the most inferior portion of the suture between the frontal and the parietal bones, and an incision made through dura and skull is carried up between the bones to the point marking the beginning of the anterior fontanel. The line of incision then leaves the suture and continues through the parietal bone near the edge of its superior and posterior margins. The incision is made about ¼ in. from the edge, leaving untouched the superior sagittal suture, the lambdoidal suture and the anterior and posterior fontanels. As the incision reaches the inferior margin of the parietal bone, it is directed slightly anteriorly through the lower edge of the parietal bone to avoid entering the cerebral sinuses underlying its posterior inferior angle.

Fig. 6–2.—Surface of the brain. **A,** normal infant delivered at term through the vagina. Skull opened by the Beneke technic. Note the close approximation of brain to skull and absence of meningeal fluid. **B,** premature infant weighing 2,000 gm with meningeal fluid normal for infant of this size.

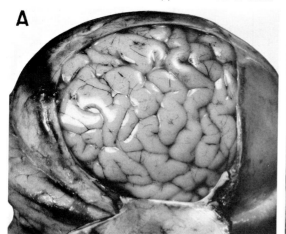
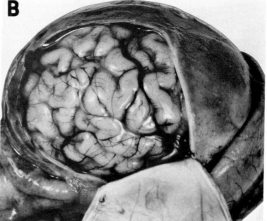

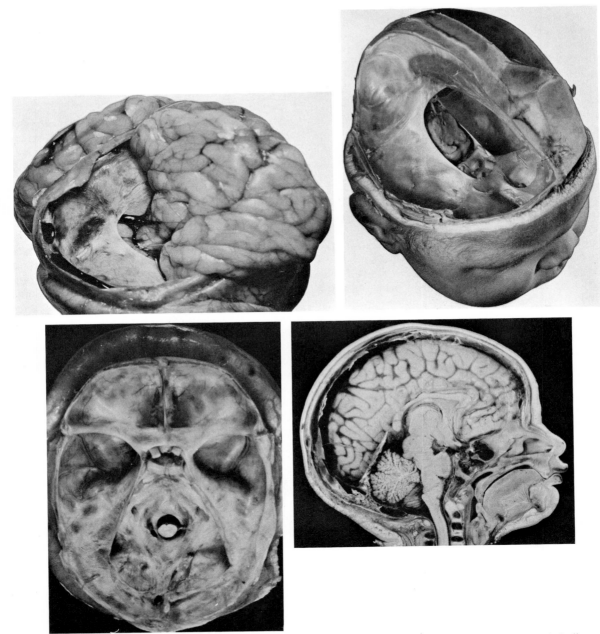

Fig. 6–3 (top left). — Great internal cerebral vein (vein of Galen). The occipital lobe is drawn forward so that the vein may be seen entering the straight sinus. Right lateral sinus is also visible at the posterior edge of the tentorium cerebelli.

Fig. 6–4 (top right). — Interior of head showing falx cerebri and tentorium cerebelli after cerebral hemispheres have been removed.

Fig. 6–5 (bottom left). — Base of the normal skull.

Fig. 6–6 (bottom right). — Sagittal section through the head of a normal, slightly premature newborn infant. Falx cerebri has been removed. Cerebral hemisphere has shrunk and drawn away from the skull as a result of fixation.

Reflexion of the parietal bone and dura permits examination of the brain surface. In the normal newborn the convolutions are well developed, and in an infant delivered at term through the vagina the quantity of meningeal fluid is less and the brain fits the skull more snugly than at any other time of life (Fig. 6–2,A). In a premature infant the convolutions are smaller and less completely developed and meningeal fluid is more copious than at term (Fig. 6–2,B). In normal full-term infants delivered through the vagina no meningeal fluid can be obtained at autopsy. In premature infants the amount recoverable depends on the length of gestation but averages 10–15 ml.

After the incision has been completed, the head is held in the palm of the left hand with the neck between the first and second finger. This permits perfect control of the head, which can be handled at will. After the surface of the brain is inspected for the character of the blood vessels, excessive fluid, hemorrhage or other abnormalities, the occipital lobe of the cerebral hemisphere is gently drawn forward, with care taken not to tear the underlying blood vessels, and the falx, tentorium and vein of Galen are examined (Fig. 6–3).

After one side has been inspected, the parietal bone is replaced to protect the brain while the opposite side is being opened in the same manner. After the outer surface of the brain and supporting structures has been inspected, the intact brain may be removed by cutting through the falx and tentorium, or the cerebral hemispheres and cerebellum may be removed separately, leaving the falx and tentorium intact (Fig. 6–4).

Unless there is specific reason for doing otherwise, the brain is preferably removed as a whole and fixed before further examination is undertaken. Its softness makes sectioning difficult in the fresh state, and better examination is ordinarily possible following fixation. Removal of the brain is most easily accomplished by placing the body in a supine position and cutting through the narrow strip consisting of superior saggital sinus and edges of the parietal bones and attached falx cerebri. The brain can then be drawn backward as the cranial nerves and basilar arteries are severed, and the cerebellum is freed by cutting the tentorium cerebelli where it is attached to the skull. The spinal cord is severed as low as possible in the spine. The removal of the brain can be expedited by removing the frontal bones after cutting them transversely, as in an adult autopsy, but this makes reconstruction of the head more difficult. A better method is to open the suture between the frontal bones. This does not interfere at all with reconstruction and very little with the accessibility of the forebrain.

The base of the skull is examined for possible defects, changes in relative size of the fossae, space between the sella turcica and foramen magnum and abnormal prominences and depressions (Fig. 6–5).

If final disposition of the body permits and it is possible to inject the vessels and fix the head, sectioning in a sagittal direction after detachment from the body may give valuable information. Hemorrhage beneath the tentorium is often shown best by this method (see Fig. 8–9). A sagittal section of a normal head is illustrated in Figure 6–6.

Spinal Cord

The spinal canal can be opened from the exterior by linear incisions through the laminae of both right and left sides of the vertebrae. The central strip containing the spines is removed and the extradural space examined (Fig. 6–7). The cord is so fragile that it gives way wherever grasped by forceps and, unless removed intact within the dura, is usually unsatisfactory for microscopic examination. The spine can also be opened from the inside of the body with short, narrow-bladed, stout scissors used to sever the pedicles of the vertebrae. After incising two or more intervertebral disks one blade is inserted into the canal and the other lateral to the pedicle. The entire cord and its coverings should be removed intact.

Thorax

The body cavities are opened by a midline incision that begins above the pubis and extends to the upper part of the thorax. From there it is directed outward toward each shoulder. The skin is reflected until adequate exposure is obtained. The abdominal viscera are inspected in situ before the chest is opened, but detailed examination is left until later. The diaphragms are palpated and the chest percussed. If the diaphragms are depressed or the chest hyper-resonant, the body should be placed under water and an opening made into each thoracic cavity. If a graduate is filled with water and inverted so that the open lower end covers the point of incision, any air escaping from the chest will rise in the graduate and the amount can be measured.

The chest plate is removed by cutting through the ribs, the line of incision being carried upward slightly medially to end at the costoclavicular junction. The organs are first examined in situ (Fig. 6–

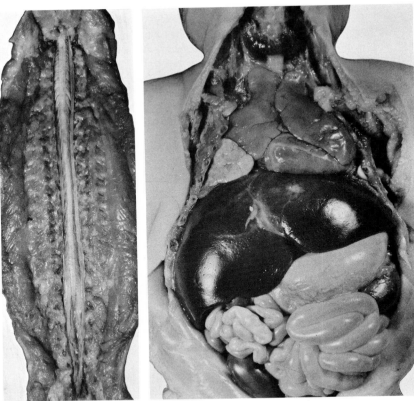

Fig. 6–7 (left).—Normal spinal cord of mature fetus exposed by severing the vertebral laminae.

Fig. 6–8 (right).—Surface view of normal viscera in chest and abdomen of a mature infant who could not be resuscitated because of anoxia from prolapsed cord. Thymus is made up of two lobes each composed of a broad basal portion lying over the heart and a lingual portion extending into the neck. Lungs are invisible except for a portion of the right lower lobe. Liver extends across the entire upper abdomen, and right lobe extends 2–3 cm below the costal margin. Stomach and small intestine were distended by air during attempts at resuscitation.

8). Then the thymus is removed by sharp dissection in order to avoid injuring the innominate vein, which runs through it or is in close juxtaposition to its posterior surface. The pericardium is then removed as completely as possible. The closer it is severed to its line of attachment, the more easily can the heart and great vessels be investigated. The next step is to identify the chambers of the heart and great vessels going to the head and upper extremities (Fig. 6–9). It is much easier to identify the vessels and the areas they supply at this time than after the heart is removed from the body. This is one of the principal reasons why dissection in situ is preferable to dissection of viscera removed in a single mass. If the great vessels are normal and enter the normal chambers of the heart, confusing compound major abnormalities are rarely present within the heart. Almost the only lesions that will

ever be found in such circumstances are interventricular septal defects or a persistent atrioventricular foramen.

At this point all of the viscera may be removed by the Rokitansky technic in a single block or the organs may be dissected in situ. Both methods begin with isolation and double ligation of the right carotid, subclavian and iliac arteries. Distally and proximally applied ties help identification and allow for greater ease of embalming. In the Rokitansky technic the tongue is then separated by cutting its attachments close to the mandible from the midline to the angle of the jaw. The pharynx is separated from the roof of the mouth by sharp dissection. The anterior portion of the tongue can then be displaced below the jaw. From this point all of the viscera can easily be removed from above downward. Only the lower end of the vagina, urethra and rec-

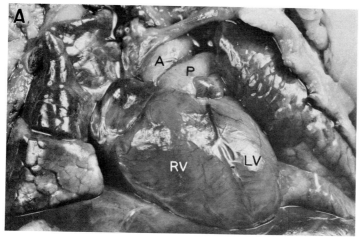

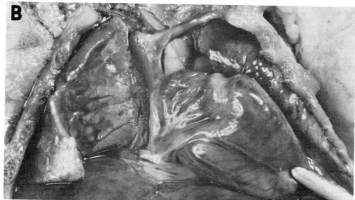

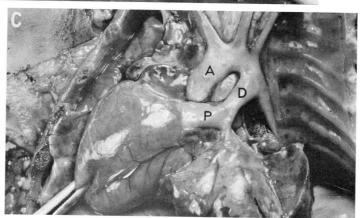

Fig. 6–9.—Heart of mature newborn infant. **A,** normal position showing right ventricle (RV) occupying most of the anterior surface, and left ventricle (LV) forming left margin. Small left auricular appendage is visible between left ventricle and pulmonary artery (P). Larger right auricular appendage is in angle between right ventricle and aorta (A). **B,** heart drawn to left to expose right atrium, inferior and superior venae cavae and innominate vein. **C,** heart drawn to right to expose great vessels: aortic arch (A), common pulmonary artery (P), ductus arteriosus (D). The three vessels arising from the arch of the aorta are the innominate, common carotid and left subclavian arteries. Note relation of origin of subclavian artery to insertion of ductus arteriosus into the aorta.

tum need be cut across. This method allows careful dissection of all organs and vessels from both anterior and posterior approaches and is especially valuable in anomalies of the esophagus, pulmonary veins, aorta and ureters. Dissection of the individual organs can be carried out in the same manner whether they are still in the body or have been removed en bloc.

The heart is removed by successively severing the inferior vena cava, pulmonary veins, superior vena cava, pulmonary artery and aorta. The interior is opened for inspection by two incisions that extend through atrial and ventricular walls on each side of the heart, leaving the septa intact. The heart is placed with the posterior surface uppermost and the atria toward the prosector. The incision is begun where the superior vena cava enters the heart, is carried downward through the atrial wall and inferior vena cava, through the tricuspid valve, along the right side of the ventricular septum (to the left side as the heart is held in the position in which it is being opened), around the apex, up the anterior portion of the right ventricular wall and ended at the cut end of the pulmonary artery. The same procedure is repeated on the left side of the heart. The incision is begun at the openings of the pulmonary veins, carried down through the mitral valve, along the left side of the ventricular septum and out at the aorta. This method of opening the heart permits adequate inspection of the valves,

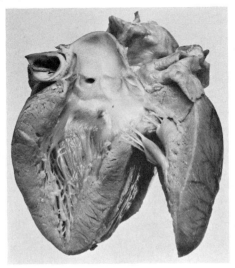

Fig. 6–10.—Heart of normal newborn infant showing cusps of aortic valve and characteristic muscle pattern of left ventricle. Origin of right coronary artery is seen behind one aortic cusp; the other is immediately to the left of the line of incision.

chambers and foramen ovale. The chordae tendineae and pectinate muscles are smaller and more evenly arranged on the left side of the septum than on the right (Fig. 6–10). This difference facilitates identification of the chambers when the heart is malformed.

The trachea is opened next, either in situ or after removal from the body. Better examination of the pharynx, larynx and trachea is possible if the tongue, trachea and lungs are removed as a unit than if they still remain in the body. This is easily accomplished by beginning removal of the tongue in the space immediately behind the anterior portion of the lower jaw and carrying the incision to both right and left around to the back of the pharynx. The esophagus can be removed with the trachea or may be temporarily left behind and removed later with the stomach and intestines.

ABDOMEN

The liver is inspected next. Before it is separated, however, the patency of the bile ducts should be established. An incision is made in the duodenum, and the papilla of Vater is exposed. Gentle pressure on the gallbladder will expel bile through the papilla. Because of the small size of the ducts this is an easier method of establishing patency than is dissecting and probing them, although experience with the latter procedures is valuable because of the occasional need for positive identification of the site of abnormalities in the extrahepatic ducts.

The spleen is removed next, and after the normal relationships of the different portions of the gastrointestinal tract have been established, the entire tract may be removed. The amount and character of the material in all portions should be recorded and the walls of the esophagus, stomach and intestines examined for ulceration, hemorrhage or other abnormalities. At birth the large bowel is normally distended to a diameter of 1.5–2 cm by meconium since evacuation does not ordinarily occur during intrauterine life in the absence of anoxia or presentation by breech. The amount of meconium averages 60 ml. The sigmoid colon is more redundant than in older individuals. Partial evacuation of the large bowel may produce irregularly distributed areas of constriction that may be mistaken for areas of stenosis. The pancreas should be dissected free from the duodenum and examined.

After the gastrointestinal tract is removed, the kidneys and adrenal glands are in full view. The ureters should be traced to their insertion into the bladder. The kidney and adrenal gland on the same side are most conveniently removed together by grasping the pelvis of the kidney. This avoids crushing the substance of either structure.

GENITAL ORGANS

The internal genital organs are inspected next. Female sex organs can be removed as a unit by cutting through the lower portion of the vagina. In the male the seminal vesicles lie on the posterior surface of the lower part of the bladder and the prostate encircles the urethra immediately below the bladder. All are easily removed.

EXTREMITIES

The extremities are carefully inspected for length, curvature, abnormal shape, protuberances, fractures and so on. The muscles are examined for hemorrhage, wasting or excessive fluid. The knee joints are severed and the lower ends of the femurs freed of soft tissue. A longitudinal section through the end of the bone can be made by cutting through the cartilage into the bone with an instrument designed to cut ribs. This will expose the junction of the cartilage and the metaphysis of the bone and will also show whether a center of ossification is present.

PLACENTA

Examination of the placenta should include weight, measurements, inspection of fetal and maternal surfaces and substance and inspection of membranes, cord and cord vessels. The length of the umbilical cord should be measured and the vessels examined for number, varicosities and rupture. The membranes should be inspected carefully, especially in case of multiple pregnancy. Microscopic sections should include fetal and maternal surfaces of the placenta, the intervillous space, decidua, peripheral membranes and umbilical cord.

TISSUES FOR MICROSCOPIC EXAMINATION

Ideally, blocks of tissue for microscopic examination are taken from all organs. Surprising changes may be found in many organs that appear normal on gross examination, and if sections are taken only from those that appear abnormal, many important and interesting lesions may be overlooked. The number of sections will, however, vary to some extent with the state of preservation of the body and with the apparent cause of death.

Sections should invariably be taken from both lungs regardless of the degree of postmortem change. The lungs retain their affinity for stains longer than most other tissues and much may be learned in spite of changes caused by advanced maceration. Other organs in the body are useless for microscopic study if maceration exists, although if syphilis is suspected, Levaditi staining for spirochetes may still be possible.

If the organs are not macerated, at least the lungs, heart, liver, kidneys, thymus and brain should be examined microscopically. Organs of internal secretion frequently show interesting changes. Petechial hemorrhages, zones of degeneration or other abnormalities are occasionally found only in localized parts of the brain, and consequently multiple sections of brain and spinal cord may be of value. Sections from the region of the lateral ventricles and the brain stem ordinarily have more pathologic interest, provided gross lesions are not present in other areas, than those from other parts of the brain. Many pathologic lesions are inevitably overlooked, however, by such cursory examination, and ideal laboratory facilities would permit serial sectioning of the entire brain.

The microscopic appearances of normal organs of newborn infants are shown in the chapters devoted

Fig. 6–11.—Normal adipose tissue from region of the adrenal gland of mature infant dying of congenital heart disease at age 3 weeks. Most cells are strongly acidophilic and contain only small amounts of fat.

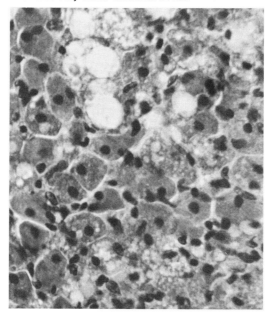

to individual organs. The degree of differentiation of adipose tissue in the fetus and young infant varies in different parts of the body. In some areas fat cells may be large and ovoid or polyhedral with small compact central nuclei. The cytoplasm may be strongly acidophilic and may contain few or no fat droplets (Fig. 6–11). In other areas the cells may consist entirely of fat and may be identical to normal adult fat cells.

FIXATIVES

Ten percent formalin when carefully buffered makes a good general fixative but when unbuffered causes much precipitation of "formalin pigment," especially in areas with many red cells. Even when buffered it causes tissue shrinkage unless special precautions are taken during infiltration with paraffin; it also may obscure fine cellular details such as some inclusion bodies. A particular advantage is good penetration of large tissue masses, a feature possessed by almost no other fixative. In definition of cellular detail and preservation of form both Zenker's and Bouin's fixatives are superior, though both require care in trimming and washing tissues. Formalin can be used for gross fat preservation but is unsatisfactory for many lipids unless calcium-cobalt mixtures are added. For preservation of most polysaccharides Rossman's fluid (absolute alcohol saturated with picric acid 90%, formalin 10%) is excellent. In cases in which special fixation and staining might be advantageous but the exact method is in doubt, quick freezing of a group of small blocks on a cryostat head with deep freeze storage in small sealed bottles has been found a helpful procedure. When removed, the tissues can be handled as if never frozen, and fixed and stained as desired.

The postmortem examination may be considered complete when (1) gross examination of the body has been finalized; (2) the microscopic findings and results of bacteriologic, serologic and chemical studies have been added to the gross findings; (3) all of these have been correlated with the history of the mother during pregnancy and confinement and of the infant during its brief span of life; and (4) the conclusions have been recorded in a suitable manner.

REFERENCES

Adair, F. L., and Potter, E. L.: Evidence of intrauterine death of the fetus, Am. J. Med Jurisprudence 2:252 1939.

Arey, J. B.: Pathologic findings in the neonatal period, J. Pediatr. 34:44, 1949.

Baar, H. S.: Postmortem examination of the newborn infant, Br. Med. Bull. 4:178, 1946.

Epstein, I. M.: Causes of death and incidence of disease in children: Review of 1,000 consecutive necropsies, Am. J. Dis. Child. 41:1363, 1931.

Lev, M.: Autopsy Diagnosis of Congenitally Malformed Hearts (Springfield, Ill.: Charles C Thomas, 1953).

Lillie, R. D.: Histopathologic Technique and Histochemistry (3d ed.; New York: McGraw-Hill Book Co., 1967).

MacGregor, A.: The pathology of stillbirth and neonatal death, Br. Med. Bull. 4:174, 1946.

Morison, J. E.: Foetal and Neonatal Pathology (3d ed.; London: Butterworth & Co., Ltd., 1970).

Potter, E. L.: Postmortem examination of stillborn and newly born infants, Arch. Pathol. 25:607, 1938.

Potter, E. L.: Importance of the postmortem examination of the fetus and newly born infant, Am. J. Clin. Pathol. 13:133, 1943.

Potter, E. L.: The pathologist's contribution to clinical interpretation of disorders of the newborn, Am. J. Clin. Pathol. 17:524, 1947.

Potter, E. L., and Adair, F. L.: Fetal and Neonatal Death (2d ed.; Chicago: University of Chicago Press, 1949).

Schaffer, A. J.: Diseases of the Newborn (2d ed.; Philadelphia: W. B. Saunders Co., 1965).

Stowens, D.: Pediatric Pathology (2d ed.; Baltimore: Williams & Wilkins Co., 1965).

7

Anoxia

Anoxia is the term used to indicate a reduction below physiologic levels of the amount of oxygen present in body tissues. It is customary to divide the causes of anoxia into four groups according to the point within the system of oxygen intake and utilization at which interference with oxygenation occurs. In *anoxic anoxia* interference is with the source of oxygen: before birth this may be caused by failure of fetal blood in the placenta to be oxygenated, as in abruptio placentae, or by inability of oxygenated blood in the placenta to pass through the umbilical cord to the fetus, as in cord prolapse; afterbirth abnormalities or immaturity of the lungs may prevent delivery of an adequate amount of oxygen to the blood. In *anemic anoxia* the source of oxygen is adequate but the amount of hemoglobin or number of erythrocytes is insufficient to transport oxygen to the tissues: before birth this may result from hemolysis of fetal cells caused by maternal isoimmunization or may follow loss of blood caused by rupture of fetal blood vessels in the cord or placenta; after birth it may be associated with anemia or hemorrhage from any cause. In *stagnant anoxia* the source of oxygen and amount of hemoglobin are sufficient but blood does not move through the vessels fast enough to permit normal transfer of oxygen to the tissues; generalized stagnation is caused by heart failure either before or after birth, whereas localized stagnation is caused by regional interference with circulation resulting from pressure on blood vessels by constriction of a part by the umbilical cord or by contraction of the cervix around a partially delivered part of the body. Stagnant anoxia is seldom a primary form of anoxia in the fetus although it may complicate either anoxic or anemic anoxia. *Histotoxic anoxia* results from a disturbance in cells that makes utilization

of oxygen impossible even though it is delivered in normal amounts: this is rare except through direct poisoning by various chemical substances; the barbiturates so commonly used in obstetrics are among the drugs stated to be capable of producing such a disturbance.

Before birth the fetus is dependent for its oxygen supply on the placenta and umbilical cord, and any interference with the function of either will be followed by anoxia. After birth, when the cord is cut, the infant is dependent on the substitution of an organ—the lungs—whose immediate function must be completely adequate if anoxia is to be prevented. Because of the multiplicity of factors that may interfere with delivery of oxygen to the fetus before birth, or with normal function of the lungs after birth, anoxia is responsible for greater loss of life in the fetal and neonatal period than is any other known agent.

Intrauterine Anoxia

The conditions that can cause anoxia before birth are (1) those that interfere with oxygenation of the fetal blood in the placenta because *(a)* the villi are separated from oxygenated maternal blood by a stagnant layer of blood, as in abruptio placentae and some cases of placenta previa, *(b)* the maternal blood lacks oxygen, as during general anesthesia when oxygen intake is reduced, *(c)* maternal blood does not circulate normally in the placenta, as in maternal shock from blood loss, rupture of the uterus or hypotension resulting from spinal anesthesia, *(d)* a large portion of the placenta is functionally inactive due to intervillous thrombosis and infarction, as in some cases of hypertension and chronic renal disease; (2) those that interrupt the course of circulation between the fetus and the placenta, as with prolapse, knots, entanglements or excessive twisting or stretching of the umbilical cord; and (3) those responsible for loss of fetal blood *(a)* into the maternal circulation, as in the fetal-maternal transfusion syndrome, *(b)* to a twin in certain cases of vascular anastomoses in the placenta or *(c)* to the outside, as in cases of a torn or ruptured vasa previa.

ABRUPTIO PLACENTAE (PREMATURE PLACENTAL SEPARATION). — At any time during the last trimester, especially in women with preeclamptic toxemia, part or all of the placenta may become detached from the uterine wall (see Fig. 3–17). If the area is small, the remaining portion of the placenta may be sufficient to oxygenate the fetal blood and the fetus may suffer no ill effects. If a large part is separated, death occurs quickly. If the separation is marginal, blood escapes into the uterus and is expelled through the cervix. If the separation does not extend to the placental margin, blood may accumulate behind the placenta over a gradually increasing surface area. Pressure on placental villi may cause compression infarcts that further reduce the space in the placenta in which fetal blood may come in contact with oxygenated maternal blood. Separation takes place in the decidual layer and the blood comes from the maternal sinuses. There is no evidence that the integrity of the fetal vessels is destroyed or that the bleeding is of fetal origin. Massive separation is often accompanied by hypofibrinogenemia, caused by precipitation of fibrin within the retroplacental clot or by release of thromboplastic and thrombolytic agents into the general circulation.

PLACENTA PREVIA. — The anoxia that may occur with placenta previa is a result of premature separation of the placenta, as it is in abruptio placentae. Attachment of the placenta over part or all of the internal cervical os does no harm to the fetus until the cervix begins to undergo changes incident to labor and delivery. If cervical effacement or retraction causes separation of the placenta, oxygenated maternal blood cannot enter the placenta. Separation occurs in the decidual layer, and blood escapes from the maternal sinuses. The fetal circulation remains intact unless disrupted by actual laceration of the placenta during delivery.

Analgesics and anesthetics. — The part played in the production of fetal anoxia by analgesics and anesthetics when administered to the mother during labor and delivery has been the subject of much investigation, but in most reports dealing with human material it is impossible to separate the effect of medication from other factors of labor and delivery. There seems to be no evidence that any drug administered in therapeutic doses interferes directly with intrauterine circulation or produces intrauterine death. Experiments on animals show that various drugs commonly used for analgesia inhibit intrauterine respiration but do not interfere with circulation, and when such animals are exposed to normal extrauterine conditions, respiration is ordinarily established immediately. The oxygen saturation of fetal blood is abnormally low only after administration of inhalation anesthetics that require pronounced reduction in the oxygen content of the maternal blood.

OBSTRUCTION TO CIRCULATION THROUGH THE UMBILICAL CORD. — At times the cord may be looped several times around the neck or an extremity or it may have a true knot without obstructing the circulation. At other times any of these conditions may cause tension on the cord and reduce the caliber of the vessels to a degree incompatible with the passage of blood. Prolapse of the cord with compression between the head of the fetus and the maternal pelvis will effectively cut off circulation almost immediately.

When heart tones disappear and fetal circulation ceases during labor or delivery without apparent reason, the cause is usually to be found in some form of compression of the umbilical cord. A loop of cord may be prolapsed into the lower pelvis and may be compressed between the presenting part and the birth canal. This is often not recognized, especially if membranes are unruptured, but should be considered whenever fetal distress is evident. It is known as occult cord prolapse. After the membranes have ruptured, contractions of the uterus may compress the cord against the body of the fetus to a degree incompatible with normal circulation. Difficulty in delivering the shoulders may lead to anoxia from prolonged compression of the cord between the abdomen of the fetus and the uterine wall. When delivery of the after-coming head is delayed, anoxia may be caused by compression of the cord between the infant's head and the maternal pelvis or by detachment of the placenta following delivery of the body of the infant.

OTHER CAUSES. — Severe compression of the chest during delivery or contraction of the cervix around the neck in breech delivery may interfere with return of venous blood from the head and may cause extreme congestion of the brain, with distention and sometimes rupture of small vessels. This may be responsible for severe cyanosis limited to the head that persists for several days. It is designated traumatic cyanosis and in a dead infant could be confused with postnatal strangulation.

The most common maternal state associated with fatal anoxia is an abnormally long labor. This is usually a result of uterine inertia or cephalopelvic disproportion. A first stage of labor of over 30 hours or a second stage of over 1½ hours, especially when associated with the use of sedatives (Lund), are both conducive to anoxia.

SYMPTOMS

The principal symptom of intrauterine anoxia is an irregularity or slowing of fetal heart rate that is unrelated to uterine contractions. Even in normal infants the heart rate is often slow during a contraction but returns to normal between contractions. With anoxia a temporary increase may precede the slowing or irregularity and may be associated with a brief period of increased fetal activity. Intestinal peristalsis is increased and the anal sphincter is relaxed when anoxia is severe. Consequently, when the head is the presenting part, the presence of meconium in the amniotic fluid is a grave sign. In breech presentation relaxation of the anal sphincter is common and meconium has no pathologic significance.

When an infant has been severely anoxic before birth but is born with the heart still beating, the skin is pale and muscle tone poor (asphyxia pallida). The skin and fingernails may be yellow because of meconium in the amniotic fluid. Respiration often cannot be established and circulation soon stops. When anoxia has been less severe, the tone and color may be moderately good and the infant may breathe spontaneously or after a short period of resuscitation (asphyxia livida).

Neonatal Anoxia

After birth other causes of anoxia come into play. Even though the circulation seems normal and the muscle tone good, and there is no evidence of intrauterine anoxia, the infant may not begin to breathe. Conditions responsible for failure to breathe after birth, in addition to those causing intrauterine anoxia, include intracranial hemorrhage with pressure on the vital centers in the brain stem; diminished space for pulmonary expansion, as with diaphragmatic hernia or pleural effusion; lack of space for oxygen in the alveoli because the lumens are filled with solid material, such as leukocytes in intrauterine pneumonia or squamous epithelial cells and other debris following excessive intrauterine respiration; tumors compressing the trachea or obstructing the larynx; hypoplasia or other malformations of the lungs; and depression of the respiratory center by excessive use of analgesic or anesthetic drugs during labor. Immaturity of the respiratory center is sometimes given as a cause of failure to breathe but this is probably rarely if ever true. The respiratory center is sufficiently developed to function very early in intrauterine life, and a fetus of only 50–100 gm, if delivered without trauma, as by hysterectomy, will make respiratory movements of sufficient depth to inflate its lungs. Breathing in a very premature infant may cease within a short time because the lungs are too immature to allow adequate oxygenation of the blood, but the cause of death in such circumstances is immaturity of the lungs, not immaturity of the respiratory center.

Anoxia may develop somewhat later from hyaline material in the lungs, pharyngeal and pulmonary infections, aspiration of mucus or gastric contents, certain types of congenital heart disease, compression of the trachea by tumors or abnormal vessels arising from the aortic arch and so on.

Pathologic Changes Associated with Anoxia

Unfortunately no specific pathologic lesions are produced when death is caused by uncomplicated oxygen deprivation. This fact is responsible for many of the discrepancies in interpretation of postmortem findings by different prosectors. When death occurs rapidly, as with abrupt compression of the umbilical cord or sudden obstruction of the trachea, no pathologic changes are necessarily produced and postmortem examination often reveals few if any abnormalities. In such circumstances it is difficult to prove pathologically that anoxia was the cause of death, and recourse must be had to a clinicopathologic diagnosis. In no other age group is it so important to have a clinical history to use in conjunction with an autopsy protocol in order to arrive at a cause of death. When specific complications known to be responsible for cutting off the fetal circulation have existed, this information should be an adequate basis for a diagnosis of anoxia if no other abnormalities that might have caused the death are found.

Severe anoxia reduces the blood pressure and at the same time injures capillary endothelium. Although no changes are noticeable if death follows immediately, blood cells and plasma escape through the injured capillary walls when there is a period of survival and the blood pressure is restored to normal. Then, hemorrhage, edema or cellular necrosis may appear.

ABRUPTIO PLACENTAE. — Premature detachment of the placenta is the one cause of fatal anoxia that produces specific changes. When placental separation interferes sufficiently with oxygenation of fetal blood to cause death, countless round, sharply circumscribed petechial hemorrhages 2–3 mm in diameter are found under the visceral pleura covering all surfaces of the lungs (Fig. 7–1). They are also usually present throughout the cortical portions of the thymus (Fig. 7–2), under the pericardium in the region of the coronary sinus on the posterior surface of the heart and along the principal coronary vessels. They may also be found under the parietal pleura on the posterior aspect of the chest, on the pleural surface of the diaphragm and in the connective tissue of the mediastinum. All vessels in the lungs are intensely engorged with blood, and small hemorrhages are usually present around blood vessels in interstitial connective tissue.

The organs beneath the diaphragm are extremely congested. The vessels at the apexes of the pyramids in the kidneys are greatly dilated and may be surrounded by local extravasations of cells. The sinusoids of the liver are distended and often appear wider than the cords of hepatic cells between which they are located (Fig. 7–3). Despite the congestion, superficial hemorrhages of the variety found in the chest are seldom visible on the organs in the abdomen.

The brain substance may be the site of hemorrhages similar to those found in the thymus and lungs (Fig. 7–4). Such hemorrhages are ordinarily

Fig. 7–1.—Hemorrhages characteristically produced by premature placental separation. **A,** hemorrhages under visceral and parietal pleura. **B,** numerous round, sharply demarcated petechiae distributed over all surfaces of thymus and lungs.

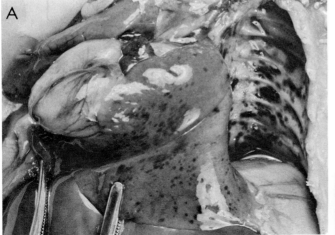

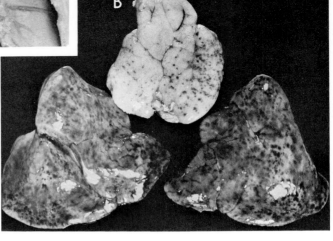

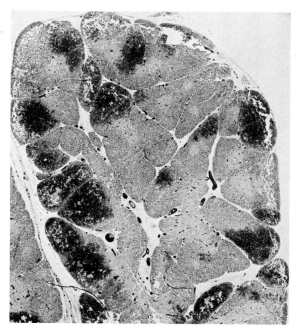

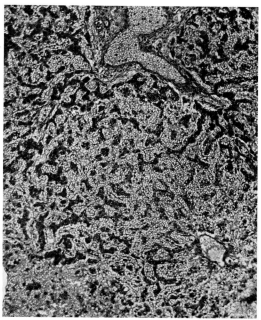

Fig. 7—2 (left). — Petechiae in cortical portions of thymus caused by anoxia from premature placental separation.

Fig. 7—3 (right). — Extreme distention of hepatic sinusoids *(light areas)* caused by anoxia from premature placental separation.

localized accumulations of cells around small blood vessels and are especially common in areas adjacent to the ventricles. Gross bleeding into the substance of the brain is rare.

UMBILICAL CORD OBSTRUCTION. — The principal reason for the difference in appearance of the body tissues following death from anoxia caused by cord compression and that caused by placental separation probably lies in the amount of placental blood continuing to enter the fetus as the heart begins to fail. When the cord is obstructed, the amount of blood in the fetus cannot increase and an extrauterine type of circulation is established while the fetus is still in the uterus; blood pressure falls quickly

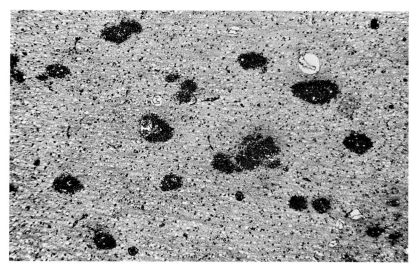

Fig. 7—4. — Petechiae in cerebral hemispheres caused by anoxia from premature placental separation.

and death occurs almost immediately, before hemorrhage can occur. When placental separation is responsible for oxygen deprivation, the uterine contractions continue to force blood from the placenta into the fetus, and consequent overloading of the circulation causes severe distention of the hepatic sinusoids and cardiac atria as the heart fails. The increased pressure in the left atrium interferes with venous return from the lungs, and the extreme venous congestion causes distention of the alveolar capillaries, interstitial and intra-alveolar hemorrhage and subpleural petechiae. Increased distention of the coronary vessels is responsible for the petechiae characteristically found in their vicinity.

OTHER CAUSES.—When death follows anoxia from causes other than placental separation, petechiae, generally smaller than those just described, are occasionally found on the thoracic organs, and a few irregular ecchymotic areas sometimes called "flame" hemorrhages may be present in the mediastinum and on the lungs. When death is due to acute obstruction of circulation through the umbilical cord, hemorrhages are ordinarily not found in any part of the body.

BRAIN

When prolonged labor or difficult delivery, especially of the shoulders, causes anoxia, the thoracic and abdominal viscera are usually normal except for severe congestion, but the leptomeninges are

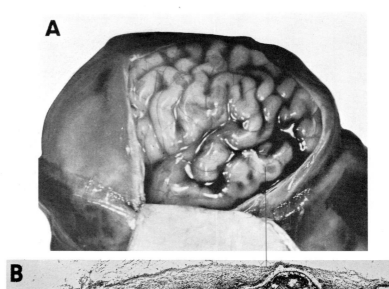

Fig. 7–5.—Mild extravasation of cells into subarachnoid space as a result of anoxia. Newborn infant weighing 1,750 gm. **A,** gross appearance. **B,** microscopic appearance.

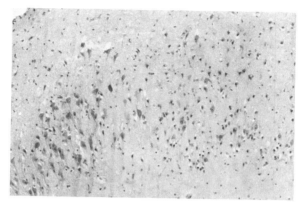

Fig. 7–6.—Portion of the hippocampal cortex of an infant who survived for 5 weeks following a postnatal attack of anoxia. On the right the total number of neuronal cells is decreased and only "ghost" cells remain. On the left the cellular pattern is normal.

often extremely congested and infiltrated by red blood cells. The cells are most numerous in the subarachnoid space; they may also be found in semilocalized areas or may form a uniform thin layer of blood over the cerebral hemispheres (Fig. 7–5) and around the cerebellum. The sulci of the cerebral hemispheres are a common site of local accumulations, which are often confused with bleeding that follows traumatic rupture of vessels, although trau-

matic hemorrhage is ordinarily subdural whereas anoxic hemorrhage is subarachnoid.

Damage to the neuronal cells and white matter of the brain secondary to anoxia or hypoxia can be recognized only if the infant survives for at least several hours after an acute or prolonged insult. Since most infants with intrauterine anoxia have no recovery period and the majority die in the first 24 hours, brains with easily recognized alterations are not commonly found. However, the infant's brain, and especially that of the premature infant, can survive anoxia better than the adult brain, and the structures that develop earliest are those in which it is easiest to recognize anoxic changes. These include the hippocampus and Ammon's horn, the dentate and amygdaloid nuclei and the Purkinje layer in the cerebellum. In these areas pyknosis and shrinkage of nuclei, loss of Nissl substance and shrinkage of cell cytoplasm may be present while other areas of the brain contain no recognizable lesions. In infants surviving more than a few days there may be a reduction in the number of nuclei and a reactive gliosis (Fig. 7–6).

When the infant is more mature and neuronal elements are better developed, alterations can be recognized more easily and repair is more obvious. When the loss of the neurons in the cortex is focal and not marked, especially in the rapidly developing brain of the premature infant, damage can be

Fig. 7–7.—Various stages of white matter necrosis in the paraventricular area of infants with severe neonatal anoxia. **A,** the area at the top is normally cellular; at the bottom, cells are absent or pyknotic and glial net is loosened. **B,** area where the glial net has broken down and the nuclei have disappeared. **C,** area where glia has responded and damaged area is being repaired.

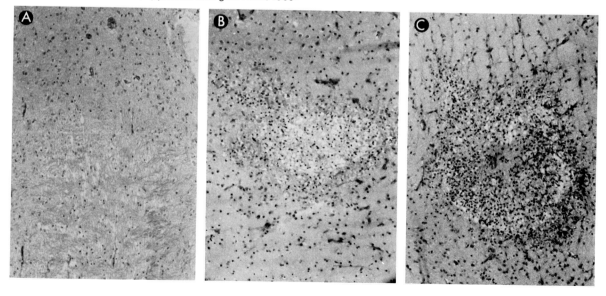

established only when meticulous cell counts indicate that too few normal cells are present.

The white matter as well as the nerve cells can be damaged by anoxia. The lesions are located in the periventricular white matter of the frontal, temporal and occipital regions. Foci of leukomalacia were described by Banker and Larroche as consisting of isolated round foci of dead cells associated with a broken glial net and an increase in the stainable fat. These foci soon undergo a reactive gliosis and can then be recognized as opaque white areas in the poorly myelinated white matter near the lateral walls of the ventricle. They may be mistaken for evidence of encephalitis (Figs. 7–7 and 7–8). Brand *et al.* described a fibrillary gliosis in the internal capsule and medulla that can be detected only by use of a specific glial stain (Holzer). They found this to be most prominent in infants over 7 days of age, and although attributed to the hypoxia of respiratory distress, it may be a response to treatment with high levels of oxygen.

The frequency with which neuronal degeneration and leukomalacia are detected in infants dying

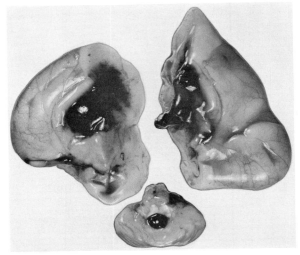

Fig. 7–9.—Hemorrhage from choroid plexus and vena terminalis into lateral ventricle and brain substance of a 900 gm infant.

Fig. 7–8.—Section from the lateral ventricle of the same infant as in Fig. 7–7,C; the ependymal cells have partially disappeared and the ventricle is focally lined by necrotic glial cells that form a net beneath the surface.

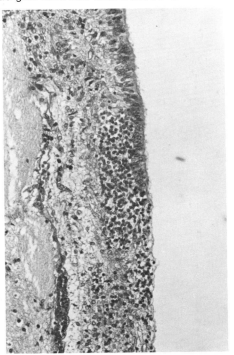

neonatally depends on the care exercised in the preparation of the tissues and the intensity of the search for such lesions. Terplan found leukomalacia in nearly 40% of infants dying with respiratory distress, and other authors have found it even more frequently when a large number of blocks or serial sections of the entire brain have been examined. Routine postmortem studies with random brain sections give a much lower yield of lesions.

Another brain lesion that may be found in asphyxiated premature infants is hemorrhage into the lateral wall of the lateral ventricles. This appears to start in the region of the tributaries of the great vein of Galen. Here large vessels in the small premature infant are surrounded by developmental zones of immature glial and neuroblastic tissue. This tissue supplies little support for the thin-walled veins in comparison to that afforded by normal adult glial tissue; thus, the wall of a vessel may rupture and blood break through into the ventricle (Fig. 7–9), or it may dissect laterally into the cerebral substance. When intraventricular hemorrhage is severe, it fills the ventricles and appears in large amounts in the subarachnoid space about the medulla, having passed through the third and fourth ventricles. In such cases the typical history is that of a 1,200–1,500 gm premature infant who, after 24–36 hours of severe respiratory distress and hypoxia, suddenly becomes jittery, convulsive and apneic. Tobin believed that necrosis in this developmental glial zone preceded the onset of hemorrhage, though this has not been the experience at the Boston Hospital for Women.

LUNGS

Additional findings often noted in a fetus dying of anoxia are the presence in the lungs of large amounts of debris derived from the amniotic fluid and a reduction in the amount of meconium in the large intestine. Although it seems probable that the fetus normally inspires amniotic fluid throughout the greater part of pregnancy (see discussion, p. 59), normal respiratory movements are shallow and only a little fluid is present in the lumens of the bronchi and alveolar ducts. When the oxygen supply is diminished, the respiratory center is stimulated and the depth of respiratory excursions increases. This draws larger amounts of amniotic fluid into all parts of the pulmonary tree. Part of the fluid inspired may be exhaled and part may be absorbed by the capillaries in the alveolar walls, but enough remains to produce visible dilatation of alveoli. If such respiratory activity is limited to the early months of pregnancy, little evidence remains after death because at that time the amniotic fluid is almost free of particulate matter. During the latter part of pregnancy, however, sebaceous material is excreted by the glands of the skin, lanugo is shed and epithelium is desquamated; when the amniotic fluid that enters the lungs contains this debris, it is left behind in high concentration as the fluid is absorbed (see Fig. 15–6).

If bacteria are present in the inspired amniotic fluid, pneumonia may develop promptly. If the fluid is sterile, small amounts of debris often appear to do no harm and may still be found in the alveoli many weeks after birth (see Fig. 15–7). Eventually it is removed by phagocytes.

OTHER ORGANS

The anal sphincter normally remains closed throughout fetal life. Only when anoxia occurs does it relax and permit expulsion of meconium from the intestine into the amniotic sac except during delivery from a breech position where meconium is sometimes present even without recognizable abnormality. At birth the large bowel is ordinarily distended with meconium; in the mature fetus the diameter averages 2–3 cm. In the presence of anoxia it is completely or partially emptied and the diameter may be reduced to a few millimeters.

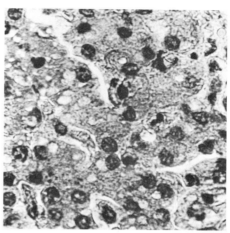

Fig. 7–10.—Liver. Intracellular anoxic vacuoles in the parenchyma, each having a small central eosinophilic mass.

Generalized edema, seen at autopsy as an increased wetness of all tissues, has been described as a characteristic of anoxia. In our experience the amount of fluid in the tissues of infants dying of anoxia has seldom been appreciably increased.

It is perhaps only an academic point to attempt to differentiate traumatic from anoxic hemorrhage in the infant who dies during labor. If the fetus were entirely uninjured neither type would occur, and consequently hemorrhage from capillaries damaged by anoxia may justifiably be considered as much a result of trauma as hemorrhage from a gross laceration of a larger vessel. To avoid making a distinction some investigators have grouped deaths from anoxia and trauma together. It seems wiser, however, to make a distinction since there is a difference in approach to prevention of intracranial hemorrhage caused by mechanical rupture of a blood vessel and that caused by anoxia.

In an occasional infant dying neonatally with prolonged severe asphyxia both fatty infiltration and so-called "anoxic vacuolation" may be found in the liver and heart (Fig. 7–10). The latter vacuoles do not stain for fat except for a small central inclusion that is eosinophilic in sections stained with hematoxylin and eosin.

Sequelae of Anoxia

Contrary to the prospective study of Keith and Norval, which showed no abnormalities in the first few years of life among 111 infants asphyxiated at birth, the retrospective study of Eastman *et al.* of the birth records of 753 patients with cerebral palsy who had no significant events after the neonatal period showed a definite correlation of spastic mono- and diplegia with severe asphyxia at birth or with an extreme degree of prematurity. Graham *et al.,* also, by following infants with severe respiratory distress or apnea, found that 40% were mentally retarded.

Even more impressive are the data from the Collaborative Maternal and Infant Health Project of the National Institute of Mental Disease and Blindness (Fisch, *et al.*). In a sample taken from survivors of the respiratory distress syndrome who weighed over 1,500 gm at birth, motor and neurologic damage was twice as frequent as in normal control subjects when all were examined at 8 months and 1 year. Evidence of neurologic damage was as high as 20% among survivors in the weight group 1,500–2,500 gm and 15% in the group over 2,500 gm.

Very late gross destructive lesions of the brain were described by Towbin and by Greenfield, which they thought resulted from perinatal anoxia. They described gross vacuolation, focal gyral atrophy, a cribriform state of partially vacuolated brain substance and uneven myelinization (status marmoratus) of the basal ganglia. Such lesions are probably unusual and far less common than less extensive and less obvious lesions, although even the latter may cause severe handicap. (See Chapter 24.)

REFERENCES

Banker, B. Q., and Larroche, J.: Periventricular leukomalacia, Arch. Neurol. 7:386, 1962.

Brand, M. M., Durbridge, T. C., Rosan, R. C., and Northway, W. H.: Neuropathological lesions in respiratory distress syndrome: Acute and chronic changes during hypoxia and oxygen therapy, J. Reprod. Med. 8:267, 1972.

Courville, C. R.: *Cerebral Anoxia* (Los Angeles: San Lucas Press, 1953).

Eastman, N. J., Kohl, S. G., Maisel, J. E., and Kavoler, F.: The obstetrical background of 753 cases of cerebral palsy, Obstet. Gynecol. Surv. 17:459, 1962.

Fisch, R. O., Grovein, H. J., and Engel, R. R.: Neurological status of survivors of neonatal respiratory distress syndrome, J. Pediatr. 73:395, 1968.

Gordan, H. R.: Fetal bradycardia after paracervical block, N. Engl. J. Med. 278:410, 1968.

Graham, F. K., *et al.*: The relationship of neonatal apnea to development at 3 years, in Neurology and Psychiatry in Childhood, Res. Publ. Assoc. Nerv. Ment. Dis. 39:159, 1962.

Greenfield, J. G.: *Neuropathology* (London: Edward Arnold Ltd., 1958).

Holzer, W.: Über eine neue Methode der gliafasern Färbung, Zeit. Ges. Neurol. U. Psych. 69:354, 1921.

Keith, H. M., and Norval, M. A.: Neurologic lesions in the newly born infant: I. Preliminary study; II. Role of prolonged labor in asphyxia and delayed respiration, Pediatrics 6:229, 1950.

Lewis, R. B., and Haymaker, W.: High altitude hypoxia, J. Aviat. Med. 19:306, 1948.

Lund, C. J.: Fetal distress during labor, Ill. Med. J. 83:96, 1943.

Moon, V. H.: Origins and effects of anoxia, Bull. N. Y. Acad. Med. 26:361, 1950.

Potter, E. L.: Respiratory disturbances in the newly born infant, Ill. Med. J. 83:100, 1943.

Rosefsky, J. B., and Petersiel, M. E.: Perinatal deaths associated with mepivicaine paracervical block in pregnancy, N. Engl. J. Med. 278:530, 1968.

Schreiber, F.: Apnea of the newborn and associated cerebral palsy, J.A.M.A. 111:1263, 1938.

Terplan, K. L.: Histopathologic brain changes in 1152 cases in perinatal and early infancy period. Biol. Neonate 11:348, 1968.

Towbin, A.: *The Pathology of Cerebral Palsy* (Springfield, Ill.: Charles C Thomas, 1960).

Windle, W. F., *et al.*: Alterations in brain structure after asphyxiation at birth. An experimental study in the guinea pig, J. Neuropathol. Exp. Neurol. 3:224, 1944.

Windle, W. F., *et al.*: Structural and functional sequelae of asphyxia neonatorum in monkeys, in Neurology and Psychiatry in Childhood, Res. Publ. Assoc. Nerv. Ment. Dis. 34:169, 1954.

Wohlwill, F.: Zur Frage der sogennanten Encephalis congenita (Virchow), Z. Neurol. Psychol. 68, I:384, 1921; 73, II:360, 1921.

Wolfe, A., and Cowan, D.: The cerebral atrophies and encephalomalacias of infancy, in Neurology and Psychiatry of Childhood, Res. Publ. Assoc. Nerv. Ment. Dis. 34:199, 1954.

8

Birth Trauma

Head

THE PASSAGE through the birth canal is the most hazardous experience to which the ordinary individual is ever subjected and it is surprising, not that there is occasional injury, but that injury does not occur more often.

Although anoxia resulting from interference with circulation during delivery is trauma in a broad sense, the term is usually limited to local mechanical injury resulting in gross hemorrhage. The head is more commonly involved than any other part of the body and death results most often from interference with vital functions as a result of increased intracranial pressure.

The reported incidence of intracranial hemorrhage has varied greatly, with earlier studies generally showing a much higher rate than more recent ones. Early investigators attributed from 20–40% of deaths among stillborn and newborn infants to intracranial injury, although some reported a figure as high as 70% or more.

In general, the higher the intrapartum mortality, the greater the percentage of deaths attributable to injury. When mortality rates decrease, trauma is usually the first condition to show a reduction. At the Chicago Lying-in Hospital the mortality rate for injury incurred during delivery was 5.6/1,000 total births from 1931–1941, when it accounted for 14% of the deaths and stillbirths, and was only 0.3/1,000 births from 1961–1966, when it was responsible for 1.7% of the deaths and stillbirths.

The survey made by the Birthday Trust in England for the month of March 1958 showed the perinatal death rate for cerebral trauma to be 1/1,000 live births, or 3.1% of all deaths (Butler and Bonham).

GENERAL ETIOLOGY

Much stress has been placed on the fact that hemorrhage is occasionally found after apparently normal noninstrumental deliveries, and in some instances an attempt seems to have been made to exonerate the physician of all responsibility for the presence of hemorrhage. Although hemorrhage may follow natural cephalic delivery, the incidence is higher in all other forms of delivery. As the judgment and technical skill of the obstetrician improve, the incidence of intracranial hemorrhage and other forms of trauma diminishes. According to Dekaban, small amounts of blood often may be found in the spinal fluid (up to 300 red cells per ml of clinically normal newborn infants, although Nasralla et al. found no more than 5 per ml in the spinal fluid of 100 newborn infants. The broadened indications for the use of cesarean section and the prevention of excessive prolongation of labor have been important factors in reducing birth trauma.

Hemorrhage found in an infant delivered spontaneously from a cephalic position is often secondary to prolongation of the second stage of labor. The judicious application of forceps following complete dilatation of the cervix may be accompanied by much less trauma to the head than would be incurred by permitting the head to deliver naturally.

At one time it was thought that hemorrhagic disease of the newborn was a common cause of intracranial hemorrhage, but if hemorrhage does occur from this cause it must be infrequent, and almost all cases of gross intracranial hemorrhage occurring during labor can be attributed to trauma.

Fatal or crippling injury is least common when labor and delivery are of moderate length, when uterine contractions increase normally in duration and intensity, when the head is the presenting part and the occiput is anterior and when the maternal pelvis is large enough for passage of the fetus. Alteration of any of these conditions increases the possibility of trauma. In our experience deliveries by version and extraction, mid and high forceps and from a breech or occiput posterior position are all associated with a higher incidence of trauma than are deliveries from an occiput anterior position, either spontaneous or aided by low or outlet forceps. This is in part because the last two types of delivery are less frequently associated with other abnormalities of labor, but it is also in part because of the mechanical factors involved in the delivery. In a labor of average length the shape of the head is slowly adjusted to the contour of the birth canal, and the dural septa are gradually put under increasing tension. A membrane that can withstand a severe strain when force is exerted gradually may rupture when the same force is applied suddenly. It is for this reason that delivery is often traumatic following the abrupt change in shape caused by (1) delivery of the head after the body has been extracted, (2) application of forceps while the head is still high in the birth canal or (3) the sudden expulsion of an unmolded head in a precipitate delivery. Kelly found that when forceps were used, the presence of hemorrhages, nerve palsies and low Apgar scores were limited to the exertion of over 55 lb of tension on the baby by the operator. With traction of less than 50 lb the incidence of injury was negligible. When labor is excessively long, mortality from anoxia is increased, but the length of labor in itself does not contribute to an increased incidence of mechanical trauma. An increase in length of labor may be associated indirectly with an increase in trauma because the same factors responsible for abnormal labor are responsible for abnormal delivery, and the incidence of injury in operative delivery by means other than outlet forceps is always increased. If labor is prolonged because of an abnormal fetal position or a disproportionately large fetal head, the likelihood of trauma is great. In some hospitals delivery by outlet forceps is semi-routine in normal labor with a cephalic presentation because of the belief that shortening the second stage of labor lessens injury to the maternal perineum as well as to the fetus. Such deliveries at the Chicago Lying-in Hospital were associated with less injury than any other variety.

It should be pointed out that, of all methods of delivery, breech extraction is by far the most hazardous to the infant. In such deliveries there is, in addition to intracranial damage, an increase in injury to long bone (Snedecor and Wilson), spinal cord (Crothers and Putnam), vertebrae (Yates) and brachial nerves. According to Towbin, in breech deliveries when the occiput is arrested under the symphysis pubis, strong traction may produce intracerebellar as well as subarachnoid hemorrhage. It may also cause herniation of the brain into the foramen magnum with injury to the cerebellum and cerebrum. Suprafundic pressure, particularly on the after-coming head, may also cause injury.

Subdural hemorrhage results most frequently from an injury to the straight sinus caused by laceration of the tentorium near its junction with the falx or by rupture of the vein of Galen. In either case blood will be found at the base of the skull around the cerebellum and brain stem. With face and brow presentations, stretching of the falx by elongation of the vertex may tear bridging veins as they enter the superior sagittal sinus from the arachnoid membrane. If this is sufficiently extensive it may cause interference with function of vital centers as a result of pressure on the medulla. At the Chicago Lying-in Hospital subdural hemorrhage has been very uncommon; when present, it has generally been limited to the region of the sylvian fissure and has appeared to result from injury to the middle cerebral vein. Rarely, the superior cerebral veins may be torn as they enter the sagittal sinus, giving rise to diffuse subdural hemorrhage.

CAPUT SUCCEDANEUM

The presenting part of the fetus is usually edematous immediately after birth, the extent of the edema ordinarily being related to the length of the second stage of labor. The presenting part of the fetus is surrounded and compressed by the uterus and, late in labor, by the cervix except in the region of the cervical opening. The part underlying the cervical orifice is under less pressure than the rest of the body and is subject to exudation of fluid and extravasation of blood into the subcutaneous tissues.

If the head is the presenting part, the area of maximal edema is usually over the vertex, and this is called a caput succedaneum (Fig. 8-1). In face presentation the subcutaneous tissues of the eyelids, cheeks, nose and lips are edematous and hemorrhagic (Fig. 8-2). Similar areas of edema and

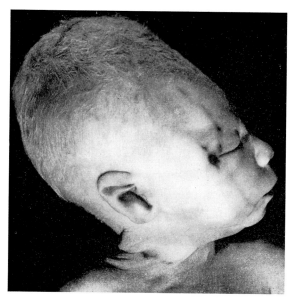

Fig. 8—1.—Head molding with caput succedaneum over vertex.

hemorrhage are present over the buttocks when the infant has been in a breech position. The scrotum or labia are also usually extremely congested and in severe cases the testes and epididymus may show extensive interstitial extravasations of blood. An arm or a leg that is prolapsed through the cervix becomes edematous and discolored. Gangrene

Fig. 8—2.—Edema and suffusion of blood into subcutaneous tissue as a result of face presentation.

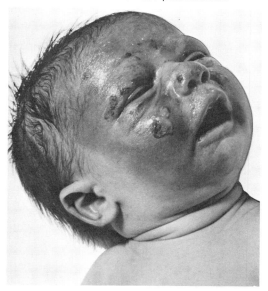

has been reported as a rare sequela to prolonged circulatory obstruction caused by constriction of the cervix around the proximal portion of a prolapsed extremity. Microscopic examination of tissue from a caput succedaneum reveals an excessive amount of fluid and a mild extravasation of blood cells around the smaller blood vessels. Generally the tissues return to normal in a few days.

CEPHALHEMATOMA

Slightly more severe injury than that producing a caput succedaneum results in the formation of a cephalhematoma. This is an accumulation of blood between the surface of a calvarial bone and its pericranial membrane. Each bone of the calvarium is completely enveloped by an individual sheath, and blood that accumulates beneath this membrane is limited in surface area to the bone involved. Blood may be present over one or both parietal bones or over the squamous portion of the occipital bone, and one, two or three individual elevations may be produced. They are easily differentiated from a caput succedaneum in a living child because they never extend over a suture line (Fig. 8–3). Bleeding in such a location takes place slowly and may not be apparent for several hours after birth.

During the first few days the blood of a cephalhematoma is fluid and the mass is soft and fluctuant. The blood eventually clots and may be absorbed slowly or become organized and eventually be converted into bone. Bony elevations disappear only as the skull increases in size and thickness. Calcium is often deposited around the outer margin of the hemorrhage and forms a thin, hard rim that may make the bone beneath the cephalhematoma seem thinner than the rest of the skull. However, the underlying bone is almost never abnormal. Similar accumulations on the inner surface of a calvarial bone are rare.

FRACTURES OF SKULL BONES

The bones of the calvarium generally contain less calcium at the time of birth than they do even a short time later. Ordinarily the amount of calcium in the skull is related to the size of the fetus, but even in very large infants the bones are somewhat compressible. This, and the fact that they are separated by membranous sutures, usually permits enough alteration in the shape of the head to facilitate its passage through the birth canal without damage to the bones themselves.

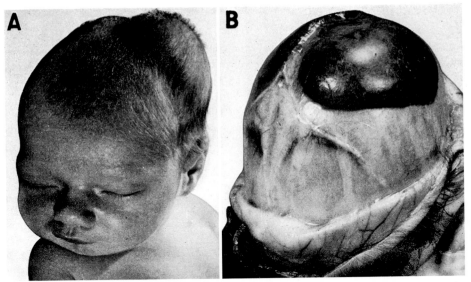

Fig. 8–3.—Cephalhematoma over left parietal bone. **A,** external view in a living infant. **B,** scalp reflected to show effect of sutures in localizing subpericranial hemorrhage in a dead infant.

As a result of pressure against the maternal symphysis pubis or the promontory of the sacrum or, more frequently, because of pressure from a forceps blade a several centimeter portion of one parietal bone may become depressed, a condition known as a depressed fracture. This is not a true fracture, for an actual break in continuity almost never occurs; it consists rather of a snapping inward of a thin resilient portion of bone (Fig. 8–4). Symptoms are seldom produced, but the depressed area is usually elevated surgically because of the fear that long-continued pressure might injure the underlying cortex.

Fig. 8–4.—Depressed fracture in right parietal bone.

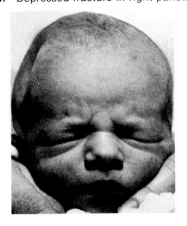

When a fracture does occur, the break is usually radial and follows a plane of cleavage. Fractures extend from the margin toward the center of the parietal bone, from the upper margin of the frontal bone down toward the supraorbital ridges and from the upper margin of the occipital bone down toward the basal portion. Only with excessive pressure does a break occur at right angles to the plane of cleavage (Fig. 8–5,A).

Fracture of the occipital bone with separation of the basal and squamous portions is a form of injury frequently mentioned in the older literature but rarely observed with modern obstetric technics. It is invariably fatal because the underlying vascular sinuses are disrupted by the separation of the two parts of the bone (Fig. 8–5). It almost never occurs except in breech deliveries and ordinarily results when traction is applied to the hyperextended spine of the infant while the head remains fixed in the maternal pelvis. The squamous portion of the occipital bone is held beneath the symphysis pubis, and if the infants's body is pulled upward, the basal portion of the occipital bone moves with the spine and separates from the squamous portion which is fixed in the pelvis. The line of separation is a suture earlier in fetal life and for this reason is weaker than any other part of the bone. If the infant's spine is not hyperextended during breech delivery at the same time at which traction is exerted, such a fracture will not occur.

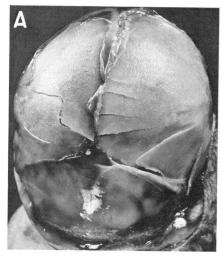
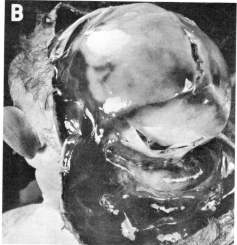

Fig. 8–5.—Severe birth trauma in infant stillborn at term. **A,** multiple skull fractures along normal planes of cleavage. The one fracture at right angles required more force for its production than did the others. **B,** fracture separating squamous and basal portions of occipital bone, responsible for hemorrhage under scalp and for laceration of cerebral sinuses with resultant massive intracranial hemorrhage.

INTRACRANIAL HEMORRHAGE

The intracranial cavity is the most common site of fatal or crippling injury. The head of the fetus is constructed in such a way that it can withstand considerable distortion at the time of birth but, despite this, certain structures may give way, causing rupture of blood vessels with resultant hemorrhage into the intracranial cavity.

LACERATION OF TENTORIUM CEREBELLI.—The brain is encased in a tough membrane—the dura mater. A midline extension of the dura grows downward from the superior sagittal suture to form a somewhat crescentic sheet separating the cerebral hemispheres and helping to hold them in place. This is the falx cerebri. In the posterior portion of the skull the falx cerebri divides into the two leaves of the tentorium cerebelli which form a roof over the cerebellum. The margins of the falx cerebri and tentorium cerebelli are reinforced with fibers designated "bands of stress" because, like the selvage on a piece of cloth, they can withstand more strain than the rest of the membrane (see Fig. 6–4).

As long as a force increases gradually and is directed toward the midline or is equally distributed on both sides of the head, there is little danger that the margin of either the falx or the tentorium will give way. If force is applied asymmetrically, one leaf of the tentorium is relaxed while the other is placed under excessive tension, and if the force is sufficient, especially if suddenly applied, the leaf of the tentorium that is under tension will rupture. A simple laceration of the anterior margin of the tentorium does no harm in itself for there are no blood vessels there. However, as the tentorium tears, the rent extends medially into the straight sinus that runs anteroposteriorly along the apex of the tentorium or laterally into the portion of the transverse sinus that lies just below the attachment of the tentorium to the dura mater. If one of these sinuses ruptures, the ensuing hemorrhage increases intracranial pressure and usually causes death (Fig. 8–6). The major bleeding is subtentorial, but a thin layer is often present over the surface of the brain in the subdural space (Fig. 8–7). The lower edge of the falx cerebri carries the inferior sagittal sinus, and rupture of the margin leads to immediate bleeding. Fortunately the tensions within the head are such that the margin of the falx seldom tears.

RUPTURE OF THE VEIN OF GALEN.—The other structure to which injury almost invariably causes death is the internal cerebral vein, commonly called the great vein of Galen. It is a confluence of the internal veins of both cerebral hemispheres and is somewhat less than 1 cm long. Arising near the posterior margin of the area in which the two cerebral hemispheres unite, it empties into the straight sinus. It is unsupported and literally hangs in space during its brief course (see Fig. 6–3). If the anteroposterior diameter of the head is abnormally increased, excessive tension may cause rupture of

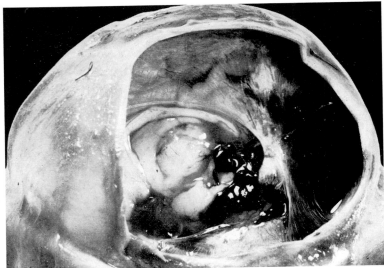

Fig. 8–6.—Intracranial hemorrhage caused by rupture of left leaf of tentorium cerebelli with extension into straight sinus.

the wall of the vein of Galen with blood loss into the space around the base of the brain and between the cerebral hemispheres (Fig. 8–8), with extension over the surface of the brain under the dura mater.

Hemorrhage from the vein of Galen or from the transverse or straight sinus is usually fatal owing to the compression of vital centers in the brain stem that results from bleeding into the subtentorial space (Fig. 8–9). The location makes surgical treatment impossible.

SUBDURAL HEMATOMAS.—Bleeding from one of the superficial cerebral vessels is a third type of gross intracranial hemorrhage. The middle cerebral artery is the vessel most commonly injured

and the blood accumulates in the subdural space most often over the temporal region on one side of the brain. This is a rare cause of death in young infants; among those born at the Chicago Lying-in Hospital between 1934 and 1966 it was observed only twice, once in an infant who died at 2 days (Fig. 8–10) and once in an infant of 5 days.

Intracranial hemorrhage occurring later in infancy originates most often from a meningeal vein. This may be associated with a history of trauma but often there is no known injury. The hemorrhage is usually more diffuse than in the newborn and is often designated internal hemorrhagic pachymeningitis. In older infants retinal hemorrhages are considered almost pathognomonic of this

Fig. 8–7.—Fatal hemorrhage from extension of tentorial laceration into lateral sinus. **A,** thin layer of blood under dura (note difference between this and asphyxial subarachnoid bleeding [see Fig. 7–5]). **B,** blood filling posterior cranial fossa and subtentorial space.

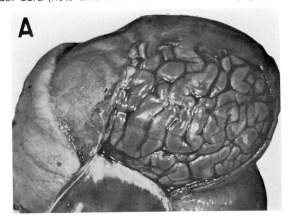

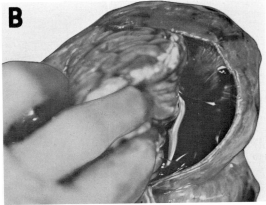

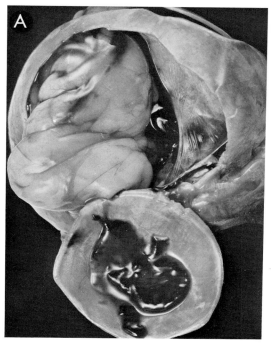

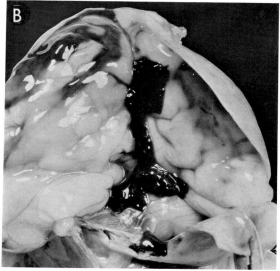

Fig. 8–8.—Rupture of vein of Galen. **A,** blood in region of vein of Galen and under dura. **B,** blood extending forward between cerebral hemispheres.

condition. Retinal hemorrhages are common in the newborn, occurring immediately after birth in 15–20%. They have no relation to intracranial hemorrhage and disappear within the first few days.

Bleeding from a meningeal vessel is usually found first in the subarachnoid space. If severe it may destroy underlying brain tissue and extend into the ventricular system. If less severe the blood may remain in the meninges and the brain may be

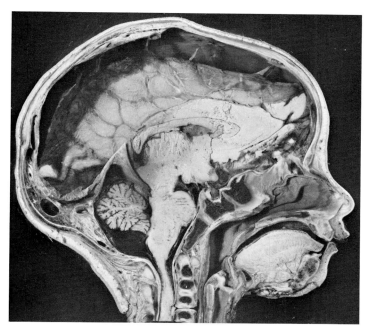

Fig. 8–9.—Sagittal section of head showing subtentorial hemorrhage compressing cerebellum. Cerebral hemisphere is discolored and shrunken as a result of prolonged fixation.

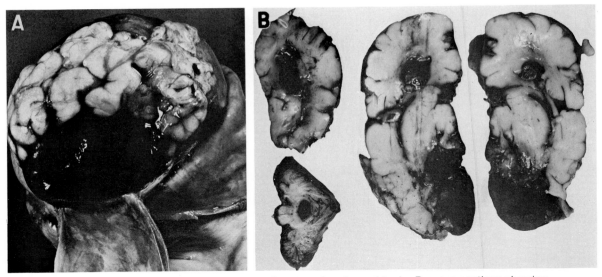

Fig. 8—10.—Massive subdural hematoma. **A,** external surface of brain. **B,** cross-sections showing destruction of brain tissue and intraventricular hemorrhage.

Fig. 8—11.—Intraventricular hemorrhage in an infant weighing 1,950 gm.

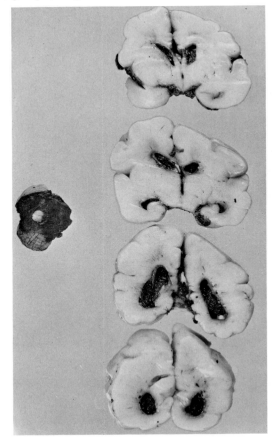

injured only as a result of pressure. When the hemorrhage is extensive, death often occurs in a short time. If the infant survives, evidence of increased intracranial pressure appears and part or all of the extremities show localizing motor and sensory disturbances. The surface of the blood clot is often converted into a layer of granulation tissue that acts as a dialyzing membrane. Fluid is drawn into the clot, increasing its size and intensifying the symptoms. By means of a needle inserted through one of the cranial sutures several milliliters of blood may be obtained on several successive days. After a short time the material removed usually changes from pure blood to blood-tinged fluid and often it disappears entirely. An undisturbed hematoma may be resorbed, but the larger ones are often invaded by capillaries and connective tissue. They become organized and are gradually converted into fibrous tissue or bone. At the Chicago Lying-in Hospital one infant who died unexpectedly at 1 month of age had no symptoms of intracranial injury but the cerebral hemispheres were covered by a thin organized hematoma containing bone.

The destruction of blood cells in a hematoma may increase the serum bilirubin sufficiently to cause deep jaundice. This must be kept in mind in the differential diagnosis of jaundice in the newborn period since subdural hematomas may exist without producing localizing symptoms.

SUBARACHNOID HEMORRHAGE.—Hemorrhage into the subarachnoid space is usually mild, consisting principally of slight extravasation of cells in the areas around the major blood vessels (see Fig. 7–5). Such hemorrhage is almost invariably a result of anoxia and is not caused by mechanical injury.

INTRAVENTRICULAR HEMORRHAGE. — Intraventricular hemorrhage may accompany traumatic hemorrhage in other parts of the head but when found alone it is usually a result of anoxia. Such injury of the choroid plexus, the vena terminalis or capillaries in the wall of the lateral ventricle may be responsible for bleeding that distends the lateral ventricles and sometimes extends through the entire ventricular system (Fig. 8–11). It passes out of the foramina of Luschka and Magendie into the subarachnoid space about the medulla and pons. The bleeding often has more than one point of origin and there may be small hemorrhages in the paraventricular white matter as well as in the developmental glial zone about the vena terminalis. This is especially true in infants on the borderline of viability. The special anatomic features of this area that account for the increased susceptibility have been discussed in Chapter 7. Small clots may be found in the region of the choroid plexus in any infant with anoxia, but they are seldom large enough to increase intracranial pressure and have no clinical significance. In rare instances the fourth ventricle may be the only site of hemorrhage and a massive hematoma may excavate the interior of the cerebellum (Fig. 8–12).

Small hemorrhages in the brain substance unaccompanied by external bleeding are seldom traumatic, usually being caused by anoxia (see Fig. 7–4).

Bleeding into the leaves of the tentorium cerebelli or falx cerebri produces no clinical symptoms. It may be found with anoxia or with other evidence of trauma and occasionally in the absence of either.

INTRACRANIAL HEMORRHAGE BEFORE ONSET OF LABOR. — Very infrequently, infants who are stillborn or die soon after birth have hemorrhagic areas in the brain that antedate birth. These areas are usually small but may be 1–2 cm in diameter. Although some fresh blood may still be present in the central portions, the periphery of the lesions is usually made up predominantly of large macrophages. Some areas contain blood pigment and others have lipoid material derived from destroyed brain tissue. The cause of such bleeding is almost impossible to prove, but it is usually attributed to rupture of an aneurysm or hypoplastic blood vessel. Porencephalic areas in older individuals have been attributed to preexisting hemorrhages that destroyed portions of the brain. The complete absorption of destroyed blood cells and brain substance is believed to leave behind the fluid-filled cystic spaces characteristic of porencephaly (see Fig. 24–33). Although this might account for some such areas, it cannot explain them all, for porencephaly may be found in stillborn infants with no evidence of hemorrhage.

Small groups of macrophages known as "gitter" cells, which are filled with lipoid material, are occasionally found around cerebral blood vessels and probably result from preexisting hemorrhage.

CLINICAL DIAGNOSIS

During the early days of the living infant it is often difficult to differentiate the effects of trauma from those of anoxia and it is usually impossible to localize an area of hemorrhage. In the surviving infant it may never be known whether gross hemorrhage was present or whether the symptoms were a result of edema, anoxia, shock or malformation. This is the principal reason for the difference of opinion concerning the cause of Little's disease—

Fig. 8–12.—Hemorrhage from choroid plexus of 4th ventricle causing distention and destruction of the cerebellum.

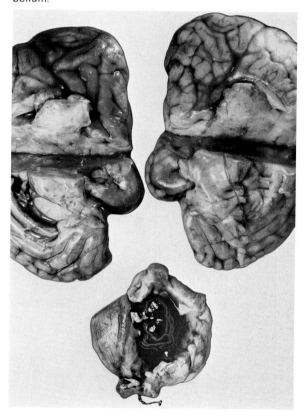

the permanent paralysis of one or more extremities dating from birth. Early investigators believed that it was almost always a result of trauma. Recent investigators have suggested that malformations of the brain are more often responsible. Even though trauma may not be the cause of all birth palsies, there is no doubt that it causes some.

The most common symptoms of intracranial hemorrhage occurring soon after birth are lethargy, somnolence, failure to respond normally to stimuli, inability to suck adequately, irregular respiration with periods of apnea and accompanying cyanosis, and irregular twitching of muscles or convulsions either localized or generalized. The anterior fontanel is often tense or bulging.

If a large amount of blood is present, especially beneath the tentorium, the infant generally dies immediately after birth or in the first 24 – 48 hours of life. In the surviving infant the hemorrhage is usually in the subdural area over the surface of the cerebral hemispheres.

Spinal puncture is often performed in an attempt to determine whether or not hemorrhage exists, and unwarranted conclusions are often based on the presence or absence of blood in the cerebrospinal fluid. The absence of blood does not preclude the possibility of intracranial hemorrhage and its presence does not prove the existence of gross hemorrhage. Fresh blood cells may be present as a result of local trauma inflicted by the spinal puncture needle, and only degenerated or crenated cells or xanthochromia of the serum should be considered significant. Even these changes may be associated with the meningeal extravasations that are a concomitant of prolonged anoxia.

An infant appears to be capable of fairly normal behavior even in the absence or destruction of cerebral hemispheres. The behavior of the average infant at birth seems to be largely a result of reflex activity involving only the centers of the spinal cord or those in the cerebellum and brain stem. In several infants reported who lived for many weeks without exhibiting recognizable abnormalities, postmortem examination disclosed an almost complete absence of cerebral hemispheres (hydranencephaly). Hemorrhage can destroy much of the brain substance without producing localizing signs in the early days of life, and when symptoms are present early they are usually caused by the transmission of pressure to the infratentorial portions of the brain. This is also one reason for the early absence of paralysis of the extremities that would be expected from local compression of the motor areas of the cerebral cortex.

Spine and Spinal Cord

The spine of the infant is rarely injured during birth or at any subsequent time except in breech delivery. It is able to withstand considerable tension, and it has been stated that elongation of 2 cm or more produces no injury as long as the direction of traction is in the straight axis of the spine. Pierson showed experimentally that 105 lb of tension will separate the spinous cervical body from its epiphysis, the most common type of serious spinal column injury. If, however, strong traction is exerted when the spine is hyperextended or if the direction of pull is lateral, fracture and separation of the vertebrae may be produced. This is most apt to occur when difficulty is encountered in extracting part of the body from the birth canal – either the shoulders in a cephalic presentation or the after-coming head in a breech presentation.

Vertebral fractures are found most frequently where the 7th cervical joins the 1st thoracic vertebra, and although any level of the cervical or upper thoracic spine may be involved, fractures are rare in other locations. With partial or temporary displacement of the vertebrae the meningeal vessels may be torn and blood may fill the spinal canal. The degree of spinal cord injury depends on the amount of vertebral displacement that takes place. If it is sufficient to cause complete transection of the cord, the portion below the level involved atrophies and there is permanent paralysis of the parts of the body supplied by nerve fibers arising below this level (Fig. 8 – 13). Even though paralysis at first seems to be complete, symptoms may be due partly to edema and hemorrhage, and their disappearance is followed by striking improvement. For the first few days after birth the legs are flaccid and immobile because of hemorrhage into the spinal cord. If injury involves the cervical region, symptoms of brachial paralysis will also be evident. Tendon reflexes and spontaneous reflex activity are absent. The bladder becomes distended and urine dribbles from it. Constipation is often severe. If improvement does not occur in a few weeks, trophic disturbances begin to appear. The muscles of the lower parts of the body atrophy, contractures and deformities develop, the skin becomes thin and ulcerates in areas subjected to pressure, and urinary infections are common. If the child survives, the lower extremities grow more slowly than the upper extremities.

Loss of sensation is often difficult to determine in young infants. It can be tested best by changes in texture. According to Buchanan, the texture below

Most infants with severe spinal cord injuries die soon after birth. Postmortem examination may reveal a fracture and separation of the vertebrae; less often, blood in the spinal canal is the only evidence of injury. If vertebrae have been dislocated, blood is usually present external to the spine in the connective tissue immediately surrounding the site of fracture (Fig. 8–14). It has been said that dislocation may be temporary, with the fracture escaping notice on postmortem examination. This seems improbable if the examination is properly made.

Hemorrhage in the spinal canal may be intra- or extradural. If the vertebrae have been displaced, the spinal cord may be partially or completely crushed in the region of the fracture. Hemorrhage within the cord may extend both above and below the point of injury. If the child survives for some time, the hemorrhagic areas may become organized and fibrotic.

At autopsy, after the brain is freed from its local attachments it may be lifted from the skull, and with gentle traction the cord may be extracted from

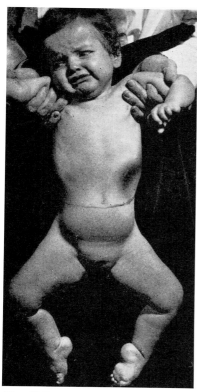

Fig. 8–13.—Child aged 1½ years with complete motor and sensory loss in lower half of body as a result of cord injury sustained at birth.

Fig. 8–14.—Fracture of spine in mid-dorsal region showing complete separation of vertebrae with hemorrhage into adjacent soft tissues. Intrapartum death.

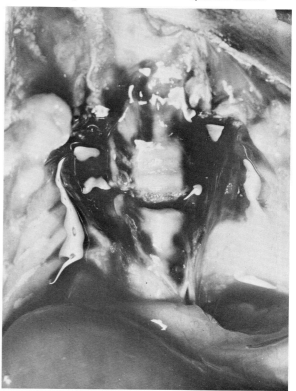

the level of transection is like that of silk, and above, like that of velvet. The injury to the sympathetic nervous system that occurs simultaneously with that to the spinal cord causes absence of perspiration below the transected area. An indelible pencil will fail to make a mark where perspiration is absent but will mark the normal skin.

If the original paralysis was due to edema and mild hemorrhage, recovery may be complete. More often, however, the injury of the nerve cells and tracts is permanent, and only partial improvement occurs. Even though the cord has been completely transected, reflex activity below the point of destruction may be reestablished after a few weeks. Then tonic spasms are common and reflexes in the lower extremities often cause permanent flexion of the hips, knees and ankles. Urine is expelled at intervals, often in association with movement of the extremities. There are no trophic disturbances, and the prognosis for survival and a moderately comfortable existence is much better than when the reflexes are permanently absent.

the spinal canal, the nerves being sheared off and left behind. This has been described as a nerveless cord, but it is of no significance and is only an artifact caused by the method of removal.

Viscera

HEART

The liver and adrenal glands are the only internal organs frequently injured. Rarely, an enlarged spleen that is ruptured or evulsed leads to fatal hemorrhage, but a spleen of normal size is almost never injured. A rare type of injury was observed at the Chicago Lying-in Hospital in a stillborn fetus delivered 2 days after the mother had fallen down a flight of stairs. Fetal movements became imperceptible a short time after the accident, and autopsy revealed blood distending the pericardial cavity (Fig. 8–15). It seems reasonable to assume that the accumulated blood interfered sufficiently with cardiac function to cause death and that it resulted from injury to the maternal abdomen.

LIVER

Although a subcapsular hematoma is the most common form of liver injury, it is seldom seen except following breech delivery. It is usually caused by pressure exerted on the liver during delivery of the head. If it follows cephalic presentations it is usually the result of trauma sustained during attempts at resuscitation. No symptoms are produced as long as the capsule remains intact but later ma-

nipulation of the infant during bathing, feeding or examination often causes the hematoma to rupture; blood escapes into the abdomen and release of pressure permits fresh hemorrhage (Fig. 8–16). The infant frequently becomes exsanguinated from loss of blood into the abdominal cavity and dies before medical aid can be obtained or a diagnosis established. Small hematomas probably disappear without rupturing, although organized clots or areas in the liver suggesting earlier injuries are almost unknown. The small unruptured hematomas occasionally found at autopsy cannot be considered a cause of death.

ADRENAL GLANDS

The central part of the fetal zone of the adrenal gland is composed of anastomosing cords of cells separated by sinusoidal spaces somewhat like those in the liver. When these are dilated, as is common with anoxia or early maceration, the central portion of the gland appears hemorrhagic on gross inspection. Even on microscopic examination this dilatation may be mistaken for hemorrhage by an inexperienced observer.

The statement made by some investigators that the adrenal glands of the newborn are always hemorrhagic is not correct, and hemorrhage into the adrenal is actually uncommon. When hemorrhage does occur, it begins in the central part of the gland and may spread to involve the entire structure. An accumulation of as much as 30–40 ml of blood may remain in the capsule, but with greater bleeding the capsule generally ruptures and blood escapes into the surrounding tissues, producing perirenal hemorrhage (Fig. 8–17). Such hemorrhage is usually unilateral although occasionally both glands are involved.

The mechanism producing adrenal hemorrhage has never been satisfactorily explained, although it is seen most often in infants delivered from a breech position and is generally thought to result from trauma inflicted on the fetal abdomen during delivery of the head. It is rarely accompanied by bleeding in other locations and there is no indication that lowered prothrombin is responsible. The cause of death in infants with such hemorrhage is not clear, especially when only one gland is involved, since insufficient blood is lost to cause death from exsanguination. It has been suggested that destruction of the adrenal gland is responsible for shock to which the infant succumbs. It is possible that involvement of a single gland is coincidental and not related to death. In older infants calcified

Fig. 8–15. — Sagittal section through heart of stillborn showing pericardium distended by blood.

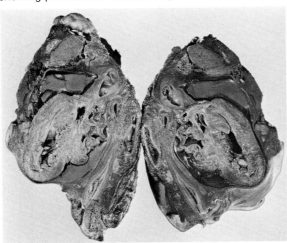

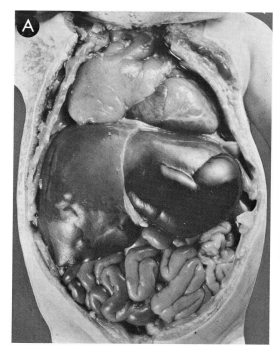
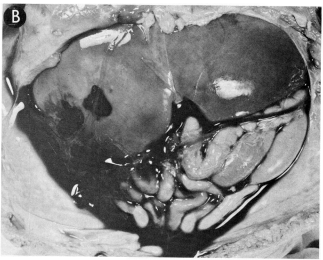

Fig. 8–16.—Subcapsular hematomas of liver. **A,** unruptured. This was not the cause of death. **B,** ruptured hematoma that produced exsanguinating intra-abdominal hemorrhage in infant 2 days of age.

areas that have resulted from earlier hematomas may distend the central portion of the gland, thus giving evidence that all adrenal hemorrhages are not fatal (Fig. 8–18).

Muscles

Muscles are rarely injured during birth. The sternocleidomastoid muscle is sometimes thought to be the site of trauma, but whether a normal muscle can be injured during delivery, whether injury is found only in hypoplastic muscles or whether the supposed injury is a malformation is not definitely known. A small mass of 1–2 cm may be discovered in the sternocleidomastoid muscle soon after birth or may be found first when the child is several days old (Fig. 8–19). It may regress and leave the muscle with normal function, it may persist without producing symptoms or it may cause permanent inclination of the head toward the affected side. Torticollis in older individuals rarely dates from birth, and injury sustained at birth seldom seems responsible for permanent inclination of the head. If injury were the cause, it could be expected to be hyperextension of the neck. Hyperextension is also believed to be the most frequent cause of injury to the brachial plexus. The fact that muscle abnormality is almost never coexistent with brachial

palsy suggests a different origin for the two conditions.

Microscopic examination of such a mass in the sternocleidomastoid muscle reveals atrophy and partial absence of muscle cells with proliferation and hyalinization of intervening connective tissue (Fig. 8–20).

Nerves

Paralysis of the face, upper extremities and, rarely, the diaphragm may be caused by injury of peripheral nerves sustained during delivery.

FACIAL NERVE

Paralysis of the facial nerve is usually unilateral and can be diagnosed from the immobility of the muscles on the affected side. The eye often remains partially open, the nasolabial fold is flattened and the mouth drawn to the opposite side (Fig. 8–21). Symptoms are aggravated during crying. If only part of the nerve fibers are involved, either the upper or lower portion of the face may escape paralysis.

Injury to the nerve is generally peripheral and usually the result of pressure exerted anterior to the ear where the nerve emerges from the skull. In

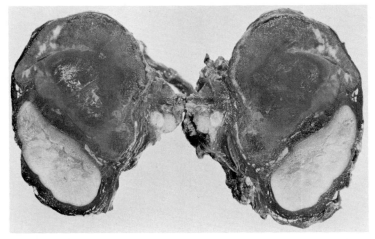

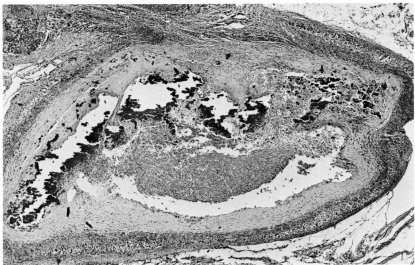

Fig. 8–17 (top).—Extension of adrenal hemorrhage into perirenal tissues. The white masses are halves of the kidney.

Fig. 8–18 (bottom).—Organized and partially calcified hemorrhage in center of adrenal gland from an infant aged 9 months.

a few reported cases it was thought to have been caused by pressure of the side of the head against the shoulder or against a bony prominence in the maternal pelvis, but most injuries result from compression of the nerve by the tip of a forceps blade. Agenesis of the nucleus of the facial nerve in the brain or hemorrhage in this area are possible but extremely rare causes of facial paralysis. Symptoms result from hemorrhage and edema in and around the nerve trunk, and nerve fibers are seldom actually lacerated. Consequently the paralysis is usually temporary, and when the edema subsides and the blood is resorbed, normal function is established. If the injury is a result of intracranial hem-

orrhage, the paralysis may be permanent, but usually the prognosis is excellent and recovery is complete within a few weeks.

Brachial Plexus

Injury to the brachial plexus may be sustained in breech deliveries when strong lateral traction is exerted on the neck in order to deliver the aftercoming head or in cephalic deliveries when similar lateral traction is exerted to extract the shoulders. Excessive digital pressure against the axilla or forceful extension and abduction of the shoulder during delivery of an arm may have the same re-

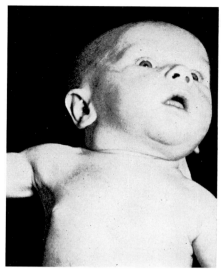

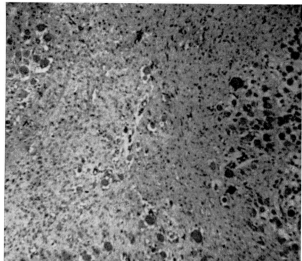

Fig. 8–19 (left).—Mass in right sternocleidomastoid muscle in an infant aged 2 months. No torticollis. (Courtesy Children's Memorial Hospital, Chicago.)

Fig. 8–20 (right).—Sternocleidomastoid muscle showing marked fibrosis and replacement of muscle by connective tissue. Same infant as in Fig. 8–19.

sult. The 5th and 6th cervical nerve roots, those most commonly injured, are responsible for paralysis of the upper arm. The 7th cervical and 1st thoracic nerves may also be involved if the injury is more severe. This increases the extent of the paralysis and the whole arm is affected. If only the lower portion of the plexus is injured, the hand alone is functionless.

Injury usually causes a laceration of the nerve sheath, and the nerve fibers become compressed by edema and hemorrhage. If the nerve fibers are torn the paralysis will be permanent. Generally, however, recovery is complete in a few weeks.

Fig. 8–21.—Paralysis of right side of face from injury to right facial nerve by tip of forceps blade anterior to the ear. (Courtesy Dr. Ralph V. Platou.)

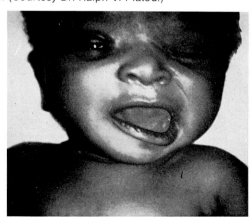

Injury to the 5th and 6th cervical roots leads to the paralysis of the muscles activating the upper arm known as *Erb's palsy* (Fig. 8–22). The affected arm is rotated inwardly at the shoulder and is held in extension and adduction. The forearm is pronated and the palm of the hand is directed posteriorly or posterolaterally. The wrist is often flexed. The paralysis is particularly evident when an attempt is made to elicit a Moro reflex since the affected arm remains motionless. Passive movement reveals absence of activity of the abductors and external rotators of the shoulders and flexors of the elbow. Unless the entire plexus is injured the infant can flex the fingers, and the grasp reflex is normal.

The phrenic nerve is derived in part from the portion of the brachial plexus injured in Erb's palsy, and paralysis of the diaphragm is occasionally associated with paralysis of the upper arm. Recurrent attacks of cyanosis are usually the first symptom to attract notice, and examination reveals decreased excursion of the affected side of the chest and shifting of the mediastinum to that side. The diaphragm seems to retract instead of descend with inspiration, and in rare cases in which the involvement is bilateral, breathing is entirely thoracic and the abdomen does not protrude. Recovery of diaphragmatic function is often slow and susceptibility to respiratory infections is great.

Paralysis resulting from injury to the lower portion of the cervical plexus is known as the *Klumpke type* (Fig. 8–23). It makes up 2–3% of all brachial palsies. The intrinsic muscles of the hand are para-

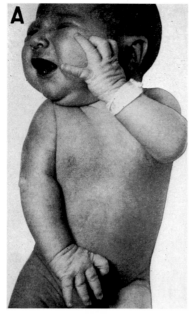
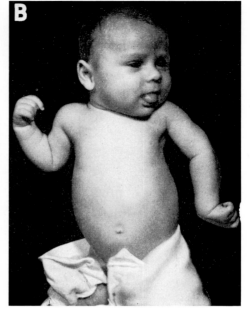

Fig. 8–22.—Erb's palsy. **A,** paralysis of right arm showing characteristic position assumed following injury to 5th and 6th cervical roots of brachial plexus. Infant aged 7 days. **B,** similar paralysis involving left arm of infant aged 3½ months.

lyzed, the long flexors of the wrist and fingers are weak and the hand is often edematous. The grasp reflex is absent. Accompanying sympathetic nerve injury may lead to constriction of the pupil and drooping of the eyelid on the affected side. Recovery is usually prompt, but if the injury is permanent the hand fails to grow properly and contractures of the fingers develop.

Fig. 8–23.—Klumpke type of brachial plexus injury. Only the lower cervical roots are involved and paralysis is limited to the hand. (Courtesy Dr. Ralph V. Platou.)

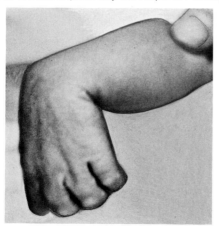

Peripheral Skeleton

CLAVICLE

The clavicles are fractured during delivery more often than any other bones. The breaks, which are located in the center or at the junction of the middle and outer third, occur most frequently in large infants whose shoulders form a temporary obstruction to delivery, although they occasionally are associated with seemingly uneventful births. Crepitation of the clavicle can be felt and activity of the affected side is reduced. The latter is most noticeable when an attempt is made to elicit a Moro reflex. Roentgen investigation may be necessary to establish a diagnosis (Fig. 8–24).

FEMUR AND HUMERUS

The femur and humerus are the only other bones ordinarily fractured during delivery. Fractures are rare with cephalic deliveries but may occur with breech presentation or during an internal version. The fractures are usually located in the middle third of the bone and are ordinarily diagonal (Fig. 8–25). There is usually marked overriding but often little or no lateral displacement. Callus forms rapidly and permanent disability is rare.

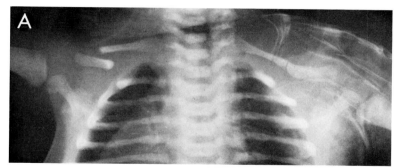

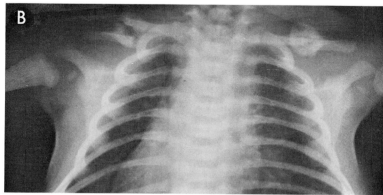

Fig. 8–24.—Bilateral fracture of the clavicles. **A,** at age 2 days right clavicle well aligned; left, severely displaced. **B,** at age 10 days callus deposited around both fractures.

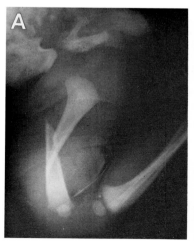
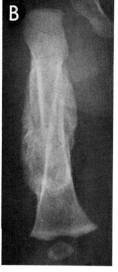

Fig. 8–25.—Fracture of right femur. **A,** at age 1 day. **B,** at age 21 days.

REFERENCES

Buchanan, D. N.: Personal communication.

Butler, N. R., and Bonham, D. G.: *British Perinatal Mortality Survey: Perinatal Mortality* (Edinburgh: E. & S. Livingstone, Ltd., 1960).

Charlewood, G. P.: Aetiology of congenital torticollis and certain associated deformities, J. Obstet. Gynaecol. Br. Emp. 54:499, 1947.

Claireaux, A. E.: Cerebral pathology in the newborn, Guys Hosp. Rep. 108:2, 1959.

Crothers, B., and Putnam, M. C.: Obstetrical injuries of the spinal cord, Medicine 7:41, 1927.

Dekaban, A. S.: *Neurology of Infancy* (Baltimore: Williams & Wilkins Co., 1959).

Everson, T. C., and Cole, W. H.: *Spontaneous Regression of Cancers* (Philadelphia: W. B. Saunders Co., 1966).

Grontoft, O.: Intracerebral and meningeal haemorrhages

in perinatally deceased infants. II. Meningeal haemorrhages, Acta Obstet. Gynecol. Scand. 32:458, 1953.

Hemsath, F. A.: Birth injury of the occipital bone with report of 32 cases, Am. J. Obstet. Gynecol. 27:184, 1934.

Holland, E. L.: Cranial stress in the foetus during labor, J. Obstet. Gynaecol. Br. Emp. 29:551, 1922.

Ingraham, F. D., and Matson, D. D.: Subdural hematoma in infancy, Adv. Pediatr. 4:231, 1922.

Kelly, J. V.: Compression of the fetal brain, Am. J. Obstet. Gynecol. 85:687, 1963.

Morgan, J. E.: Calcification in cephalohematoma of the newborn infant, Am. J. Obstet. Gynecol. 48:702, 1944.

Nasralla, M., Gawronska, E., and Hsia, D. Y. Y.: Studies on the relation between serum and spinal fluid bilirubin during early infancy, J. Clin. Invest. 37:1403, 1957.

Norman, R. M.: Atrophic sclerosis of the cerebral cortex associated with birth injury, Arch. Dis. Child. 19:111, 1944.

Paine, R. S.: Neurologic conditions in the neonatal period, Med. Clin. North Am. 8:576, 1961.

Pierson, R. C.: Spinal and cranial injuries of the baby in breech deliveries, J.A.M.A. 92:217, 1929.

Rubin, A.: Birth injuries: Incidence, mechanisms and end results, Obstet. Gynecol. 23:218, 1964.

Schwartz, P. H.: Birth Injuries of the Newborn (Darien, Conn.: Hafner Publishing Co., 1961).

Smith, L. H.: Blood in the cerebrospinal fluid of newborns, Am. J. Obstet. Gynecol. 28:89, 1934.

Snedecor, S. T., and Wilson, H. B.: Some obstetrical injuries to long bones, J. Bone Joint. Dis. 31A:378, 1949.

Towbin, A.: Spinal cord and brain stem injury at birth, Arch. Pathol. 77:620, 1964.

Yates, P. O.: Birth trauma to the vertebral arteries, Arch. Dis. Child. 34:43, 1959.

INFECTIOUS AGENTS may cause pathologic processes at any time before or after birth, but for the first few weeks following conception, during the period of organogenesis, specific diseases in the sense that they occur later in life do not exist in the fetus. Since blood vessels are rudimentary and leukocytes are not yet being formed, congestion and leukocytosis are never present. Disease is manifested only as a local or general alteration in rate of cell division or maturation and can be identified only when deviations from normal growth patterns are produced. Consequently, malformation or death is the only evidence of disease that can be found in the first 8–10 weeks of intrauterine life.

The first abnormal location in which leukocytes can be observed is the lumen of the pulmonary tree. They may be present there before alveoli begin to develop, and in a fetus as young as 16–18 weeks, weighing only 150–200 gm, polymorphonuclear leukocytes occasionally fill the bronchi and respiratory ducts. In slightly older fetuses they are common (Fig. 9–1). It would be interesting to know the specific circumstances responsible for the presence of leukocytes at this early age.

Are the conditions the same as those that would cause such an exudation at a later age? Can one assume that bacteria have entered the lung by aspiration of infected amniotic fluid and that the

Fig. 9–1.—Lung of 700 gm fetus with leukocytes in respiratory ducts. This is the location of the earliest leukocyte infiltration. An interstitial inflammatory exudate is also present.

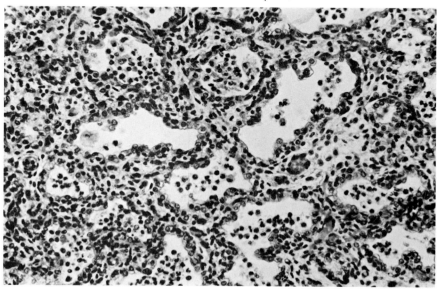

presence of such cells is further proof that the fetus breathes at this age and that the defensive mechanisms of the body are already functioning as they do in a mature individual? Or are cells aspirated directly from the amniotic sac and of maternal rather than fetal origin?

Antenatal Infection

Before birth the only possible route by which harmful substances can reach the fetus is through the uterus. They may enter through the uterine arteries, and as blood circulates through the placenta, bacteria or other noxious agents may penetrate the covering of the villi and enter the fetal bloodstream. It has often been assumed that the covering of the villi has a protective function and exerts a selective action that permits only certain substances to pass from maternal to placental circulations. It seems probable, however, that the protective nature of the villous surface has been overrated and that most bacteria, viruses or parasites in the general circulation of the mother can pass the "placental barrier" and enter the fetal circulation. Whether or not a maternal disease caused by bacteria will be transmitted to the fetus depends largely on whether it is associated with bacteremia.

Theoretically, bacteria can enter the blood circulating in the villi directly from the wall of the uterus without going first into the general maternal circulation. Thus, if the uterus were the site of an acute or chronic infection, direct fetal bacteremia might be produced. In the early weeks of development bacteria have also been described as possibly entering the fetal blood in the villi by first invading the uterine cavity through the lumens of the fallopian tubes or the cervix and penetrating the decidua vera that covers the surface of the chorionic vesicle exposed to the uterine cavity. Such sources of entrance are rare if they exist at all, and bacteria in the blood of the young fetus almost always have their origin in maternal bacteremia.

The older fetus may become infected by contamination of amniotic fluid by bacteria that pass from the cervix either through the intact chorionic and amniotic membranes or into the amniotic sac after the membranes have ruptured. Since amniotic fluid covers the surface of the infant and is inspired and swallowed, bacteria in the fluid may affect the skin, lungs or gastrointestinal tract or may enter the short eustachian tube. Bacteria may also invade the umbilical cord or be found in the blood vessels near the chorionic surface of the placenta and give rise to severe local leukocytic infiltration into amnion, chorion and umbilical cord (see Fig. 3–33). Skin lesions are occasionally present at birth, and swallowed bacteria have been thought responsible for ulceration of the stomach or intestine. Otitis media has been attributed to bacteria present in amniotic fluid, and aspiration and infection in the lungs may be found in conjunction with infection of the middle ears and sinuses. The ears may be affected more often than the lungs though clinically recognized infection is less frequent. Ziai and Haggerty found that 19 of 58 infants with neonatal meningitis also had otitis media when examined at autopsy, the otitis presumably being the source of the meningitis. However, the lungs appear to be more susceptible to bacteria in the amniotic fluid than any other structure, and evidence of infection is usually limited to the pulmonary system. This is true even when fetal blood vessels in the cord and placenta are extensively involved. The liver rarely gives evidence of infection, and if pneumonia were the result of bacteremia, the liver as well as the lungs would be affected.

It has been shown that bacteria are generally present in the amniotic fluid within 6 hours of the onset of labor even when membranes are intact, and following rupture of membranes they are usually present in a much shorter time even though labor has not begun. However, even in the absence of labor, coitus or interference by medical attendants, the amniotic fluid may remain sterile for a long but unpredictable time following large or small tears in the membranes. The fetus becomes infected in relatively few instances of premature rupture of the membranes or long labor, but when pneumonia does originate before birth it is usually preceded by one or both of these conditions. When aspiration of infected fluid leads to infection of the lungs, leukocytes are diffusely distributed in most of the potential air spaces. The involvement is fairly uniform because of the presence of amniotic fluid in all parts of the pulmonary tree. Epithelial cells from the skin surface and other debris are intermixed with leukocytes, but fibrin usually is not present. In the pneumonia that follows aspiration of amniotic sac contents, the infecting organisms are overwhelmingly those of the intestinal tract. Since not all inflammation of the placental membranes or umbilical cord is accompanied by demonstrable bacterial infection, simple aspiration of inflammatory cells must be distinguished from true aspiration pneumonia. In the latter instance inflammatory cells are usually encountered in the peribronchial tissue and alveolar walls as well as in the alveolar spaces.

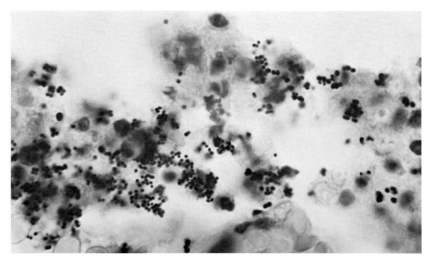

Fig. 9–2.—Staphylococci in alveolar exudate in an infant dying of pneumonia at 4 days of age.

It seems probable that any variety of bacteria, virus or parasite in the maternal blood can at least occasionally pass through the placenta and produce disease in the fetus. In such circumstances the liver is often the site of the principal lesion since blood from the placenta comes to this organ first.

Intranatal Infection

Since the period of labor is included in the intrauterine life of the fetus, almost any of the statements made in the preceding section may apply equally well to this interval. Bacterial contamination of the amniotic fluid is more common during labor than earlier, and pneumonia is observed more often after birth as a result of bacterial infection acquired during labor than it is before birth as a result of an earlier infection. In a few reported cases pneumonia was believed to have been caused by pneumococci transmitted from the maternal blood before or during labor, but such a source of infection is rare, and almost all pulmonary infections in the 1st week of life are caused by aspiration of colon bacilli, fecal streptococci or other enteric organisms (Fig. 9–2) present in infected amniotic fluid.

Meningitis, like aspiration pneumonia, because of the time of onset and the nature of the offending organisms, appears related to contamination during passage through the birth canal. One half of the cases of neonatal meningitis reported by Ziai and Haggerty were in infants under 2 weeks of age; in these cases enteric organisms were frequently isolated, and complications such as prolonged labor, prolonged rupture of the membranes and maternal fever were often present. In the infants over 2 weeks of age such complications were absent, beta-hemolytic streptococci were more commonly isolated and streptococcal pneumonia was more often present.

Neonatal Infection

In 1946 Dr. Agnes MacGregor wrote that infection was a major cause of perinatal death and that it became increasingly important in postnatal life. In her study, infection was responsible for only 3.2% of prenatal deaths, but rose to 30.7% in the first 3 days of life and to 65% in infants who died after that time. These figures from Scotland are fairly old now, and contemporary data show a marked reduction in pneumonia as a cause of early death. For a 5-year period ending in 1966 at the Chicago Lying-in Hospital, pneumonia accounted for only 7% of the deaths among all neonates over 1,000 gm who died in the first 2 weeks of life, and there were no deaths from infection at other sites. For a 5-year period ending in 1969 at the Boston Hospital for Women, among autopsied liveborn infants of more than 20 weeks' gestation, pneumonia accounted for 13.5% of all deaths and 95% of those from infection.

BACTEREMIA.—Bacteremia in the first few days of life is probably more common than is generally recognized. Much of the so-called inanition or dehydration fever so often noted in the 1st week is probably actually due to bacteremia. A study at the Chicago Lying-in Hospital revealed bacteria in the blood of most infants during the period of fever. Usually the defenses of the body are adequate and the organisms do not remain in the blood for more than a brief period; only rarely do they become pathogenic and give rise to septicemia.

SEPTICEMIA.—The newborn is especially susceptible to septicemia for reasons not entirely clear. Antibodies of the 19S class such as are found in gram-negative organisms like *Escherichia coli* do not cross the placenta, but those of the 7S type do. Premature babies have a phagocytic defect, demonstrated by the "skin window" technic of Rebuck and Crowley, but this is not true of full-term infants. The initial infection may be in the umbilicus or gastrointestinal tract but the lungs are the most common site. The symptoms of septicemia are not specific, but the infant usually seems acutely ill. Disinclination to nurse, progressive weight loss, nervous excitability and convulsions are typical. The temperature and leukocyte count are usually elevated but may be subnormal. Severe icterus is often present. In premature infants elevation of the indirect bilirubin may cause kernicterus. The latter is usually an unexpected observation at autopsy and is rarely diagnosed during life since neither the neurologic signs nor the bilirubin levels are sufficiently abnormal to attract attention. The prognosis is poor, many infants dying within 1 week or 10 days of birth. When the umbilicus is the source of infection, evidence can usually be found in this region on both gross and microscopic examination, and pneumonia may be present if the original infection is in the lungs. However, occasionally there may be no evidence of localization, and few pathologic lesions other than petechiae and ecchymotic hemorrhages on serosal surfaces may be found at autopsy. In some studies beta-hemolytic streptococcus was the organism most frequently found in the blood in neonatal sepsis, with the gram-negative organisms, *E. coli* and *Aerobacter aerogenes,* ranking second (Eickhoff *et al.*).

OMPHALITIS.—In modern hospitals omphalitis is infrequent, but in earlier days and even now in some parts of the world it is a common cause of neonatal death. If asepsis is not practiced, organisms may enter the bloodstream directly through the cut end of the umbilical cord vessels or pass through the walls of the vessels into the tissues surrounding the umbilicus. If there is extension into the local tissues, the periumbilical area becomes red and edematous (Fig. 9–3), and the stump of the cord has a foul odor. Pus may exude from around the

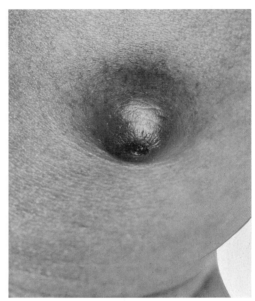

Fig. 9–3.—Mild acute omphalitis. Infant aged 7 days.

cord or from the navel after the cord has dropped off. Such an infection, if not properly treated, may spread to involve much of the abdomen, and the tissues around the navel may become necrotic. In the preantibiotic era septicemia was the usual endresult, which sometimes occurred even though the umbilicus seemed to be only mildly infected. Organisms may travel in the vessel wall or the thrombosed lumen of the umbilical vein and produce local hepatitis or be carried by the bloodstream into the pulmonary and systemic circulations. Although pneumonia usually results from aspiration of infected amniotic fluid, some cases are caused by infections of the umbilical stump, as are also some cases of meningitis, pyoarthritis, myocarditis and so on. In many instances the infant dies of septicemia before localization occurs.

TETANUS.—In some parts of the world it is still the custom to put street dust or manure on the newly cut cord. In such localities not only is the incidence of septicemia high but tetanus is frequent. The organisms, *Clostridium tetani,* like those of diphtheria, remain localized but a powerful exotoxin acts on the central nervous system and symptoms begin to appear 6–14 days after birth. The early symptoms are nonspecific and include hyperirritability and difficulty in swallowing. Nervous manifestations begin with mild twitching and soon develop into extreme tonic spasms involving the entire body. The jaws become fixed and cannot be pried open, the body maintains a boardlike rigidity with back arched, lower limbs extended, arms either extended or tightly flexed and fists clenched. The facial expression is fixed, with the eyes tightly closed, forehead wrinkled and contraction of muscles causing a characteristic sardonic grin. The mortality has been high for treatment was almost entirely unsuccessful until the use of tracheotomy and hyperbaric oxygen began. The organisms produce no specific pathologic lesions although the anoxia resulting from the cardiac and respiratory depression caused by the severe tonic spasm may produce scattered ecchymosis in the thoracic viscera.

PNEUMONIA DUE TO RESUSCITATION.—This is another hazard to which the infant is exposed immediately after birth. With mouth-to-mouth breathing or the attempted expansion of the lungs by someone blowing into a tracheal catheter, there is always a possibility of pulmonary infection. Fortunately, in a modern hospital such procedures are rarely used. However, improperly sterilized resuscitation instruments or contaminated water in the reservoirs of incubators in newborn nurseries have been sources of endemic Pseudomonas and Klebsiella infections of the brain, lung and kidney (Bassett *et al.*). Pneumonia from such a source of infection is usually peribronchial in distribution.

Infection in the 1st Year of Life

The majority of deaths from such causes as premature birth, difficult delivery and malformation take place before the end of the 1st month. Thereafter, infections become the most important cause, even though they are numerically less common than in the 1st month.

In the United States in 1967 there were 3,615 deaths from pneumonia and 388 from intestinal infections in infants under 1 month of age, whereas during the last month of the 1st year there were only 112 from pneumonia and 35 from intestinal infections. They accounted for 7% of infant deaths during the 1st month and almost 25% during the 12th month. In the 12th month pneumonia, upper respiratory infections, malformations and accidents, the four major causes of death, all accounted for an equal number of deaths.

Viral Infections

RUBELLA (GERMAN MEASLES).—The fact that viruses are easily propagated in embryonic tissue has been known for many years, but not until 1942, when Gregg found an association between rubella in early pregnancy and congenital defects of the eyes and heart, was it recognized that virus diseases might be the cause of certain malformations. Following an epidemic of rubella in Australia, Gregg originally reported 78 infants with congenital cataracts, 68 of whose mothers had had rubella early in pregnancy. In all but 16 infants the cataracts were bilateral and in at least 44 there was some clinical evidence of cardiac malformation. Further investigations by Gregg, Swan *et al.* and others soon established the fact that, in the Australian epidemic, women who contracted rubella during the first 2 months of pregnancy almost invariably gave birth to defective children; when the disease occurred later the infant was less often affected, although eye defects were observed in a few instances following its occurrence in the 3d month and ear defects after its occurrence in the 4th month.

According to the Australian investigators, children born following maternal rubella contracted early in pregnancy were often small, poorly nourished and difficult to feed. They were particularly subject to three varieties of defects: cataracts involving the central part of the lens, ear defects producing deaf-mutism because of the almost complete loss of hearing occasioned by a sacculo-ocular type of degeneration, and cardiac disturbances resulting from an interventricular septal defect or patency of the ductus arteriosus. Late eruption of the teeth and abnormalities in enamel production were also reported. Microcephalus and other abnormalities were described in infants with eye or ear defects. Heart disease was rare without accompanying eye or ear malformations. Most of the cataracts were found in children whose mothers had had rubella in the 2d month of pregnancy, and most of the ear abnormalities occurred when the disease was contracted late in the 2d or in the early part of the 3d month.

Since the one in Australia, more recent rubella epidemics in Sweden and the United States have greatly increased our knowledge of the incidence, nature and distribution of the lesions. It is now recognized that maternal rubella in the 1st trimester of pregnancy causes an increased frequency of abortions and stillbirths. The infants that are born alive are small for length of gestation and are thought to have fewer cells per organ than normal infants. The presence of congenital cataract has been amply confirmed, but retinitis has been found almost as often and deafness now seems to be the most common defect. The ductus arteriosus is often patent and other heart lesions include pulmonary

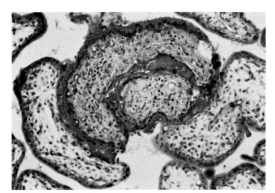

Fig. 9–4.—Placental villi of an aborted fetus with proved rubella infection showing 2 villi with a mild mononuclear infiltration and necrobiosis of the syncytial layer and connective tissue.

stenosis, focal thickening of the coronary artery walls and of the aortic wall in areas of elastic tissue destruction (Campbell).

The histopathology of the early lesions in the lens, ear and heart are chiefly destructive, with necrosis and failure of normal proliferation of affected cells, rather than primarily teratogenic (Esterly and Oppenheimer). Thus, defects of the interventricular septum can be correlated with focal myocardial necrosis. The lesions of rubella characteristically lack evidence of inflammation except in the placenta, where infiltration of lymphocytes appears to be of maternal origin (Fig. 9–4). A rubella syndrome is now recognized that includes thrombocytopenia, myocarditis, hepatosplenomegaly, jaundice, pneumonia and an abnormal radiologic appearance of the long bones. The liver changes have not been well described but include cellular swelling and vacuolization with giant cell formation. In several instances biliary atresia has been present. The lungs are the site of interstitial pneumonia, with infiltration of mononuclear cells responsible for thickening of the alveolar walls. The lesion of the long bones chiefly affects the meta-

physis of the femur, producing radiolucence, linear streaking and irregularity of the metaphyseal epiphysis. Histologically, the metaphysis is normally cellular, but little osteoid is laid down. Table 9–1, from Tondury and Smith, gives a good indication of the distribution of rubella lesions in the young fetus. The virus has been isolated from many affected fetuses.

MUMPS (EPIDEMIC PAROTITIS).—Mumps has been observed in early pregnancy on several occasions without resulting fetal malformations, although a few cases leading to a malformation have been reported. An attempt has been made to correlate positive skin tests with endocardial fibroblastosis but most investigators deny any relationship (Eichenwald and Schinefield).

Although parotid swelling, which may be associated with nonspecific parotitis, has been observed soon after birth, no virologically proved mumps has been demonstrated in newborn or young infants.

Fig. 9–5.—Smallpox in a young infant. **A,** face. **B,** leg. (Courtesy Prof. C. H. Hu and Dr. Robert A. Moore.)

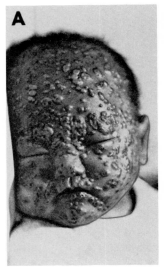
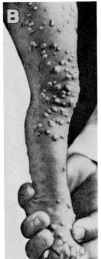

TABLE 9–1.—FREQUENCY AND DISTRIBUTION OF ABNORMALITIES IN FETUSES WITH RUBELLA*

GESTATIONAL AGE AT TIME OF ONSET OF MATERNAL RUBELLA (Weeks)	NUMBER OF FETUSES	PERCENTAGE ABNORMAL	PERCENTAGE OF FETUSES WITH ABNORMALITY IN SPECIFIC ORGANS			
			EYE LENS	HEART	EAR	SKELETAL MUSCLE
0–4	20	80	35	65	12	25
4–8	31	58	48	45	13	16
8–11	6	66	66	50	0	0

*From Tondury, G., and Smith, D. W., J. Pediatr. 68:967, 1966.

VARIOLA (SMALLPOX).—Smallpox may be contracted during intrauterine life although it does not appear to produce fetal malformations. Infants have been born with active or healed skin lesions or have developed lesions soon after birth, depending on the time of the maternal infection (Fig. 9–5). The lesions in the lung, liver, adrenal gland and placenta consist largely of necroses (Fig. 9–6). There is an interstitial nephritis, and confluent pustules in the skin have acute granulation tissue in the underlying dermis. The placenta may have syncytial degeneration and intervillous thrombosis in addition to necrosis.

VACCINIA.—During pregnancy this may produce a lethal infection of the fetus. In 16 case reports assembled by Green *et al.* in which the mothers had been vaccinated at 3–24 weeks of pregnancy, the fetuses died either in utero or soon after birth. The lesions were described as similar to those of variola but the fetuses were often macerated and structur-

al details lost. In one case described subsequently by Aitkens *et al.* in which the mother was vaccinated at 15 weeks' pregnancy, fetal movements stopped at 21 weeks and a macerated fetus of 205 gm was delivered at 23 weeks. White lesions were detected in the liver, heart, lungs and serosa of the small intestine, which were the site of necrosis and calcium deposit. Vaccination of the mother during pregnancy presents a real hazard to the fetus.

VARICELLA (CHICKENPOX).—Antenatal infection with varicella has been recorded in both stillborn and liveborn infants (Garcia; Oppenheimer). In a stillborn fetus large, sharply circumscribed areas of necrosis infiltrated by mononuclear cells were found in the placenta, lungs, kidneys, liver, pancreas and other organs, in addition to the lesions in the skin (Fig. 9–7). In the living newborn infant, as in older children, a papulovesicular rash soon follows conjunctivitis. The rash consists of intraepithelial vesicles that are caused by cellular degener-

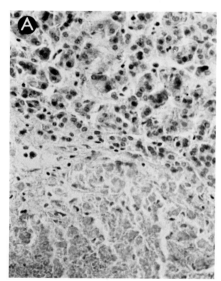
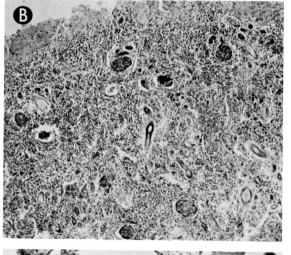
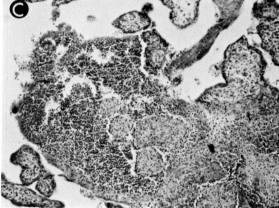
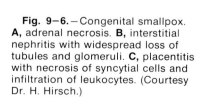

Fig. 9–6.—Congenital smallpox. **A,** adrenal necrosis. **B,** interstitial nephritis with widespread loss of tubules and glomeruli. **C,** placentitis with necrosis of syncytial cells and infiltration of leukocytes. (Courtesy Dr. H. Hirsch.)

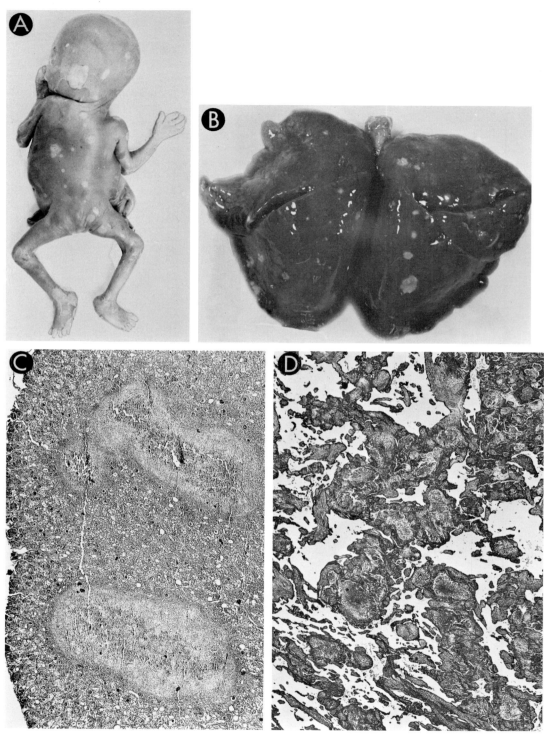

Fig. 9–7.—Chickenpox in 16-week fetus. **A,** diffusely distributed circumscribed skin lesions. **B,** lungs, with grossly visible circumscribed areas of necrosis similar to those found in all organs. **C,** kidney, with similar areas of necrosis. **D,** placenta with multiple areas of necrosis and leukocytic infiltration. (Courtesy Dr. Aparecida Garcia.)

ation and become filled with leukocytes (Fig. 9–8, A). With extension of the process the stratum germinativum disappears and the corium becomes, involved. In some fatal cases small foci of degeneration have been present in the liver and spleen. Intranuclear inclusions may be found in these areas as well as in the skin, esophagus (Fig. 9–8, B), stomach, intestines, lungs, pancreas, adrenal glands, kidneys and Hassall's corpuscles of the thymus. Both Johnson and Cheathem *et al.* found that the endothelial cells of the capillaries and blood vessels often contained inclusions and that such areas were often the site of thrombosis and hemorrhage.

Maternal immunity to both smallpox and chickenpox confers only a temporary immunity on the infant and thereafter the infant is highly susceptible.

HERPES ZOSTER.—Herpes zoster has been reported in at least 10 newborn infants. Pinpoint vesicles have been described more commonly in the sciatic and sacral areas than in any other location. The infection is usually mild and not accompanied by other clinical manifestations. Dorsal root ganglia of the affected nerves contain inclusions but the virus cannot be distinguished from that responsible for varicella.

ACUTE ANTERIOR POLIOMYELITIS.—When the disease in the mother occurs in the 1st trimester, the frequency of abortion appears to be increased, although if the fetus is not aborted, no abnormalities are discernible in the infant at birth. However, if the mother is in an acute stage of the disease at the time, the infant may contract the disease shortly before or after delivery.

Barsky and Beale isolated poliomyelitis type I virus from the meconium of three stillborn fetuses whose mothers had had an acute infection at the time of delivery; however, no pathologic changes attributable to the virus were found in the fetuses at autopsy. Several cases of the disease have been observed in the immediate newborn period, and Bates found almost 60 cases reported before 1955 with symptoms occurring in the 1st month. He reported one infant with symptoms at birth. Two cases were reported by Baskin *et al.* with death on the 7th and 14th days of life, respectively. In the first case the mother was acutely ill at the time of delivery. The infant had fever on the 3d day of life (minimal incubation period usually 5 days), became rapidly worse and before death on the 7th day was extremely flaccid and breathed irregularly. In the second case the mother had symptoms of acute po-

Fig. 9–8.—Chickenpox in an infant aged 4 months. **A,** intradermal vesicle. **B,** intranuclear inclusions in esophageal epithelium. (Courtesy Dr. Eleanor Humphreys.)

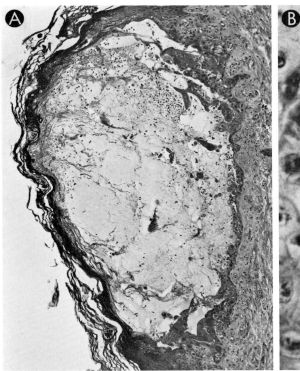
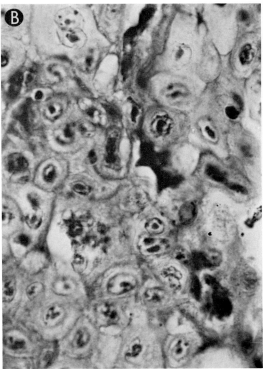

liomyelitis on the 2d day after delivery and the infant had a fever on the 8th day, flaccidity of extremities on the 9th day and died on the 14th day following development of marked flaccid quadriplegia and inability to swallow.

Pathologic changes in these infants were characteristic of those found in older individuals with anterior poliomyelitis. The ganglion cells of the anterior horns of the spinal cord were almost entirely absent and those of the lateral and posterior columns showed foci of degeneration. All parts were infiltrated by inflammatory cells. The basal nuclei and motor areas of the brain also were irregularly degenerated and infiltrated by leukocytes. Perivascular cuffing of blood vessels by lymphocytes was present throughout the brain. The cardiac muscle of one infant showed multiple areas of degeneration. Since immunization against poliomyelitis is now possible, it is hoped that prepregnancy immunization will prevent the crippling effects of the disease in the newborn as well as the older child.

RUBEOLA (MEASLES).— Measles may be transmitted from mother to fetus. If the mother is exposed late in pregnancy, she and the infant may develop the disease simultaneously some time after delivery or the infant may be born with a well-developed exanthem. Dyer reported 24 cases of measles complicating pregnancy. Of nine infants born while the mother had the disease, six were at or near term, and of these, three had measles at birth or contracted it within 2 days. None died. Since passive immunity derived from the mother lasts for about 6 months, measles seldom causes death in the first months of life. Denton, summarizing the pathology of 100 fatal cases in older children, found no specific changes in the tissues; the deaths were primarily due to secondary bacterial infections. Syncytial giant (Warthin-Finkeldy) cells are formed in lymphoid tissue and in the lungs (giant cell pneumonia) only early in the disease or in instances of abnormalities of the immunologic defense system.

CYTOMEGALIC INCLUSION DISEASE (SALIVARY GLAND VIRUS INFECTION).— Salivary gland virus is a species-specific virus found widely in laboratory animals as well as in animals in the wild state. It is also common in man, the infection taking one of four forms: (1) that of adults, with absence of symptoms and limitation of pathologic changes to salivary glands; (2) that of children or adults, with spread to lungs or intestine, in the presence of debilitating disease from other causes or with acquired or induced immunologic deficiencies; (3) that of infancy or early childhood, with involvement of

lungs or intestine, with death from either the viral infection or associated disease; and (4) that of the fetus, with production of a generalized, usually fatal disease.

Infection occurring as a result of intrauterine transmission of the virus is, clinically, one of the important forms of the disease. Isolation of the virus from the cervix of pregnant women has been accomplished in a number of cases, and a significant fraction of some population groups harbors the virus in the genital tract. Fortunately, the fetuses are rarely involved. At the Boston Hospital for Women, cytomegalic inclusion cells were identified in the cervix of a pregnant woman and the virus was subsequently isolated from the same source. Her infant was delivered normally and without recognizable disease.

The virus is responsible for prenatal destruction of erythrocytes, which causes a hemolytic anemia and stimulates production of erythrocytes in normal and abnormal locations in the body, producing a disease similar to Rh-erythroblastosis. The early jaundice, widespread ectopic erythropoiesis, indirect hyperbilirubinemia and erythroblastemia are the same in both conditions. Purpuric hemorrhages in the skin are more commonly present at birth in cytomegalic inclusion disease than in erythroblastosis, and anemia may not be as severe but progresses rapidly in the early days of life. Death usually occurs before or soon after birth. More mildly affected infants who survive suffer from gradual progression of the disease with jaundice, hepatomegaly and chronic encephalitis, the latter leading to microcephaly and mental deficiency.

The characteristic pathologic findings are single large, sharply marginated, dark-staining inclusion bodies in the enlarged nucleus of enlarged cells. They are constantly present in great numbers in the kidney, especially in convoluted tubules, and almost always in portal bile ducts in the liver. They are also frequently present in bronchial epithelium, and desquamated into the alveoli of the lungs, and in the pancreas; they have been observed occasionally in most other organs (Fig. 9–9). Although erythropoiesis is ordinarily severe in liver, spleen, kidneys and other organs, necrosis or other evidence of local response is generally limited to the brain and liver. When mildly affected, the infant may present clinical features of neonatal hepatitis (Weller and Hanshaw). In such cases the liver contains parenchymal multinucleated giant cells but only rare inclusions. With severe involvement the subependymal zone of the lateral ventricles may show diffuse areas of necrosis, cellular infiltra-

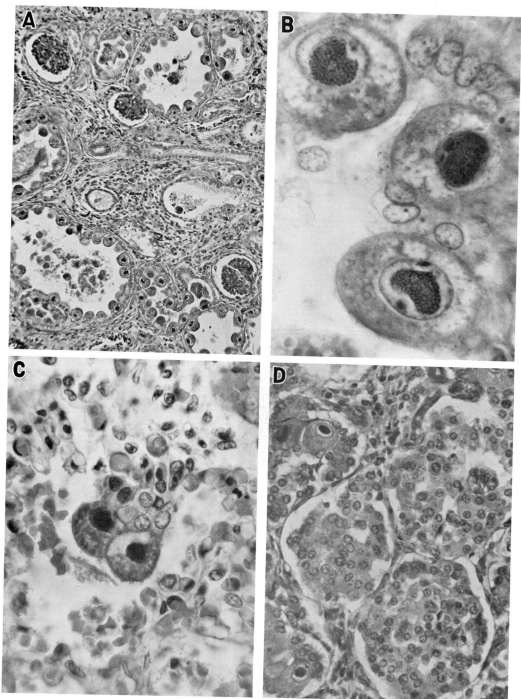

Fig. 9–9.—Cytomegalic inclusion disease. **A,** cells lining convoluted tubules of the kidney have large intranuclear inclusions, margination of the nuclear chromatin and granularity of the cytoplasm. **B,** high power view of cells with inclusions. **C,** lung showing similar cells in alveoli. **D,** pancreas with similar cells in acinar epithelium. (Courtesy Drs. D. F. Cappell and M. N. McFarlane.)

tion and calcification. Cells with typical inclusions may be found in these areas or they may be present as isolated cells in otherwise normal tissue. The ventricles are often dilated, and in the only case observed at the Chicago Lying-in Hospital, several hundred milliliters of fluid had to be removed from the head before delivery could be accomplished. The location of the calcification in the walls of the lateral ventricles is characteristic, and the diagnosis can sometimes be made by x-ray examination of the head.

Since the abnormal cells in the renal tubules are often desquamated and passed in the urine, examination of urine sediment will usually reveal them for several weeks after birth. They have been observed in gastric washings, probably having their origin in swallowed bronchial secretions. The virus has been demonstrated in the urine for as long as 26 months after birth.

The placenta of affected infants is often greatly enlarged and is similar in gross and microscopic appearance to that in erythroblastosis fetalis (Fig. 9–10). Occasional large cells with cytoplasmic inclusions have been recognized in the villi.

Similar cells have not been found in association with any other virus. In older children they may be present in the salivary glands without producing symptoms, a fact responsible for the name. They have been reported in the lungs in association with *Pneumocystis carinii* or other infections and in intestinal mucosa of children and adults suffering from intestinal infections.

Medearis' table indicates the clinical frequency and anatomic distribution of the lesions in disseminated cytomegalic disease in newborn infants (Table 9–2).

HERPES SIMPLEX. — Bass in 1952 described the first case of what appears to have been a fatal generalized herpes simplex virus infection in a young infant. He had not seen a similar histologic appearance previously and did not know its cause but commented that "if one were forced to select the etiologic agent from a group of well-established filtrable viruses, the herpetic virus would be favored as the most probable causative factor in this singular disease." Zuelzer's subsequent isolation of the virus from infants with identical lesions proved his supposition to be correct.

Although capable of causing only minor epithelial infections in adults, a fatal viremia may occur in young infants, especially prematures. The virus may enter through the umbilicus, conjunctiva, skin or mucous membranes, usually during delivery, although in a few cases transplacental infection has been established (Mitchell and McCall). Spread from other sources seems much less likely, particularly since it has been established that herpes genitalis and the disseminated disease in the newborn are of a similar antigenic type (type II) but are different from the usual perioral strain (type I). The site of original infection may not be apparent and symptoms do not develop until the virus has propagated in the liver and other organs.

Zuelzer described the clinical picture in the newborn as having a characteristic onset at 5–7 days of age with fever or hypothermia, icterus, lethargy, vomiting, dyspnea, cyanosis and rapidly developing circulatory collapse. Thick yellow mucus often collects in the throat, and bleeding may occur because of hypoprothrombinemia due to liver insufficiency or to disseminated intravascular coagulation. The spleen and liver are always enlarged. The presence of skin or mucous membrane lesions together with the other symptoms suggests a diagnosis of septicemia.

Older infants may develop viremia following herpetic stomatitis, but the visceral lesions are limited in distribution and the disease is less severe than in the newborn.

In the newborn with fatal disease, lesions are most often found in the liver, adrenals, lungs, brain, esophagus, tongue and colon; less often they are present in the spleen, lymph nodes, stomach, bone marrow, conjunctivae, pharynx and heart (Wheeler and Huffines). The liver is enlarged and generally riddled with pale yellow, firm, necrotic nodules 1–6 mm in diameter. These may become confluent and almost the entire liver may become necrotic. Affected cells first show swelling, reduced affinity for acid stains, reticulation and vacuolization, which is followed by disintegration of the cytoplasm and disruption of the cell membrane. The reticulum framework and endothelium of the sinus-

Fig. 9–10.—Placenta of macerated fetus with cytomegalic inclusion disease showing infection and foci of stromal calcification.

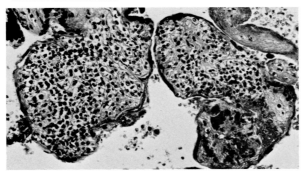

TABLE 9–2.—CLINICAL AND PATHOLOGIC CHARACTERISTICS
OF 42 NEWBORN INFANTS WITH CYTOMEGALIC
INCLUSION DISEASE*

SYMPTOMS	No.	%
Hematologic abnormalities	31	74
Jaundice	30	71
Hepatosplenomegaly	26	62
Prematurity	23	55
Central nervous system abnormalities	16	38

SITE OF INCLUSIONS	No.	%
Kidney	37	88
Liver	33	79
Lung	29	69
Pancreas	24	57
Thyroid	18	43
Brain	10	24
Salivary gland	8	19

*Modified from Medearis, D. N., Jr., Pediatrics 19:467, 1957.

oids and larger vessels become necrotic. The devastated areas may involve part of a single lobule or many lobules (Fig. 9–11, A). There is no cellular reaction, but a large share of the marginal cells contain intranuclear inclusions. These may be large, sharply circumscribed, acidophilic, slightly granular masses surrounded by a clear zone inside the nuclear membrane (Fig. 9–11, B), or, in less recently affected cells, the entire nucleus may be occupied by the inclusion. The cytoplasm of the affected cells is sometimes increased in amount and may contain small acidophilic granules.

The lesions in the adrenal glands are similar to those in the liver. They often extend from the medulla to the surface, are sharply delineated, have complete necrosis of cells and stroma and are surrounded by cells with inclusions (Fig. 9–11, C). Lesions in the brain consist of widespread, discrete areas of necrosis especially common in the basal ganglia and brain stem. There is usually little cellular reaction, and cells containing inclusions are found at the margins of the necrotic areas. Occasionally the brain is the only organ in the body to be affected. Cells with inclusions have also been found in sympathetic ganglia (Fig. 9–12).

COXSACKIE INFECTION.—In older children and adults Coxsackie virus infections have been reported as epidemic pleurodynia (Bornholm disease) or have been recognized as sporadic cases. The symptoms are usually mild and short-lived, and the disease is never fatal. It may be manifested only as a nonspecific febrile illness or may be accompanied by aseptic meningitis, myalgia and, rarely, pericarditis.

The symptoms in young infants are more severe than in adults, as is true of many viral infections, especially if contracted antenatally or during delivery. Among 54 cases summarized by Kibrick and Benirschke 45 infants had myocarditis, clinically or pathologically, 12 of whom recovered. All of 29 autopsied had histologic evidence of myocarditis, 76% had meningoencephalitis, 11% had pancreatitis and 16% had adrenal involvement. Fever, feeding difficulty and lethargy were the most common symptoms, with respiratory and cardiac disturbances occurring in about one half and evidence of central nervous system irritation, hepatosplenomegaly and sudden collapse in one third. Meningitis was found in several infants who had no suggestive symptoms, which indicates that it occurs more often than clinical observation would suggest.

Coxsackie virus, group B, type 4 was most commonly isolated although a few cases were caused by types 2 and 3. Isolation was accomplished by animal inoculation; an unexpected finding in connection with inoculation with type 4 virus was severe destruction of anterior horn cells indistinguishable from poliomyelitis. This seems to verify the original impression that Coxsackie virus in man is capable of producing poliomyelitis-like lesions associated with muscle weakness.

The lesions in the liver are usually striking; they vary from irregular areas of mild necrosis, most often located near the central vein, to a widespread

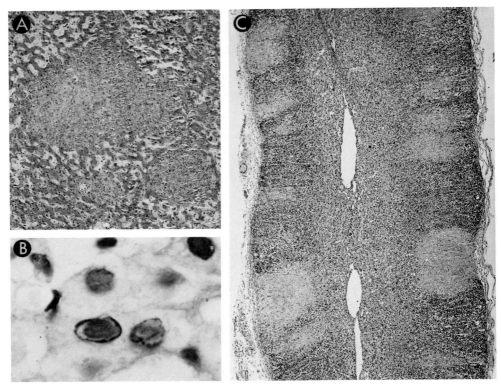

Fig. 9—11.—Herpes simplex virus infection. **A,** liver with circumscribed nonreactive zones of necrosis. **B,** characteristic intranuclear inclusion body with margina-tion of the nuclear chromatin. **C,** adrenal gland with zones of necrosis. (Courtesy Dr. Philip Graff.)

devastating necrosis in which only a few cells immediately adjacent to the portal areas remain unaffected (Fig. 9–13, A). The necrotic areas are less well circumscribed than those of herpes infections, the adrenal glands are less often involved and inclusions are usually absent.

Fig. 9—12.—Herpes simplex virus infection showing sympathetic ganglion with intranuclear inclusions.

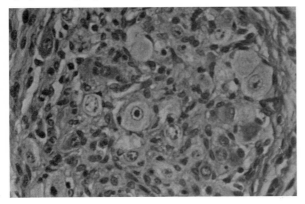

Since myocarditis, which is rare in young infants, has been found in nearly every case of proved Coxsackie infection, it might be justifiable to consider every case of myocarditis in the newborn to be due to this cause until proved otherwise. The lesion is focally destructive and is accompanied by an infiltration of mononuclear cells (Fig. 9–13, B).

INFLUENZA. — Placental transmission of the influenza virus was described as a cause of morbidity and mortality in fetuses and newborn infants by Maksimovich and Kornyushenko. They isolated the virus from the lungs of infants whose mothers had had the disease shortly before delivery as well as from some whose mothers presented no clinical evidence of infection and were considered to have had a latent form of the disease. Symptoms were nonspecific, consisting principally of respiratory distress. Microscopic changes, which were limited to the lungs, consisted of atelectasis, congestion and mild leukocytic infiltration. Occasionally there were hyaline membranes in the alveoli, and in slightly older infants, bronchial epithelium showed areas of hyperplasia. Eosinophilic cytoplasmic

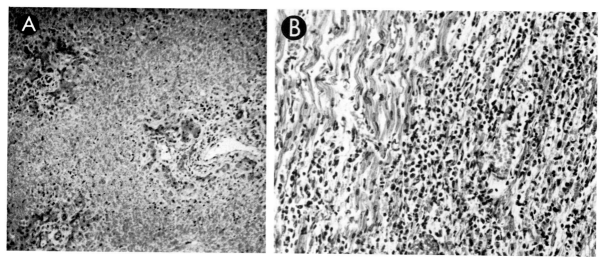

Fig. 9–13.—Coxsackie B infection in the newborn. **A,** liver with devastating necrosis. **B,** severe myocarditis with mononuclear infiltration. (Courtesy Dr. Kurt Benirschke.)

bodies and basilar nuclear inclusions similar to those reported in adults were found in cells lining the bronchi and alveoli.

When pregnant mice were inoculated with influenza virus Group A strain PR$_8$, the virus was regularly isolated from the decidua and lungs of the fetuses and newborn animals. It was postulated that viremia in the mother is associated with fixation of the virus in the decidua, secondary passage into the amniotic fluid and infection of the lungs

Fig. 9–14.—Inclusion blennorrhea. **A,** diffuse inclusion. **B,** small initial inclusion body. **C,** large inclusion adjacent to nucleus. (Courtesy Dr. Phillips Thygeson.)

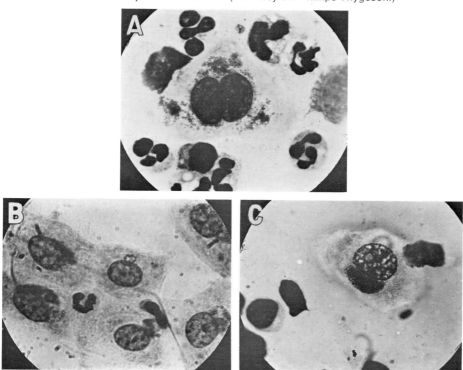

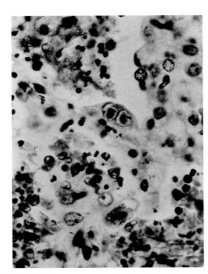

Fig. 9—15.—Virus pneumonia in infant aged 2 weeks. Two cells with typical inclusion bodies in wall of an alveolus. (Courtesy Dr. Ernest W. Goodpasture.)

arising from inhaled viral particles. According to Maksimovich and Kornyushenko, the virus can be demonstrated regularly in cells from the lungs by the use of acridine-orange.

Coffey and Jessup, in a prospective, controlled study of mothers who contracted influenza during pregnancy, found twice as many congenital malformations among their offspring as in those of control mothers without the disease. Anencephaly and spina bifida were encountered most frequently; these observations were made in Ireland where these malformations are more common than in the United States. As might be expected, malformations were proportionately highest in those mothers who contracted the disease in the 1st trimester of pregnancy.

INCLUSION BLENNORRHEA. — This is an acute conjunctivitis that may affect infants as well as adults. Caused by a virus of the psittacosis – lymphogranuloma venereum group, it is believed to be transmitted to the fetus from the mother during delivery. Thygeson and Mengert found a high correlation between this form of conjunctivitis in newborn infants and the presence of identical inclusion bodies in the cervical squamous epithelium of the mother. In the mother the disease is usually symptomless. The incubation period of the conjunctivitis is 5–10 days, onset is abrupt and the rapidly developing infection especially involves the lower lid. The acute stage lasts 10–14 days then gradually becomes less intense. It is self-limiting and never produces blindness, but the conjunctiva may not return to normal for many months. According to Thygeson and Mengert, biopsy material taken at the onset of the disease shows round cell infiltration and great increase in the thickness of the conjunctiva. The infectious units are elementary bodies with an individual diameter of about 0.25 μ. They may be free in the exudate but are more often observed in masses in the superficial layers of the conjunctival epithelium (Fig. 9–14). They are morphologically identical to those of trachoma although, according to Julianelle and co-workers, the

Fig. 9—16.—Diffuse, presumably viral, pneumonia with a mononuclear exudate in a newborn. *Inset,* intranuclear inclusion body in an alveolar cell of same lung.

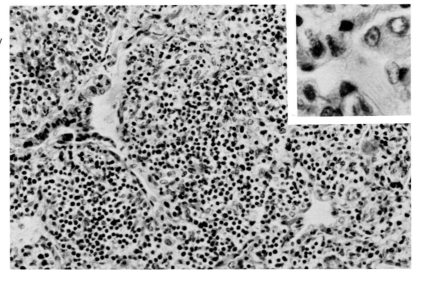

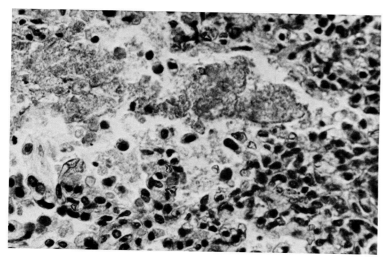

Fig. 9–17.—Adenovirus infection of the lung with hyperchromatic, hyperplastic nuclei and intra-alveolar masses of necrotic cells.

virus of inclusion blennorrhea of the newborn manifests itself in the adult as swimming pool conjunctivitis and is unrelated to trachoma. The disease in the newborn may be differentiated from gonorrhea by delay of onset for a week or more after birth, the presence of a pseudomembrane, the absence of gonococci and the presence of cellular inclusions. The finding of inclusion bodies is pathognomonic since trachoma never affects newborn infants.

VIRAL PNEUMONIA.—Although many atypical pneumonias of children and adults are thought to be caused by viruses, inclusion bodies have rarely been identified. Goodpasture and co-workers reported several cases of pneumonia in infants whose lungs contained large acidophilic intranuclear inclusions following measles or whooping cough. They also reported inclusions in a 2-week-old infant who had had no other known disease. The nuclei were not appreciably enlarged but the inclusions were centrally placed and surrounded by a clear zone, and chromatin was condensed around the nuclear membrane (Fig. 9–15). An identical picture was described by Chany *et al.* and Sohier *et al.* in fatal adenovirus infections in young infants. Both groups described penetrating necrosis of the lung parenchyma and of the tracheal and bronchial epithelium. Sohier *et al.* also described lesions in the heart, kidney tubules and brain. Most fatal cases are in the very young. Suggestive lesions were observed in a 2-day-old premature infant (Fig. 9–16) delivered at the Boston Hospital for Women, whose placenta had marked inflammation of the membranes. In cases of adenovirus, intra-alveolar necrosis and large atypical cells may be the main histologic features (Fig. 9–17).

Adams reported a few cases in which cytoplasmic inclusions were found in the bronchial epithelium of the lungs in association with generalized pneumonitis (infection of the air sacs, bronchi and trachea). The infection was attributed to a virus because of the presence of a few inclusions. These, described as round or oval, sharply circumscribed acidophilic masses often associated with local proliferation of bronchial epithelium, were identified in throat smears as well as in sections of tissue obtained at autopsy. The disease was stated to occur both sporadically and epidemically in both premature and full-term infants. No virus was identified.

Bacterial Infections

Colon bacilli, streptococci and staphylococci, by passage through the gastrointestinal tract, lungs or skin, may all produce sporadic or epidemic disease during infancy. In the last few years staphylococci that are resistant to antibiotics have become an important hazard to infants in newborn nurseries and to those recently discharged. Most of the cases follow colonization of the skin by a virulent, often antibiotic-resistant "hospital strain" (Beaven and Bussey). The frequency of staphylococci as a cause of pneumonia early in life was emphasized by the isolation of this organism in 60% of lung punctures from affected infants under 2 years of age (Mimica *et al.*). The pneumonia is frequently accompanied by abscesses, pneumatocele and empyema. Epidemics of diarrhea may be due to contamination of milk or water by many different organisms.

TYPHOID FEVER.—Abortion or stillbirth is report-

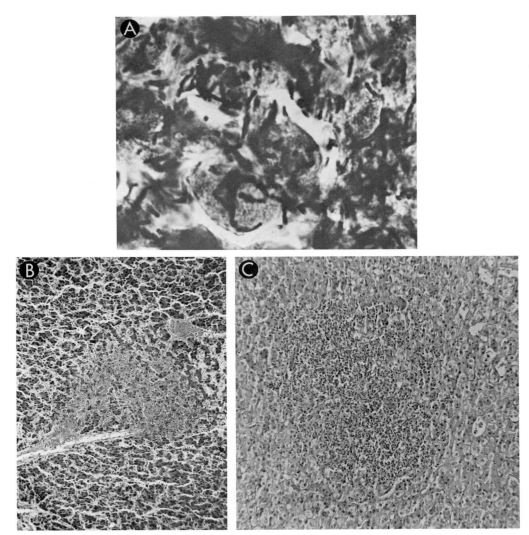

Fig. 9–18.—Listeriosis. **A,** pleomorphic organisms shown in silver stain from same area as *B*. **B,** liver from 17-day-old infant with areas of necrosis without leukocytic infiltration. **C,** liver from 5-day-old infant showing localized leukocytic infiltration. This is interpreted as an older lesion than that shown in B. (**A** and **B,** courtesy Dr. Rita Cardosa; **C,** courtesy Dr. K. Aterman.)

ed to occur in about half of the women who have typhoid fever during pregnancy. The reasons generally given are the ill effects of high maternal temperature or toxins in the maternal blood, although at times fetal septicemia can be demonstrated by recovery of organisms from the blood of the fetus. Intestinal lesions are not ordinarily produced. An infant born alive with the disease is usually feeble and generally dies in a short time. In about half of the pregnancies the fetus does not seem to be affected by the maternal disease although its Widal reaction may be positive.

Typhoid fever is rare in early infancy but, when present, is generally in the form of septicemia without intestinal lesions.

PARATYPHOID, SHIGELLA AND SALMONELLA.—Infections with all of these organisms have been observed in newborn infants whose mothers had the infection when they were born. Infants may recover although they often die of septicemia produced by these bacteria. Salmonella meningitis may appear in early infancy with no overt diarrheal symptoms (Smith and Landing). It carries a high mortality, and residual neurologic damage is common in survivors.

HEMOPHILUS INFLUENZAE.—This organism is the

most common cause of bacterial meningitis in infants (Smith and Landing). It produces destructive lesions in the brain through its tendency to cause vascular thromboses but may also produce diffuse neuronal damage or local suppurative encephalitis. Mortality is high. It may also cause otitis media and lower respiratory tract infections.

LISTERIOSIS.—*Listeria monocytogenes* affects wild and domestic animals as well as man throughout the world, and although it is assumed that the disease in man is transmitted from animals, the manner of infection is not known. The disease occurs at all ages and has been classified into six types, one of which is granulomatous sepsis of the newborn. The child is infected in utero or during delivery by a mother who harbors the bacteria but remains clinically well. In a case observed by Aterman, identical organisms were obtained from the maternal vagina and the fetus.

L. monocytogenes is a motile, pleomorphic grampositive rod 2–3 μ long and 0.5 μ wide and is strongly argentophilic (Fig. 9–18, A). Animal inoculation or fluorescent antibody technic is required for positive identification.

The infant may be stillborn or may die soon after birth. Symptoms are not specific and the commonly associated meningoencephalitis may lead to a diagnosis of birth injury or a disturbance secondary to intrauterine anoxia. Treatment is with sulfonamides and antibiotics, but the mortality rate in recognized cases is about 30%.

At autopsy the characteristic gross findings are granulomatous areas of necrosis in the meninges (Fig. 9–19) and occasionally in the brain, with innumerable small yellow foci of necrosis in the liver, spleen, adrenal glands and lungs. On microscopic examination miliary foci of necrosis may be found in almost all organs. In early stages the lesions may be free of leukocytes and consist only of areas of necrosis having a peculiar coagulated appearance (Fig. 9–18, B), but in later stages they are gradually infiltrated by mononuclear and polymorphonuclear cells (Fig. 9–18, C). The same granulomatous lesions are found occasionally in the placental villi and membranes in cases of disseminated disease.

DIPHTHERIA.—Löffler's bacilli are often present in the vagina of women with diphtheria. The infant may contract the disease during passage through the vagina and should be treated prophylactically if the mother has diphtheria at delivery. If the infant becomes infected, the throat, umbilicus or vulva may be coated with a firm white membrane from which organisms can be recovered. Death may occur through suffocation or pneumonia if the upper airway is involved, but if the umbilicus is the principal site of infection, a toxic myocarditis may cause death; this may be recognizable pathologically only if the heart muscle is stained for fat.

GONORRHEA.—Ophthalmia neonatorum is caused in most instances by the gonococcus, although the virus of inclusion blennorrhea and bacteria, including pneumococci, staphylococci, streptococci and Morax-Axenfeld diplobacilli, are occasionally responsible. While contamination of the eye with vaginal mucus containing gonococci is the usual source of infection, in a few reported cases the organisms were believed to have been transmitted through the placenta because of the presence of gonococcic septicemia or the occurrence of the disease following delivery by cesarean section.

Gonorrheal ophthalmia can usually be prevented by the instillation of a silver solution or penicillin ointment into the eyes immediately after birth.

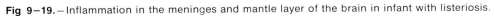

Fig 9–19.—Inflammation in the meninges and mantle layer of the brain in infant with listeriosis.

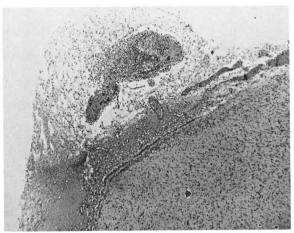

Organisms that are not destroyed penetrate the conjunctival epithelium and cause congestion, edema and purulent exudation. In severe cases the cornea becomes ulcerated and blindness results. The diagnosis is established by growing the organisms in appropriate culture media. In smears made directly from the exudate the organisms appear as large intracellular gram-negative diplococci of characteristic coffee-bean shape. They must be differentiated from staphylococci which, after ingestion by leukocytes, lose their ability to retain the gram stain and appear gram-negative (Hansman).

Gonorrheal arthritis has been observed soon after birth both with and without a conjunctival infection.

Infections are now rare in the United States because of regulations requiring the instillation of prophylactic solutions into the eyes immediately after birth. Chemical conjunctivitis may follow the use of such drugs, especially if the eyes are not properly washed following instillation. Such conjunctivitis must be differentiated from that caused by gonococci. The secretion is usually serous, is of shorter duration and does not contain organisms.

BRUCELLOSIS. – The organisms of undulant fever often cause abortion in cattle but there is little evidence that they do so in man. The fetus is infected only when the maternal disease is in an early stage and few such cases have been observed in human beings during pregnancy. Williams reported a woman living in Malta in whom the disease developed in the 8th month of pregnancy. One month later she delivered an infant whose temperature promptly rose to 103 F and whose blood contained agglutinins in a titer of 1:500. There was no contact between mother and infant after delivery and the infant recovered. Hagebusch and Frei reported recovering organisms from abortuses and also from colostrum. They believed that infection of the child before birth or during delivery was possible and was more severe and more difficult to treat than milk-borne infections acquired later in life. Other investigators reporting cases in very young infants have also considered the possibility of intrauterine infection, although it could rarely be proved because the infants had postnatal contact with the mothers. When the disease appears later in infancy, the course is relatively benign.

TUBERCULOSIS. – There are few cases in which tubercle bacilli are known to have been transmitted through the placenta and to have produced tuberculosis in the fetus. In most of those that have been substantiated the mother had fulminating pulmonary or miliary tuberculosis and usually died of the disease soon after delivery. The rarity of congenital tuberculosis is doubtless a result of the infrequency with which tubercle bacilli are present in the maternal blood except when the disease is extremely severe.

When tuberculosis does exist in the fetus, lesions are usually disseminated throughout the body. It has been suggested that bacteria might be present in the amniotic fluid and that aspiration of infected fluid by the fetus might result in lesions primary in the lungs, but in most instances the umbilical vein is the site of entry and the liver is the organ most severely involved. Tubercles may be several millimeters in diameter. They may be similar to those found at other age periods, consisting of giant cells, epithelioid cells and lymphocytes, but are more often "soft tubercles" with foci of necrosis and little tissue reaction. Occasionally, true caseation may be present.

Since the disease is rarely evident at birth, placentas of affected infants have seldom been examined but the infection has been described as beginning in an intervillous space as a thrombus containing Mycobacterium tuberculosis with later development into a necrotic tubercle. If the fetal vessels draining the area become thrombosed, the disease might not reach the fetus, a fact that would explain the reportedly greater frequency of placental than fetal tuberculosis.

Most infants reported to have had tuberculosis have survived several months, and their contact with the mother or any other tuberculous person after birth must be excluded before the infection can be assumed to be of prenatal origin.

Tuberculosis in the 1st year of life is now very rare due to effective detection and control programs in maternal health clinics. When the young infant is infected by someone in his environment, discovery of the disease is often delayed because specific symptoms are absent. Because of the relative lack of immunity in young infants a diffuse spread throughout the lung parenchyma of tuberculous pneumonia and the development of generalized miliary tuberculosis are relatively more common than in older individuals. In miliary tuberculosis these are widely disseminated in the lungs, liver, spleen, lymph nodes, bone marrow and central nervous system. Occasionally, symptoms of meningitis are the first evidence of the disease. The widespread nature of the disease is usually responsible for early death.

LEPROSY. – The organisms of leprosy may be found in the placenta and umbilical cord, but if they reach the fetus they seem to be effectively destroyed. A negligible percentage of infants separated from their mothers immediately after delivery develop the disease. None of the reported cases of congenital leprosy has been supported by careful bacteriologic examination. It has been reported that in over 1,000 births at the Culion leper colony there were no cases of congenital leprosy. The earliest lesion observed was a white macule in an infant 8 months of age, which became positive for *Mycobacterium leprae* 10 months later. King and Marks reviewed 52 pregnancies of patients with leprosy and found aggravation of the disease in 18 of 23 patients not receiving sulfone and in only 6 of 23 on maintenance doses of sulfone. No fetuses were affected.

Other Infections

SYPHILIS.— Congenital syphilis results from infection of the fetus with *Treponema pallidum* before birth. The mother must be infected before the disease can be acquired by the fetus, although it is possible for impregnation and infection to take place at the same time. The organisms are highly motile, are $10-15\ \mu$ long and consist of $10-15$ spirals. The rotary movement made possible by their shape aids in their passage from the maternal circulation through the walls of the villi into the fetal circulation. Since the liver is the first organ with which they come in contact, it is the first and often the most severely affected organ. Organisms can be demonstrated there more constantly than in any other part of the body (Fig. 9–20).

Infection of the fetus seems to occur rarely before the 5th month of pregnancy. This conclusion is based on two pieces of evidence. First, the incidence of abortion is no greater among syphilitic than nonsyphilitic women, and organisms are rarely demonstrable. Second, if antisyphilitic treatment is begun before the 5th month of pregnancy the child is usually normal at birth.

Whether or not the child of a syphilitic woman will be affected depends largely on the stage of the maternal infection at the time of conception and on the treatment during pregnancy. A woman who has been adequately treated before conception and is not reinfected during pregnancy will give birth to a normal child. A woman who has active syphilis at the time of conception or acquires an infection during pregnancy and is not treated will usually have an affected child. In a study including women in all stages of the disease Roberts reported an incidence of infected infants of only 2.2% among 1,459 mothers thought to have been treated adequately during pregnancy, 16.4% among 996 inadequately treated, and 38% among mothers receiving no therapy.

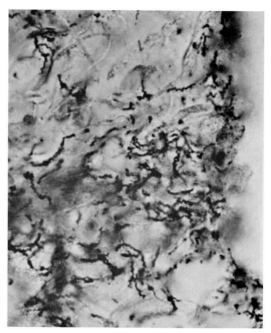

Fig. 9–20.—*Treponema pallidum* in fetal liver.

Syphilis may cause intrauterine death of the fetus during the last trimester of pregnancy, the infant may be born alive with symptoms of the disease, or clinical manifestations of the disease may not appear until after birth.

If the fetus dies in utero the degree of maceration at birth is directly related to the length of time it was retained before delivery. Maceration was formerly considered a priori evidence of syphilis, but since it always follows intrauterine death, there is no direct relation between maceration and syphilis.

Early severe intrauterine syphilitic infections are often associated with anasarca, and the external appearance of the infant may be identical to that of the hydropic form of erythroblastosis. Even in the absence of edema, syphilis and erythroblastosis may be confused on clinical inspection of the child as well as on postmortem examination. Both conditions may be responsible for anemia, the presence in the circulation of immature red blood cells, excessive erythropoiesis in extramedullary areas and enlargement of the spleen and liver.

Microscopic examination usually permits differentiation of the two conditions because the lymphocytic infiltration and visceral fibrosis so constantly associated with fatal forms of congenital syphilis are not found in erythroblastosis. A positive Wassermann reaction of the maternal blood in syphilis and the demonstration of Rh antibodies in the maternal blood in erythroblastosis are additional means of differentiation.

In liveborn infants the extent of the disease varies greatly. There may be no demonstrable symptoms and it may be impossible to establish a diagnosis at the time of delivery. It has been reported that syphilis cannot be diagnosed at birth in as many as 40% of infants subsequently shown to have the disease. The Wassermann reaction of cord blood or blood taken from an infant soon after birth is usually the same as that of maternal blood since the reagins responsible for a positive reaction pass through the placenta and are present in fetal blood in a concentration only slightly lower than in the maternal blood. However, in an unaffected infant the titer gradually decreases after birth whereas in an affected infant it rises, and the diagnosis can usually be established before 20 weeks of age.

The first symptoms do not appear until the 2d month of life in the majority of affected infants (Wechselbert and Schneider). The first evidences of the disease may be purulent rhinitis, skin eruptions, hepatosplenomegaly and anemia. Skin and bone changes are observed less often than previously, possibly because of earlier treatment. In children or in adults maculopapular skin lesions or condylomas, osteochondritis or enlargement of the spleen and liver are often found in well-established cases.

The symptoms described as characteristic of syphilis under the name of Hutchinson's triad are notched, peg-shaped teeth, interstitial keratitis and periostitis, but they do not appear until after the newborn period.

The typical syphilitic change at any age is visceral fibrosis, but at no other time is it so widespread as when the infection occurs before birth. It is most severe in the liver and pancreas, although spleen, kidney, adrenal glands and lungs are also usually involved. The heart may be the site of infection. Extramedullary erythropoiesis simulating that of erythroblastosis is often found in the liver, spleen, kidneys and other organs. The placenta is usually large as a result of villous hypertrophy, and the blood vessels in the villi are often moderately sclerotic. An increase in Hofbauer cells and foci of tissue necrosis and mononuclear cell infiltration are common with severe infections. The walls of the blood vessels of the cord may show peripheral necrosis and leukocytic infiltration, and organisms may be demonstrable in scrapings of the intima.

GRANULOMA VENEREUM. — The organism of granuloma venereum, *Donovani granulomatosis,* has caused the death of infants whose mothers had the disease (Scott *et al.*). Hester reported a 40% mortality rate among the fetuses of affected mothers. Skin lesions in the infants begin as papules that later ulcerate. They are well-vascularized granulomas consisting of monocytes with vacuolated foamy cytoplasm containing bacillary bodies. Suppuration does not occur, though the skin reacts by elongation of rete pegs. Destruction of bone may take place, followed by a fusiform periosteal reaction.

VIBRIO FETUS. — While this common cause of abortion in sheep and cattle has long been recognized as venereally spread, Eden has reported eight cases related to pregnancy and the perinatal period in human beings. The male ordinarily becomes infected by eating contaminated meat and harbors the organisms in the testes. The female acquires the infection through coitus. During pregnancy it may cause suppuration and necrosis of fetal membranes with resultant abortion, or later it may produce meningoencephalitis in the fetus or newborn. The mother appears capable of transmitting the infection even in the absence of symptoms of the disease.

CHAGAS' DISEASE (SOUTH AMERICAN TRYPANOSOMIASIS). — Caused by *Trypanosoma cruzi* and transmitted by bites of reduviid bugs, this disease occurs in the acute form in children under the age of 2 years and has been observed in newborn infants as a result of placental transmission, organisms having been found in the fetal vessels in the villi (Fig. 9–21). The disease occurs in many parts of South America and Mexico but has not been reported in the United States. In the acute form fever, conjunctivitis, lymphadenopathy and generalized edema are common. The spleen, liver and sometimes the thyroid are enlarged. Death may occur during the acute stage, or the disease may become chronic or heal spontaneously. In older children and adults the disease does not pass through an acute phase but is chronic from the beginning. The organism can invade any part of the body, and symptoms depend largely on the part involved.

The lesions of acute Chagas' disease are granulomas composed of polymorphonuclear leukocytes and histiocytes containing organisms in the leishmanial form. When the lesions are more chronic they are fibrotic, the cells are largely lymphocytes and scattered among them are histiocytes that may be filled with organisms.

In fatal cases parasites may be found, especially in neuroglia in the brain and in cardiac and skeletal muscles. They are usually accompanied by a severe inflammatory reaction sometimes associated with local necrosis.

MALARIA. — From the reported investigations it

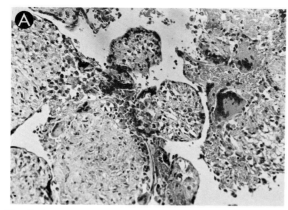

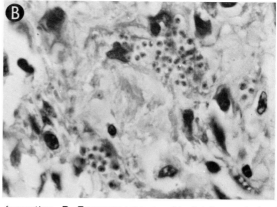

Fig. 9–21.—Placenta of fetus with Chagas' disease. **A,** area of necrosis, leukocytic infiltration and giant cell formation. **B,** *Trypanosoma cruzi* in fetal vessels in villi. (Courtesy Dr. Rita Cardosa.)

seems proved that, although uncommon, malarial infection of the fetus is possible. The disease seems to be more conducive to fetal infection when contracted by foreigners during short residence in a malaria-infested region than in native women. During active stages of the disease the stroma of the placenta contains many macrophages and lymphocytes, and many of the maternal blood cells circulating between the villi contain malarial parasites. It has been suggested that the principal cause of fetal death is lack of normal oxygen-bearing maternal erythrocytes. Other possible causes are absorption of toxic substances from a massively infected placenta and the stimulation of premature labor by high maternal temperature. Wickramasuriya found malarial parasites in cerebral vessels and abnormal pigment in the spleen and liver in six fetuses. All were caused by the estivo-autumnal variety of *Plasmodium falciparum*. This organism has been responsible for most of the fetal infections reported. Newborn infants have no characteristic lesions and diagnosis is based on the finding of organisms in the blood. Infants born to malarial mothers are often of low birth weight despite the absence of intrinsic pathology.

TOXOPLASMOSIS. — Toxoplasmosis is an infectious disease caused by protozoa of the genus Toxoplasma that affects cats, dogs, sheep, rabbits, guinea pigs and other animals as well as man. It was not recognized as pathogenic for man until 1939, when the first cases were described by Wolf *et al.* Since then many cases have been reported. Three types are recognized: (1) a congenital form with onset in utero, manifested chiefly as fetal or neonatal encephalomyelitis, often fatal within the first few weeks but sometimes asymptomatic until later in infancy or childhood; (2) an acute febrile type in adults associated with lymphadenopathy; (3) a latent infection in children and adults recognized only from the presence of neutralizing antibodies in the serum.

The four principal symptoms of the congenital form of the disease, sometimes called the tetrad of toxoplasmosis, are (1) hydrocephalus or microcephalus; (2) chorioretinitis that has a special predilection for the macular region; (3) convulsions or other evidence of involvement of the nervous system; and (4) roentgenographic evidence of cerebral calicification. Skin rash, purpura, prolonged jaundice, hepatosplenomegaly and extramedullary hemopoiesis are also common; these have sometimes led to confusion with erythroblastosis.

The disease has been recognized in stillborn infants and immediately after birth in liveborn infants. The central nervous system is the most constant site of involvement at this age period, and microcephalus, anencephalus and hydrocephalus have all been observed. The head may appear normal at birth but increases rapidly in size in the first few days of life. When the course is less rapid the head may not enlarge, but patients who survive the early stages usually have mildly progressive hydrocephalus associated with mental retardation.

The first sign of chorioretinitis, which affects three fourths of those with the disease, is the presence of small hemorrhages in the retina that gradually become converted into flamelike yellow-white areas bordered by or studded with black pigment. Although they may be found anywhere in the fundus, they have a special predilection for the macular region. Vision is impaired and searching nystagmus is usually present. Many investigators consider such lesions pathognomonic for toxoplasmosis. Cerebral calcification in the form of small granules scattered through the brain only rarely can be identified by x-ray in the newborn, but it soon becomes more pronounced and is easily seen in about one third of affected infants at 6–8 weeks of age (Couvreur and Desmonts).

The Toxoplasma organisms are round, piriform or crescentic with a distinct nuclear membrane and a clear homogenous cytoplasm. They are 4–7 μ long and 2–4 μ wide in blood smears, but in tissues

they are considerably smaller. As obligate intracellular parasites they enter a cell, undergo multiplication and, when virulent, cause cell rupture with liberation of the organisms. When less virulent, multiplication continues, the cell nucleus disappears and the resulting organism-packed cell is known as a pseudocyst (Fig. 9–22). Such cells are rarely observed in granulomatous areas and are usually found in otherwise normal tissue.

On postmortem examination the brain shows more striking changes than any other organ. The

Fig. 9–22.—Toxoplasma. **A,** isolated pseudocyst in the brain. **B,** macrophage in lung, filled with organisms. **C,** cardiac muscle containing organisms. (**B** and **C,** courtesy Drs. H. R. Pratt-Thomas and W. M. Cannon.)

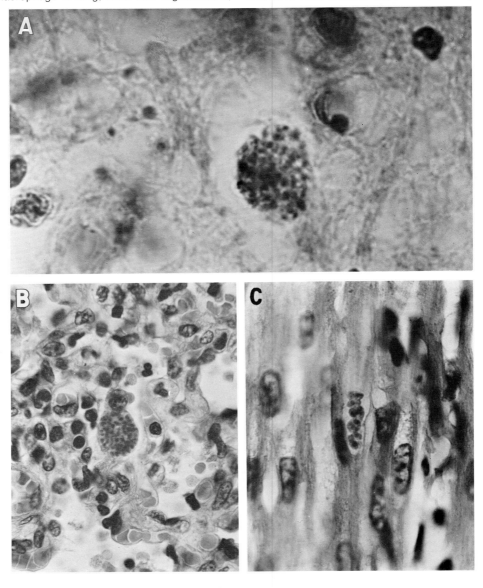

external surface is usually the site of multiple discrete, necrotic yellow nodules measuring from a few millimeters to more than 1 cm in diameter. Similar lesions may also be present in the substance of the brain; occasionally they are limited to this portion and are not visible on the surface. The subependymal regions are often severely affected, and hydrocephalus, which is often present, is generally a result of blockage of the outlets of the ventricular system by granulation tissue or necrotic debris.

Microscopic examination usually reveals granulomas in all portions of the brain. They may be of microscopic size and consist of only a few epithelioid cells and lymphocytes (Fig. 9–23), or they may be large with central areas of necrosis and peripheral cellular infiltration. Free and intracellular parasites are usually numerous, although at times they are found with great difficulty. Varying amounts of calcium are present. The lesions in the eyes begin with acute vasculitis followed by necrosis and infiltration of mononuclear cells, plasma cells and occasional eosinophils. As necrosis contin-

ues, calcium is deposited and organization takes place.

Toxoplasma organisms have been described in many other parts of the body and may be found in areas where no cellular response is visible. The reported distribution has varied greatly, and although organisms have been observed in myocardium, adrenal glands, lungs, subcutaneous tissue, testes, ovaries, pancreas, stomach, kidneys and liver, they have been found in only a few of the sites in any one case.

In the active acute stage of toxoplasmosis it seems doubtful if the brain is ever involved without other organ involvement. In older, chronic or, more especially, inactive cases the specific lesions disappear in the peripheral tissues on healing yet leave recognizable hydrocephalus, calcification and scarring with persistent pseudocysts in the brain.

When the fetus is infected, Toxoplasma pseudocysts can be found frequently in the cord and membranes of the placenta but less often in the villi. In the cord and membranes there is no cellular reaction.

Fig. 9–23 (left).—Granuloma in brain in toxoplasmosis. (Courtesy Dr. Wolf W. Zuelzer.)
Fig. 9–24 (right).—*Histoplasma capsulatum* in macrophages and reticuloendothelial cells of spleen. Infant aged 6 months. (Courtesy Dr. Clayton Loosli.)

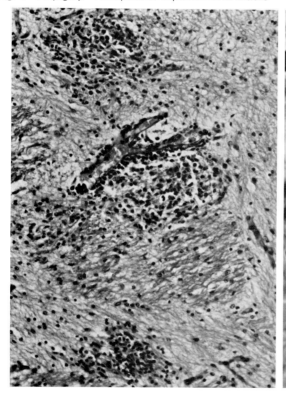
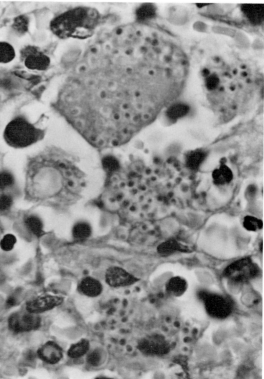

HISTOPLASMOSIS.—Infection by *Histoplasma capsulatum* may occur at any age, and although death has not been reported in infants under several months of age, the onset of symptoms immediately after birth in a few infants suggests a possible intrauterine transmission.

The disease, which attacks the reticuloendothelial system, is ordinarily generalized in infants and most of the viscera are involved. The course is characterized by irregular fever, enlargement of the spleen and liver, emaciation, anemia and leukopenia. Diagnosis often may be confirmed by demonstration of organisms in the sternal marrow or in blood cultures. After death, organisms are often found in reticuloendothelial cells and macrophages in the spleen, liver, lungs, myocardium, adrenal glands and kidneys. In older individuals small granulomas with necrotic centers and peripheral calcification are common but they have rarely been observed in young infants.

A benign form of the disease localized to the lungs appears to be endemic in much of the United States. It is demonstrable on roentgen examination of the chest or by skin tests in many individuals who do not have clinical symptoms. The disease is probably present in many pregnant women and, like toxoplasmosis, possibly may be responsible for the disease in the fetus even though unsuspected in the mother.

In tissues *H. capsulatum* is seen as an oval yeast-like body, 1–5 μ in diameter, with a sharply defined, clear, colorless capsule and a central dark-staining chromatin mass sometimes possessing a round vacuole (Fig. 9–24). On culture in Sabouraud's medium it may occur as a yeast form but is more often seen as white, cottony mycelium with microscopic septate hyphae or filaments bearing small, piriform chlamydospores.

COCCIDIOIDOMYCOSIS.—Few cases of this condition have been reported in infants, but Christian *et al.* observed one infant who died at 29 days following several days' illness characterized by progressive dyspnea, cyanosis and nonproductive cough. The mother had had a granuloma of the right calcaneus in which organisms had been demonstrated but it was thought to have healed before she became pregnant. At autopsy the lungs of the infant were covered with multiple yellow nodules. The lesions produced by coccidioidomycosis are granulomas, with irregular giant cells and lymphocytes often surrounding single large endospores 20–60 μ in diameter (see Fig. 3–31). Christian *et al.* reviewed 14 patients under 1 year of age and found bone involvement, with osteomyelitis the most frequent lesion; meningitis was occasionally present. In very young infants pulmonary lesions alone are usually not lethal. Although the fetus is usually spared when there is maternal involvement, rare cases of placental involvement have been reported (Baker).

CANDIDIASIS.—Thrush, an infection of the mouth caused by *Candida albicans,* when found in newborn infants is often secondary to maternal vaginal infection. Invasion of the amniotic cavity with infection of umbilical cord, placental membrane and

Fig. 9–25.—Thrush. Mycelia and conidiophores of *Candida albicans* in esophagus associated with widespread involvement of the intestinal tract responsible for death. (Courtesy Dr. Eleanor Humphreys.)

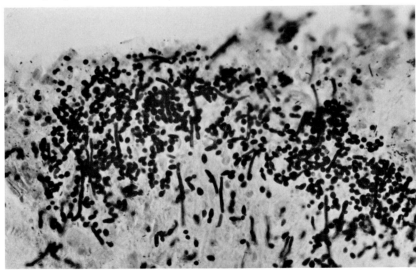

skin has been recorded several times. The organisms can be identified by the characteristic mycelia and conidiophores (Fig. 9–25). The latter are oval structures found separately or attached to mycelial threads.

The tongue, palate, pharynx and inner surface of the cheeks are irregularly covered by a thick white membrane (see Fig. 18–9) that can be detached only by also removing the epidermis and leaving a raw bleeding surface. It is usually limited to the buccal cavity but may spread into the esophagus and occasionally into the lower parts of the gastrointestinal tract. Ulceration with perforation of the intestinal lesions has been reported. When the mother is known to be infected, prophylactic treatment of the infant's mouth will ordinarily prevent the disease.

ASPERGILLOSIS. — Allen and Anderson listed three patients under 1 year of age with this condition. Two of these cases were primary and one was believed to be secondary to the administration of steroids. The skin had papules and ulcers; granulomas were present in the mediastinum, liver and, with cavitation, in the lungs.

REFERENCES

Adams, J. M.: Primary virus pneumonitis with cytoplasmic inclusion bodies, J.A.M.A. 116:925, 1941.

Aitkens, G. H., *et al*: A case of foetal vacinia, Med. J. Aust. 2:173, 1968.

Allen, G. W., and Anderson, D. W.: Generalized aspergillosis in an infant 18 days of age, Pediatrics 26:452, 1960.

Aterman, K.: Personal communication.

Baker, R. L.: Pregnancy complicated by coccidioidomycosis, Am. J. Obstet. Gynecol. 70:1033, 1955.

Barsky, P., and Beale, A. J.: Transplacental transmission of poliomyelitis, J. Pediatr. 51:207, 1957.

Baskin, J. L., Soule, E. H., and Mills, S. D.: Poliomyelitis in the newborn: Pathologic change in 2 cases, Am. J. Dis. Child. 80:10, 1950.

Bass, M. H.: Diseases of the Pregnant Woman Affecting the Offspring, in Dock, W., and Snapper, I. (eds.): *Advances in Internal Medicine* (Chicago: Year Book Medical Publishers, Inc., 1952), Vol. 5.

Bassett, D. C. J., Thompson, S. A. S., and Page, B.: Neonatal infections with *Pseudomonas aeruginosa* associated with comtaminated resuscitation equipment, Lancet 1:781, 1965.

Bates, T.: Poliomyelitis in pregnancy, fetus and newborn, Am. J. Dis. Child. 90:189, 1955.

Beaven, D. W., and Bussy, A. F.: Staphylococcal pneumonia in newborns, Lancet 2:211, 1956.

Bernstein, J., and Evans, A.: Sepsis and jaundice in early infancy, Pediatrics 29:873, 1962.

Bernstein, J., and Wong, J.: The pathology of neonatal pneumonia, Am. J. Dis. Child. 101:350, 1960.

Campbell, E. P.: Chickenpox in a 12 day old infant, Am. J. Dis. Child. 57:1408, 1939.

Carruthers, D. C.: Congenital deaf-mutism as sequela of a rubella maternal infection during pregnancy, Med. J. Aust. 1:315, 1945.

Chany, C., Lipine, P., Lelong, N., Le Tan Vinh, O. O., Satge, P., and Virat, J.: Severe and fatal pneumonia in infants and young children associated with adenovirus, Am. J. Hyg. 67:367, 1958.

Cheathem, W. J., Weller, T. F., Dolan, T. F., and Dauer, J. C.: Varicella: Report of two fatal cases with necropsy, virus isolations and serological findings, Am. J. Pathol. 32:1015, 1956.

Christian, J. R., Sarre, S. G., Piers, J. H., Salazar, E., and de Rosario, J.: Pulmonary coccidioidomycosis in a 21 day old infant, Am. J. Dis. Child. 92:66, 1956.

Coffey, V. P., and Jessup, W. J. E.: Maternal influenza and congenital deformities, Lancet 2:935, 1959.

Copeman, P. W. M., and Wallace, H. J.: Eczema vaccinatum, Br. Med. J. 2:906, 1964.

Couvreur, J., and Desmonts, G.: Congenital and maternal toxoplasmosis: Review of 300 cases, Dev. Med. Child. Neurol. 4:519, 1962.

Denton, J.: The pathology of measles, Am. J. Med. Sci. 169:531, 1925.

Dyer, I.: Measles complicating pregnancy, South. Med. J. 33:601, 1940.

Eichenwald, H. F., and Schinefield, H. R.: Viral infections in fetus, premature infants, newborns, Adv. Pediatr. 12:249, 1962.

Eickhoff, T., Klein, G. O., Daly, K., Ingall, D., and Finland, M.: Neonatal sepsis and other infections due to Group B beta hemolytic streptococci, N. Engl. J. Med. 271:1221, 1964.

Esterly, J. R., and Oppenheimer, E. H.: Pathological lesions due to congenital rubella, Arch. Pathol. 87:380, 1969.

Evans, M. W.: Congenital dental defects in infants subsequent to maternal rubella during pregnancy, Med. J. Aust. 2:225, 1944.

Farber, S., and Wolbach, S. B.: Intranuclear and cytoplasmic inclusions ("protozoan-like bodies") in salivary glands and other organs of infants, Am. J. Pathol. 8:123, 1932.

Feldman, H. A.: Toxoplasmosis, N. Engl. J. Med. 279:1370, 1432, 1968.

Frenkel, J. K., and Friedlander, S.: *Toxoplasmosis* (Public Health Service Publication no. 141) (Washington, D.C.: U. S. Department of Health, Education and Welfare, 1951).

Garcia, A.: Personal communication.

Goodpasture, E. W., *et al*: Virus pneumonia of infants secondary to epidemic infections, Am. J. Dis. Child. 57:997, 1939.

Green, D. M., Reid, S. M., and Rhaney, K.: Generalized vaccinia in the human foetus, Lancet 1:1296, 1966.

Gregg, N. M.: Rubella during pregnancy of the mother with its sequelae of congenital defects in the child, Med. J. Aust. 1:313, 1945.

Gregg, N. M., Bevis, W. R., Haseltine, M., Mochrin, A. E., Vickery, D., and Meyers, E.: The occurrence of congenital defects in children following maternal rubella, Med. J. Aust. 2:122, 1945.

Hagebusch, O. E., and Frei, C. F.: Undulant fever in children, Am. J. Clin. Pathol. 11:497, 1941.

Hansman, D.: Personal communication.

Haymaker, W., Girdany, B. M., Stephens, J., Lillie, R. D., and Fetterman, G.: Cerebral involvement with advanced periventricular calcification in generalized cytomegalic inclusion disease of the newborn, J. Neuropathol. Exp. Neurol. 13:562, 1954.

Hendren, W. H., and Haggerty, R. H.: Staphylococcal pneumonia in infancy and childhood, J.A.M.A. 108:6, 1958.

Hester, L. S., Jr.: Granuloma venereum of cervix and vulva, Am. J. Obstet. Gynecol. 63:312, 1951.

Hood, M.: Listeriosis: Report of 10 cases, Am. J. Clin. Pathol. 28:18, 1947.

Horley, J. F.: Congenital tuberculosis, Arch. Dis. Child. 27:167, 1952.

Hoyne, A. L., and Brown, R. H.: Staphylococcic meningitis: Rarity in newborn. Review of the literature; report of a 3 day old infant with recovery, Arch. Pediatr. 65:175, 1948.

Jelliffe, E. F.: Low birth weight and malarial infection of the placenta, Bull. W.H.O. 38:69, 1968.

Johnson, H. N.: Visceral lesions associated with varicella, Arch. Pathol. 30:292, 1940.

Julianelle, L. A., Harrison, R. W., and Lange, A. C.: Studies on the infectious agent of inclusion blennorrhea, Am. J. Pathol. 14:579, 1938.

Kagan, B. M., et al.: Meningitis in premature infants, Pediatrics 4:479, 1949.

Kibrick, S., and Benirschke, K.: Severe generalized disease (encephalohepatomyocarditis) occurring in newborn period and due to infection with Coxsackie virus, group B: Evidence of intrauterine infection with this agent, Pediatrics 22:857, 1958.

King, J. A., and Marks, R. A.: Pregnancy and leprosy: A review of 52 pregnancies in 26 patients, Am. J. Obstet. Gynecol. 76:438, 1958.

Kluge, R. C., Wicksman, R. S., and Weller, T. H.: Cytomegalic inclusion disease of newborn, Pediatrics 25:35, 1960.

Korones, S. B., Ainger, L. E., Monie, G. R. G., Roone, J., and Sever, J.: Congenital rubella syndrome study of 22 infants with myocardial damage, Am. J. Dis. Child. 110:434, 1965.

Lowenstein, E.: Congenital tuberculosis, Am. Rev. Tuberc. 51:225, 1945.

Lucchesi, P. F., La Boecatta, A. C., and Peale, A. R.: Varicella neonatorum, Am. J. Dis. Child. 73:44, 1947.

MacDonald, A. M., and MacArthur, P.: Foetal vaccinia, Arch. Dis. Child. 28:311, 1953.

MacGregor, A.: The pathology of stillbirth and neonatal death, Br. Med. Bull. 4:174, 1946.

MacGregor, A. R., and Henderson, J. L.: Intestinal thrush, Arch. Dis. Child. 17:168, 1942.

Maksimovich, N. A., and Kornyushenko, N. P.: On intrauterine transmission of influenza virus, Pediatria 38:33, 1960.

Marsden, J. P., and Greenfield, C. R. M.: Inherited smallpox, Arch. Dis. Child. 19:309, 1934.

Medearis, D. N., Jr.: Cytomegalic inclusion disease, Pediatrics 19:467, 1957.

Medearis, D. N., Jr.: Human cytomegalovirus infection, Bull. Johns Hopkins Hosp. 114:181, 1964.

Michaels, R. H., and Mellin, G. W.: Prospective experience with maternal rubella and associated congenital malformation, Pediatrics 26:200, 1960.

Mimica, I., et al.: Lung puncture in the etiological diagnosis of pneumonia, Am. J. Dis. Child. 122:278, 1971.

Mitchell, J. E., and McCall, F. C.: Transplacental infection by herpes simplex virus, Am. J. Dis. Child. 106:207, 1963.

Moosy, J., and Geer, J. C.: Encephalitis, myocarditis and adrenal cortical necrosis in Coxsackie B3 virus infection, Arch. Pathol. 70:614, 1960.

Naidoo, P., and Hirsch, H.: Prenatal vaccinia, Lancet 1:196, 1963.

Nelson, J. S., and Wyatt, J. P.: Salivary gland virus disease, Medicine 38:223, 1959.

Oppenheimer, E. H.: Congenital chickenpox with disseminated visceral lesions, Bull. Johns Hopkins Hosp. 74:240, 1944.

Oppenheimer, E. H.: Congenital syphilis in newborn infant: Clinical and pathological observations in recent cases, Johns Hopkins Med. J. 129:63, 1971.

Paige, B. H., Cowen, D., and Wolf, A.: Toxoplasmic encephalitis: V. Further observations of infantile toxoplasmosis: Intrauterine inception of diseases, visceral manifestations, Am. J. Dis. Child. 63:474, 1942.

Potter, E. L.: Placental transmission of viruses, Am. J. Obstet. Gynecol. 74:505, 1957.

Rebuck, J. W., and Crowley, J. H.: A method of studying leukocytic functions, Ann. N. Y. Acad. Sci. 113:575, 1964.

Rudolf, A. J., Singleton, E. B., Rosenberg, M. F., Singer, D. B., and Phillips, C. A.: Osseous manifestations of congenital rubella syndrome, Am. J. Dis. Child. 110:428, 1965.

Scott, C. W., Harper, D. M., Jason, R. F., and Helweg, E. B.: Neonatal granuloma venereum, Am. J. Dis. Child. 85:308, 1953.

Seeliger, H. P. R.: Listeriosis (New York: Hafner, 1961).

Shinefield, H. R., and Townsend, T. E.: Transplacental transmission of western equine encephalomyelitis, J. Pediatr. 43:21, 1953.

Shuman, H. H.: Varicella in newborn, Am. J. Dis. Child. 58:564, 1939.

Signey, A. G., and Bruce, R. D.: Umbilical diphtheria, Arch. Dis. Child. 6:43, 1931.

Smith, E. S.: Salmonella meningitis in infancy, Am. J. Dis. Child. 88:732, 1954.

Smith, J. F., and Landing, B. H.: Mechanisms of brain damage in H. influenzae meningitis, J. Neuropathol. Exp. Neurol. 19:248, 1960.

Sohier, R., Chardonnet, Y., and Prunieras, M.: Adenovirus, Prog. Med. Virol. 7:253, 1965.

Sonnenschein, H., Clark, H. L., and Taschdjian, C. L.: Congenital cutaneous candidiasis in premature infant, Am. J. Dis. Child. 99:81, 1960.

Sussman, M. L., Strauss, L., and Hodes, H. L.: Fatal Coxsackie group B virus infection in the newborn, Am. J. Dis. Child. 97:483, 1959.

Swan, C., Tostevin, A. L., and Black, G. H. B.: Final observation on congenital defects in infants following infectious diseases during pregnancy, with special reference to rubella, Med. J. Aust. 2:889, 1946.

Thygeson, P., and Mengert, W. F.: The virus of inclusion conjunctivitis: Further observations, Arch. Ophthalmol. 15:377, 1936.

Tondury, G., and Smith, D. W.: Fetal rubella pathology, J. Pediatr. 68:867, 1966.

Wechselberg, K., and Schneider, J. D.: Morbidity and clinical features of congenital syphilis in infancy. Dtsch. Med. Wochenschr. 95:1976, 1970.

Weller, T. H., and Hanshaw, J. B.: Virological and clinical

observations on cytomegalic inclusion disease, N. Engl. J. Med. 266:1233, 1962.

Wheeler, C. E., and Huffines, W. D.: Primary disseminated herpes simplex, J.A.M.A. 191:455, 1964.

Whipple, D. V., and Dunham, E. C.: Congenital syphilis, J. Pediatr. 12:386, 1938.

Wickramasuriya, G. Q. W.: Some observations on malaria occurring in association with pregnancy, J. Obstet. Gynecol. Br. Emp. 42:816, 1935.

Williams, E. M.: Mediterranean fever: Infection in utero, J. Royal Army Med. Corps 9:59, 1907.

Wolf, A., Cowen, D., and Paige, B. H.: Toxoplasmic encephalomyelitis, Am. J. Pathol. 15:657, 1939.

Ziai, M., and Haggerty, R. J.: Neonatal meningitis, N. Engl. J. Med. 259:314, 1958.

Zuelzer, W. W.: Infantile toxoplasmosis with report of 3 new cases, including two in which the patients were identical twins, Arch. Pathol. 38:1, 1944.

Zuelzer, W. W., and Stulberg, C. S.: Herpes simplex virus as cause of fulminating visceral disease and hepatitis in infancy, Am. J. Dis. Child. 83:421, 1952.

10

Inborn Errors of Metabolism Involving Multiple Organ Systems

THE DESIGNATION inborn errors of metabolism was first used by Garrod in 1908 for a small number of diseases including alkaptonuria, cystinuria, pentosuria and albinism, which he described as having certain common characteristics. They often occur in more than one member of a family, can often be identified in early infancy, are relatively benign and compatible with a normal life expectancy and are especially common in consanguineous marriages. He postulated that inherited enzyme deficiencies might be responsible for interference with normal metabolism of certain substances and that these substances would then be excreted without further alteration.

In the years that have elapsed since Garrod's speculations, improvements in chemical methods and in knowledge concerning enzymatic function have made it possible to place a host of disorders in this category, and they are only a part of those that will eventually be included. Many are less benign than those of Garrod's original group and many cannot be detected in early infancy, but the concept of inherited enzymatic deficiencies responsible for metabolic alterations remains firm.

Most of these conditions are inherited in a mendelian recessive manner with the disease fully expressed only in the homozygous state. In some instances heterozygotes can be identified because they exhibit mild forms of the disease; in other instances they appear entirely normal. In a few cases genes responsible for these diseases are dominant or sex-linked. Since penetrance and expression of genes may vary, there is always the possibility that inheritance may not seem uniform and that clinical manifestations may vary.

A classification of inborn errors of metabolism may emphasize one or more aspects of a disease process according to the interests of the classifier. Thus, some authors may choose the principal chemical constituent involved, such as carbohydrate, amino acid, protein or lipid, as the identifying feature, others may choose the organ system chiefly affected, and yet others may make a division on the basis of structural abnormalities or the physiologic system involved, e.g., immunologic, pigment metabolism or energy system.

We have chosen an arbitrary grouping of individual disorders, based largely on custom, that includes errors in carbohydrate, amino acid and lipid metabolism, followed by diseases with abnormal intracellular storage of various substances. This is in full realization that all such transmissible disorders have alteration in the genetic code or in its transmission as their basis and that the demonstrable absence of a specific enzyme may be the unique identifying feature in many.

In this chapter only those generalized multiorgan disturbances that can be recognized in the 1st year of life will be discussed. Others that affect only a single organ or related organs (such as skin or bone disorders or immunoglobulin deficiencies) will be taken up in the appropriate chapters.

Errors Affecting Carbohydrate Metabolism

GLYCOGEN STORAGE DISEASE. — Six forms of disturbance in glycogen synthesis and breakdown are now well recognized (Hers). Three others have been proposed but are represented by only a few cases.

The five well-delineated forms that can be recognized in the 1st year of life are described below.

Glycogen storage disease of the liver and kidney (type I) (von Gierke's disease, hepatonephromegalic form of glycogen storage disease) is due to a lack of glucose-6-phosphatase (Fig. 10–1). The failure of glucose to be formed in the normal manner leads to hypoglycemia, acidosis and ketosis; amino acids are lost by their conversion to glucose, and lipid stores are constantly mobilized as a result of hypoglycemia. The disease makes itself apparent in the first months of life by enlargement of the liver, vomiting, acidosis and failure to grow.

The liver and kidney are the only organs directly affected in this form of the disease. An excessive amount of glycogen and fat are present in the parenchymal cells of the liver and the cells of the proximal convoluted tubules in the kidney. These substances in the renal tubules are thought to inhibit amino acid reabsorption from the tubular lumen and to cause amino-aciduria. The wastage of protein by conversion to glucose and the loss of amino acids in the urine lead to growth retardation as well as bone decalcification and fracture. Elevated levels of serum lipids and cholesterol give rise to skin xanthomas. High serum uric acid levels may result in symptoms of gout. Glucose tolerance tests display elevated curves, and galactose loads cause an increase in serum lactic acid because of the failure of galactose to convert to glucose. Glucagon and epinephrine tolerance tests fail to show the usual rises in glucose levels. The enzyme defect can be demonstrated during life in white blood cells obtained from the buffy coat of the peripheral blood.

At autopsy the liver and kidneys are enlarged, the former being as much as three to four times the normal size. The liver is pale, firm and smooth without evidence of fibrosis. The liver cells have centrally placed nuclei surrounded by a large amount of clear cytoplasm rich in glycogen. In many cells fatty vacuoles can also be demonstrated (Fig. 10–2, A). The glycogen stains normally and disappears promptly on exposure to salivary diastase or amylase, although it may be unusually resistant on autolysis at room temperature. The lipid is in the form of neutral fat. The cells of the proximal convoluted renal tubules are also large and contain both glycogen and fat; those of the distal convoluted tubules are little involved (Fig. 10–2, B). Electron microscopic observations fail to show

Fig. 10–1.—Diagram of major pathways of glycogen synthesis and degradation. Key: 1, hexokinase; 2, phosphoglucomutase; 3, UDPG + (uridine diphosphoglucose transglucosidase); 4, amylo-1-4, 1-6 transglucosidase; 5, phosphorylase; 6, amylo-1-6 glucosidase; 7, glucose-6-phosphatase; 8, alpha glucosidase. (Modified from Field, F.: Glycogen Deposition Diseases, in Stanbury, J. [ed.]: The Metabolic Basis of Inherited Disease [New York: McGraw-Hill Book Co., 1966], p. 171.)

A SIMPLIFIED SCHEMA OF THE FORMATION AND DEGRADATION OF GLYCOGEN

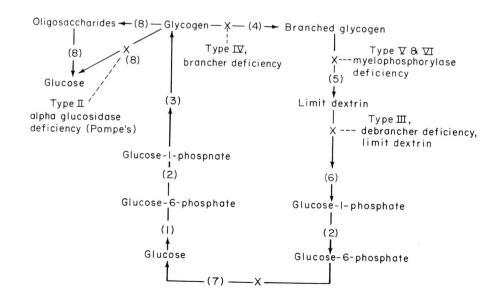

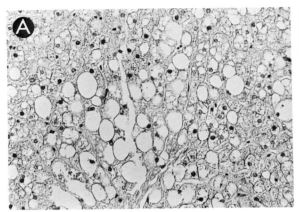
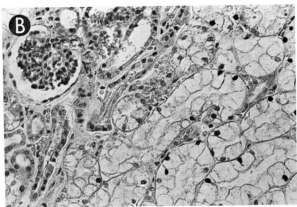

Fig. 10–2.—Glycogen storage disease, type I (von Gierke's disease). **A,** liver. Hepatic cells show a generalized increase in glycogen and localized infiltration of fat. **B,** kidney. Cells of proximal convoluted tubules are enlarged by presence of glycogen. (Courtesy Dr. G. Vawter.)

unusual features of glycogen formation even though the amount is increased.

This disease is inherited in an autosomal recessive manner. In affected individuals the enzyme is completely absent; no partial forms indicating heterozygosity have been recognized. Despite this, some patients survive to adult life, presumably through adaptive utilization of other metabolic pathways. This disorder is responsible for about 30% of all cases of glycogen storage diseases.

Generalized glycogenosis (type II) (Pompe's disease, glycogen storage disease of the heart) is caused by an absence of the enzyme alpha-glucosidase, which removes glucose from the outer chain of the glycogen molecule (see Fig. 10–1). It produces ab-

normalities in nearly all parts of the body but is often first recognized because of cardiac failure associated with marked enlargement of the heart. Vomiting, anorexia and failure to grow are also common early symptoms. Because of the peripheral muscle involvement hypotonia is marked and the tongue is often enlarged.

The clinical diagnosis can be confirmed by the finding of large amounts of glycogen in circulating leukocytes or in biopsies of voluntary muscle. Response to epinephrine, glucagon, glucose and galactose loads is normal. Survival beyond the first years of life is uncommon.

At autopsy the heart is enlarged and pale and the ventricular walls are thickened. The endocardi-

Fig. 10–3.—Glycogen storage disease, type II (generalized glycogenosis). **A,** heart muscle filled with glycogen. With hematoxylin-eosin stain the cells appear enlarged and empty. (Courtesy Dr. G. Vawter.) **B,** skeletal muscle in which fibers show dense basophilic masses and clear glycogen-containing areas. (Courtesy Dr. A. J. MacAdams.)

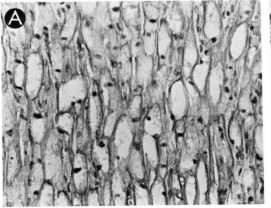
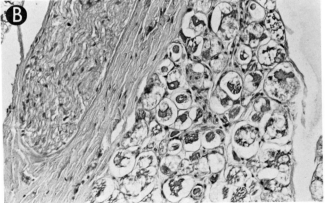

al thickening and pallor that are often present must be distinguished from those found in congenital endocardial sclerosis. The muscle cells of the heart and peripheral voluntary and smooth muscle contain large central vacuoles filled with glycogen, and myofibrils are dispersed to the periphery (Fig. 10–3, A). Changes are especially prominent in the tongue and diaphragm. Glycogen can also be demonstrated in the kidneys, liver, adrenal, reticuloendothelial system, vascular endothelium and brain. In the kidneys the deposition is primarily in the loops of Henle and collecting tubules, which distinguishes this variety from type I. Fat deposition is not a prominent feature. In the peripheral muscle some of the periodic acid-Schiff-positive material displays red metachromasia when stained with toluidine blue and is visible as central basophilic masses with other stains (Fig. 10–3, B). This material is diastase resistant and may not be glycogen inasmuch as glycogen proper is promptly removed by saliva or malt diastase. Since some of the glycogen may be lost after alcohol fixation, fixation in Rossman's fluid followed by an alcoholic periodic acid-Schiff (PAS) oxidation sequence may be required to demonstrate all of the glycogen. In this form of the disease glycogen is present in membrane-bound sacs, thought to represent lysosomes, in the liver parenchyma and muscle cells as well as being free in the cytoplasm (Fig. 10–4).

This disorder accounts for less than 5% of all cases of glycogen storage disease. Among the cases described 12 have occurred in siblings in 7 families.

In *limit dextrin or debrancher defect (type III)* the absent enzyme is the debrancher enzyme amylo-1-

Fig. 10–4.—Glycogen storage disease, type II. Electron photomicrograph showing dense lysosomal masses filled with glycogen. (Courtesy Dr. G. Hug.)

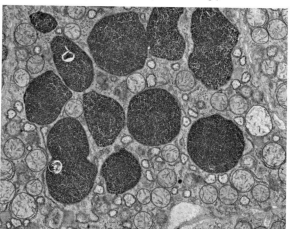

6-glucosidase (see Fig. 10–1). Glycogen can be broken down as far as the first branched chain where the 1-6 linkage occurs. As a result of the defect abnormal glycogen with shortened or absent outer glucose chains can often be isolated during fasting. Because of the patient's inability to provide adequate amounts of glucose on demand, the signs and symptoms are similar to those of type I. Although symptoms may appear as early as 1 year of age, they are milder and may not be recognized until increasing weakness and enlargement of the liver become apparent in the early teens. The liver cells are clear because of increased amounts of glycogen. Although glycogen may constitute as much as 14% of the liver by weight, it is usually in smaller masses than in types I and II. Unlike those of type I, the cells appear normal on routine staining even though an increase in glycogen can be demonstrated in heart and peripheral muscle. Fat in the liver may be increased, especially in the periportal areas.

Hers believed that two different forms of the disease exist, with the enzyme defect present in both liver and muscle in one and in the liver only in the other. The meager data available suggest that the combined defect has an autosomal recessive distribution. About one third of all cases of glycogen storage disease fall into this category.

In *brancher defect (type IV) (Andersen's disease, glycogen storage disease with cirrhosis)* there is a postulated defect in the brancher enzyme amylo-1-4, 1-6 glucosidase that is responsible for formation of glycogen with excessively long outer chains and a few branch points (amylopectin). This glycogen is less soluble in water than normal glycogen.

Most cases occur in the 1st year of life and are characterized by a greatly enlarged liver, ascites and jaundice. The liver exhibits multilobular cirrhosis with some proliferation of bile ducts. The liver cells are enlarged and contain a crystalline form of glycogen that stains blue with iodine and gives a positive PAS and Hale colloidal iron reaction (Fig. 10–5). It is digested slowly and incompletely with diastase or by autolytic degradation. The Kupffer cells of the liver; glial cells of the brain; reticuloendothelial cells of the heart, spleen, bone marrow and lymph nodes; and many macrophages in the connective tissue contain a similar form of glycogen. The kidney parenchyma and the voluntary muscle are uninvolved.

In the few cases described so far all of the patients have had affected siblings, which suggests an autosomal recessive inheritance. Until 1962 only 76 cases had been reported. Death usually occurs before the age of 2 years.

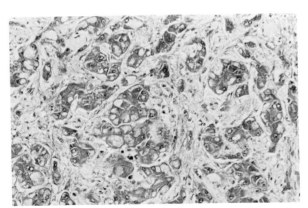

Fig. 10–5.—Glycogen storage disease, type IV (brancher defect), with cirrhosis. Dense crystalline masses of stored diastase-resistant material are present in the liver cells. Macrophages in the dense connective tissue also contain glycogen.

Myelophosphorylase deficiency (type V) (McArdle-Schmidt-Pearson disease), which has not been described in the very young, causes pain, stiffness and weakness on exercise. Increase in glycogen is limited to peripheral muscle.

Unlike other forms of glycogen storage disease, *hepatophosphorylase deficiency (type VI)* may be a partial defect. The disorder results in defective removal of outer and inner glucose chains, but there is no difficulty with splitting at the branch points. The liver parenchymal cells are enlarged by an increased deposit of glycogen and encroach on liver sinusoids. They are surrounded by prominent reticulum but there is no real increase in fibrous tissue. Since phosphorylase is deficient in the liver only, the muscle and other organs are normal. Fat in the liver may be increased but has no characteristic distribution. Although the most common form of glycogen storage disease, accounting for about 35% of all cases, it may be the hardest to diagnose with certainty because of variability in the intensity of the defect and because other forms of glycogen storage disease may show secondarily low levels of phosphorylase activity. The liver enzyme must be at least 75% deficient to allow a positive diagnosis.

MAURIAC'S SYNDROME.—Occurring in poorly controlled, very young diabetic patients, this syndrome presents with obesity, dwarfism, ketosis, acidosis and a greatly enlarged liver containing as much as 12% glycogen. The disorder might be confused pathologically with type I glycogen storage disease except that the proximal convoluted tubules are not affected.

Additional forms of abnormal glycogen metabolism were described by Hug *et al.* However, the cases reported are as yet isolated examples, and more data are required for certain identification.

GALACTOSEMIA.—In this familial disease affected individuals lack the enzyme responsible for conversion of galactose to glucose. This enzyme, galactose-1-phosphate uridyl transferase, facilitates the reaction:

$$\text{galactose-1-phosphate} + \text{uridyl} \\ \text{diphosphoglucose} \rightarrow \text{uridyl diphosphogalactose} \\ + \text{glucose-1-phosphate}$$

Since absence of the enzyme results in an inability to convert galactose to glucose, an increased amount of galactose-1-phosphate is found in the blood and tissue. This substance is thought to be the toxic metabolite.

Infants with galactosemia fail to thrive and are subject to attacks of hypoglycemia and vomiting. Hepatomegaly, ascites, jaundice and diarrhea soon develop, and cataracts, liver cirrhosis and mental deficiency follow if lactose is not withdrawn from the diet. Laboratory tests show hypoglycemia, galactosemia, galactosuria and amino-aciduria. The amino-aciduria is renal in origin and secondary to resorption difficulties.

The enlarged liver contains much fat, which is often distributed in isolated nodule-like groups of cells (Fig. 10–6, A). Early in life the liver cells arrange themselves about bile canaliculi in a characteristic pseudoacinar pattern with the fat at the periphery of the cell (Fig. 10–6, B). Stasis of bile in the canaliculi and bile ducts is responsible for the high serum bilirubin levels. Hepatocellular damage becomes less severe after a few months, but in untreated patients Laennec's cirrhosis may develop, with individual lobules of fairly regular size being isolated by bands of collagen (Fig. 10–6, C). Proximal convoluted tubules in the kidney are distended, at times severely enough to be confused with renal cystic disease (Fig. 10–6, D).

Infants dying in the first few days of life in whom galactosemia is suspected because an older sibling has had this diagnosis may show no abnormality except an excessive amount of fat in the liver. In spite of the fact that the presence of galactose in the diet is thought to be responsible for clinical symptoms, the existence of such an abnormality at birth or soon after suggests that other factors may have been operating prenatally. Three such cases were studied at the Chicago Lying-in Hospital.

Early in life the brain is said to be only edematous, and late changes have not been well described. Crome reported a case with marked gliosis,

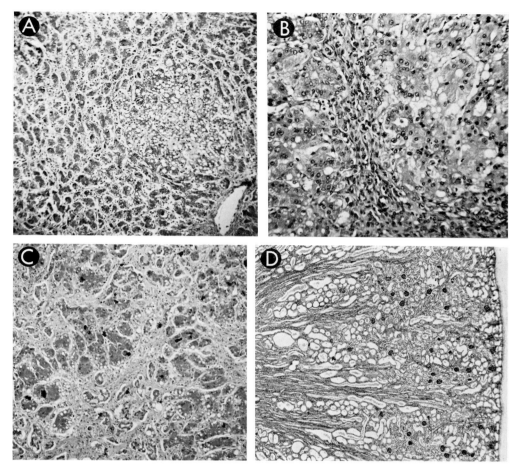

Fig. 10–6.—Galactosemia. **A,** liver with mild diffuse increase in intralobular connective tissue, mild diffuse deposit of fat, pseudoacinar structures and circumscribed nodule of liver cells with greatly increased fat.· **B,** liver with pseudoacinar structures and periportal fibrosis. **C,** liver in later stage, with marked increase in intralobular fibrosis, fat droplets in characteristic location at periphery of cells, distention of many pseudoacini with bile. **D,** kidney with characteristic distention of proximal convoluted tubules.

scarring of the white matter and deficiency of the globus pallidus suggestive of kernicterus, but there may have been additional causative factors.

Inheritance is by an autosomal recessive gene. Heterozygotes among the parents and siblings of an affected infant have reduced activity of the enzyme in their red cells and can be fairly well identified although there is some overlap with noncarriers. Examination of the urine of all newborn infants for galactose could eliminate the mental deficiency and death otherwise associated with this disorder.

FRUCTOSE INTOLERANCE.—This condition, similar in many ways to galactosemia, results from a lack of the fructose-1-phosphate splitting enzyme, aldolase. As in galactosemia, phosphate ester accumulates in the tissues. When fruits or foods containing fructose or sorbitol are present in the diet, the infant fails to thrive and is subject to vomiting, jaundice, hepatomegaly, amino-aciduria and albuminuria. Associated hypoglycemia is due in part to a block in release of glucose from the liver and in part to comprehensive binding of phosphates by fructose.

In severe cases ascites, edema and splenomegaly may be present. The liver is large, smooth and filled with fat; it may show a slight fibrosis and the same pseudoacinar pattern that is found in the liver cell cords in galactosemia. It may return to normal within 1 or 2 years after complete withdrawal of fructose from the diet. Two patterns of inheritance have been suggested, one recessive and one dominant. Three families have been described in which it seemed dominant, and a recent survey identified 18 families in which it seemed recessive (Froesch).

Errors Affecting Amino Acid Metabolism

PRIMARY OXALOSIS AND HYPEROXALURIA. — Symptoms of oxalosis and hyperoxaluria may arise in the 1st year of life as they did in a series of all ages gathered by Hockaday. However, only 3 of his patients succumbed during the 1st year of life. The first symptom may be failure to thrive or the passage of oxalate stones. Deposition of calcium oxalate in the kidney leads to swelling, then scarring and shrinkage, of the renal parenchyma with ultimate failure of renal function.

Although oxalates are deposited in the myocardium, liver, thyroid, adrenal, pancreas, thymus and lumens of the epididymal tubules, there is little accompanying tissue damage. The kidney is the only organ ordinarily injured. Refractile crystals of calcium oxalate are found in the lumens of the proximal convoluted tubules (Fig. 10–7) and in the media and adventitia of the renal vessels. The crystals are doubly refractile, yellow and globular with radiating spicules. They can be identified by x-ray diffraction or simple chemical tests such as exposure to sulfuric acid before and after incineration: before incineration characteristic calcium sulfate deposits are formed; after incineration sulfuric acid liberates carbon dioxide from the calcium carbonate coming from the burned calcium oxalate. Interstitial renal fibrosis and pyelonephritis are caused

Fig. 10–7. — Oxalosis. Kidney with intra- and extratubular masses of oxalate crystals. (Courtesy Dr. C. Witzleben.)

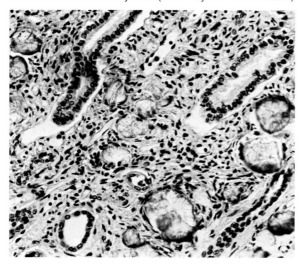

by tubular blockage with oxalate crystals. The end-result is a small kidney with a thickened renal capsule and depressed scars produced by tubular atrophy and fibrosis. Because of the calcium oxalate deposits, nephrocalcinosis can be identified during life by the presence of radiodensities. Glomeruli are normal except for periglomerular sclerosis.

The biochemical defect appears to be, at least in part, a block in the action of the transaminase, allowing the transformation of glycine to glyoxylate but preventing the reversal of the process. This results in an increase in the glyoxylate pool and a three- to eightfold increase in the excretion of oxalate.

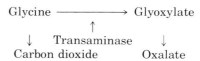

That the enzymatic defect is not limited to the kidney has been demonstrated by the prompt precipitation of oxalate in a normal kidney transplanted to an affected host.

The abnormality is usually inherited through an autosomal recessive gene; homozygotes are detected by the increased excretion of oxalate that follows a glyoxylate load. A dominant form of inheritance is also suggested by the finding of the disease in three generations of one family (Wyngaarden and Elder).

PHENYLKETONURIA. — This genetic defect, caused by an autosomal recessive gene, was identified only 35 years ago when Følling described 10 mentally deficient patients who excreted excessive amounts of phenylpyruvic acid. It was subsequently found that the livers of such patients were deficient in phenylalanine hydroxylase. This deficiency increases the levels of phenylalanine in the serum to as much as 30 times the normal amount. For reasons not understood the disturbed phenylalanine levels are associated with a deficiency in cerebral cerebrosides and cholesterol.

Untreated, the homozygous bearer of the defect develops signs of mental retardation and later has epileptic seizures; the skin and hair may be lighter in color than that of nonaffected siblings. These changes are caused by the block in conversion of phenylalanine to tyrosine.

Not all affected infants have easily demonstrable pathologic lesions, but in the majority the brain weight is reduced to about 40% of normal and there is evidence of diffuse failure of myelinization accompanied by astrocytic gliosis. The myelin loss may be most marked in infants dying in the first 2 years of life (Fig. 10–8). Crome described cases that appeared to have widespread myelin breakdown with formation of sudanophilic gitter cells similar to those found in Schilder's leukoencephalopathy.

The disease may be detected by chromatographic study of the serum for phenylalanine or the urine for phenylketone soon after the introduction of milk or other proteins containing phenylalanine into the diet. Since the chief source of phenylalanine is ingested protein, the high serum level can be controlled by rigorous elimination of this amino acid from the diet. Infants carried on such a regime for the first few years of life, until brain myelinization is complete, develop normally and can then be allowed a less restricted diet.

TYROSINEMIA. – Patients with the autosomal recessively inherited trait of tyrosinemia have many of the clinical characteristics of those with cystinosis. In these cases there is a high level of tyrosine in the plasma, and the urine contains tyrosine as well as p-hydroxyphenyl-lactic-pyruvic acid and p-hydroxyphenyl-lactic-acetic acid. The exact enzyme defect has not been identified although p-hydroxyphenylpyruvate oxidase is absent from the liver.

In the very young, dehydration, acidosis and amino-aciduria are caused by defects in tubular resorption. In children over 16 months of age, resistant rickets, phosphaturia, glycosuria and generalized amino-aciduria are common.

All patients described so far have had cirrhosis of the liver accompanied by marked but often focal fatty changes, increased reticulum and a variable degree of central necrosis. Death from liver failure has been reported. In a few fatal cases hepatomas have been present. The cells of all renal tubules are

Fig. 10–8. – Phenylketonuria. Myelin stain of an adolescent brain with focal areas of pallor (failure of myelinization). (Courtesy Dr. P. Yakovlev.)

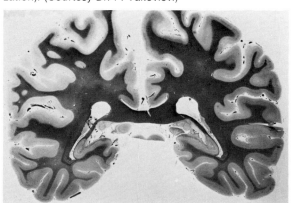

irregularly enlarged, degenerated and filled with eosinophilic droplets. These changes become progressive in the more chronic forms of the disease. The glomeruli are unaffected.

CYSTINE STORAGE DISEASE, LIGNAC-FANCONI DISEASE, NEPHROTIC-GLYCOSURIC DWARFISM. – The multiplicity of names attached to this disorder, or group of disorders, indicates the complexity of its identification. At present the view of Bickel *et al.* appears reasonable; they believe that in most patients with the general findings of resistant rickets, osteoporosis, glycosuria and amino-aciduria adequate study will reveal cystine crystals in the tissues. This requires proper sampling, adequate fixation in absolute alcohol and observation under crossed Nicol prisms of tissues that have never been exposed to water. Some investigators (e.g., de Toni) still believe that two syndromes exist, the first consisting of rickets with gluco-amino-phosphate diabetes, and the second being the same condition plus cystine deposition in the tissues. In either case the signs and symptoms are very similar. In the young infant they are malnutrition, vomiting, fever, acidosis, polyuria and dehydration. They can be found as early as the 4th month and before the appearance of a full rachitic state.

The defect appears to be essentially a failure of tubular resorption; thus, glycosuria and severe amino-aciduria, deficient ammonia formation and potassium losses in the urine are to be expected. When cystine storage is marked, the amino acids in the urine consist largely of cystine, lysine, arginine and ornithine; at times the other substances may be excreted in amounts greater than cystine.

The cystine crystals are widely distributed in the body, principally in the reticuloendothelial system. The reticuloendothelial cells of the spleen, the Kupffer cells of the liver and the medullary cords of the lymph nodes are most severely involved (Fig. 10–9). The lymph nodes may be preferable to bone marrow for identification since crystals are often absent in bone marrow smears although they are present in aspirated whole marrow. Slit lamp examination of the cornea for the presence of cystine crystals is an excellent method of establishing the diagnosis.

Early in the disease the kidneys may be enlarged and pale with the chief alteration being in the tubular cells, which are large and contain increased amounts of fat. They may show vacuolation beneath the nucleus similar to that found in potassium deficiency. The tubular membranes and the capsular membranes of Bowman's spaces are thickened. Later in the disease glomerular scarring,

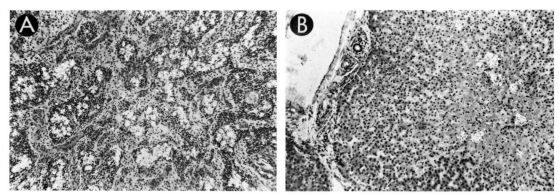

Fig. 10–9.—Cystinosis with crystals in reticuloendothelial cells photographed under polarized light. **A,** lymph node. **B,** liver. (Courtesy Dr. K. Aterman.)

tubular atrophy and interstitial inflammation may be present (Fig. 10–10). Cystine crystals are often absent, but when present, are usually in interstitial tissue or glomeruli. Cystine crystals can be stained by use of the de Golantha technic for uric acid in alcohol-fixed tissues. Electron microscopic studies by Spear *et al.* showed the presence of sulfur-containing granules in addition to cystine crystals. Microdissection of the renal tubules usually reveals shortening of proximal convoluted tubules and the "swan neck deformity," which consists of narrowing of the tubule for a short distance from the glomerulus (Darmady and Stranack). The liver ordinarily contains fat as well as cystine crystals.

The rachitic bones have wide uncalcified zones of osteoid around the trabeculae, and secondary hyperparathyroidism due to renal failure may be responsible for osteoporosis and osteitis fibrosa cystica.

Fig. 10–10.—Cystinosis. Kidney showing epithelial crescents, glomerular sclerosis, hyalinization and mild diffuse cellular infiltration of the interstitium of the kidney.

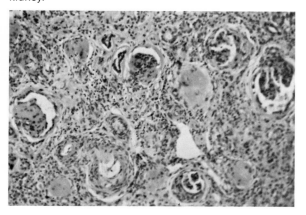

If death occurs in the early stages of the disease, it is most often due to acidosis and dehydration resulting from tubular defects. Later, as glomerular and tubular degeneration destroy progressively greater portions of the kidneys, more common forms of renal insufficiency are encountered.

This rare disease is associated with parental consanguinity but has not been described in siblings.

MAPLE SUGAR URINE DISEASE, BRANCHED CHAIN KETONURIA.—This disorder derives its name, and was first identified, because of the peculiar odor of the urine in four siblings who died early in infancy (Menkes *et al.*). Dancis and Lively gathered 18 reports of infants with this defect, which consists of a block in the oxidative decarboxylation of the branched chain amino acids leucine, isoleucine and valine. The exact enzyme lacking in the five steps required in the process is not known and the defect may not be the same in all cases. Affected infants eat poorly, have a high-pitched cry and are lethargic and alternately hypo- and hypertonic. Convulsions are common and respiratory disturbances lead to early death.

In all cases high levels of the three branched amino acids and the three keto-acids are found in the plasma and urine respectively. The white matter of the brains of patients who die in infancy is poorly myelinated, but neurons are intact. In some cases there is a glial response with astrocytosis and an increase in oligodendroglia. The viscera (described by Silberman *et al.*) have been normal except for one infant with hepatosplenomegaly.

Errors Affecting Lipid Metabolism

BETA-LIPOPROTEIN DEFICIENCY.—Though the underlying mechanism responsible for this disorder is the absence of a serum protein fraction, the result is a disturbance in lipid metabolism. Since protein is absent from the serum, transport of lipid fractions in the bloodstream is impaired and the observable disturbances arise from failure of removal of fats or delivery of fats to various organ systems for incorporation and use.

Steatorrhea, often the first sign of the disease, may occur as early as 2–4 months after birth. This is followed by ataxia, intention tremor and nystagmus, which are similar to the findings in Friedreich's ataxia. The deep reflexes are absent and muscle weakness is pronounced. Serum triglyceride and cholesterol levels are low. The red blood cells are abnormal, and small elevations on them produce "burr cells" or acanthrocytes as a result of abnormal lipid composition of the cell wall.

The intestinal cells contain fat even after an 18–24-hour fast, and intestinal biopsy reveals no fat in the lacteals after a fatty meal. Removal of fat is blocked by the absence of beta-lipoprotein carrier in the serum.

The nervous system displays loss of myelin in the posterior columns, the cerebellar spinal tracts and the peripheral nerves. Anterior horn cells and cerebellar nuclei (molecular layer and Purkinje cells) are reduced in number.

FAMILIAL HYPERILIPOPROTEINEMIA.—Of the five types included in this general disorder only two need be considered here since three forms have not been recognized in the 1st year of life.

Type I, Buerger-Grütz disease, is distinguished by massive chylomicronemia when the diet is normal, with some decrease when it is fat-free. The fundamental defect is the absence of tissue lipoprotein lipase.

The first symptoms are skin eruptions, which may appear as early as 4 months after birth and are followed by hepatosplenomegaly by the age of 7 months. By the age of 7 years increased intake of fat often gives rise to attacks of abdominal pain of unknown cause. Serum levels of lipids and cholesterol are extremely high.

Some of the reticuloendothelial cells in the liver, spleen and lymph nodes are usually converted into foam cells by their increased fat content, and some of the liver parenchymal cells may be similarly involved. Pancreatitis may be present in older infants. The pattern of inheritance is autosomal recessive.

Type II, hyperlipoproteinemia, which is more common than type I, is recognized because lipid- and cholesterol-filled histiocytes are present in tendons, conjunctivae, eyelids and endothelium. By 1 year of age these deposits may form noticeable masses. Levels of cholesterol and beta-lipoprotein

in the blood are 2–10 times normal. Symptoms of coronary heart disease often begin in midchildhood and cause death in early adolescence.

This condition is caused by a recessive gene, and both heterozygotes and homozygotes are affected; the former may have only abnormal chemical values while the latter develop symptoms.

Errors Affecting Cell Function as a Result of Abnormal Intracellular Storage

CONGENITAL AMAUROTIC FORM OF TAY-SACHS DISEASE.—Of the six forms of Tay-Sachs disease only the infantile congenital form, often known as amaurotic familial idiocy, begins in the 1st year of life. Symptoms usually begin at about 6 months of age and progress steadily until death at 1–4 years. Pathologic changes are limited to the nervous system.

The presenting signs are listlessness, weakness, developmental retardation and feeding difficulties. These may be followed by an inattentive gaze and hyperacusis with subsequent development of seizures, general brain deterioration, a cherry red spot in the macula, blindness and deafness.

If death occurs before 2 years of age, the head may be enlarged, the gyri irregularly pale and swollen and the ventricles decreased in size. When death occurs later, the gyri are thin, the sulci deep and gaping and the ventricles enlarged as a result of loss of myelin in the periventricular areas. The cerebellum and brain stem also undergo atrophy.

In early stages the nerve and ganglion cells are swollen and filled with a sudanophilic material that causes displacement of the nucleus to the axon hillock (Fig. 10–11). Macrophages filled with neu-

Fig. 10–11.—Tay-Sachs disease. Brain with swollen neuronal cells. (Courtesy Dr. F. Gillis.)

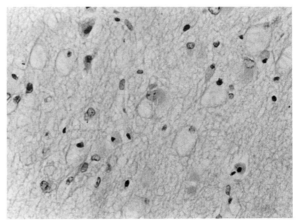

tral fat and called gitter cells, crowd the perivascular areas. Later, demyelinization and glial hyperplasia are common. The material in the neurons is sudanophilic and positive for PAS and Luxol fast blue. The perivascular gitter cells contain mostly neutral fat, but an increase in gangliosides, cholesterol and phosphatides can be demonstrated. Electron photomicrographs of the neurons show the presence of many lipid-filled laminated structures which, on analysis, yield the elements listed above (Fig. 10–12). The only stored lipid that appears specific for the disease is oxyl-sphingosine-triose acetyl neuraminic acid. A histochemical reaction for neuraminic acid (Bial's reaction) is sometimes positive. Because peripheral neuronal cells as well as cells of the central nervous system are involved, rectal biopsy aids in establishing the diagnosis.

A positive PAS reaction and Luxol fast blue deposits have been recognized in the cytoplasm of the neurons of a fetus as early as at 21 weeks' gestation (Adachi *et al.*).

The disease is inherited in an autosomal recessive manner, but no clinical indication of the heterozygous state has been detected. It affects people in all parts of the world but is 100 times more common among Jews than any other group, 90% of all affected individuals in the western world being of Jewish descent. The defect has been identified by Okeda and O'Brien as an absence of hexosaminidase A.

Sandhoff's disease closely resembles Tay-Sachs disease both clinically and in the pathologic changes in the brain, but in Sandhoff's disease lipid is present in occasional macrophages in the viscera and in renal tubular cells. Hexosaminidase A and B are nearly lacking, while in Tay-Sachs disease only A is nearly absent.

Fig. 10–12.—Tay-Sachs disease. Electron photomicrograph of the characteristic membranous bodies within the cells. (Courtesy Dr. B. Volk.)

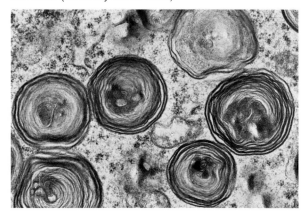

INFANTILE GAUCHER'S DISEASE.—Gaucher's disease is characterized by the storage of glucosyl ceramide and accompanied by a deficiency of a glucocerebroside hydrolase (Brody *et al.*). Although a disease of nearly all ages, the variety that begins in the 1st year of life is more acute, is accompanied by a poorer prognosis and is the only one that frequently involves the central nervous system.

As in Tay-Sachs disease, the first signs—failure to grow normally and develop normal motor skills, anemia, lymphadenopathy and hepatosplenomegaly—appear at about 6 months of age. They are followed by strabismus, irregular respiration, a high-pitched cry, absent Moro reflex and opisthotonos. Serum acid phosphatase is elevated. The joints of the long bones may show destructive lesions as well as a characteristic Erhlenmeyer flask deformity caused by thinning of the bony cortex and widening of the metaphysis.

The essential lesion is an accumulation in enlarged, crinkled reticuloendothelial cells of a slightly sudanophilic, PAS-positive substance that stains best on frozen sections or chromated tissues that have been embedded in paraffin. This helps to prevent extraction of the lipid materials by the fat solvents used in dehydration and clearing. Such cells are found in abundance in the liver (Fig. 10–13, A), spleen (Fig. 10–13, B), lymph nodes, bone marrow, lamina propria of the intestine and alveolar spaces of the lung. The "crinkles" or "folds" that are typical of the Gaucher cells in the viscera are brought out especially well by phosphotungstic acid staining of chromated tissues. Electron microscopy shows them to be collections of tubules of fairly uniform size within membrane-lined spaces in the cytoplasm (Fig. 10–13, C).

Only in the infantile form of Gaucher's disease is the brain involved. Here the lesions are diffuse yet focal. The pyramidal cells of the cortex and neurons of the hippocampus, basal ganglia and brain stem are enlarged and stain in a manner similar to typical Gaucher cells although they lack the characteristic crinkling. Other cells that may be present in perivascular areas that are crinkled are thought to be derived from macrophages. There may also be a mild loss of cells (Fig. 10–14). Although an increase in phospholipid and glycolipid can be demonstrated in the viscera, especially the spleen, they are not increased in the brain.

Three separate modes of inheritance appear possible for this disorder: the infantile form involving the brain seems to be autosomal recessive, while the other forms have been reported as both dominant and recessive. It is most common in Jewish females.

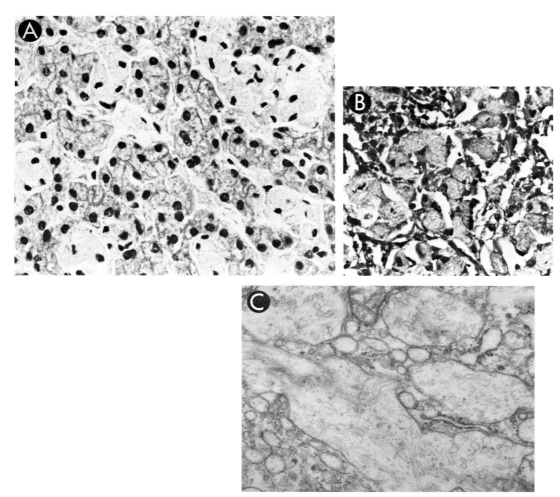

Fig. 10–13.—Gaucher's disease. A, liver with histiocytes distending the sinusoids. (AFIP Reg. No. 5310474.) B, spleen with large histiocytes in the splenic pulp. (Courtesy Dr. G. Vawter.) C, electron photomicrograph of a splenic Gaucher cell showing the tubules within membranes that are distinctive of Gaucher's disease. (Courtesy Dr. E. Fisher.)

Fig. 10–14.—Infantile Gaucher's disease. Brain stem with markedly swollen cells. (Courtesy Dr. G. Vawter.)

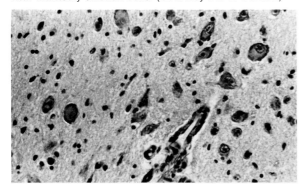

In older patients the viscera and one or many bones may be involved. All affected cells have an almost identical appearance at all ages, except in the brain where no neuronal cells have the typical crinkly pattern seen peripherally.

NIEMANN-PICK DISEASE; SPHINGOMYELIN LIPIDOSIS.—Unlike most diseases of metabolic origin, Niemann-Pick disease may produce death in utero; it also differs from most of the other cerebral lipidoses in that symptoms may appear in the first weeks of life. The presenting sign is often persistent jaundice caused by direct reacting bilirubin, which becomes evident in the neonatal period. The abdomen usually enlarges during the next few months; this is accompanied by inanition, and the patient fails to develop normally. Bronchitis and broncho-pneumonia are common. A cherry red spot is often found in the macula on ophthalmoscopic examination of the retina. Late in the disease mental deterioration and stiffness of the extremities become prominent features. In nearly 85% of the patients the disease progresses rapidly, and death from bronchopneumonia occurs before the end of the 2d year.

At autopsy the liver and spleen are enlarged. The sinusoids of both organs are filled with large round to oval cells with centrally placed round nuclei, or multiple nuclei, surrounded by foamy cytoplasm. The parenchymal cells of the liver are also foamy, the appearance in both instances caused by the presence of large amounts of sphingomyelin and cholesterol (Fig. 10–15). Foam cells are also often found in lymph nodes, bone marrow and alveoli of the lungs, less often in kidney glomeruli and nerve

ganglia. Fat vacuoles are present in monocytes of the peripheral blood.

The affected cells are faintly sudanophilic and PAS-positive in formalin-fixed tissue. Baker's acid hematein, the Smith-Dietrich stain and Landing's phosphomolybdic stain are positive, as would be expected from the excessive phospholipid (as sphingomyelin). Since cholesterol is also increased in the tissues, the Schultz stain for this element is also positive. Changes in the brain are almost indistinguishable from those of Tay-Sachs disease.

In the late stages the brain is decreased in weight, the gyri are narrow and the sulci gaping; the neuronal cells are enlarged, pale and degranulated, the axon hillock is swollen and intracellular fibrils are lost (Fig. 10–16). The major nerve tracts have a decreased amount of myelin but the loss is less severe than in Tay-Sachs disease.

Placentas of fetuses and infants with Niemann-

Fig. 10–15.—Niemann-Pick disease showing characteristic histiocytes filled with a granular lipid material.

A, lymph node. **B,** spleen. **C,** liver. **D,** lung (AFIP Reg. Nos. 5310461, –60, –63 and –58.)

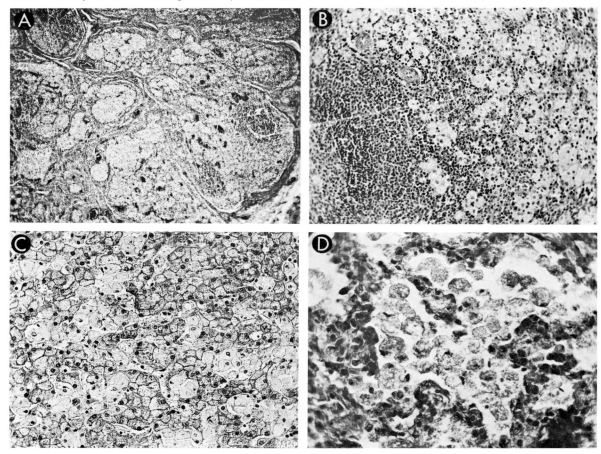

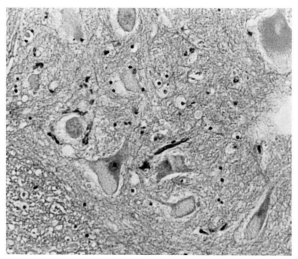

Fig. 10–16. — Niemann-Pick disease. Spinal cord showing markedly swollen neuronal cells. (Courtesy Dr. F. Gillis.)

Pick disease have been described as containing numerous typical foam cells among the Hofbauer cells. Except for one case of Tay-Sachs disease diagnosed in a 21-week fetus, no other congenital metabolic disturbance has been described as a cause of fetal death or as having a distinctive placental lesion.

Sphingomyelin, which appears to be the most actively accumulated lipid in this disease, is increased in the liver, spleen and lymph nodes.

Crocker *et al.* suggested four inheritance patterns in Niemann-Pick disease but the one thought to be responsible for the disease as it occurs in early infancy is the homozygous state of a recessive gene. In this group the ratio of affected to total infants in a single sibship is greater than 50%; 38% are of Jewish descent (Fredrickson).

LIPOGRANULOMATOSIS. — In 1957 this hereditary metabolic defect was first described in detail by Farber *et al.* in three cases; 17 additional cases have been recorded in the intervening years.

The disease may begin in the 1st month of life with a hoarse cry, loud respiration and pain and limitation of motion in all joints. The child fails to grow and develop normally, the joints become immobilized in flexion, and fever is often present later in the course of the disease. Mental deterioration, areflexia and loss of sight and hearing usually precede death, which usually results from respiratory infection or inanition in the first few years of life.

The primary alteration in the disease is the infil-

tration of many tissues with masses of foam cells, the appearance of which results from the presence of multiple small droplets in histiocytes. They are accompanied by local destruction and a granulomatous reaction. Lesions are present in the heart valves. The lung alveoli are filled with foam cells and the alveolar walls are greatly thickened (Fig. 10–17, A). Foam cells are abundant in the sinusoids of the lymph nodes (Fig. 10–17, B) and spleen. Tendon sheaths are infiltrated, and infiltration of the joint capsules leads to the fibrosis and pannus formation responsible for restricted mobility (Fig. 10–17, C). Cells in subcutaneous tissue produce palpable skin nodules. The liver and bone marrow are usually spared although portions of bones near the joints may be destroyed. Neurons are chiefly affected in the spinal cord, medulla and basilar areas of the brain and less affected in the cerebral cortex. The neuronal cells are swollen and degranulated, the nucleus is displaced and the axon hillock swollen (Fig. 10–17, D).

The foam cells and the enlarged neurons are Sudan-, PAS- and Hale-positive, indicating the presence of fat and mucopolysaccharides. The storage material has not been completely identified but is considered to be a glycolipid.

GENERALIZED GANGLIOSIDOSIS, FAMILIAL NEUROVISCERAL LIPIDOSIS. — Such cases have been reported in the past as "visceral Tay-Sachs" or "Hurler's variant," but it now seems fairly obvious that they are a distinct entity. Two different forms of the disease have been identified: the first, with a very early onset, has more of the features that suggest Hurler's disease, while in the second, with an onset at about 8 months, viscera are spared and bones are chiefly affected (Suzuki *et al.*).

This syndrome is marked by the onset of edema, ascites and respiratory difficulty in the first weeks of life. Hepatosplenomegaly is usually present early. A constant feature is the development of kyphosis with narrowing and wedging of the lumbar vertebrae in a manner similar to that seen in Hurler's disease. The long bones are shortened, coarsely trabeculated and thickened and the medullary cavity is expanded. Cherry red spots have been seen in the macular areas in several cases. Mental retardation is common and blindness is occasionally present. Alder-Reilly granules (basophilic cytoplasmic granules) appear in the granulocytes and lymphocytes of the peripheral blood.

The liver, spleen, bone marrow, thymus, lymph nodes and lamina propria contain lipid-filled foamy histiocytes (Fig. 10–18, A), and the parenchymal cells of liver, pancreas and thyroid are some-

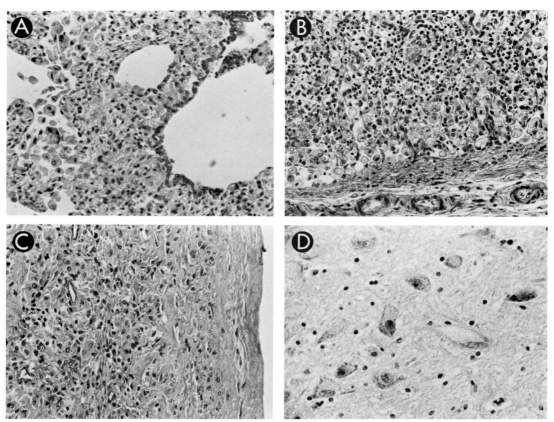

Fig. 10–17.—Lipogranulomatosis with foam cells. **A,** lung. **B,** lymph node. **C,** joint synovia. **D,** basal ganglia of the brain. (Courtesy Drs. G. Vawter and S. Farber.)

times vacuolated. The glomerular epithelium has a distinctive swelling of nonvacuolated cells (Fig. 10–18, B). Neurons of brain and peripheral ganglia are enlarged and faintly PAS-positive but not metachromatic. Sudan-black-positive material is present exclusively in the histiocytes of the liver and spleen. The glomerular epithelium is PAS- and Hale-positive. The histochemical reactions suggest the presence of a glycolipid; chemically the stored material has been reported to be a ganglioside and the defect has been identified as a lysosomal deficiency of beta-galactosidase (O'Brien).

The hereditary pattern has not been established; cases have been observed in Jews, Negroes and Italians.

THE GENETIC MUCOPOLYSACCHARIDOSES. — Of the five members of this group brought together by McKusick only types I and II have a sufficiently early onset to be considered in infants under 1 year of age.

Type I, Hurler's disease (gargoylism, Hurler-

Pfaundler's disease), is the most common member of the group. It usually begins after only a few months of normal life. The presenting symptoms are musculoskeletal with progressive stiffness of the joints and development of a gibbus. Rhinitis and noisy breathing appear early. In the fully developed disease the infants have a typical and unique appearance with prominent frontal ridges, abnormal nasal bones, corneal clouding, hyperexpanded chest, enlarged liver and spleen, umbilical hernia, broad hands, coarse fingers and a lanugo type of hair on the skin (Fig. 10–19). Roentgenograms reveal short wide bones with decreased trabeculation and expanded medullary cavities, beaked lumbar vertebrae and an enlarged sella turcica.

The parenchymal and reticuloendothelial cells of the enlarged liver and spleen and the cells of the proximal convoluted tubules of the kidneys have vacuoles that surround the nucleus symmetrically. Similar cells are also present in cardiac valves, myocardium, blood vessel walls, meninges and cor-

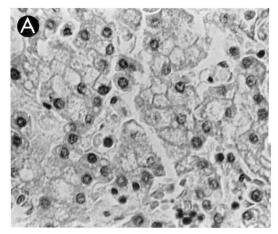

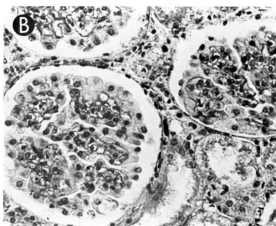

Fig. 10–18.—Familial neurovisceral lipidosis. **A,** liver. The cells are vacuolated, but the contained material is neither neutral fat nor glycogen. **B,** kidney showing swelling of epithelial cells in a renal glomerulus.

nea. The corium of the skin may have diffuse deposits of extracellular mucopolysaccharide that can sometimes be felt below the skin surface. Infiltration of the meninges may cause hydrocephalus. In the central nervous system the neurons are swollen (Fig. 10–20), the nuclei displaced and the neurofibrils lost. Changes are also present in the glial cells but are less marked than in the neural elements. Rarely, demyelinization is present (see also Chapter 24).

Since the stored material is soluble in nearly all aqueous fixatives and partially soluble in alcohol, special precautions are needed for its demonstration. The most effective fixatives are Rossman's

Fig. 10–19.—Hurler's disease. **A,** infant aged 6 months. The father made the diagnosis at birth, stating that the infant appeared exactly the same as had an older affected sibling. **B,** siblings with Hurler's disease. The one on the left is the child shown in A.

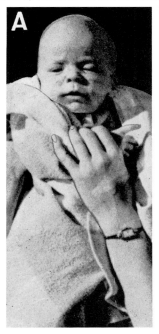

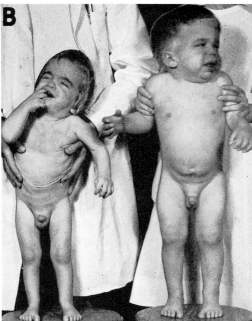

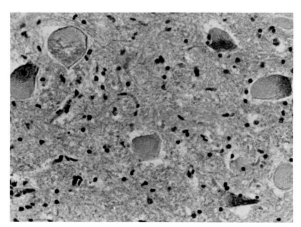

Fig. 10–20. — Hurler's disease. Spinal cord with swollen vacuolated neuronal cells. (Courtesy Dr. G. Vawter.)

(absolute alcohol saturated with picric acid, 10% formalin and 2% glacial acetic acid added by volume) or Lindsay's (dioxane saturated with picric acid, formaldehyde 10% and glacial acetic acid 2% by volume). When properly fixed and stained, the stored material is PAS- and Hale-positive and brilliantly metachromatic with toluidine blue. The principal and characteristic material stored is a combination of chondroitin sulfate B and heparitin S, both of which are complex polysaccharides containing active sulfate groups that give the metachromasia. The fact that lipids can be demonstrated in the brain and in some chondrocytes gave rise to the name lipochondrodystrophy, but since the chief and characteristic materials are mucopolysaccharides, the term mucopolysaccharidosis is the preferred designation.

Inheritance is consistent with an autosomal recessive pattern.

Type II, Hunter-Hurler syndrome, has many of the features of type I with the same stored material and géneral pathologic findings. However, it develops more slowly and is marked by greater deafness, longer life and less clouding of the cornea. It is inherited through a sex-linked recessive gene and is more common than the simple recessive form designated as type I.

Among the other genetic mucopolysaccharidoses are *Morquio's* disease, which is discussed in Chapter 25. *San Fillipo's* and *Scheie's* diseases, which have an onset after the 1st year of life, will not be considered here.

Other inborn errors of metabolism are reviewed in the chapters dealing with the individual organs chiefly involved.

REFERENCES

Adachi, M., Torri, J., Schneck, L., and Volk, B. W.: The fine structure of fetal Tay-Sachs disease, Arch. Pathol. 91:48, 1971.

Alvord, E. C., Stevenson, L. D., Vogel, F. S., and Engel, R. L., Jr.: Neuropathological findings in phenylpyruvic oligophrenia (phenylketonuria), J. Neuropathol. Exp. Neurol. 9:298, 1950.

Banker, B. Q., Miller, J. O., and Crocker, A. C.: The Cerebral Pathology of Infantile Gaucher's Disease, in Aronson, S. M., and Volk, B. W. (eds.): *Cerebral Sphingolipidoses* (New York: Academic Press, 1962), p. 73.

Bell, L. S., Blair, W. C., Lindsay, S., and Watson, S. J.: Lesions of galactose diabetes, Arch. Pathol. 49:393, 1950.

Bickel, H., Barr, H., Astley, R., Douglas, A. A., Finch, E., Horns, H., Harvey, C. C., Hickmans, E. M., Smallwood, W. C., Smellie, J. M., and Teell, C. G.: Cystine storage disease with aminoaciduria and dwarfism (Lignac-Fanconi), Acta Paediatr. Scand. (supp.) 90:1, 1952.

Bloom, W.: The histogenesis of essential lipid histiocytosis (Niemann-Pick's disease), Arch. Pathol. 6:828, 1928.

Brody, R. O., Kenfer, J. R., and Shapiro, D.: Metabolism of cerebrosides. II. Evidence of an enzymatic defect in Gaucher's disease, Biochem. Biophys. Res. Commun. 18: 221, 1965.

Burne, J. C.: Niemann-Pick's disease in a fetus, J. Pathol. Bacteriol. 66:473, 1953.

Cardiff, R. D.: A histochemical and electron microscope study of skeletal muscle in Pompe's disease, glycogenosis II, Pediatrics 37:249, 1965.

Crocker, A. C., Cohen, J., and Farber, S.: The Lipogranulomatous Syndrome, in Aronson, S. M., and Volk, B. W. (eds.): *Inborn Disorders of Sphingolipid Metabolism* (Oxford: Pergamon Press, 1967).

Crocker, A. C., and Farber, S.: Niemann-Pick's disease: A review of 18 patients, Medicine 37:1, 1958.

Crome, L.: A case of galactosemia with pathological and neuropathological findings, Arch. Dis. Child. 37:415, 1962.

Crome, L.: The association of phenylketonuria with leukodystrophy, J. Neurol. Neurosurg. Psychiatry 25:149, 1962.

Dancis, J., and Lively, M.: Maple Syrup Urine Disease (Branched Chain Ketonuria), in Stanbury, J. B. (ed.): *The Metabolic Basis of Inherited Disease* (2d ed.; New York: McGraw-Hill Book Co., 1966), p. 353.

Darmady, E. M., and Stranack, F.: Microdissection of the nephron in disease, Br. Med. Bull. 13:21, 1957.

de Toni, G.: Renal rickets with phospho-gluco-amino renal diabetes, Ann. Paediat. 187:42, 1956.

Dorfman, A.: Heritable Disorders of Connective Tissue: The Hurler Syndrome, in Stanbury, J. B. (ed.): *The Metabolic Basis of Inherited Disease* (2d ed.; New York: McGraw-Hill Book Co., 1966), p. 963.

Diezel, P. B., and Martin, K.: Maple syrup urine disease, with familial occurrence, Arch. Pathol. Anat. 337:425, 1964.

di Sant Agnese, P. A., Andersen, D. H., Mason, A. H., and Bauman, W. A.: Glycogen storage disease of the heart, Pediatrics 6:402, 1950.

Farber, S., Cohen, J., and Uzman, L. L.: Lipogranulomatosis — a new lipoglycoprotein "storage" disease, J. Mt. Sinai Hosp. 24:816, 1957.

Field, R. A.: Glycogen Deposition Diseases, in Stanbury, J. B. (ed.): *The Metabolic Basis of Inherited Disease* (2d ed.; New York: McGraw-Hill Book Co., 1966), p. 141.

Følling, A.: Uber Auscheiding von Phenyl brenztraubensaure in den Harn als Stoffwechsel anomalie in Verbindung mit Imbezillitat, Z. Physiol. Chem. 227:169, 1934.

Forbes, G. B.: Glycogen storage disease, J. Pediatr. 42: 645, 1953.

Fredrickson, D. S.: Cerebral Lipidoses, Gaucher's, in Stanbury, J. B. (ed.): *The Metabolic Basis of Inherited Disease* (2d ed.; New York: McGraw-Hill Book Co., 1966), p. 565.

Fredrickson, D. S., and Lees, R. S.: Familial hyperlipoproteinemia, in Stanbury, J. B. (ed.): *The Metabolic Basis of Inherited Disease* (2d ed.; New York: McGraw-Hill Book Co., 1966), p. 429.

Froesch, R.: Essential Fructosuria and Hereditary Fructose Intolerance, in Stanbury, J. B. (ed.): *The Metabolic Basis of Inherited Disease* (2d ed.; New York: McGraw-Hill Book Co., 1966), p. 124.

Garancia, J. C.: Type II glycogenosis, Am. J. Med. 44:289, 1968.

Gentz, J., Jagenburg, R., and Zetterstrom, R.: Tyrosinemia, J. Pediatr. 66:670, 1965.

Ghadimi, H.: Diagnosis of inborn errors of metabolism, Am. J. Dis. Child. 114:433, 1967.

Globus, J.: Amaurotic familial idiocy, J. Mt. Sinai Hosp. 9:451, 1942.

Halversen, J. L., Pande, H., Løsen, A. C., and Gjessing, L. R.: Tyrinosis, Arch. Dis. Child. 41:238, 1966.

Henderson, J. L., MacGregor, A., Thannhauser, S. J., and Holden, R.: Pathology and biochemistry of gargoylism, Arch. Dis. Child. 27:230, 1952.

Hers, H. G.: Glycogen storage disease, Adv. Metab. Disord. 1:2, 1964.

Hockaday, T. D. R., Clayton, J., Frederick, E. W., and Smith, L. H., Jr.: Primary hyperoxaluria, Medicine 43: 315, 1964.

Hsia, D. Y.: *Inborn Errors of Metabolism* (2d ed.; Chicago: Year Book Medical Publishers, Inc., 1966).

Hug, G., Garancis, J. C., Schubert, W. K., and Kaplan, S.: Glycogen storage disease: Types II, III, VIII and IX, Am. J. Dis. Child. 111:457, 1966.

Isselbacher, K.: Galactosemia, in Stanbury, J. B. (ed.): *The Metabolic Basis of Inherited Disease* (2d ed.; New York: McGraw-Hill Book Co., 1966), p. 178.

Isselbacher, K., Scheig, R., Plotkin, G. R., and Caulfield, J. B.: Congenital beta-lipoprotein deficiency, Medicine 43:347, 1964.

Jervis, G. A.: Gargoylism (lipochondrodystrophy), Arch. Neurol. Psychiatry 63:681, 1950.

Jordan, S. W.: Electron microscopy of Gaucher's cells, Exp. Mol. Pathol. 3:76, 1967.

Lagunoff, D., Ross, R., and Benditt, E.: Histochemical and electron microscopic study in a case of Hurler's disease, Am. J. Pathol. 41:273, 1962.

Lamy, M., Dubois, R., Rossier, A., Frezul, J., Loeb, H., and Blancher, G.: La glycogenese par deficiencie en phosphorylase hepatique, Arch. Fr. Pediatr. 17:14, 1960.

Landing, B. H., and Freiman, D. G.: Histochemical studies on the cerebral lipidoses and other cellular metabolic disorders, Am. J. Pathol. 33:1, 1957.

Landing, B. H., Silverman, F. S., Craig, J. M., Lahey, M. E., and Chadwich, D. L.: Familial neurovisceral lipidosis, Am. J. Dis. Child. 108:503, 1964.

Levin, S.: Specific skin lesion in gargoylism, Am. J. Dis. Child. 99:444, 1960.

Lindsay, S., Reilly, W. A., Gotham, T. J., and Skahan, R. J.: Gargoylism, II: Study of the lesions and clinical review of 12 cases, Am. J. Dis. Child. 76:239, 1948.

Lough, J., Fawcett, J., and Wiegensberg, B.: Wolman's disease: An electron microscopic, histochemical and biochemical study, Arch. Pathol. 89:103, 1970.

Lynn, R., and Terry, R. D.: Lipid histochemistry and electron microscopy in adult Niemann-Pick's disease, Am. J. Med. 37:987, 1964.

MacDonald, A. M., and Shanks, R. A.: Hypophosphatasia, Arch. Dis. Child. 32:304, 1957.

Maker, J. A., Epstein, F. H., and Hand, E. A.: Xanthomatosis and coronary heart disease, Arch. Intern. Med. 102:437, 1958.

McKusick, V.: Mucopolysaccharidosis, in *Heritable Disorders of Connective Tissues* (St. Louis: C. V. Mosby Co., 1966).

McKusick, V. A.: The relative frequency of the Hurler and Hunter's syndrome, N. Engl. J. Med. 283:853, 1970.

McKusick, V. A.: The genetic mucopolysaccharidoses, Medicine 46:445, 1965.

Menkes, J. H., Hurst, P. L., and Craig, J. M.: A new syndrome: Progressive familial cerebral dysfunction associated with an unusual urinary substance, Pediatrics 14: 462, 1954.

Morrison, R. M., Urich, H., and Lloyd, O. C.: The neuropathology of infantile Gaucher's disease, J. Pathol. Bacteriol. 72:121, 1956.

O'Brien, J. S.: Generalized gangliosidosis, J. Neurol. 75: 167, 1969.

Okeda, S., and O'Brien, J. S.: Tay-Sachs disease: Generalized absence of a beta D-N-acetyl-hexosaminidase component, Science 165:698, 1969.

Patrick, A. D., and Lake, B. D.: Acid lipase deficiency in Wolman's disease, Nature 222:1067, 1969.

Royer, P., Lastendet, I. H., Habib, R., Lardinois, R., and Desbuquois, B.: L'intolerance hereditaire au fructose, Bull. Mem. Soc. Med. Paris 115:805, 1964.

Sidbury, J. B., Jr., Mason, J., Burns, W. B., and Reubner, B. H.: Type IV glycogenosis. Report of a case proven by characterization of the glycogen and studied at necropsy, Bull. Johns Hopkins Hosp. 111:157, 1962.

Silberman, J., Dancis, J., and Feigin, I.: Neuropathological observations in maple syrup urine disease, Arch. Neurol. 5:351, 1961.

Sobreville, L. A., Goodman, M., and Kane, C. A.: Demyelinating central nervous system disease, macular atrophy and acanthrocytosis, Am. J. Med. 37:821, 1964.

Spear, G. S., Slusser, R. J., Tousimis, A., Taylor, C. G., and Schulman, J. D.: Cystinosis. An ultrastructural and electron-probe study of the kidney with unusual findings, Arch. Pathol. 21:206, 1971.

Suzuki, I., Crocker, H. C., and Suzuki, K.: GM 1 gangliosidosis, Arch. Neurol. 24:58, 1971.

Townsend, E. H., Jr., Mason, H. H., and Strong, P. S.: Galactosemia and its relation to Laennec's cirrhosis, Pediatrics 7:760, 1951.

Wolfe, H. J., and Cohen, R. B.: Non glycogen polysaccharide storage in glycogenosis. Type II (Pompe's disease), Arch. Pathol. 86:579, 1968.

Wyngaarden, J. B., and Elder, T. D.: Primary Hyperoxaluria and Oxalosis, in Stanbury, J. B. (ed.): *The Metabolic Basis of Inherited Disease* (2d ed.; New York: McGraw-Hill Book Co., 1966), p. 189.

11

Malformations

THE FREQUENCY and importance of malformations as a cause of death or handicap are difficult to assess because of variation in the definition of the term and the fact that they are often not discovered on casual physical examination.

Three of the problems of definition are (1) whether enzymatic disturbances producing the large group of conditions known as inborn errors of metabolism should be included, (2) whether the abnormality must be visible at birth and (3) whether the defect must be a result of primary disturbance in embryonic development or whether it may be secondary to changes such as those caused by prenatal rubella or toxoplasmosis. Warkany summarized the various points of view and reasonably concluded that "congenital anomalies" should be used to include all abnormalities of behavior, function and structure known to be present at birth, while "malformations" should include all *gross* structural abnormalities present at birth regardless of cause.

Malformations may be single or multiple, internal or external, major (capable of causing handicaps or death) or minor, primary or secondary, familial or sporadic, limited to certain ethnic groups or of equal frequency in all populations, and of known or unknown cause. Those not visible at birth and manifesting themselves only months or years later would be excluded on the basis of Warkany's strict definition.

Through the ages the cause and significance of malformations have prompted innumerable speculations. Superstitions such as belief in the importance of astrologic events, maternal impressions and the work of witches were slow to die even after the elaboration of the microscope, the establishment of cells as units of growth and the discovery of embryologic processes.

In modern times it has been realized that both heredity and environment play a role in the production of malformations, i.e., the genetic and chromosomal components of the germ cells and the milieu in which they develop. Until the thalidomide tragedy, however, the importance of the environment as related to the development of the human fetus was not fully appreciated in spite of the earlier demonstration by many investigators of the role it plays in the development of laboratory animals.

At present some malformations are recognized as being caused by genetic or chromosomal abnormalities, by environmental disturbances such as the presence in the mother of certain diseases or drugs, or in some instances by genes that manifest themselves only under certain environmental conditions.

Incidence

Statistics on the prevalence of malformations vary greatly, even in similar population groups. An example of this is evident in comparing the incidence of malformations found by most investigators with that from a prospective study by McIntosh *et al.* who made a determined effort to bring to light all definable malformations by repeated follow-up examinations and free use of roentgenograms. This group gave an incidence of 13.6% for fetuses dying in utero, 23.3% for those dying intrapartum and 29.6% for infants dying in the first 30 days of life. Of those living more than 30 days, 7% had malformations. In contrast to this, Stevenson *et al.,* whose data were taken from retrospective study of the records of stillborn and newborn infants at discharge in an obstetric hospital, reported an incidence of 15.9% among stillbirths, 13.2% among infants dying in the first 10 days of life and 1.7% among those who were discharged from the hospital at more than 10 days of age. For all births the incidence of malformations was 2.7%. In this study no special effort was made to discover malformations.

Some malformations vary greatly in different races—e.g., postminimus in negroes—or in the same race in different parts of the world—e.g., anencephalus. To have significance the location and the conditions surrounding collection of data must be known.

Malformations of Genetic or Chromosomal Origin

Malformations may result from the presence of genes responsible for the unusual development of certain structures. Such genes have been transmitted from a parent who harbored them because of mutation or previous transmission. Genes from one parent may be sufficient to cause the abnormality (dominant), or similar genes from both parents may be required (recessive). When abnormalities are largely limited to one sex, the responsible genes are said to be sex-linked. A few abnormalities occur principally in one sex—e.g., anencephaly in females and bilateral renal agenesis in males—in the absence of recognized genetic disturbance and with the cause unknown. Mutations producing some changes in genes appear to be rare, while others, such as those for achondroplasia, are common. Mutant genes are subsequently transmissible, and all inherited abnormalities are probably originally a result of mutation.

Disturbances caused by genetic abnormalities most often involve a localized part of the body (syndactyly, polydactyly) or a particular variety of tissue (achondroplasia), although a few that have been described as pleotrophic affect various organs or tissues. If a certain gene always produces the malformation, penetrance is said to be high. If the phenotypic changes accompanying the presence of a gene are always the same, expressivity is described as high (Fig. 11–1).

Chromosomal abnormalities came to be recognized as causes of malformations when it was learned that, by the use of certain technics, chromosomes within cells could be studied individually. Methods used for the identification of chromosomes consist of growing cells in tissue culture, adding colchicine in order to arrest mitosis at the metaphase, then placing them in hypotonic saline solution in order to cause swelling and separation of

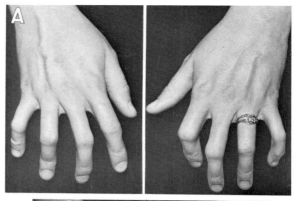

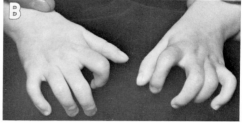

Fig. 11–1.—Contractures of fingers caused by dominant genes of high penetrance and expressivity. **A,** mother. **B,** daughter.

chromosomes, and finally staining and squashing. By this means it is possible to observe all chromosomes in a cell and categorize them according to shape and size (Fig. 11–2). Chromosomes have been numbered and placed in groups designated by letters as follows:

A = 1–3	D = 13–15
B = 4–5	E = 16–18
C = 6–12	F = 19–20
	G = 21–11

The sex chromosomes, X and Y, are considered separately and not numbered. Various abnormalities such as fragmentation, ring formation and adherence of abnormal parts have been identified, but by far the most common is the presence of one too few or too many chromosomes. The differences in numbers are believed to result from nondisjunction of chromosomes during meiotic division of a primitive germ cell or the first mitotic division of the zygote. Turner's syndrome is the condition most often associated with one too few and trisomy D, E or G with one too many chromosomes. If the chromosomal abnormality occurs after the first zygote division, a state of mosaicism exists in which some somatic cells have normal and some abnormal chromosomes.

A search for chromosomal abnormalities as a

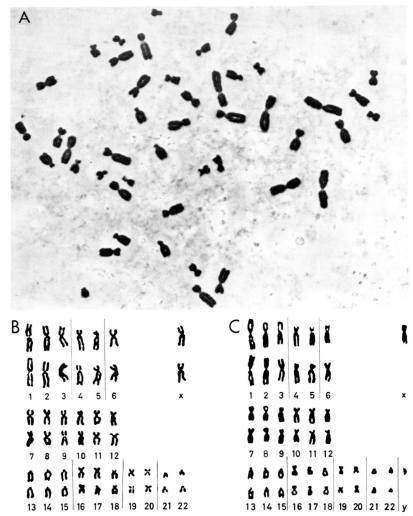

Fig. 11–2.—A, squash preparation of human cell. (Courtesy Dr. A. Levan and T. C. Hsu.) **B** and **C,** idiograms of human mitotic chromosomes rearranged by Tijo and Puck from photographs previously published by them. Present numbering was agreed upon by a committee of specialists in 1960. Arrangement based on size of chromosome and position of centromere. **B,** human female; **C,** human male. (Courtesy Dr. T. T. Puck.)

cause of malformations is most rewarding if children with multiple, seemingly unrelated abnormalities are investigated. Among the earliest diseases in which chromosomal abnormalities were found were those with an abnormal number, e.g., trisomy of chromosome 21 in Down's syndrome, the absence of one of the two X chromosomes in Turner's syndrome, and the presence of an extra X chromosome added to the XY already present in Klinefelter's syndrome. Down's syndrome, which produces severe mental retardation, is discussed here only

briefly and at more length in Chapter 24 (Central Nervous System). Turner's and Klinefelter's syndromes, which produce major changes in gonadal development, are discussed in more detail in Chapter 23 (Reproductive Organs and Breast).

Some of the other conditions, in which malformations are widespread throughout the body without special predilection for any one site, are included here.

DELETION OF A SEX CHROMOSOME.—Absence of an X chromosome from an XY combination seems to prevent development of the zygote, since no material, even from early conceptuses, has ever been found with a YO karyotype. Absence of an X chromosome from an XX combination, giving an XO karyotype, produces *Turner's syndrome* in which absence of germ cells from the ovaries is the outstanding characteristic. In infants, edema of the lower extremities and an excess of skin at the back of the neck are strongly suggestive of this syndrome. Less commonly observed chromosomal changes that produce the same abnormalities are mosaics in which XO cells are combined with XX, XY, XYY and XXX cells (see Chapter 23).

ADDITION OF SEX CHROMOSOMES. — The most common of these is the addition of one X to the normal XY combination, yielding 47 chromosomes all with an XXY constitution. This produces Klinefelter's syndrome, which is characterized by testicular hypoplasia and a eunuchoid appearance. Because of a lack of somatic abnormalities in infancy the diagnosis is seldom made at this time. Other karyotypes that have been found in Klinefelter's syndrome include an additional Y chromosome and as many as 3 additional X chromosomes.

TRISOMY C. — Juberg *et al.* in 1970 reported the first infant with an extra chromosome in the C group to be born alive at term. The major abnormality was the presence of large bilateral cystic kidneys of the Potter type II. Since such kidneys are nonfunctioning in utero, a characteristic Potter facies was present. In addition there were cleft palate, hyperextensible joints and bilateral hip dislocation. The infant weighed 2,200 gm at 38 weeks' gestation and died 1 hour after birth.

TRISOMY D_1 (13 – 15). — Abnormalities in the 13 – 15 group have been widely reported, and affected infants have had malformations of different kinds and degree. Those considered especially characteristic and most often present are arhinencephalus (cyclops and cebocephalus with their accompanying eye and nasal defects), cleft lip and palate, capillary hemangiomas, congenital heart defects (especially ventricular septal defects and patent ductus arteriosus), polydactyly and flexion deformities of thumbs and fingers. Mild cystic disease of the kidneys of Potter type III, umbilical hernias or omphalocele and other minor abnormalities of the intestinal tract are moderately common. Most affected infants die within a few months of birth. None of these abnormalities is constantly present and the same constellation may be found with a normal chromosomal pattern. Chromosomal abnormalities other than a simple

trisomy have been described in a few cases.

TRISOMY E 16 – 18). — This syndrome is characterized by a multiplicity of malformations involving variable organ systems, many abnormalities being relatively minor. The infants are usually underweight at birth and the skin is lax, giving a malnourished appearance. Usually the face is triangular because of a broad cranium and a receding chin, the sutures are wide, the occiput is elongated and the ears stand out from the head, are less upright than normal and are often of unusual shape. Minor skeletal abnormalities are almost always present, with flexion contractions being by far the most common, as they are in trisomy D_1. Short or abnormal sternum, limited hip abduction, rocker bottom feet and syndactyly are also often seen. Cardiac defects are among the most common visceral abnormalities. As in trisomy D_1, ventricular septal defect and patent ductus arteriosus are the most frequent cardiac defects. Malformations of the brain such as those producing cyclops and cebocephalus are rare, but the brain is not normal and the few patients who survive the 1st year are mentally retarded.

Gastrointestinal and urogenital malformations are less common than in trisomy D_1. Death usually occurs within a few months of birth.

TRISOMY 21 (MONGOLISM, DOWN'S SYNDROME). — This syndrome is associated with 47 chromosomes and trisomy of chromosome 21 (G) in over 90% of cases. In the remainder of cases only 46 chromosomes are present, and the abnormality consists of fusion of a small acrocentric chromosome to one of the D chromosomes (D/G) or to a small 21 or 22 chromosome (G/G). The presence of an acrocentric chromosome in a cell may be inherited, and in siblings suffering from Down's syndrome this variety of chromosomal abnormality is usually responsible. The principal changes associated with the abnormality are severe mental retardation and a diagnostic facies. Accompanying abnormalities that are present with varying frequency are brachycephaly, increased width of the lower part of the face, epicanthic folds, Brushfield's spots on the iris, abnormal helix of the ear, in-curved little finger, simian creases in the palm of the hand, increased space between first and second toes and a cardiac defect usually consisting of an atrioventricular ostium.

PARTIAL DELETION OF THE SHORT ARMS OF CHROMOSOME 4. — This defect gives rise to a syndrome characterized by hypertelorism, beaked nose, exophthalmos, hypospadias, cryptorchid testes and bilateral inguinal hernias. Muscular hyperreactivity with twitching begins before 9 months of age (Leão *et al.;* Lejeune *et al.*).

PARTIAL DELETION OF THE SHORT ARM OF CHROMOSOME 5. — This has been identified in association with multiple congenital anomalies of face, skin and growth patterns and is characterized by moon face, micrognathia, microcephaly, hypertelorism and low implantation of the ears (Gordon and Cooke). The infants are small, mentally deficient and have a high-pitched mewing cry *(cri du chat)*. The viscera are usually normal, but in one instance autopsy revealed the absence of the spleen and one kidney as well as malrotation of the large bowel.

RING CHROMOSOME IN THE 1–5 GROUP. — This has been reported in at least 46 cases (Wolf *et al.*). Affected infants, who are retarded microcephalic dwarfs with elfin facies and low-set ears, respond to exogenous growth hormone. No data are available on possible visceral abnormalities.

TRANSLOCATION DEFECT INVOLVING CHROMOSOME 3 AND THE B GROUP. — Affected infants are hypotonic and have a small head, cleft lip and palate, small mandible, low-set ears and coloboma (Walzer *et al.*). They may have transposition of the aorta and subcapsular renal cysts. Six infants have been described in whose families other members have been affected also.

Malformations of Environmental Origin

Alterations in manner of development have been produced in laboratory animals in many ways but few investigators provide explanations for the way in which malformations are produced in man. Many chemical agents will produce such disturbances in laboratory animals but only thalidomide has produced them with any frequency in man. X-ray has produced heritable kidney abnormalities in rats but only microcephaly in human beings. Antigen-antibody reactions have produced various malformations experimentally, but erythroblastosis, a common disease resulting from such a cause, is rarely accompanied by malformations. Viruses and other infectious agents present serious problems in some animals because of the frequency with which they produce abnormalities in the offspring, but in man the only such agent of consequence is the rubella virus, with Toxoplasma and the virus of cytomegalic inclusion disease much less frequent offenders. Maternal diseases other than infections have not been indicted with certainty although severe maternal diabetes mellitus seems to be associated with some increase in malformations of off-spring. The incidence of babies born with malformations is greater among lower than among higher socio-economic groups, a fact that has not been adequately explained. It is known that the absence of certain vitamins or amino acids from the diet may produce malformations experimentally, but such extreme deficiences almost never occur in man. Hypoxia is known to produce malformations both experimentally in animals and under certain conditions in human beings. Placenta previa, which is sometimes accompanied by a reduced placental oxygen supply, is associated with a slightly greater frequency of malformations. In twin pregnancies a fetus receiving blood from only a small portion of the total placenta, or one whose umbilical vessels arise directly from the cord of its twin, may be severely malformed (Fig. 11–3).

A situation that is doubtless also true in man was demonstrated experimentally by Andersen, who showed that the frequency of a certain type of hernia could be greatly increased in some animals by eliminating certain basic substances from the diet in early pregnancy. All experimental and clinical evidence leads to the conclusion that most malformations are similarly a result of an interplay of genetic and environmental factors.

THALIDOMIDE. — This is the only substance ever known to have had a damaging effect on large numbers of infants; it is thought to have produced malformations in almost 7,000 infants during the 4–5-year period it was available. This soporific drug, when taken between the 27th and 45th days of pregnancy, can produce skeletal and visceral abnormalities. The arms, which are most often involved, are affected in about 80% of cases. The degree of involvement varies; there may be no more than shortening or absence of a thumb, or an entire arm may be absent with only a suggestion of fingers attached directly to the shoulder girdle. In severe cases both arms and legs may be phocomelic. The pinna of the ears may be hypoplastic or, rarely, the ears may be absent. Visceral anomalies are infrequent, but aplasia of the gallbladder and appendix, atresia of the duodenum and a bicornuate uterus have been observed.

The compound appears to act on tissues that contain large amounts of glycogen such as rapidly growing cartilage cells. This may account for the severe involvement of the long bones. Thalidomide fulfills three of the characteristic features of the action of teratogenic agents: (1) The lesion produced is dependent upon the time of exposure, involvement of the legs resulting from a later exposure than that of the arms. (2) The agent may be

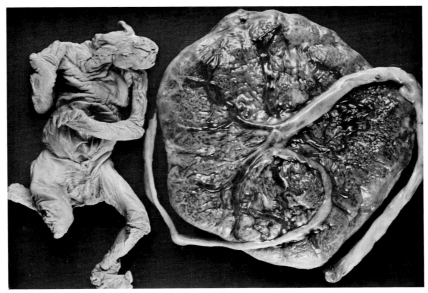

Fig. 11–3.—Anencephalic monster with vessels of its umbilical cord anastomosing with those of its normal monozygotic twin.

harmless to a mother in doses that injure the fetus; no known maternal toxicity has been described. (3) The degree of anomaly appears to be dose-dependent. Unlike many teratogenic agents, the dose difference between lethal and teratogenic levels is large, and this may account for so many children being affected before the relationship between thalidomide and malformations was appreciated.

OTHER CHEMICAL AGENTS.—Among the agents used for tumor therapy are chemicals that are proved teratogens in human beings. Aminopterin, which has been used for therapeutic abortion despite its high maternal toxicity, when given in less than abortifacient doses has produced infants with hydrocephaly, meningoencephalocele, cleft palate, cleft lip, small mandible, low-set ears and abnormal extremities (Warkany). Other reported teratogens of this general class are 6-mercaptopurine and Myleran.

Certain progestins administered to the mother late in pregnancy were described by Wilkins as responsible for genital anomalies in female infants. The malformations, consisting principally of an enlarged clitoris and fused labia, are thought to result from the androgenic properties of the compounds. Such effects might be predicted in view of the general susceptibility of the female external genitalia to androgens.

X-RAY.—Of the physical agents capable of producing anomalies, ionizing radiation is the only one that has been demonstrated in human beings.

(Hicks and D'Amato). The rapidly dividing neuroblasts of the paraventricular regions of the brain are particularly susceptible. Damage to these at critical times leads to a deficit in total neural tissue, particularly the cerebral cortex, with resultant microcephaly. This condition was found in a few infants whose mothers were exposed to an atomic bomb explosion and received high but not lethal radiation at a critical time in pregnancy. Therapeutic radiation of the pelvic organs has been shown to have a similar effect.

INFECTIOUS AGENTS.—The only infectious agent proved to be teratogenic in man is the rubella virus. Rubella infection may cause severe generalized damage to the developing fetus, but true malformation is limited to the heart, as distinguished from destructive effects, which include microcephaly, deafness and cataract formation. The most common cardiac lesions are patent ductus arteriosus and pulmonary stenosis, while those somewhat less common are atrial and ventricular septal defects and malformations of the aortic arch such as stenosis and coarctation (Cooper).

MATERNAL DISEASE.—The unusually high frequency of congenital anomalies observed at the Boston Hospital for Women among infants of diabetic mothers may well be another example of the effect of environment on the conceptus. Since diabetes itself may be in part an inherited disease, it is difficult to separate the components. The observation that anomalies in infants of diabetic mothers are more frequent in more severely affected mothers suggests that the teratogenic state is dose-dependent and hence environmentally controlled. Observations at the Chicago Lying-in Hospital failed to confirm an increased frequency of malformations in infants of diabetic mothers, but it is possible that the mothers were less severely affected than those at the Boston Hospital for Women.

Syndromes of Combined Genetic and Environmental Origin

The malformations that have an incidence of at least 1/1,000 total births (such as cleft lip, cleft palate, pyloric stenosis, clubfeet, congenital hip dysplasia, spina bifida, anencephaly and congenital cardiac defects) have genetic and family patterns with much in common. Carter thought that their inheritance patterns strongly suggest a polygenic inheritance interacting with environmental factors. Many malformations doubtless fall into this category including those such as neurofibromatosis and osteogenesis imperfecta in which the manifestations are variable.

Recklinghausen's neurofibromatosis is a disturbance inherited through a dominant gene that, like achondroplasia, has a high mutation rate. It has been observed repeatedly in as many as three to four generations (Borberg). The manifestations are extremely variable, even within families. The lesions most commonly present at birth are macrodactyly (see Fig. 25–91, B) and *café au lait* spots on the skin. Others observed at birth include neurofibromas, buphthalmos, macroglossia, scoliosis, pathologic fractures and pseudarthrosis (Warkany). The occasional presence of these conditions in the newborn infant indicates that the fetus is susceptible to malformation resulting from the presence of the gene, but the fact that many individuals at a later time show only some of the possible abnormalities indicates that both before and after birth environmental factors must play a role in the manifestation of the potential disorders.

Osteogenesis imperfecta is another inherited condition with variable manifestations. The three cardinal abnormalities are fragile bones, blue sclerae and middle ear deafness. They may be of any degree, especially the fragility of the bones, and any or all may be present at birth or may appear in later life (see page 562).

Syndromes of Unknown Origin

Several syndromes have been described in which certain internal and external malformations have been present but no organ has been predominantly involved and no cause has been postulated. In others, various malformations are present that at first glance seem to be unrelated but on further study are found to be directly related to the principal malformation. One of the best examples of this is the pulmonary hypoplasia, clubfeet and facies that accompany renal agenesis.

Other syndromes with no definitely established cause but in which there has been an occasional attempt to show a genetic background include the following:

LENZ MICROPHTHALMIA SYNDROME. — This is associated with microphthalmia, microcephaly, skeletal and dental defects, hypospadias, cryptorchidism and renal dysgenesis.

MECKEL SYNDROME (DYSENCEPHALIA SPLANCHNOCYSTICA). — This syndrome, as described by Opitz and Howe, seems entirely nonspecific, and it appears that almost any malformation may be included although those involving kidneys, head, heart and digits are said to be the most common. At the Chicago Lying-in Hospital, among 120 fetuses and infants with type II cystic kidneys (fatal renal dysgenesis), 34 had malformations of the central nervous system. Most of these fetuses and infants also had malformations in other parts of the body, including the heart, and 18 had malformed hearts without recognized malformations of the central nervous system. Abnormalities of digits and other parts of the body were common in both groups. Many infants have been seen without renal malformations but with malformations in several organ systems, and it seems questionable whether categorizing such variable abnormalities as belonging to a particular syndrome is warranted.

ZELLWEGER'S CEREBROHEPATORENAL SYNDROME. — This is an unusual combination of extreme hypotonia, mental retardation, characteristic facies, leukoencephalomyelopathy, pigment deposition in the liver and mild cystic involvement of the kidneys. Two siblings were the only cases reported with suspected genetic transmission.

BECKWITH'S SYNDROME. — This has now been described by enough investigators to be established as a definite entity. Beckwith originally described an infant with an umbilical hernia, macroglossia, visceral hypertrophy especially involving the kidneys and cytomegaly of the adrenal glands. These still remain the outstanding characteristics of the syndrome (Fig. 11–4) but some infants subsequently reported have had hemihypertrophy, hyperinsulinism from island cell hyperplasia in the pancreas, an increase in bone age and rate of growth, and clitoral hypertrophy (Roe *et al.;* Sotelo-Avila and Singer).

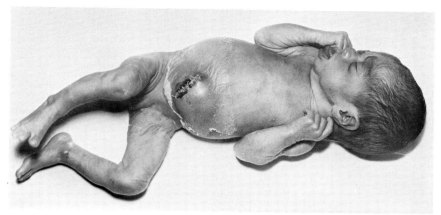

Fig. 11–4.—Beckwith's syndrome in newborn infant. Note macroglossia and umbilical hernia.

As in most syndromes, any of these conditions may be found separately or in combination with other abnormalities. The reason for this particular combination is unknown. The syndrome is not incompatible with survival but most affected infants described have died in the early months of life.

REFERENCES

Andersen, D. H.: Effect of diet during pregnancy on incidence of congenital hereditary diaphragmatic hernia in the rat: Failure to produce cystic fibrosis in the pancreas by maternal vitamin A deficiency, Am. J. Pathol. 25: 163, 1949.

Beckwith, J. B.: Macroglossia, omphalocele, adrenal cytomegaly, gigantism and hyperplastic visceromegaly, Birth Defects (Original Article Series) 5:188, 1969.

Borberg, A.: Clinical and genetic investigations into tuberous sclerosis and Recklinghausen's neurofibromatosis, Acta Psychiatr. Neurol. 71:239, 1951.

Carter, C. O.: Genetics of common disorders, Br. Med. Bull. 25:52, 1969.

Childs, B., and Sidbury, J. B., Jr.: Survey of genetics as it applies to medicine, Pediatrics 20:177, 1959.

Conference on Congenital Malformations: Symposium, J. Chronic Dis. 10:83, 1959.

Congenital malformations: Symposium, Pediatrics 19:719, 1957.

Cooper, L. Z.: Rubella: A preventable cause of birth defects, Birth Defects 4:23, 1968.

Dumers, K. W., Jr., Gaskill, C., and Kitzmiller, N.: Le cri du chat (crying cat) syndrome, Am. J. Dis. Child. 108: 553, 1964.

Ferguson-Smith, M. A.: Karyotype-phenotype correlations in gonadal dysgenesis, J. Med. Genet. 2:142, 1965.

Gordon, R. R., and Cooke, P.: Facial appearance in cri du chat syndrome, Dev. Med. Child Neurol. 10:69, 1968.

Hecht, F., et al.: The number 17-18 (E) trisomy syndrome, J. Pediatr. 63:605, 1963.

Hicks, S. P., and D'Amato, C. J.: Effects of ionizing radiation on mammalian development, Adv. Teratol. 1:195, 1966.

Hoefnagel, D., and Benirschke, K.: Dyscephalia mandibulo-oculo-facialis, Arch. Dis. Child. 40:57, 1965.

Hsia, D. Y.: Human Developmental Genetics (Chicago: Year Book Medical Publishers, Inc., 1968).

Juberg, R. C., Gilbert, E. F., and Salisbury, R. S.: Trisomy C in an infant with polycystic kidneys and other malformations, J. Pediatr. 76:598, 1970.

Leão, J. C., et al.: New syndrome associated with deletion of short arms, chromosome # 4, J.A.M.A. 202:434, 1967.

Lejeune, J., et al.: Partial deletion of short arms of chromosomes. Differentiation of a new syndrome, Sem. Hôp. Paris 40:1067, 1964.

Lenz, W.: Chemicals and Malformations in Man, in Fishbein, M. (ed.): Second International Conference on Congenital Malformations (New York: International Medical Congress, 1964), p. 263.

Lewis, A. J.: The pathology of 19 trisomy, J. Pediatr. 65: 258, 1964.

Marin-Padilla, M., Hoefnagel, D., and Benirschke, K.: Anatomic and histopathologic study of two cases of D_1 (13–15) trisomy, Cytogenetics 3:258, 1964.

McIntosh, R., et al.: The incidence of congenital malformations: A study of 5,964 pregnancies, Pediatrics 14:505, 1954.

Migeon, B. R., and Whitehouse, D.: Familial occurrence of the somatic phenotype of Turner's syndrome, Johns Hopkins Med. J. 120:178, 1967.

Nishimura, H.: Chemistry and Prevention of Congenital Anomalies (Springfield, Ill.: Charles C Thomas, 1964).

Opitz, J. M., and Howe, J. J.: The Meckel Syndrome (Dysencephalia Splanchnocystica, the Gruber Syndrome), in Birth Defects: Original Article Series, 5:167 (New York: The National Foundation-March of Dimes, 1969).

Polani, P. E.: Autosomal imbalance and its syndromes, excluding Down's, Br. Med. Bull. 25:81, 1969.

Polani, P. E., et al.: A mongol girl with 46 chromosomes, Lancet 1:721, 1960.

Rabinowitz, J. G., et al.: Trisomy 18, esophageal atresia, anomalies of radius and hypoplastic thrombocytopenia, Radiology 90:488, 1967.

Rhode, R. A., Hodgman, J. E., and Cleland, R. S.: Multiple congenital deformities in the E_1 trisomy (16–18) syndrome, Pediatrics 33:258, 1969.

Roe, T. F., et al.: Beckwith's syndrome: Extreme organ hyperplasia, Pediatrics 52:372, 1973.

Snodgrass, G. J. A. I., *et al.:* D (13–15) trisomy syndrome—analysis of 17 examples, Arch. Dis. Child. 41: 250, 1964.

Sotelo-Avila, C., and Singer, D. B.: Syndrome of hyperplastic fetal visceromegaly and neonatal hypoglycemia (Beckwith's syndrome), Pediatrics 46:240, 1970.

Stevenson, S. S., Worcester, J., and Rice, R. G.: 677 Congenitally malformed infants and associated gestational abnormalities, Pediatrics 6:37, 1950.

Sutten, H. E.: *An Introduction to Human Genetics* (New York: Holt, Rhinehart, and Winston, 1965).

Walzer, S., *et al.:* New translocation syndrome 3/B, N. Engl. J. Med. 275:290, 1966.

Warkany, J.: *Congenital Malformations* (Chicago: Year Book Medical Publishers, Inc., 1971).

Warkany, J., Beaudry, P. H., and Hornstein, S.: Attempted abortion with aminopterin, malformation of the child, Am. J. Dis. Child. 97:274, 1959.

Warkany, J., Passarge, E., and Smith, L. B.: Congenital malformations in autosomal trisomies, Am. J. Dis. Child. 112:502, 1966.

Wilkins, L.: Masculinization of the female fetus due to use of orally given progestins, J.A.M.A. 172:1028, 1960.

Willis, R. A.: *Borderlands of Embryology and Pathology* (London: Butterworth & Co., Ltd., 1958).

Wolf, C. B., *et al.:* Ring 1 chromosome and partial dwarfism, J. Pediatr. 71:719, 1967.

Yakovlev, A.: Pathoarchitectonic studies of cerebral malformation. III. Arrhinencephalydes, J. Neuropathol. Exp. Neurol. 18:22, 1959.

12

Tumors

General Survey

IT IS IMPOSSIBLE to differentiate sharply between tumors present at birth and other types of congenital malformations. Since the latter include all abnormalities in tissue differentiation that arise during intrauterine development, tumors must be included in this category. Nevertheless, it is interesting to try to isolate a group of malformations that resemble lesions that in adults are ordinarily included under the heading of neoplasms.

A tumor, according to most concepts, is a mass of cells that proliferates without relation to pattern or rate of growth of the part in which it is located and is capable of independent growth after the inciting agent has stopped acting. The last part of the definition in large measure limits the tissue overgrowths present at birth that can be correctly diagnosed as congenital tumors to those that are malignant, since after birth most others grow at the same rate as the rest of the body.

The following discussion describes many more conditions than a strict definition of the word tumor would permit and includes all masses of tissue that have grown in locations or amounts that diverge from the normal pattern of development and that do not duplicate, partially or completely, any normal structure of the body. This eliminates such overgrowth of tissue as double ureters, accessory spleens and duplication of the intestinal tract; however, it is not as easy to draw the line in other areas. There is no sharp distinction between a parasitic fetus and a superficially located teratoma, nor is it easy to decide whether a small digitus postminimus should be called an accessory digit or a tumor.

A mixed tumor or teratoma may rarely have a remarkable resemblance to a fetus and there may be difficulty in differentiating such abnormal growths from the malformations that result from abortive attempts at twinning.

A special problem exists in the microscopic distinction between benign and malignant neoplasms in tumors that have arisen before birth. All cell proliferation takes place rapidly in utero, and it is often impossible to tell by examination of tissue immediately after birth whether the cells have been growing independently with the complete lack of restraint characteristic of malignancy or whether their growth, although abnormal, has been subject to the same restraining influences as the rest of the body.

The multiplication of all cells in normal tissue is limited. The genetic propensity for growth is such that a certain size, once reached, is maintained without further increase. If mutations change the genetic potentialities, or if the environment is altered, such limitation may be lost and a malignant tumor produced.

No tumor of the adult ordinarily grows as rapidly as does the normal embryo. Especially in the early stages of development, normal embryonic cells may have some of the characteristics of neoplastic cells. While many malignant cells have abnormal chromosome numbers, and in mitosis with triploidy and tetraploidy may appear very abnormal, others, even with demonstrable aneuploidy, may not have abnormal mitotic figures demonstrable in routine sections. Consequently, abnormal mitoses cannot always be used to distinguish malignant from benign tumors.

It is often only from knowledge of the postnatal course of a tumor that definite proof can be obtained of its malignancy. Neuroblastomas are usually considered malignant, but some have been observed in which neuroblasts differentiated postnatally into mature ganglion cells and did not behave as would those of a malignant tumor. Neuroblastomatous tissue has been found widely distributed throughout the liver and abdominal cavity at birth and has sometimes been considered of metastatic origin. However, since neuroblasts are normally present in the liver and other parts of the embryo, it is more probable that these cells are subject to the same stimulus responsible for the more massive local proliferation considered as the primary tumor but are of local origin rather than disseminated from the principal tumor.

One very malignant-appearing tumor in the forearm of an infant at birth involved both the ulna and radius; roentgen examination revealed only small portions of the proximal and distal ends of the bones remaining (Fig. 12–1). The tumor was composed of extremely immature fibroblasts, many

Fig. 12–1.—Spindle cell sarcoma of forearm removed immediately after birth. No bone present except small masses near wrist and elbow. Child survived following simple amputation.

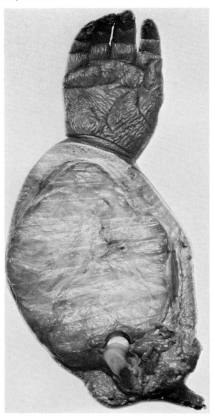

of which were in mitosis, and there seemed little doubt of its malignancy. The forearm was disarticulated at the elbow and the child was well several years later. Was this a malignant tumor cured by simple amputation?

Even among the congenital tumors that Wells in his extensive study accepted as being malignant there were many in which evidence of malignancy was limited to the histologic appearance. Of several neuroblastomas seen at the Chicago and Boston Lying-in Hospitals only two caused death by uncontrolled growth and widespread dissemination before birth. Tumors that are not histologically malignant may cause death shortly after birth because of their location. We have observed one hemangioma, one pheochromocytoma and several lymphangiomas and sacral coccygeal teratomas that caused death even though histologically benign.

CHORISTOMAS.—This term was used by Albrecht for a tissue histologically normal for an organ or part other than the one in which it is located. He included particularly those masses that are large enough to produce pressure symptoms, but the term can include all aberrant tissue equally well.

Cells that appear normal except for their location may come from many organs and may be found in many different parts of the body. At times they are included in adjacent tissues as a result of slight displacement. Thyroid cells may be found in the thymus, thymic tissue in the thyroid, splenic tissue in the pancreas and so on. Sometimes they are far removed from their point of origin. Cells resembling those of the normal adrenal gland may be found in lungs, liver, testis and ovary. Multiple areas of tissue resembling brain were found in the lungs of two anencephalic monsters at the Chicago Lying-in Hospital and have been reported by other investigators. Since anencephalic monsters are the only fetuses in which such lesions have been found, it seems probable that at some time during early intrauterine life brain tissue undergoes disruption, which is responsible for both the anencephalus and the presence of brain tissue in the amniotic fluid. Aspiration of amniotic fluid permits implantation of nerve cells in the lungs, where, finding the environment satisfactory, they proceed to grow.

Aberrant cells may also be distributed diffusely throughout an organ in such a way that their presence seems to result from a directional disturbance in the growth of local tissue rather than from implantation of foreign cells. The Chicago Lying-in Hospital collection includes one fetus whose right lung contained striated muscle distributed throughout the greater part of one lobe. Blood vessels were increased in size and no normal alveolar ducts or alveoli had been formed although bronchi and bronchioles were present. The long axes of the muscle fibers, which extended in all directions, were separated by blood vessels and small masses of cells resembling abortive attempts at alveolar formation. The muscle cells were mature and cross-striations were visible everywhere (see Fig. 15–38).

HAMARTOMAS.—This term has come to be applied especially to excessive localized overgrowths of cells in which the degree of maturation is similar to that found in the rest of the organ but the pattern assumed by the cells is not related to the normal tissue. Adenomas of the liver and rhabdomyomas of the heart are among the tumors most commonly placed in this group, although all hemangiomas, lymphangiomas, pigmented nevi and neurofibromas are often included. Cystic disease of the lung and liver as well as type I cysts of the kidney might well be included with those localized proliferations of cells that maintain a normal degree of differentiation but show an altered pattern of growth.

TERATOMAS.—Teratomas form another group of congenital tumors. According to Willis:

They arise from foci of plastic pluripotential embryonic tissue which has escaped from the influence of the primary organizer during early embryonic development, this escape being in some way related to disturbances emanating from the invaginated organizing tissues of the primitive streak and so affecting median or paramedian parts in close relationship to these tissues. The affected primordium as it grows shows no effect of a primary organizer, but differentiates in accordance with its own labile determinations, producing a variety of tissues foreign to the part from which they grow.

Willis believed that the overwhelming majority of well-studied teratoid tumors can be distinguished easily either as teratomas or abortive fetuses, but he admitted that in rare cases differentiation may be very difficult.

MALIGNANT TUMORS.—Continued growth without maturation of certain cells that are normally present during embryonic development but that usually mature after birth is responsible for many of the malignant congenital tumors. Wilms' tumors are derived from metanephric blastema that has lost its propensity for differentiation but not for growth. Neuroblastomas of the adrenal gland come from cells that arise in the neural crest and wander into the gland early in embryonic life. Normally these cells differentiate into chromaffin tissue, but occasionally the transformation fails to take place, and proliferation without differentiation produces a neuroblastoma.

Other tumors that occur predominantly in the first years of life and have certain features of embryonic growth include embryonic sarcomas, orchioblastomas, hepatoblastomas and medulloblastomas of the brain. Some teratomas of the sacrococcygeal and retroperitoneal regions can be included with those having an overgrowth of embryonic components that fail to mature. The cells of many sarcomas resemble immature fibroblasts and are probably also a result of failure of maturation coupled with an excessive stimulus for growth.

In 1940 Wells published the results of an investigation of all cases that had been reported in the literature as congenital malignant tumors for which he was able to locate the original descriptions. He found that many had been copied by one author from another and that often there was nothing in the original report to indicate that a particular tumor was malignant or had been present at birth. Among the cases investigated there were only 255 tumors present at birth that he thought might have been malignant. These he divided into 66 that seemed definitely, 66 probably and 123 possibly malignant.

The largest group—about half of the total number—was composed of sarcomas: spindle cell, round cell, angiosarcoma, myxosarcoma and fibrosarcoma. They were primary in bone, muscle, connective tissue, skin, brain, orbit, parotid, vulva, prostate, bladder, pancreas and intestine. Neuroblastomas made up the next largest group and Wilms' tumor the third.

Wells found four cases of placental transmission of malignant tumors from mother to fetus: one carcinoma from a mother with bronchogenic carcinoma, one lymphosarcoma and two melanosarcomas. The only instance in which the placenta was known to have contained tumor tissue was in one of the cases of melanosarcoma. Since then other cases have been reported, including one by Horner in which there were placental metastases from a cystadenocarcinoma of the ovary (Fig. 12–2). The child was normal. Horner also reviewed the literature and found a total of 11 cases with placental metastases. The tumor was present in only one of the children.

Wells found five cases in which a choriocarcinoma arising in the placenta was transmitted to the fetus and caused its death. In two of these the mother was normal. This is not surprising since choriocarcinoma may be present in the full-term placenta and be cast off at delivery without producing maternal involvement.

No instance of carcinoma was listed by Wells

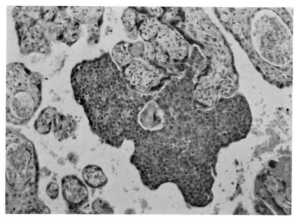

Fig. 12—2.—Placenta with villi and a mass of cells, metastatic from a carcinoma of the ovary. The infant was normal. (Courtesy Dr. Edward Horner.)

among the definitely accepted tumors arising in the fetus, and only one, a carcinoma of the liver, among the probable tumors. This finding is almost as valid today as it was 30 years ago, although carcinoma of the thyroid has been recorded in 12 newborns, and a variety of carcinomas including those of the pancreas, uterine cervix and choroid plexus have been found in the 1st year of life.

Several other malignant tumors have been recorded that caused death: medulloblastomas, astrocytomas, ependymomas, papillary carcinomas of the choroid plexus, spongioblastomas of the cerebral cortex, retinoblastomas, rhabdomyoblastomas, angiosarcomas, melanomas associated with giant (bathing trunk) nevi and a few connective tissue tumors.

The tumors generally classified as malignant that have been observed at birth at the Chicago Lying-in Hospital include four neuroblastomas limited to adrenal glands, one involving an adrenal gland and the liver, one arising next to the adrenal gland with widespread dissemination, one containing multiple neuroblastomas, ganglioneuromas and neurinomas, two early Wilms' tumors, one myelogenous leukemia causing death at 4 days and one lymphatic leukemia causing death at 6 weeks. Immature cells were present in several teratomas, but there is no proof that these would have been clinically malignant had the child survived.

BENIGN TUMORS.—The benign tumors most often present at birth are hemangiomas, lymphangiomas, pigmented nevi and teratomas. If cysts and rests resulting from malformations of the branchial cleft were to be included with tumors, these would be the most common of all. However, they are so definitely a result of maldevelopment that it seems preferable to place them with malformations rather than tumors.

Hemangiomas

Hemangiomas are observed in newborn infants more often than any other variety of tumor. They may be single or multiple and are extremely variable in extent. After birth they may remain the original size, grow with the body or exhibit a more rapid growth. Many of those in the skin are not noticed until the child is a few weeks old. The majority regress after a limited period of growth and most disappear by the end of the 2d year. Although at times they are very cellular (hemangioendothelioma) and show little elaboration into recognizable vascular structures, those present at birth rarely prove to be malignant. The skin is the most common site of hemangiomas, although they may be found in mucous membranes, deep connective tissue or internal organs such as the liver, heart and brain. Cutaneous hemangiomas are occasionally associated with similar lesions in the brain, liver or other organs. Hemangiomas in the region of the distribution of the trigeminal nerve may be associated with vascular anomalies of the choroid coat of the eye, the pia covering the brain, and the brain itself in the area beneath the involved skin. Known as the Sturge-Kalischer-Weber syndrome, this is associated with other symptoms such as congenital glaucoma and buphthalmos, local thickening of the skull, atrophy of the body on the side opposite the cutaneous hemangioma, paralysis, aphasia, jacksonian epilepsy and mental retardation. As early as the latter part of the 1st year slowing of the circulation may cause calcification near the cerebral surface; on x-ray examination this gives characteristic double-contoured opacities that come from calcific deposits about small vessels in two adjacent gyri and not from calcification of individual vessels.

The hemangiomas of von Hippel-Lindau disease (cerebellar-retinal hemangiomatosis) may be present in early life, but symptoms are rarely recognizable until the 2d decade. The vascular lesions may be single or multiple, capillary, cavernous or composed of solid hemangioendothelial masses. They may involve the skin, cerebellum, retina, spinal cord and liver. Adenomas or cystic disease of the pancreas, liver and kidney may also be present. The disease is familial in about 20% of cases.

Patients with the Maffucci-Hast syndrome have

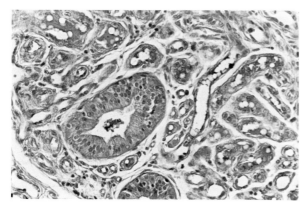

Fig. 12–3.—Capillary hemangioma of the salivary gland.

enchondromas at birth; capillary, cavernous or solid hemangiomas in the skin and subcutaneous tissue develop before puberty.

Landing and Farber listed seven separate but overlapping forms of hemangiomas:

CAPILLARY HEMANGIOMAS.—These consist of anastomosing capillaries, the lumens of which are lined by a single layer of endothelial cells (Fig. 12–3). A thin sheet of such anastomosing vessels lying in the dermis produces a pink to purple, noncompressible area on the skin surface and forms no tumor mass. Such is the nevus flammeus (Fig. 12–4) or port wine stain (nevus vinosus) (Fig. 12–5) often seen on the face or back of the neck. When such a proliferation involves a solid organ, the shape of the organ is not changed although it may be en-

larged. A *glomus tumor* is a special form of such a capillary hemangioma located predominantly on the ligaments and periosteum of the bones of the hands. Stout recorded seven cases in the 1st year of life, three known to have existed at birth. The component capillaries of glomus tumors have prominent, regularly arranged pericytes with a prominent reticulum pattern that may extend for a short distance into the surrounding tissue. Such tumors are characterized by intense localized pain in older people but not in young children. These tumors are benign.

CAVERNOUS HEMANGIOMAS.—These hemangiomas have larger vascular spaces than do the capillary hemangiomas and are compressible because of the large amounts of blood they contain. Those involving the skin are raised above the general skin level and often have a warty granular surface (Figs. 12–6 and 12–7). The raised vascular nevi such as strawberry nevi (Fig. 12–8) contain mixtures of cavernous and capillary nets. In general, the vascular channels vary greatly in size and extent, and on rare occasions may involve extensive portions of the body (Fig. 12–9).

The liver is the internal organ most often the site of a cavernous hemangioma. The extent of involvement may vary from a few millimeters to several centimeters. If superficial, trauma incident to delivery may cause rupture of some of the outermost channels, and fatal intra-abdominal hemorrhage may result. If it is deep in the liver, the tumor may never be discovered.

HEMANGIOENDOTHELIOMAS.—These tumors are

Fig. 12–4 (left).—Nevus flammeus involving left eyelid and forehead. Infant aged 3 days.

Fig. 12–5 (right).—Nevus vinosus involving left cheek and forehead. Infant aged 2 days. Hemangiomas in this location are often associated with hemangiomas of the underlying meninges and brain.

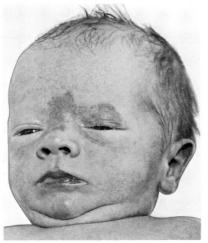

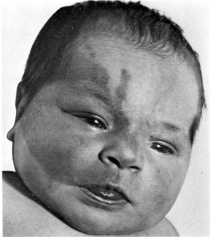

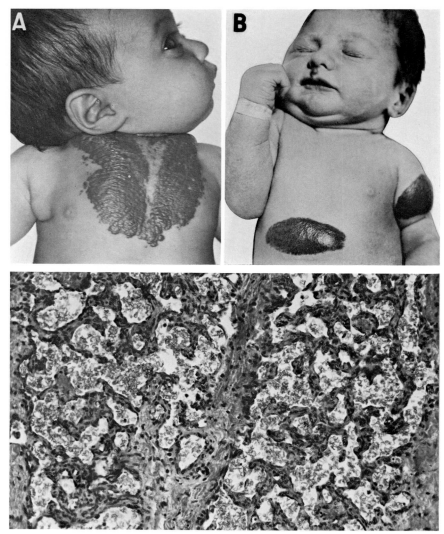

Fig. 12–6 (top).—A, raised hemangioma with multiple small excrescences involving anterior chest wall. (Courtesy Dr. Ralph V. Platou.) **B,** multiple hemangiomas having smooth cushionlike surfaces.

Fig. 12–7 (bottom).—Cavernous hemangioma of skin showing anastomosing endothelial-lined channels.

grossly firmer and paler than the two preceding forms of hemangiomas. They consist of lobules and masses of immature endothelial cells, some lining patent blood-containing spaces and some forming solid sheets. There is not much variation among the cells although mitoses usually may be found without difficulty. The cells and constituent vessels are distributed closely among normal muscle or parenchymal elements of the part involved. Most of the endothelial cells are intimately associated with reticulum fibers although no connective tissue is present in the most cellular portions of the tumor

(Fig. 12–10). Thrombosis and organization occur as in other forms of hemangiomas.

Malignant forms of endothelial vascular tumors, while rare in infancy, do occur in liver and soft tissues. Here the cells have larger and more variable nuclei and less cytoplasm. Local dissemination and metastases are common. Kaposi's sarcoma, a variably malignant tumor of the skin in which there is both capillary and connective tissue proliferation, is rare in infancy, and Stout could find only a single case in this age period. Hemangioendotheliomas of the liver are found chiefly in infants under 6

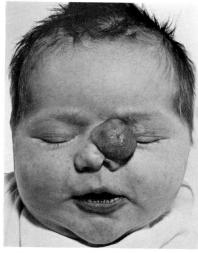
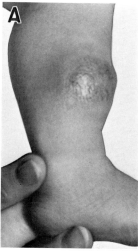
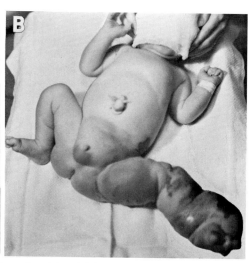

Fig. 12–8 (left).—Hypertrophic endothelial hemangioma, often called a strawberry mark.

Fig. 12–9 (right).—Deep-seated cavernous hemangioma. **A,** localized lesion on right leg. **B,** generalized hemangioma involving left leg, buttocks and lower abdomen, composed of greatly dilated vascular spaces and responsible for local gigantism. Death at 10 days.

months of age; 87% were in this age group in a series gathered by Dehner and Ishak. (See Chapter 20 for further discussion.)

HEMANGIOPERICYTOMAS.—These tumors consist of small discrete vascular channels with well-defined walls two to five layers thick, and prominent radially arranged reticulum nets. The walls are surrounded by more loosely arranged pericytes with a less prominent reticulum net around each cell. Such tumors are most often found in the subcutaneous tissue and are usually unencapsulated, rubbery and grayish white. Stout gathered 10 examples of benign hemangiopericytomas that were first noted at birth. Malignant variants have not been found at birth but have been observed among older children. They are more cellular with frequent mitotic figures and less reticulum.

VENOUS ANGIOMAS.—These consist of large endothelial-lined channels that may have smooth muscle in their walls. They may involve a large body area such as an extremity. Whether they should be considered as tumors or malformations may be open to question.

SCLEROSING HEMANGIOMAS.—These consist of varying proportions of endothelial cells, endothelial-lined channels, fibroblasts, giant cells and macrophages; the latter may contain hemosiderin or fat or both. They occur almost exclusively in the dermis of the skin, where they appear as 1–2 cm firm, slightly raised, circumscribed brownish discolorations; they are often mistaken for pigmented nevi. They are believed to represent the scarred end-stage of a capillary or hemangioendotheliomatous hemangioma. They occur at all ages and have been recognized in the first years of life.

ARTERIOVENOUS ANGIOMAS.—These tumors bear more resemblance to malformations than to true tumors. Two congenital arteriovenous angiomas involving the arteries and the large venous sinuses of the brain, both of which were associated with cardiac failure, were reported by Silverman *et al.*

Lymphangiomas

LYMPHANGIOMA SIMPLEX.—Although small superficial lymphangiomas are rare, they occur in

Fig. 12–10.—Hemangioendothelioma of skin, showing solid sheets of cells with occasional vascular channels.

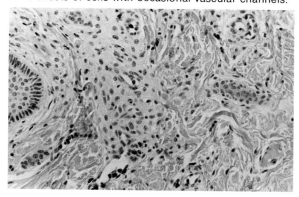

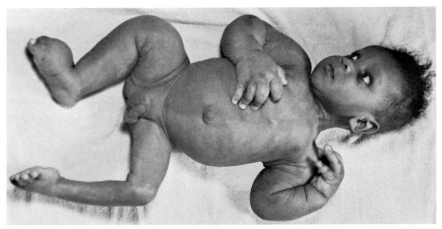

Fig. 12–11.—Diffuse lymphangiectasis involving both upper extremities and right leg. (Courtesy Children's Memorial Hospital, Chicago.)

any area, the most common locations being the skin of the neck, upper parts of the extremities and mucous membranes of the mouth. They usually appear grossly as groups of colorless, thick-walled spaces 0.5–2 cm in diameter. Microscopically, the spaces are lined by a single layer of endothelial cells surrounded by a combination of connective tissue and smooth muscle. They are often considered malformations rather than tumors since they lack evidence of independent growth.

LYMPHANGIECTASIS.—This condition is usually visible at birth as a diffuse swelling of part or all of an extremity without other symptoms (Fig. 12–11). It is not progressive and remains limited to the

area of original involvement. The skin and deep fasciae are normal, but between them the space is unusually wide and is spongelike in appearance as a result of increase in connective tissue and size of lymph spaces. Microscopic examination reveals large lymphatic channels lined by a single layer of endothelial cells and separated by normal connective tissue and blood vessels.

More rarely, diffuse cystic dilatation of lymphatic channels involves widespread portions of the body. One infant was seen at the Chicago Lying-in Hospital who appeared normal on external examination except for mild generalized edema. This appearance was caused by diffuse dilatation of lymphatic chan-

Fig. 12–12.—Cystic lymphangiomas (hygromas). **A,** unilocular tumor of the left side of the neck. Infant aged 4 days. **B,** multilocular tumor involving both sides and anterior part of the neck. Infant aged 4 weeks. (Courtesy Dr. Charles D. Kimball.)

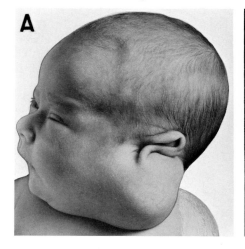
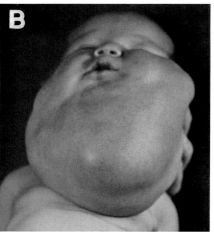

nels in subcutaneous tissues and between muscle bundles. Many of the dilated channels were visible grossly as small cysts 1–5 mm in diameter.

CYSTIC LYMPHANGIOMAS (HYGROMAS).—The use of the terms cystic and cavernous lymphangioma varies, and there is probably little reason to distinguish between the two conditions. However, the term cystic lymphangioma, or hygroma, has been applied especially to large single or slightly multilocular fluid-filled cavities most often located on one side of the neck (Figs. 12–12 and 12–13). Occasionally they are multiple and may be found in other locations. Bilateral hygromas of the neck associated with widespread lymphangiectasis are not uncommon in aborted fetuses (Fig. 12–14). Hygromas are thin-walled and filled with clear, straw-colored fluid, lined by a single layer of flat endothelial cells and surrounded by varying amounts of connective tissue and smooth muscle (Figs. 12–15 and 12–16). They are not compressible and are not visibly connected to lymphatic channels. They may increase in size after birth because of increased secretion of fluid. Evacuation of the fluid gives only temporary reflief, and unless the wall is completely destroyed the fluid will reappear.

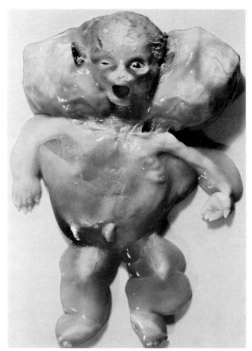

Fig. 12–14.—Fetus with cystic lymphangiomas of neck and generalized lymphangiectasis of subcutaneous tissue.

Fig. 12–13.—Multiple cystic lymphangiomas involving right side of neck, right axillary region and mediastinum, present since birth. Infant aged 6 months. (Courtesy Dr. Rustin McIntosh.)

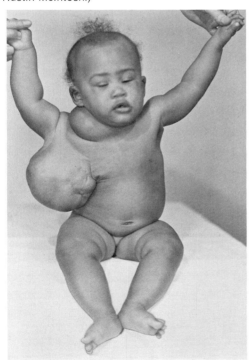

CAVERNOUS LYMPHANGIOMAS.—These tumors have also been called hygromas, but they differ from those just described in that they are composed of innumerable cystic spaces. The individual cysts are ordinarily only a few millimeters in diameter but larger tumors may attain a diameter of several centimeters. The cystic spaces, which are lined by endothelial cells, are separated by varying amounts of connective tissue (Fig. 12–17). They occur most often on the trunk, forearms, calves and backs of the hands and feet. Three observed at the Chicago Lying-in Hospital in infants at or near term were large bulky tumors involving the chest, shoulder and upper arm (Fig. 12–18). Two of these were on the right and one on the left side. Another was a more localized tumor on the left side of the upper back (Fig. 12–19).

Goetsch, who studied the origin of cavernous lymphangiomas, on the basis of observations in 12 cases concluded that they were due to a sequestration of lymphatic tissue in early embryonic life. Those in the cervical region were thought probably to be derived from primitive jugular sacs that failed to join the lymphatic system in a normal way. Peripheral extension was explained as a result of the development of fibrillar sprouts from the margins

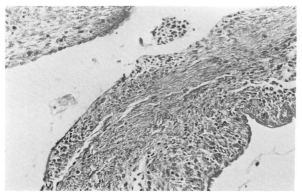

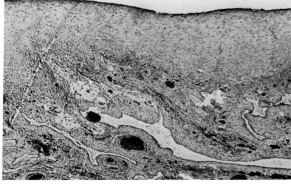

Fig. 12—15 (left). — Photomicrograph of cystic hygroma showing endothelial-lined channels with some endothelial proliferation.

Fig. 12—16. (right). — Cystic hygroma with dense collagenous wall and small dilated lymphatic channels nearby.

of existing cystic spaces. These spaces secrete lymphlike fluid that causes local distention and formation of additional gradually enlarging cysts. As the walls of older cysts become thick and fibrotic, the tumors appear to be composed of endothelial-lined spaces separated by connective tissue. Large numbers of lymphocytes also may be present.

At birth these tumors usually appear to have destroyed or prevented the development of muscles and other structures in the involved areas. They are almost never encapsulated and surgical removal is usually impossible.

Pigmented Nevi

The term nevus is used in a broad sense to include all abnormal growths in the skin but in a more restricted sense is limited to tumors containing nevus cells. Since most nevus cells contain melanin, the majority of true nevi are pigmented, the color varying from light brown to black. It has been estimated that they are present in the skin of at least 90% of the adult population. Although they are congenital, melanin may not develop immediately and they may not become visible until months or years after birth.

Many varieties of nevi have been described, the differences depending on the degree of elevation and the texture of the skin over the surface. Some are covered by soft downy hair. Many descriptive terms such as macular, nodular, pedunculated, diffuse and hairy have been used to indicate outstanding characteristics.

Although pigmented nevi are common among

Fig. 12—17. — Cavernous lymphangioma. **A,** cut surface showing innumerable cystic cavities of all sizes. **B,** photomicrograph showing lymphatic channels separated by small amounts of connective tissue.

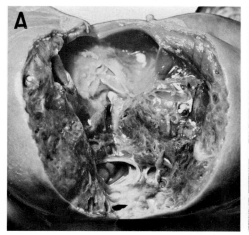

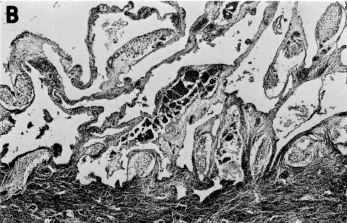

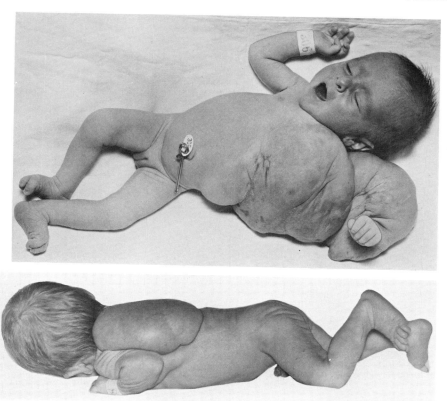

Fig. 12–18 (top).—Cavernous lymphangiomas involving chest, back and arm, the most common site of such tumors. Infant aged 5 days. Death followed unsuccessful attempt at removal.

Fig. 12–19 (bottom).—Cavernous lymphangioma on left side of back.

adults, they are not often visible at birth. Those observed most often among newborn infants involve large portions of the skin. The surface is rough and verrucous (Fig. 12–20) and the color is dark brown or black. Frequently they are covered by fine short hairs. They may be located on the trunk, face or extremities. When present on the trunk, countless other small nonelevated nevi are usually scattered over the surrounding skin. Lesions on the extremities are more often single.

Pigmented nevi contain nevus cells in the connective tissue beneath the epidermis. The cells, which are triangular or polyhedral, are arranged in small groups isolated by narrow connective tissue fasciculi. Some contain melanin. The amount of melanin both in normal skin and in nevi increases after birth and causes deepening of the color of the nevi or makes them visible for the first time.

Nearly all nevi seen at birth are benign and grow only as the body grows, but a few have been reported that were considered to have been malignant even before birth. Jensen gathered three cases of congenital malignant melanoma and 10 cases in children that arose as giant hairy nevi similar to one observed by Sweet and Connerty (Fig. 12–21). These giant hairy nevi contain nevus cells, Schwann cells and dermal melanocytes as well as Meissner's corpuscles and Verocay bodies (Fig. 12–22). In these hairy nevi the hair is always black, even in blond patients. Among 55 patients with giant hairy nevi gathered by Reed *et al.*, 20 had leptomeningeal involvement. All 20 had scalp or posterior midline involvement, yet only 13% were considered to have a truly metastatic malignancy. It seems probable in many cases, as is true in Sturge-Weber's disease, that there is simultaneous involvement of the skin and meninges. Also as in Sturge-Weber's disease, epilepsy and mental deficiency may be a prominent part of the clinical picture. If the brain itself is infiltrated, the decision as to the presence of malignancy is often difficult. In one striking case reported by Sweet and Connerty

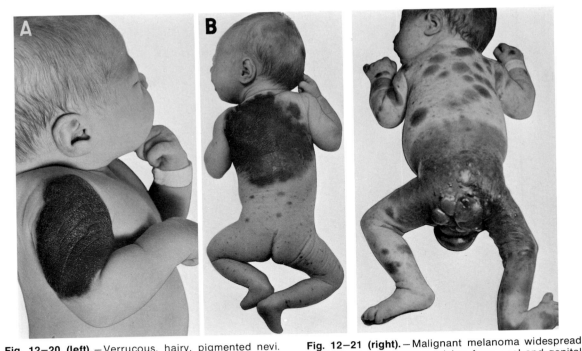

Fig. 12–20 (left).—Verrucous, hairy, pigmented nevi. **A,** lesion localized to upper arm. **B,** large lesion on upper back with multiple small flat pigmented nevi over rest of body.

Fig. 12–21 (right).—Malignant melanoma widespread over the body with tumor arising from anal and genital region. Tumor cells were also present in the brain and liver. (Courtesy Drs. Lewis K. Sweet and H. V. Connerty.)

there were widespread, darkly pigmented, moderately indurated, elevated cutaneous lesions on the head, trunk and all extremities, the largest of which were covered by hair. A diffuse gray-brown lesion covered the diaper region and extended down the right leg to below the knee. The external genitalia were replaced by large fungating growths, and similar masses arose from the perineal and perianal regions. During the infant's 17 days of life the color deepened perceptibly. Autopsy revealed numerous nonpigmented nodules of tumor tissue in the liver and masses of tumor cells containing pigment in the pons and cerebral cortex (Fig. 12–22, C) as well as in the subcutaneous tissue and in tumor masses arising from the perineal region. Because of the structure of some of the perineal tumors the question arose as to whether the diagnosis should have been congenital nevus developing into a malignant melanoma or neurofibromatosis complicated by neurogenic sarcoma and congenital nevi. A somewhat similar case was reported by Wilcox titled "Melanomatosis of the Skin and Central Nervous System in Infants" because of the association of a large nevus that covered the skin from the upper portion of the thighs almost to the costal margin, with melanin-filled nevus cells in the brain and meninges.

Teratomas

Although teratoma is defined as a true tumor composed of multiple tissues foreign to, and capable of growth in excess of, those characteristic of the part from which it is derived, it is sometimes difficult to make a distinction between teratomas and structures that result from abortive attempts at twinning. Many investigators have tried to explain all teratomas on the basis of modified twinning resulting from such processes as isolation of blastomeres, fertilization of a polar body, parthenogenetic development of an ovum and so on. An even progression can be traced from normal twins to conjoined twins, parasitic twins and fetal inclusions. At this point careful studies will reveal a break in the progression from an oriented, longitudinal, partially symmetrical structure of a twin to the jumbled, disordered, irregular growth of a teratoma in which one, two or three tissues predominate and others, such as organized skeletal muscle, liver, lung and intestinal lumens, are completely absent.

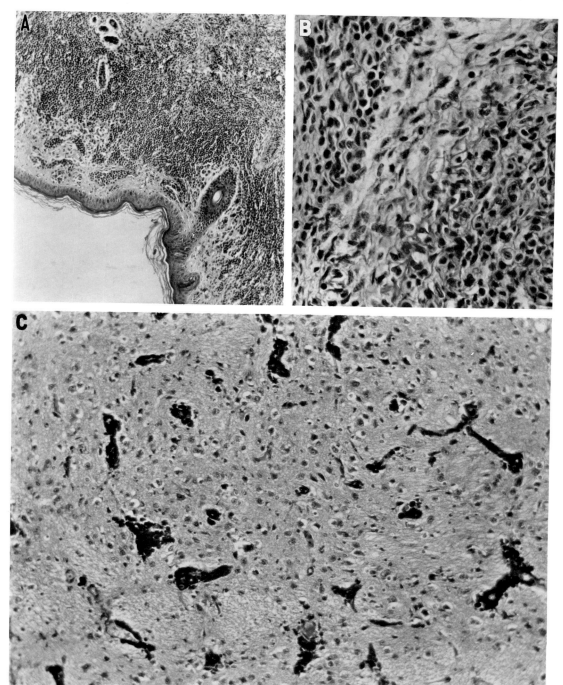

Fig. 12–22.—Malignant melanoma from infant shown in Fig. 12–21. **A,** nevus cells in subcutaneous tissue. **B,** nevus cells in malignant melanoma in peritoneum. **C,** pigmented nevus cells in brain. (Courtesy Drs. Lewis K. Sweet and H. V. Connerty.)

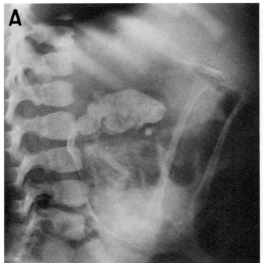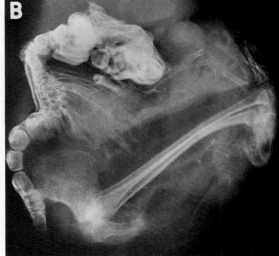

Fig. 12—23.—Roentgenogram of retroperitoneal teratoma resembling a fetus in 15-month-old child. **A,** before removal from abdomen. **B,** after removal. (Courtesy of Dr. H. E. Hoeven.)

The proper allocation of questionable masses requires careful dissection and mapping of the parts, consideration of their interrelationship, the degree to which they are organized and their growth potential. Despite the seeming progression from twins to teratomas, Willis and others have been vehement in their denial of a relationship. The distinction is based particularly on the fact that teratomas are capable of independent growth, whereas structures correctly included under malformations are limited in their potentiality for growth to a rate similar to the part of the body they resemble.

Fig. 12—24.—External surface of tumor shown in Fig. 12–23. **A,** before removal of outer covering. **B,** after removal of outer covering.

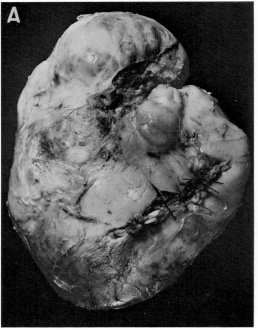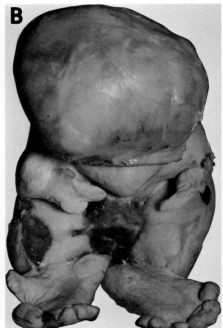

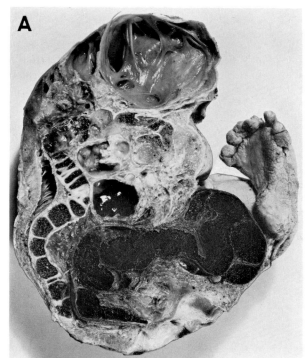

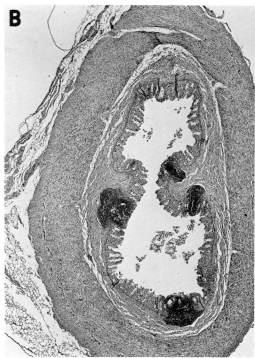

Fig. 12–25.—Tumor shown in Fig. 12–23. **A,** sagittal section showing well-developed spine, spinal nerves, base of skull and cystic brain. The large black convoluted structure is intestine filled with blood. **B,** cross-section of intestine showing presence of all muscle layers. Auerbach's plexus appears identical with that of normal intestines.

Specimens such as one from an infant delivered by Dr. H. D. Hoeven and one described by Kimmel *et al.* are excellent examples of the difficulty encountered in classifying certain tissue masses. The specimen of Dr. Hoeven was removed from the abdominal cavity of a boy aged 15 months whose mother had noticed it only 2–3 months before removal. It was attached only to the renal vessels, from which it derived its blood supply. Preoperative x-rays had shown what appeared to be an anencephalic monster in the abdominal cavity of the infant, which impression was confirmed after its removal (Figs. 12–23 to 12–25). The outer surface was covered with waxy lamellae, removal of which revealed two arms, two legs, a trunk and a head. The spine was composed of multiple well-formed vertebrae. No calvarium was present but a cystic area containing nerve tissue was situated above an irregular bony mass resembling the base of the skull. Tissues simulating lung, cardiac muscle and other organs were present in small amounts. The only well-developed organ was the intestine, which was complete, with all muscle layers, mucosa and Auerbach's plexus. The lumen of the intestine was filled with blood and, before microscopic examination, was thought to be a large blood vessel.

The specimen described by Kimmel *et al.* was the brain of a stillborn fetus that contained within its substance five structures resembling partially developed embryos (Figs. 12–26 and 12–27). In none were all of the arms, legs, trunk and head present, but there were identifiable parts of a body present in each and portions of a vertebral column were present in several. Average length of the embryos was 1–2 cm, and the bones contained more calcium than would be normal for embryos of this size. Degeneration of the brain made it impossible to ascertain their blood supply.

Teratomas have been observed in many locations at birth, but particular sites of predilection are the presacral and precoccygeal regions and the neck (Fig. 12–28). Other reported locations are the brain, pineal body, retroperitoneal tissues, anterior mediastinum, interior of the heart and pleura, pharynx, thyroid, base of the skull, spine, pelvis and subcutaneous tissues. Dermoid tumors of the eye have also been observed. Sites of those studied in young infants at the Chicago Lying-in Hospital

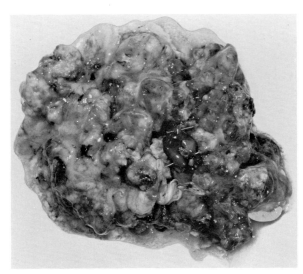

Fig. 12–26.—Brain of newborn infant that contained five abnormal embryos, one of which is shown beneath two pins. (Courtesy Drs. Donald L. Kimmel and J. Robert Willson.)

Fig. 12–27.—Five irregularly developed embryos (teratomas) removed from brain pictured in Fig. 12–26. Roentgenograms showed well-developed bones and vertebrae in several of the embryos. (Courtesy Drs. Donald J. Kimmel and J. Robert Willson.)

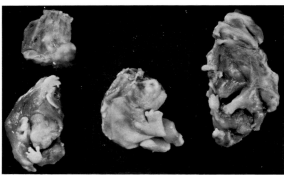

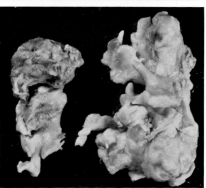

include the thyroid gland, pineal gland, pharynx, retroperitoneal tissues, pre- and postsacral areas and conjunctiva of the eye.

Since most teratomas and dermoid cysts of the ovary are not discovered until after puberty, several writers have concluded that such ovarian tumors have a different origin from those in other locations. Before the age of 12, teratomas form the most common ovarian tumor, with the youngest recorded at about age 4 years. Teratomas of the testis occur more commonly at younger ages. In a series of tumors of the testis in children described by Abell and Holtz nearly one third were recognized in the 1st year of life.

Teratomas are composed of tissues derived from each of the three layers of the embryonic disk (Fig. 12–29). Entodermal components are the least common, but at times intestinal or gastric mucosa is remarkably well developed and may be surrounded by muscle layers that are complete even to Auerbach's plexus. Ectodermal components, especially brain tissue, make up a large portion of most teratomas that are present at birth and are more prominent in these than in such tumors discovered later in life. This is especially true of the sacral and coccygeal groups. The tissue of these tumors for the most part resembles glia, although ganglion cells and cavities lined by cells simulating ependyma and choroid plexus are common. Epidermis and dermal structures including hairs and sebaceous and sweat glands are generally present, and there may be fairly well-developed teeth (Fig. 12–30). Varieties of epithelium include columnar, pseudostratified, stratified, ciliated and nonciliated, secretory and nonsecretory. Glands in addition to those derived from the skin include salivary, thyroid, pancreas, adrenal and others. Tissues resembling kidney, lung and sex organs are rare. Mesodermal components such as fat, cartilage, bone and muscle are present in almost all congenital teratomas.

SACROCOCCYGEAL TERATOMAS.—Many of these tumors are attached to the inner or outer surface of the sacrum and coccyx (see Fig. 12–28; Fig. 12–31), but others arise from the soft tissues of the pelvis. They are present at the lower end of the trunk, sometimes separating the legs and at other times extending posteriorly from the spine. If they extend into the abdominal cavity, it is usually only for a short distance and the bulk of the tumor is exterior (Fig. 12–32, A). Teratomas are usually easily shelled out of the lower pelvis but may be attached to the coccyx more firmly. They are generally large, often measuring 15–30 cm or more in diameter at birth, which indicates an origin early in intrauter-

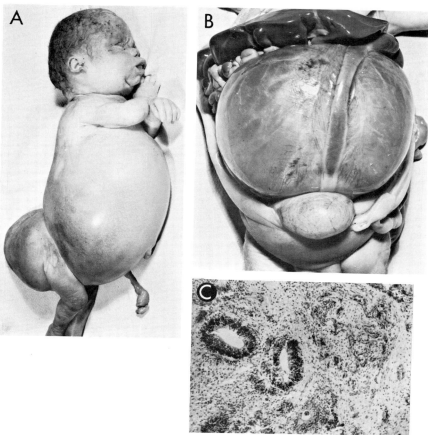

Fig. 12–28. — Newborn infant with combined pelvic and retroperitoneal malignant teratoma. **A,** external appearance. **B,** large tumor with overlying sigmoid colon. Bladder is distended as a result of urethral obstruction. **C,** primitive structures including neural rosettes mixed with more mature glial tissue.

ine life. Many are composed principally of tissue resembling brain (Fig. 12–32, B), but elements from all germ layers are usually present. They may be confused clinically with myelomeningoceles, although the latter usually occur at a higher level and are less solid.

The majority of these tumors are evident at birth and most of the remainder become evident in the 1st year of life. A few are associated with malformations of the lower spine. According to Willis, girls are affected four times as frequently as boys.

Among 103 cases of sacrococcygeal teratomas reported by Donnellan and Swenson 30 were malignant; the malignant components were carcinoma in 22, sarcoma in five, rhabdomyosarcoma in three and hemangioendothelial sarcoma in one. Five of the 30 had distinct metastases and 29 were locally invasive. They found that the malignant tumors were largely intrapelvic while the more benign

tumors tended to be limited to the sacral and perineal area. In their series only 8 of 79 (10%) diagnosed at birth were malignant, while among those discovered after the first 2 months of life, 22 of 24 (93%) were malignant. The most common presenting complaint in their series, in addition to the mass, was obstruction of the bowel or urinary tract; this was present in 79% of the malignant cases but in only 6.8% of the benign cases.

TERATOMAS OF THE NECK. — These tumors are usually found in intimate relation to the thyroid gland, even though evidence that they arise from the thyroid is usually lacking. In one case reported from the Chicago Lying-in Hospital a large mass in the right side of the neck was almost completely covered by a thin layer of thyroid tissue (Fig. 12–33). Like the teratomas of the coccygeal region they are overwhelmingly congenital in origin, 72 of 79 such teratomas reported by Silberman and Mendel-

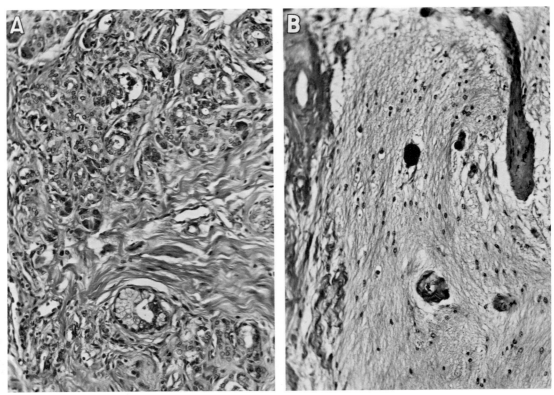

Fig. 12–29.—Sacral teratoma. **A,** area showing numerous tubular glands embedded in connective tissue. **B,** glial tissue with small mass of young bone.

Fig. 12–30.—Abdominal teratoma showing well-developed teeth embedded in bone with adjacent epithelial-lined cavities.

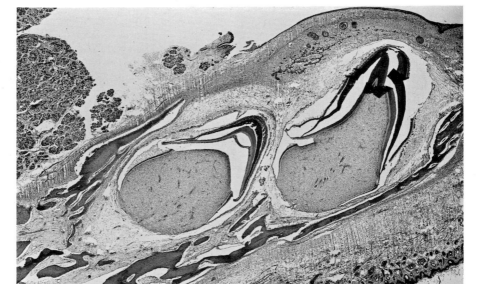

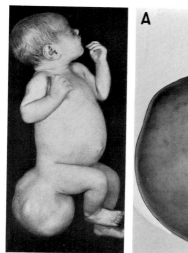
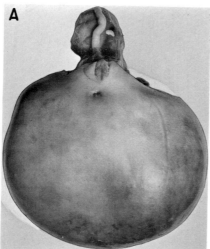
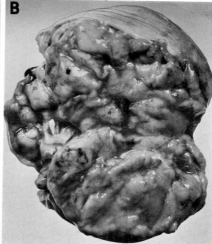

Fig. 12—31 (left).—Teratoma arising from posterior part of sacrum.

Fig. 12—32 (right).—Teratoma that arose from pelvis and extended down between the legs. **A,** exterior, showing small mass that extended into pelvis. Vaginal orifice, anus and rectum are also visible. **B,** cut surface showing cavity filled with tissue resembling brain. (Courtesy Dr. Edward J. Shalgos.)

Fig. 12—33.—Teratoma in region of right lobe of thyroid gland in a stillborn infant. **A,** view showing location of tumor. **B,** external surface showing small appendage consisting of left lobe of thyroid. Right lobe was thinned out over surface of tumor. **C,** cut surface showing intermixture of solid and cystic areas composed of multiple tissues derived from all three germ layers.

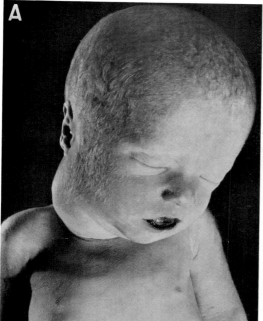
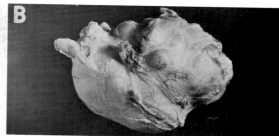
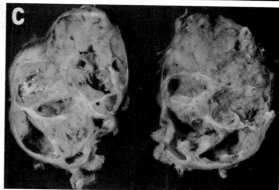

son being present at birth. Brain tissue is the most frequent component, but cartilage, bronchial epithelium and ependymal-lined cysts are common. Malignant varieties have not been described. Respiratory obstruction is the most frequent finding in addition to the mass.

PHARYNGEAL TERATOMAS (EPIGNATHI).—Arising from the soft or hard palate in the region of Rathke's pouch, these tumors vary greatly in size. They generally fill the buccal cavity and extend out through the mouth, although they may arise from the upper surface of the sphenoid bone and extend into the cranial cavity (Fig. 12–34). Rarely, an isthmus of tissue extends through the sphenoid bone connecting inner and outer masses of tumor tissue. Tumors of the base of the skull and hard palate differ only in the direction of their growth. Some of the tumors extending out of the mouth contain fairly well-differentiated structures resembling fetal parts and have been described as parasitic fetuses and designated epignathi. They actually belong to the group of teratomas and are quite different from the parasitic fetuses found in asymmetrical double monsters.

TERATOMAS IN OTHER LOCATIONS.—Teratomas have been observed in many additional locations. They are usually found in or near the midplane of the body and have not been reported in the face (except the eye) or the extremities. Most of those in the brain have arisen from the pineal body or the base of the skull. Dr. Ralph Platou observed one under the scalp near the region of the posterior fontanelle (Fig. 12–35) and another had a visible digit as a component part of a tumor that arose from the back (see Fig. 13–39).

MEDIASTINAL TERATOMAS.—These are often intrapericardial, or even intracardial. Fourteen such cases were gathered by Williams, five of which were in infants under 4 months of age; in 11 that were dissected, tissues from all three germ layers were present. The usually pedunculated masses were attached to the base of the great vessels or the atrioventricular valves.

Retroperitoneal teratomas usually lie in the posterior portion of the abdomen but above the pelvis. According to Wooley, they comprise about 5% of all childhood tumors. Like those in the sacrococcygeal region, they are usually discovered in the 1st year of life. They may be either uni- or bilateral. Only about 15% have a malignant component; this is most often carcinomatous.

Dermoid tumors of the eye have been described

Fig. 12–34.—Pharyngeal teratoma (epignathus) with great distortion of facial region. **A,** lateral view of body surface. **B,** sagittal section through midline showing extent of tumor. (Specimen courtesy Dr. S. B. Silverman.)

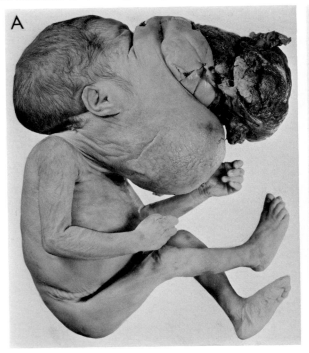
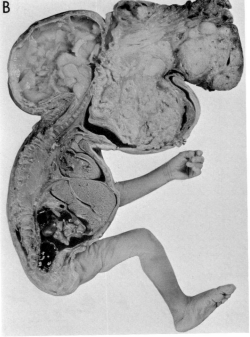

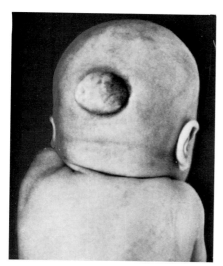

Fig. 12–35.—Teratoma of back of head. (Courtesy Dr. Ralph V. Platou.)

as arising from the conjunctiva at the margin of the iris. They are not true teratomas inasmuch as they ordinarily consist only of ectoderm and mesoderm.

Miscellaneous Solid Tumors

CONGENITAL RHABDOMYOMAS OF THE HEART.— These are among the tumorlike masses most often listed as hamartomas. They may exist as single subendocardial tumors distending the wall of the chamber in which they are located and unassociat-ed with abnormalities in other parts of the body (Fig. 12–36), or they may consist of multiple small tumors, in which case they are often associated with other disturbances in development. In many individuals the rhabdomyomas of the heart are part of the general syndrome of tuberous sclerosis with involvement of the brain and other organs (Fig. 12–37). Renal cysts or adenomas as well as malformations of the meninges, pancreas, palate and so on may also be present. The tumors are of-ten 1–2 cm in diameter and usually extend into the cavity of the heart. They are characterized by large vacuolated "spider" cells that contain abundant glycogen and often show radial extensions with transverse striations of their peripheral cytoplasm (Figs. 12–38 and 12–39). They are usually multi-ple, consisting of numerous small areas, some of which are visible only microscopically, or less often the myocardium is diffusely affected with no dis-crete lesions.

ADENOMAS OF THE LIVER.—This term has been used somewhat inaccurately for cavernous heman-giomas of that organ but is more properly limited to nodular hyperplasia of hepatic parenchyma in which normal liver structure is faithfully repro-duced. In the latter, bile capillaries are rarely pres-ent although structures resembling bile ducts have been described and cords of cells may radiate from structures resembling central veins.

ADENOMAS OF THE PANCREAS.—In one infant at the Chicago Lying-in Hospital an adenoma of the pancreas was present adjacent to the duodenum. It was sharply circumscribed, 1 cm in diameter and

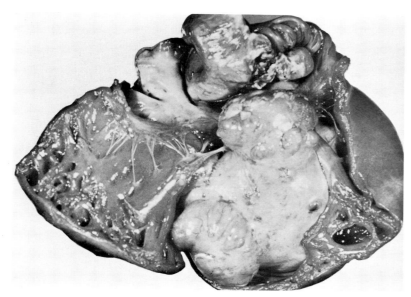

Fig. 12–36.—Single subendocardial rhabdomyoma not associated with identifiable tuberous sclerosis.

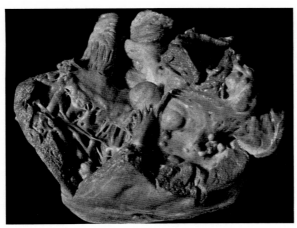

Fig. 12–37.—Rhabdomyoma of heart. Gross tumors are visible beneath the endocardium. Child, with tuberous sclerosis, died at age 6 months. (Courtesy Dr. Sidney Farber.)

composed of wide interlacing bands of cells with plump oval nuclei and poorly demarcated cell boundaries (Fig. 12–40.) No islet tissue was present, and the tumor was thought to have arisen from acinar epithelium.

LIPOMAS.—Congenital lipomas have been found on the surface of the body in various locations but they are especially common on the back in the interscapular, lumbar and gluteal regions and on the extremities, especially the palmar and plantar surfaces (Fig. 12–41). They have also been found in the region of the sucking pad. Those on the extremities are usually simple masses of adipose tissue. In other locations they are often irregular in consistency and contour and may be complicated by telangiectasias, fibromas and the presence of bone, cartilage or masses of calcium. They may be encapsulated but often merge gradually with surrounding tissues. The cells usually do not differ from those of normal fat.

Malignant liposarcomas were described by Stout in two newborn infants and in several infants later in the 1st year of life. The nuclei were large and anaplastic and the fat cells contained numerous small vacuoles characteristic of embryonal fat.

Cysts

Most cysts found in the thorax or abdomen can be explained as malformations resulting from abnormal budding of the entodermal tube. Those in the thorax are usually in the posterior mediastinum. They can be divided into three groups according to the variety of epithelial lining: bronchial, gastric or intestinal. *Bronchogenic cysts,* which are present most often at the bifurcation of the trachea, are lined by tall columnar cells similar to those on the major bronchi (Fig. 12–42). They may produce pressure symptoms in early infancy or go unrecognized for many years. *Gastric* and *enteric cysts,* usually located behind the pleura, are lined by epithelium resembling that of the stomach or intestine. They are often several centimeters in diame-

Fig. 12–38.—Rhabdomyoma of heart showing typical "spider cells." Child, with tuberous sclerosis, died at 22 days of age. See Figs. 24–23 and 24–24 for illustrations of other lesions found in this infant.

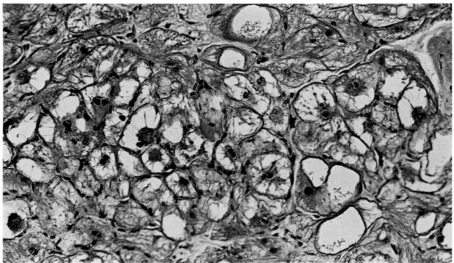

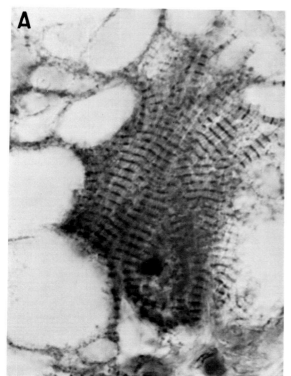

Fig. 12–39.—Rhabdomyoma of heart (same case as Fig. 12–38). A, cells showing characteristic muscular striations. B, cells containing large amounts of glycogen. Best carmine stain. (Courtesy Dr. Sidney Farber.)

Fig. 12–40 (left).—Adenoma of pancreas. Inset, tumor 7 mm. in diameter. Photomicrograph showing irregular masses of polyhedral cells separated by connective tissue. Stillborn fetus.

Fig. 12–41 (right).—Lipoma in subcutaneous tissue over left side of sacrum, present at birth.

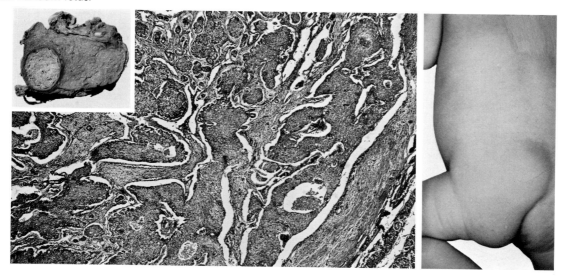

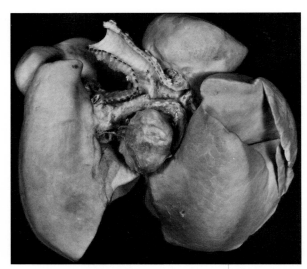

Fig. 12–42.—Cyst at bifurcation of trachea lined by a single layer of mucus-secreting cells. Stillborn fetus. Such cysts may cause asphyxia by pressure on the bronchi.

ter at birth and usually produce symptoms of pressure in early life.

Cysts in the abdominal cavity that correspond to those in the thorax are usually located in the mesentery and are closely attached to the normal bowel. The cyst and bowel are often enclosed within a common muscular coat. They are usually categorized as duplication of the intestine.

Follicular cysts of the ovary may rarely be 2 cm or more in diameter. These also are not true neoplasms but result from excessive accumulation of fluid in follicles that normally are not more than 1–2 mm in diameter.

Cysts of the urachus, kidneys, liver, lungs, pancreas and other organs are all considered malformations and discussed in appropriate chapters.

Neuroblastomas

Neuroblastomas have been called sympathicoblastomas, sympathogoniomas and gangliosympathicoblastomas, the specific name depending on the variety and degree of differentiation of the cells composing the tumor. They were commonly regarded as sarcomas until Wright in 1910 brought together the cases reported up to that time and stated his reasons for believing that they originate from cells of the embryonic nervous system. Since then they have been recognized as coming from neuroblasts that arise in the neural crest and normally migrate downward to form ganglion cells and chromaffin tissue.

They are the malignant tumors most commonly found at birth. In Wells' survey of the world's literature he listed 53 arising in the adrenal gland and 10 arising in other sites as possible, probable or acceptable congenital tumors.

Those in the adrenal gland vary from a few millimeters to several centimeters in diameter. They may be solid or cystic (Fig. 12–43). The cortical tissue of the adrenal gland usually persists and may surround the tumor or be visible only on one surface, while the rest is so attenuated that it cannot be distinguished on gross examination.

The solid portions of the tumors are red-brown, firm and somewhat granular in appearance. They are composed of small cells with poorly demarcated boundaries whose round or oval hyperchromatic nuclei are proportionately large in relation to total cell volume (Fig. 12–44). Fine fibrils either form a delicate interlacing network between the cells or are found in areas almost devoid of cells. Rosettes consisting of a small, pale, finely granular central area surrounded by a petal-like arrangement of cells are common. Hemorrhagic necrosis and calcification are often present in larger tumors.

Metastases have been reported most often in the liver, orbit and bones, those in the liver generally occurring in younger age groups than those in other locations.

In one 3,925 gm stillborn fetus delivered at the Chicago Lying-in Hospital the liver was enormously enlarged, weighing 390 gm. Liver parenchyma was almost entirely replaced by islands of neuroblasts separated by sinusoidal endothelium. The adrenal glands, although not appreciably enlarged, showed replacement of the fetal zone by cells similar to those in the liver, but the definitive cortex was uninvolved. Small islands of tumor cells were also present in the lungs and kidneys.

One extra-adrenal neuroblastoma seen at the Boston Lying-in Hospital was associated with clinical and pathologic evidence of norepinephrine release including flushing, extreme tachycardia and pulmonary edema. Unfortunately the blood pressure was not taken. Pathologically, there was massive hemorrhagic necrosis in the liver and complete necrosis of the fetal fat due to lipolytic activity of the secretion. No metastases were present.

Strauss and Driscoll reported neuroblastomas in two infants with simultaneous involvement of the placentas. The neuroblasts in the placentas were almost entirely within blood vessels, especially vil-

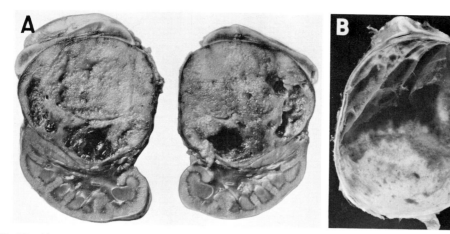

Fig. 12–43.—Neuroblastomas. **A,** solid tumor 4 cm in diameter with areas of necrosis. Death from pulmonary hemorrhage at age 4 days. **B,** cystic tumor 2.5 cm in diameter lined by typical neuroblast cells. Newborn; death from intracranial hemorrhage.

lous capillaries. The placentas were histologically immature and greatly hypertrophied, and the appearances suggested erythroblastosis due to Rh incompatibility (Fig. 12–45).

According to Stowens, the distinctions sometimes made among neuroblastomas, sympathogoniomas and sympathicoblastomas, which relate to increasing immaturity of cells, have no significance regarding the behavior of the tumor.

Stowens gave a useful summary of the prognosis of neuroblastomas based on their location. He pointed out that in eight of 14 survivors with neuroblastomas in the 1st year of life the tumor was discovered during a routine physical examination, that the tumors arose between adrenal and kidney and that several were attached to the renal pelvis. He also indicated that maturation to more adult forms (ganglioneuromas) was rare in the adrenal area as compared to the mediastinum. deLorimer found a 2-year survival in 62% of affected infants less than 1 year of age at onset but in only 21% of those in the 2d year of life. Even in the presence of metastases, 46% of those under 1 year of age at discovery lived for 2 years, although few survived beyond this time. Stowens gave about a 30% survival rate for 5 years when the onset was in the 1st year of life.

Spontaneous regression of neuroblastomas is not a rare occurrence. Everson and Cole collected 29 such instances. In some of these, as in the famous case of Cushing and Wolbach, there was maturation of the tumor; in other instances there was spontaneous degeneration and disappearance. Bo-

lande *et al.* pointed out that this behavior is largely limited to neuroblastomas in very young infants (a mean age of 3 months in Everson and Cole's series). They also found that infants with tumors in the 1st year of life have a 2-year survival rate of 35%, in contrast to 19% in the 2d year and 5% after that. When neuroblastomas were present at birth, the cure rate was about 70%. Similar trends have been observed among congenital sacral-coccygeal teratomas and retinoblastomas.

GANGLIONEUROMAS.—The 10 congenital malignant tumors of nervous origin found by Wells were all in areas other than the adrenal: he included four in the brain, five in the sympathetic ganglia and the one case of Potter and Parrish in which there was a congenital neuroblastoma-ganglioneuroma with widespread involvement of the peripheral nerves, sympathetic ganglia, adrenal glands and other organs (Fig. 12–46).

Ganglioneuromas of the adrenal area are seldom found in early life. In Stowens' series of tumors of the sympathetic system the youngest child with a combination tumor (neuroblastoma-ganglioneuroma) was 4 years of age. Most such tumors are in the sympathetic ganglia and are composed largely of immature undifferentiated cells. Only one besides the case of Potter and Parrish (Fig. 12–47) was stated to have contained ganglion cells. Ganglioneuromas, for the most part tumors of older children and adults, are more highly differentiated than neuroblastomas.

The case reported by Potter and Parrish is important in establishing a relationship not only be-

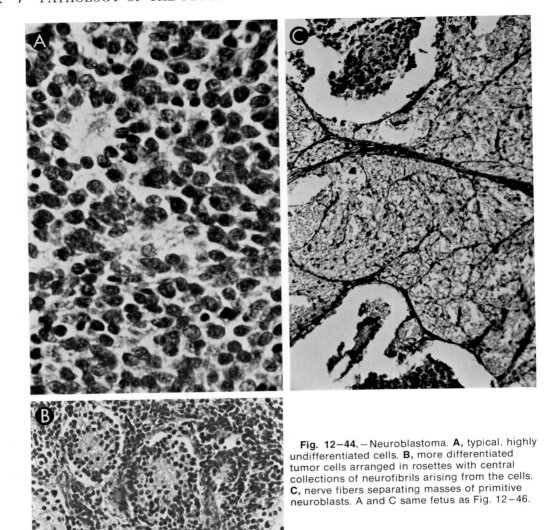

Fig. 12–44.—Neuroblastoma. **A,** typical, highly undifferentiated cells. **B,** more differentiated tumor cells arranged in rosettes with central collections of neurofibrils arising from the cells. **C,** nerve fibers separating masses of primitive neuroblasts. A and C same fetus as Fig. 12–46.

tween neuroblastomas and ganglioneuromas but between tumors composed of these cell types and those made up of typical Schwann cells. In Potter and Parrish's case diffuse hypertrophy of all peripheral nerves had also occurred (Fig. 12–48). Except for the brain, the state of which was not known because of craniotomy during delivery, all tissue of nervous origin had undergone neoplastic hyperplasia and the liver was studded with innumerable small masses of neuroblasts.

Since in the ganglioneuromas of older children there is a gradual degeneration and loss of ganglion cells, it seems probable that some of the me-diastinal neurofibromas of adults originate as ganglioneuromas in childhood.

The frequency with which small collections of neuroblasts are found in the adrenal glands in random sections of newborn infants suggests that maturation and cessation of growth of potentially lethal tumors is a relatively common occurrence. Many such collections of cells have been observed both at the Chicago and Boston Lying-in Hospitals (Fig. 12–49). Such collections of cells have been observed frequently in infants with trisomy 18. Since these infants die soon after birth, their significance in this condition is unknown (Bove *et al.*).

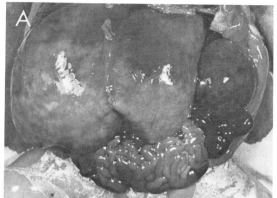 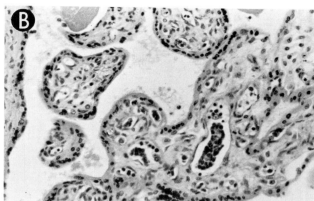

Fig. 12—45.—A, disseminated neuroblastoma in enlarged liver and spleen in a 2,420 gm full-term stillborn fetus. **B,** photomicrograph of villi of greatly enlarged placenta showing the large numbers of primitive neuroblasts in fetal vessels. No invasion of the chorionic tissue was found. (Courtesy Drs. L. Strauss and S. Driscoll.)

A congenital *pheochromocytoma* several centimeters in diameter lying just above the adrenal gland and without metastases was observed at the Boston Lying-in Hospital. Death was secondary to metabolic alterations with extensive necrosis in the areas of fetal fat. None of these tumors has previously been observed at birth.

Wilms' Tumor
(Metanephroblastoma)

Wilms' tumors arise in the kidney as a result of the abnormal proliferation of metanephric blastema. Differentiation may proceed in the direction of nephrons or connective tissue or both. The pattern

Fig. 12—46.—Neuroblastoma, ganglioneuroma and neurinoma in stillborn fetus weighing 1,385 gm. **A,** multiple nodules of neuroblastic tissue in liver and neurinoma of bladder. **B,** tumors in both adrenal glands with extension across upper abdomen. **C,** massive involvement of nerve trunks and sympathetic ganglions.

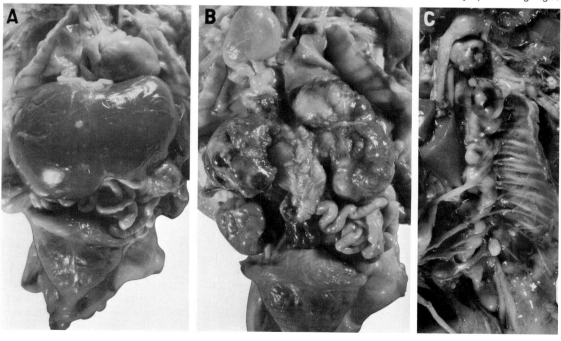

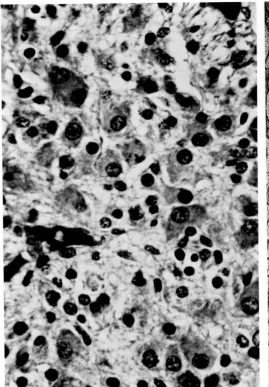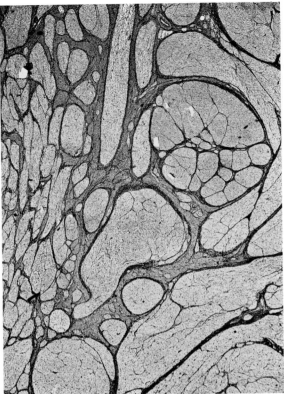

Fig. 12—47 (left).—Tumor in sympathetic ganglion showing ganglion cells in varying stages of differentiation. (Same fetus as Fig. 12—46.)

Fig. 12—48 (right).—Neurinoma of bladder showing

masses of Schwann cells resembling nerve trunks separated by connective tissue. Ganglion cells were present in some areas. (Same fetus as Fig. 12—46.)

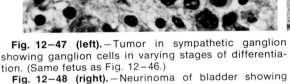

Fig. 12—49.—Adrenal gland of mature newborn infant with individual and clumped neuroblasts lying in sinusoids of fetal cortex.

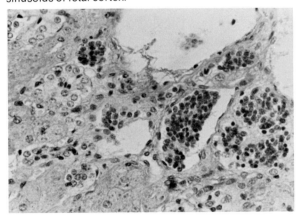

most frequently encountered is a mixture of undifferentiated cells, tubules, connective tissue and derivatives of the latter such as fat, cartilage and smooth and striated muscle (Fig. 12—50). In newborn infants the tumors are usually composed exclusively of connective tissue and are benign, in contrast to those found in children a few years older, which are highly malignant. Small zones of proliferated but undifferentiated blastema, designated in situ tumors, are occasionally encountered in very young infants; they are believed to be the source of tumors manifested clinically at a few years of age. (For more complete discussion see Chapter 22.)

Tumors and Malformations

There are a number of tumor-malformation combinations that appear to be more than coincidental. The most striking of these is acute leukemia associated with Down's syndrome. In addition there may

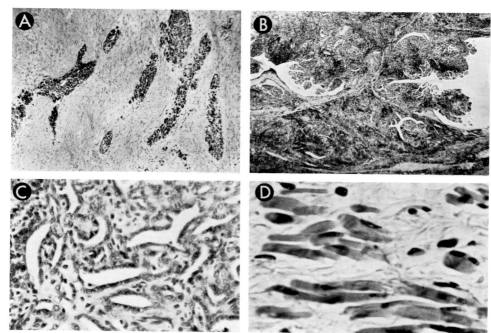

Fig. 12–50. — Wilms' tumors, showing variability in histologic pattern. **A, B** and **C** from same case. **A,** connective tissue with islands of undifferentiated cells. **B,** small cystic cavities with differentiation of papillary structures and pseudoglomeruli. **C,** irregular tubule formation. **D,** tumor consisting largely of myxomatous connective tissue and striated muscle.

be a myeloblastic response in this condition at birth that usually disappears with continued survival. The leukemic process does not become manifest until late childhood. The incidence in Down's syndrome is 18 times that in the general population. Other tumors are also more common.

Leukemia and lymphomas have been found more often than in the general population in Klinefelter's syndrome, in some metabolic disorders such as agammaglobulinemia and ataxia-telangiectasia and in some blood dyscrasias such as Bloom's syndrome, Chediak-Higashi disease and Fanconi's aplastic anemia.

In situ Wilms' tumors are among the many abnormalities occasionally found in association with trisomy 18.

REFERENCES

Abell, M. D., and Holtz, F.: Testicular neoplasms in infants and children, Cancer 16:965, 1963.

Albrecht, D. P. G.: Hamartomas, Verhandl. Deutsch. Path. Gesellsch. 7:153, 1904.

Anderson, D. H.: Tumors of infancy and childhood, Cancer 4:890, 1951.

Arnheim, E. E.: Retroperitoneal teratomas in infancy and childhood, Pediatrics 8:309, 1951.

Arnstein, L. H., Boldrey, E., and Naffziger, H. C.: A case report and survey of brain tumors during the neonatal period, J. Neurosurg. 8:315, 1951.

Arrick, M. S.: Stem cell lymphoma of the newborn, Arch. Pathol. 42:104, 1946.

Beckwith, J., and Perrin, E.: In-situ neuroblastoma: A contribution to the natural history of neural crest tumors, Am. J. Pathol. 43:1089, 1963.

Bhasken, S. N., and Lilly, G. E.: Salivary gland tumors of infancy, J. Oral Surg. 21:305, 1963.

Bigelow, N. H., Klinger, S., and Wright, A. W.: Primary tumors of the heart in infancy and early childhood, Cancer 7:549, 1954.

Bill, A. H., and Sumner, D. S.: A unified concept of lymphangioma and cystic hygroma, Surg. Gynecol. Obstet. 120:79, 1965.

Bodian, M.: Neuroblastoma, Pediatr. Clin. North Am. 6:449, 1959.

Bolande, R. P., Brough, A. J., and Izant, R. J.: Congenital mesoblastic nephroma of infancy, Pediatrics 40:272, 1967.

Bove, K. E., Koppler, H., and McAdams, J. E.: Nodular renal blastoma, Cancer 24:323, 1969.

Cushing, H., and Wolbach, S. B.: The transformation of a malignant paravertebral sympathicoblastoma into a benign ganglioneuroma, Am. J. Pathol. 3:203, 1927.

Dargeon, W. H.: *Tumors of Childhood: A Clinical Treatise* (New York: Paul B. Hoeber, Inc., 1960).

Dehner, L. P., and Ishak, K. G.: Vascular tumors of the liver in infants and children, Arch. Pathol. 92:101, 1971.

deLorimer, A. A., Bragg, K. U., and Linden, G.: Neuroblastoma in childhood, Am. J. Dis. Child. 118:441, 1969.

Donnellan, W. A., and Swenson, O.: Benign and malignant sacrococcygeal tumors, Surgery 64:834, 1968.

Edmondson, H. A.: Differential diagnosis of tumors and tumor-like lesions of liver in infancy and childhood, Am. J. Dis. Child. 91:168, 1956.

Everson, T. C., and Cole, W. H.: *Spontaneous Regression of Cancers* (Philadelphia: W. B. Saunders Co., 1966).

Farber, S.: Congenital rhabdomyoma of the heart, Am. J. Pathol. 7:105, 1931.

Favera, B., Johnson, W., and Ito, J.: Renal tumor in the neonatal period, Cancer 22:845, 1968.

Goetsch, E.: Hygroma colli cysticum and hygroma axillare, Arch. Surg. 36:394, 1938.

Gross, R. E.: Sclerosing hemangiomas, Am. J. Pathol. 19: 533, 1946.

Gross, R. E., Farber, S., and Martin, L.: Neuroblastoma sympatheticum. Study and report of 217 cases, Pediatrics 23:1179, 1959.

Gross, R. E., Clatworth, W., Jr., and Meeker, I. L., Jr.: Sacrococcygeal teratomas in infants and children, Surg. Gynecol. Obstet. 92:341, 1951.

Gwinn, J. K., Dockerty, M. B., and Kennedy, R. B.: Presacral teratomas in infancy and childhood, Pediatrics 10: 239, 1955.

Horner, E. N.: Placental metastases, Obstet. Gynecol. 15: 566, 1960.

Jensen, A. R., Martin, L., and Longino, L.: Digital neurofibrosarcoma in infancy, J. Pediat. 51:560, 1957.

Kaufman, S. L., and Stout, A. P.: Hemangiopericytoma in children, Cancer 13:695, 1960.

Kaufman, S. L., and Stout, A. P.: Histiocytic tumors (fibrous xanthoma and histiocytoma) in children, Cancer 14:469, 1961.

Kaufman, S. L., and Stout, A. P.: Lipoblastic tumors of children, Cancer 12:912, 1959.

Kimmel, D. L., Mayer, E. K., Peall, A. R., Winhorne, L. W., and Gotwales, J. E.: Cerebral tumor containing five human fetuses. Anat. Rec. 106:141, 1950.

Kohout, F., and Stout, A. P.: Glomus tumor in children, Cancer 15:555, 1961.

Krivit, W., and Good, R. A.: Simultaneous occurrence of mongolism and leukemia, Am. J. Dis. Child. 91:289, 1957.

Landing, B. L., and Farber, S.: Tumors of the Cardiovascular System, in *Atlas of Tumor Pathology* (Washington, D. C.: Armed Forces Institute of Pathology).

Lawrence, W., Jr., Jegge, G., and Foote, F. W., Jr.: Embryonal rhabdomyosarcoma, Cancer 17:361, 1964.

McCollum, D. B., and Marin, L.: Hemangiomas in infancy and childhood: 6479 cases, Surg. Clin. North Am. 36: 1647, 1956.

Marsden, H. B., and Steward, J. K.: Tumors in children, Recent Prog. Cancer Res. 3:37, 1968.

Masson, P.: Pigmented nevi as tumors of nervous origin, Ann. Anat. Pathol. 3:416, 657, 1926.

Mosberg, W. H., Jr.: Spinal tumors diagnosed during the 1st year of life, J. Neurosurg. 8:220, 1951.

Nash, A., and Stout, A. P.: Malignant mesenchymomas in children, Cancer 14:534, 1960.

Neel, H. B., and Pemberton, J. D.: Branchial cysts and fistulas, Surgery 18:276, 1945.

Olken, H. G.: Congenital gastro-enteric cysts of the mediastinum, Am. J. Pathol. 20:997, 1943.

Potter, E. L.: Teratoma of the thyroid gland, Arch. Pathol. 25:689, 1938.

Potter, E. L., and Parrish, J. M.: Neuroblastoma, ganglioneuroma and fibroneuroma in a stillborn fetus, Am. J. Pathol. 18:181, 1942.

Priebe, C. J., and Clatworth, H. W., Jr.: Neuroblastoma: Evaluation of the treatment of 90 children, Arch. Surg. 95:538, 1967.

Reed, W. B., Becker, S. W., Sr., Becker, S. W., Jr., and Nickel, W. R.: Giant pigmented nevi, melanoma and leptomeningeal melanocytosis, Arch. Dermatol. 91:100, 1965.

Shanklin, D. R., and Sotelo-Avilla, C.: In-situ tumors in fetuses, newborns and young infants, Biol. Neonate 14: 286, 1969.

Silberman, R., and Mendelson, I. R.: Teratoma of the neck, Arch. Dis. Child. 35:159, 1960.

Silverman, B. K., Breck, T., Craig, J. M., and Nadas, A. S.: Congestive failure in the newborn caused by cerebral A-V fistula, Am J. Dis. Child. 89:539, 1955.

Skov-Jensen, T., Hastings, J., and Lambrethsen, E.: Malignant melanomas in children, Cancer 19:620, 1966.

Smith, C. A.: Massive cervical hemangio-endothelioma in a newly born infant, Am. J. Dis. Child. 55:125, 1938.

Stevens, D.: Neuroblastoma and related tumors, Arch. Pathol. 63:451, 1957.

Stout, A. P.: Fibrosarcoma in infants and children, Cancer 15:1028, 1962.

Stowens, D.: Neuroblastoma and related tumors, Arch. Pathol. 63:451, 1957.

Strauss, L., and Driscoll, S.: Congenital neuroblastoma involving the placenta. Report of two cases, Pediatrics 34:23, 1964.

Sweet, L. K., and Connerty, H. V.: Congenital melanoma: Report of cases in which antenatal metastasis occurred, Am. J. Dis. Child. 62:1029, 1941.

Tech, T. B., Steward, J. K., and Willis, R. A.: The distinctive adenocarcinoma of the infant testis, J. Pathol. Bacteriol. 60:147, 1960.

Wells, H. G.: Occurrence and significance of congenital malignant neoplasms, Arch. Pathol. 50:535, 1940.

Wilcox, H. B., and Wollstein, M.: Mediastinal teratoma in an infant, Am. J. Dis. Child. 41:89, 1931.

Wilcox, J. C.: Melanomatosis of skin and central nervous system in infants, Am. J. Dis. Child. 57:391, 1939.

Williams, G. E. C.: Teratoma of the heart, J. Pathol. Bacteriol. 82:281, 1962.

Willis, R. A.: *The Pathology of Tumors of Childhood* (Springfield, Ill.: Charles C Thomas, 1962).

Willis, R. A.: *The Borderline of Embryology and Pathology* (London: Butterworth & Co., Ltd., 1958).

Winship, T., and Rosvoli, R.: Childhood thyroid cancer, Cancer 14:739, 1961.

Wooley, M. M.: Teratomas in infancy and childhood, Z. Kinderchirurg. 4:289, 1967.

Yates, P. O.: Tumors of the central nervous system in children, J. Clin. Pathol. 17:418, 1964.

13

Multiple Pregnancies and Conjoined Twins

Multiple Pregnancies

TWINS ARE BORN in the United States in 1.61% of all pregnancies, triplets in 0.01189% and quadruplets in 0.00203% according to Strandskov, who analyzed 28,000,000 births that took place in the United States from 1922 to 1936. The frequently quoted statement that twins are born once in every 89 pregnancies, triplets in 89^2 and quadruplets in 89^3 is only a rough approximation and, except for twins, gives a figure lower than the actual incidence.

The number of pregnancies in which four or more infants have been delivered has increased in the last few years owing to the use of follicle-stimulating hormone for the treatment of infertility. Although until 1940 Newman was able to find reports on seemingly authentic cases of only 45 quintuplets and four sextuplets, many more would now be available. It is questionable whether septuplets have ever been observed.

The frequency of twins varies in different races. In the United States, in 1964, Negroes had twins in 1.37% and whites in 0.95% of live births. In Japan the frequency of twins is only half that in the United States. In Nigeria, Nylander and Corney found a frequency in the vicinity of 5% of total births. The differences in frequency are dependent on the differences in numbers of fraternal twins, the incidence of identical twins being the same in all groups—0.39% of births in white and Negro populations in the United States and about the same in Nigeria.

In the United States infants are of the same sex in slightly less than two thirds of twin pregnancies. The frequency of males is slightly less than in single pregnancies, a tendency that becomes exaggerated with the increase in number of children per pregnancy. The percentage of males in the United States for single pregnancies is 51.59, for twins 50.85, for triplets 49.54 and for quadruplets 46.48. The cause for this is unknown unless it is possible that the female-producing zygote has a greater tendency than the male-producing zygote to divide into twins, triplets or quadruplets.

Multiple pregnancies are of two varieties, monovular and polyovular. Monovular pregnancies result from the division of a single fertilized ovum, polyovular from fertilization of two or more simultaneously shed ova. The proportionate number of monovular (monozygotic) and binovular (dizygotic) twins varies from one population to another since the tendency for binovular twinning appears to be determined by one or more recessive genes that affect the frequency of multiple ovulation. In certain populations, as in the Nigerian blacks, the incidence of multiple ovulation is very high. This increases the number of dizygotic twins and changes the relative frequency of the two varieties. The frequency of twinning among children of dizygotic female twins is greater than that among those of dizygotic male twins.

Polyovular pregnancies are more frequent after the second pregnancy and in older women. With the use of ovulation-inducing agents, either synthetic (clomiphene) or natural (extracts of postmenopausal urine and chorionic gonadotropin), superovulation may occur and artificially change the proportion of monovular and binovular twins.

Since polyovular pregnancies result from the simultaneous fertilization of two or more ova, it is not uncommon to find two or even three corpora lutea of the same age in one ovary or distributed between the ovaries. As many as seven corpora lutea may be found in one ovary after stimulation with extracts of postmenopausal urine. Since a single follicle occasionally contains two ova, it is possible to have twins from two ova even in the presence of a single corpus luteum. When more than two fetuses coexist in the uterus, each may be derived from a separate ovum, all may come from one ovum, or they may be a result of combined monovular and polyovular twinning.

Infants derived from separate ova are no more closely related than any other siblings. They may be of the same or different sex and may show any degree of similarity or dissimilarity in appearance.

Monovular multiple pregnancies result from the abnormal development of a single zygote. In some instances the initiation of twinning must occur at the time of the first cell division or during the morula stage. Then the first two blastomeres or the two portions of a divided morula would develop in the same way as would two fertilized eggs, and each embryo would be surrounded by a complete chorionic vesicle. From the appearance of the placentas at birth differentiation from two-ovum twins would be impossible, and to determine zygosity it would be necessary to resort to examination of the infants.

More often monovular twinning is initiated slightly later while the inner cell mass is differentiating. The blastocyst is then already established and the twins are consequently enclosed in a single chorionic vesicle. Either the primitive mass divides completely or two centers of growth originate sufficiently far apart on the germinal disk to permit normal development of two embryonic areas. In such instances each embryo is surrounded by an individual amniotic sac and the sacs are contained in a single chorionic membrane.

In a few instances twinning is initiated still later, after the ectodermal plate and amniotic sac are already formed. The appearance of two primitive streaks on the single ectodermal plate results in the development of two embryos within a single amniotic sac.

The cause of monovular multiple pregnancy is thought to be most probably a retardation of growth in the early stages of development. Monovular twinning occurs frequently in many species of animals and can be produced at will by various

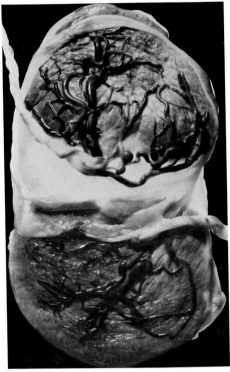

Fig. 13–1.—Separate twin placentas each complete with its own amnion and chorion. Outer surfaces of chorionic membranes were adherent because of crowding in the uterus from presence of two fetuses. Membranes transilluminated to show separation of placentas. Cord of upper placenta is velamentous in insertion.

methods, each of which acts by retarding cellular differentiation at a critical period of growth. Stockard, who found that reducing the temperature of an egg or decreasing its oxygen supply would produce such changes, attributed the effect to lowering the rate of metabolic activity. Different degrees of twinning depend on the time at which an experiment is carried out, and with the same inciting agent Stockard found it possible to produce disturbances that led to the development of two normal individuals, to the production of conjoined twins with varying degrees of duplication and to the development of single monsters. Newman suggested that possible causes of monovular twinning in the human being may be (1) understimulation of the ovum due to a defect in the development-stimulating mechanism of the sperm, (2) late placentation related to the failure of the corpus luteum to prepare the endometrium properly and (3) the inheritance of twinning as a recessive character.

Form of the Placentas

It is easy from gross examination of the placenta to determine whether each fetus was contained in an individual chorionic membrane or whether the chorionic membrane was common to two or more fetuses with separation only by the amniotic sacs. No additional information concerning the number of chorionic membranes can be gained by microscopic examination.

When two or more ova are fertilized, or when the first blastomeres of a single fertilized egg separate and each implants in a different part of the uterus, the placentas remain separate and no connection exists (Fig. 13–1). Each placenta is continuous with its own chorionic membrane, as in single pregnancies, and each contains a single amniotic sac.

When two or more ova or separated blastomeres implant near one another in the uterine wall, the close approximation of the chorionic vesicles is responsible for intermingling of contiguous villi. As villi increase in number and length, they often become so completely intertwined that no line of demarcation is visible either in the substance or on the maternal surface, and the appearance is that of a single placenta. Inspection of the fetal surface, however, will invariably reveal the chorionic membranes crossing the placenta between the points at which the cords are attached. The thin transparent amniotic membranes are only loosely adherent to the chorionic membranes and are easily separated. If a membrane is still present after the amnions have been removed, it is invariably composed of the two adherent thicker, more opaque chorionic membranes (Fig. 13–2, A). These usually are easily separated where they extend above the placenta but cannot be detached from it because they are continuous with the chorionic plates. It is not necessary to separate the two chorionic membranes to establish their duality; if there is one in this location there is always another. Such a placenta is designated dichorionic diamniotic.

When a single ovum gives rise to a twin pregnancy and the twinning is initiated during the morula stage, it results in a fused placenta with two chorionic and two amniotic membranes similar to the last variety described above. Consequently, when two chorions are present, regardless of whether the placentas are fused or separate, a decision as to whether twins are identical or fraternal cannot be made from inspection of the placenta and must rest on other findings.

At the Chicago Lying-in Hospital 36.2% of monozygotic twins had dichorionic placentas, among

Fig. 13–2.—Fused placentas viewed from the fetal surfaces. **A,** dichorionic diamniotic placenta. The fused chorionic membranes cross the center of the placenta. Amniotic sacs are separated from chorionic membranes and rolled inward slightly to show the central membrane (two fused chorions) persisting after the amnions were removed. May be from one or two ova. **B,** monochorionic diamniotic placenta after removal of amniotic sacs. Absence of central partition always indicates origin from one ovum.

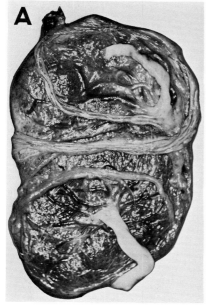

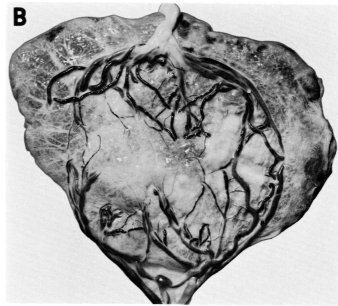

which 16.8% were from monozygotic pregnancies (Potter). In the hospital at Ibadan, Nigeria, where the frequency of dizygotic pregnancies is so much greater, 49.6% of monozygotic twins had dichorionic placentas; among these dichorionic placentas only 3.9% were monozygotic.

When single-ovum twinning is initiated early in the inner cell mass stage, the blastocyst has already been formed; as a result there will be only one placenta and chorionic membrane, but contained within it will be two amniotic sacs, each surrounding a fetus. When the placenta is examined and, after delivery, the two amniotic membranes removed, a smooth unbroken surface remains between the cords (Fig. 13–2, B). This is positive evidence of a single chorion and of monozygotic twins. Microscopic examination shows an unbroken chorionic membrane with the outer surfaces of the amnions in juxtaposition. This is a monochorionic diamniotic placenta (Fig. 13–3, B),

in contrast to the fused double chorionic membrane lying between the amniotic sacs in the dichorionic diamniotic placenta (Fig. 13–3, A).

When twinning is initiated after the ectodermal plate and amniotic sac have been established, both fetuses lie within a single amniotic membrane covered externally by the chorionic membrane. This is known as a monochorionic monoamniotic placenta (Fig. 13–4). Since no membrane separates the cords, they are always somewhat intertwined, and many such pregnancies terminate in abortion because of obstruction to fetal circulation (Figs. 13–5 and 13–6). When the fetuses reach the stage of viability, intertwining is less hazardous because the turgor in the vessels lessens the probability of tightening of knots in the cords.

RELATIVE FREQUENCY OF MONOZYGOUS AND DIZYGOUS TWINNING. — Weinberg's rule has been used for many years to calculate the percentage of twins that are monozygotic and dizygotic in any group in

Fig. 13–3.—Photomicrographs of placental membranes. **A,** dichorionic diamniotic placenta. Junction of the fused placenta showing fused chorionic membranes in which degenerated villi can still be seen. The amniotic sac of each twin is visible on lateral surfaces of the chorionic tissue. **B,** monochorionic diamniotic placenta. Approximation of amniotic sacs showing absence of chorionic membranes between them.

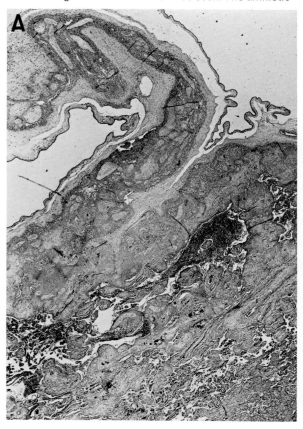
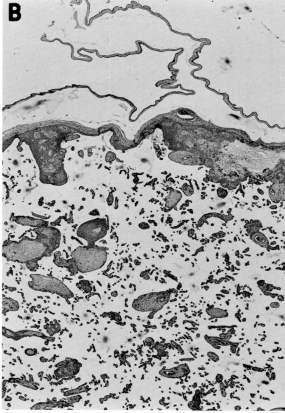

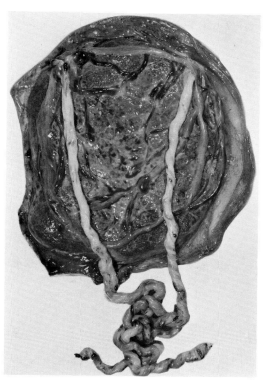

Fig. 13—4.—Monochorionic monoamniotic placenta. Placenta of one-ovum twins, both contained in the same amniotic sac. Intertwining of umbilical cords often causes fetal death. In this instance both twins survived.

which the sex of the twins is known. Inasmuch as the fertilization of two eggs should result in the chance production of an equal number of twins of like and unlike sex, any excess of like-sexed twins should come from single eggs. Weinberg's rule states that the number of monozygotic twin pregnancies equals the total number of twin pairs minus twice the number of pairs in which the twins are of unlike sex.

In order to obtain information as to whether a specific pair of twins is homozygous or heterozygous, the placenta and the children themselves must be examined. All those with monochorionic placentas can be recognized immediately as monozygotic twins and those of unlike sex as dizygotic twins. Some of those with dichorionic placentas will also be monozygotic and some of those with dichorionic placentas will be monozygotic. For these last two groups a wide variety of heritable alleles may be useful in determining zygosity. The blood groups, haptoglobins, secretor status, presence of certain enzymes, distribution of isoenzymes and examination of fingerprints may all be useful. The

survival of exchanged homografts between twins as an indicator of monozygosity has been suggested as the ultimate test, but its value in infancy has been questioned because of the difficulty of making any graft survive in young infants.

With the use of Weinberg's rule on two groups of twins in the United States studied by Potter (293 pairs) and Benirschke (250 pairs) and one in Ibadan, Nigeria, by Nylander and Corney (455 pairs) the frequency of monozygotic twinning was found to be 39%, 43% and 14%, respectively. By examination of the placentas, 23%, 31% and 4% respectively could be established as definitely monozygotic because they had monochorionic placentas. Because of differences in sex and/or blood or other characteristics, Potter established 57% of her group and Nylander and Corney 86% of their group as definitely dizygotic. From a combination of Weinberg's rule and the number of monochorionic placentas, 56% of Benirschke's group appeared probably to be dizygotic. Since in Potter's group 77% had dichorionic placentas and only 57% could be established as definitely dizygotic, it can be supposed that approx-

Fig. 13—5.—Monochorionic monoamniotic twin pregnancy resulting in abortion because of cord entanglement.

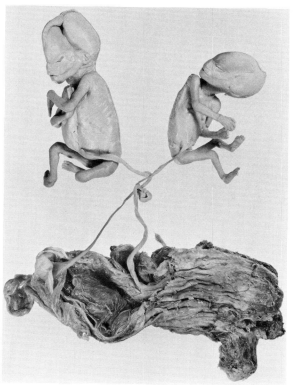

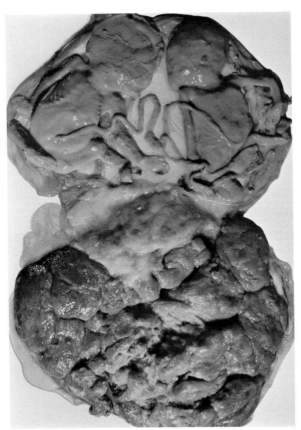

Fig. 13—6.—One-ovum triplet pregnancy. Monochorionic diamniotic triplet placenta. The two macerated fetuses with cords intertwined were contained in a single amniotic sac and attached to a completely hyalinized portion of the placenta. The one living infant (not shown) was in a separate amniotic sac. Placenta and chorionic membrane were single.

imately 20% of all twins were derived from one ovum and had dichorionic placentas. Similarly obtained figures for Benirschke are 13%, for Nylander and Corney 4%. Thus, among Potter's twins those with dichorionic placentas had five times the probability of being derived from a single ovum as did those described by Nylander and Corney. Not only is the frequency of dizygotic twinning much higher in Nigeria than in the United States, but there is also a much greater probability that twins with dichorionic placentas will have come from two ova.

TRIPLETS.—Triplets' placentas may originate from one, two or three ova. One placenta and chorionic membrane indicates one-ovum triplets, but the fetuses may be contained in one, two or

three amniotic sacs. In the specimen of aborted triplets shown in Figure 4–6 a separate amniotic sac surrounds each fetus. In the specimen shown in Figure 13–6 two fetuses were in a single amniotic sac and the third, liveborn, triplet (not shown) was in a separate amniotic sac. All were enclosed in a single chorion. To produce the latter appearance, changes responsible for twinning must have taken place early in the inner cell mass stage; then one of the two areas thus produced must have redivided after the ectodermal plate and amniotic cavity had been established, while the other developed as a single fetus in a separate amniotic sac. The probability that triplets were derived from two eggs would be found in the combination of a single placenta complete with its amniotic and chorionic sacs and a second placenta with two amniotic sacs and only one chorionic membrane (Fig. 13–7). In general, triplet and quadruplet placentas are subject to the same interpretation as are those of twins when the number of ova from which they may have arisen is being considered.

Fig. 13—7.—Triplet pregnancy, probably from two ova. One placenta was separate and complete with chorionic membrane and amniotic sac. The other had a single chorion and two amniotic sacs. Abortion at 18 weeks.

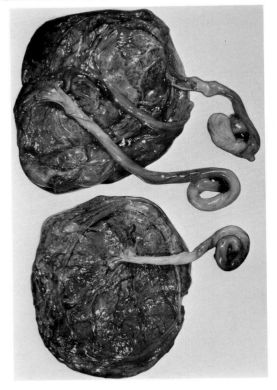

UMBILICAL CORD ATTACHMENT.—The umbilical cords of monovular twins are ordinarily attached to their appropriate portions of the placenta. Occasionally they arise very close together, or one may actually be inserted into the other with resultant direct fusion of the major blood vessels. This may be true even in the presence of two amnions but does not occur with two-ovum twins. In all cases observed at the Chicago Lying-in Hospital in which one cord inserted into the other, the fetus with the secondarily attached cord was severely malformed. Communications between the large placental blood vessels supplying different fetuses (Fig. 13–8) or between the small vessels of the villi are common with monovular twins. They are rare with two-ovum twins.

If one cord is attached peripherally and is supplied by only one small portion of the placenta, the inadequate size of the capillary bed may be responsible for malformation or fetal death (Fig. 13–9).

RATE OF GROWTH

The placentas may be of approximately equal size, or one may be larger than the other. Combined placental weight in relation to combined fetal weight is about the same as for single infants, and the ratio of placental to fetal weight is the same for monochorionic and dichorionic placentas (Potter).

The rate of intrauterine growth is approximately the same for twin and single fetuses. It has been suggested that a twin infant is actually more mature than a single infant of the same weight, but this does not generally seem to be the case. In a study conducted at the Chicago Lying-in Hospital the gestational age of twin infants was found to be slightly less than that of single infants of equal weight. The average menstrual age for twin infants with a combined weight of 5,000–6,000 gm was 270 days while for single infants of 2,500–3,000 gm it was 277 days.

Twins may show striking differences in size. When the larger infant weighs more than 2,000 gm the average difference is 500 gm. Infants of excessive size are rare; the largest infant among 1,140 twins born at the Chicago Lying-in Hospital weighed 3,940 gm. Its twin weighed 3,370 gm. The greatest combined weight was 7,440 gm. The greatest difference in birth weight of living infants was 995 gm. In 1938 Mathieu was able to find only 20 reported cases with a combined weight of 7,000 gm or more. The largest infant in his series weighed 4,650 gm and its twin 4,150 gm. The greatest reported difference was 850 gm.

Many twin pregnancies end prematurely. Among 249 twin pregnancies at the Chicago Lying-in Hospital only 18.5% ended more than 280 days after the last menstrual period, whereas in a group of 4,418 consecutive single pregnancies 52.6% ended after 280 days.

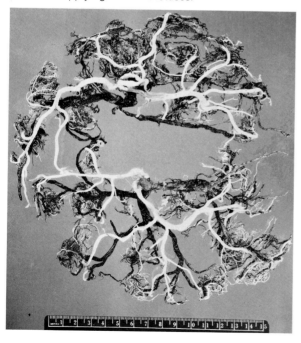

Fig. 13–8.—Monochorionic twin placenta prepared by injection and corrosion showing anastomosis of two large superficial veins coming from portions of the placenta supplying different fetuses.

COMPLICATIONS OF PREGNANCY

Palpation of the abdomen can ordinarily identify the number of fetuses in the uterus. In the presence of hydramnios or excessive adipose tissue roentgen examination may be necessary (Fig. 13–10).

Maternal complications are more frequently encountered in twin than in single pregnancies, especially preeclampsia, postpartum hemorrhage and polyhydramnios. Preeclamptic toxemia has been associated with about 8% of all pregnancies at the Chicago Lying-in Hospital but with about 25% of twin pregnancies.

FETAL AND INFANT MORTALITY

In a study conducted at the Chicago Lying-in Hospital total mortality for twins was 15.6%, or 8.2% if infants under 1,000 gm were excluded. The

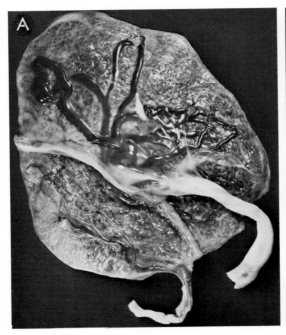

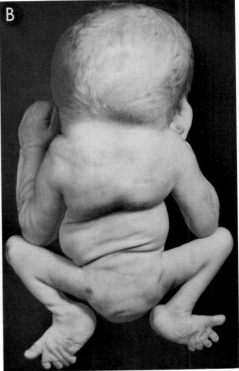

Fig. 13–9.—Twin pregnancies with one normal and one severely malformed infant. **A,** dichorionic placenta with smaller portion supplying the abnormal twin. **B,** abnormal twin with multiple anomalies including renal agenesis and absence of lumbar and lower thoracic segments of the spine.

principal reason for the higher mortality in twin than in single pregnancies is the larger number of small premature infants in the former group. When mortality rates within individual 500 gm weight groups are compared, the differences are statistically insignificant in all groups.

The incidence of malformations incompatible with life seems to be somewhat higher in twin than

Fig. 13–10.—Prenatal roentgenograms of multiple pregnancies. **A,** twin pregnancy. **B,** triplet pregnancy. **C,** quadruplet pregnancy.

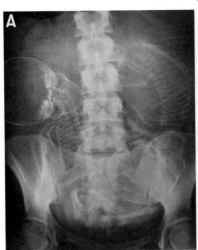

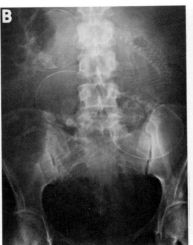

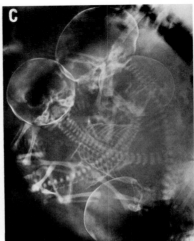

in single pregnancies. Among 1,134 twins born at the Chicago Lying-in Hospital 10 died because of malformations. This is twice the frequency of fatal malformations found among single infants in this hospital. In no instance was malformation the cause of death of both twins despite the fact that some were monozygotic. Prematurity with pulmonary hyaline membranes and atelectasis was responsible for the majority of neonatal deaths among twins, and anoxia or unknown causes for most of the stillbirths. These causes are the same as for single infants of similar weights.

Opinions as to whether the twin who is born first or second has a better chance of survival have varied. It has been suggested that the second twin is less subject to trauma than the first since it does not participate in dilating the birth passages. On the other hand, it is more subject to anoxia because of the possibility of placental separation following the reduction in uterine size that follows the birth of the first twin. In most studies mortality for first twins has been slightly lower than for second twins, although both Benirschke and Potter found them to be about the same if macerated fetuses were excluded. If one twin is alive and the other has been dead long enough to become macerated, the live twin is more often delivered first. Of 31 macerated twin fetuses in the Chicago Lying-in Hospital series, 21 were delivered second.

Mortality in relation to type of placenta was studied by both Benirschke and Potter (Table 13–1). Both concluded that premature delivery was the principal cause of death in all groups, and Potter found that because of the increased number of premature births among twins it accounted for a mortality of 42.5/1,000 twin births compared to 0.9/1,000 total births. She also found that in twins mortality was slightly higher for males (11.7%) than females (9.4%), for twins of like sex (12.2%)

than unlike sex (7.3%), for second-born (11.8%) than for firstborn (9.3%) and for twins with monochorionic placentas (13.2%) than dichorionic placentas (9.6%).

Among 116 cases of monoamniotic twins collected by Hertig and his co-workers only 63 twins survived. In 74 cases both twins were stillborn and in 21 cases one was stillborn. The majority of monoamniotic twin pregnancies observed at the Chicago Lying-in Hospital have resulted in abortion and death of young fetuses because of cord entanglement. Even with severe entanglement, however, both twins may survive.

Abnormal Twin Pregnancies

Most plural pregnancies consist of two fetuses, both in the uterine cavity and of fairly similar size at the time of delivery. On rare occasions one fetus is present in the uterus while a second develops in a fallopian tube, or, if both are in the uterus, one may become blighted while the other develops normally.

If one fetus dies, it is retained until the living fetus is delivered. If the embryo dies in the first 6 or 8 weeks of pregnancy, the amniotic sac at term may resemble a cyst on the fetal surface of the placenta of the living twin. The embryo will be greatly degenerated but can usually still be identified. Although most cysts on the placental surface are a result of local changes in the chorion, the possibility that the pregnancy originated as twins should be kept in mind whenever a cystic area is discovered.

After the death of a fetus the amount of fluid in the amniotic sac within which it is contained reduces and sometimes almost completely disappears. If the fetus is retained a sufficient length of time, much of the fluid in the body tissues is absorbed, the tissues become firmer and "mummified" and

TABLE 13–1.—Frequency of Different Varieties of Placentas and Mortality for Each Variety

	Benirschke, 1961 250 Twin Pairs		Potter, 1963 567 Twin Pairs	
	Frequency %	Mortality %	Frequency %	Mortality %
Monochorionic, monoamniotic	1.2	50	0.2	0
Monochorionic, diamniotic	29.6	25	20.6	13.2
Dichorionic, fused	34.0	8.2	33.8	8.3
Dichorionic, separate	35.2	9.6	42.1	10.0
Fused placentas, membranes unknown	–	–	3.3	26.3
Totals	100.0	(14.2)	100.0	(10.6)

the body is compressed against the uterine wall by the living fetus. Such a flattened fetus is known as a fetus papyraceus.

Because the portion of placenta belonging to the dead fetus may be smaller than would be expected to result only from cessation of growth, occasionally death appears to follow primary inadequacy in the development of placental tissue. Villi belonging to a dead fetus slowly degenerate. Following cessation of fetal circulation the maternal blood gradually stops circulating, fibrinoid material is deposited between the villi, and cellular degeneration takes place. Calcium may be deposited in the decidua and the stroma of the major villi but is rarely found in the terminal villi. The dead fetus and placenta are sterile until onset of labor and they may remain in the uterus many months without producing any ill effect. Kindred found that one twin was blighted with equal frequency whether the placentas were dichorionic or monochorionic. However, for reasons he could not explain, there was an increased frequency of one blighted monochorionic twin born to primiparous women and to women 30–35 years of age.

TWIN TRANSFUSION SYNDROME. — With monochorionic twins careful observation or injection of the placental vessels with plastic material or colored solutions will often demonstrate artery-vein, artery-artery or vein-vein anastomoses. Littlewood believed that while superficial anastomoses in the chorionic plate may be of any type, the majority of deep anastomoses are arteriovenous.

Among 100 monochorionic placentas, Scatz was able to identify 60 arterial, 2 venous and 30 arteriovenous anastomoses, with only 8 placentas showing none. Arteriovenous anastomosis is the only harmful variety and may be associated with the twin transfusion syndrome. It is possible for blood volume to remain balanced by flow in different directions in different cotyledons, but if the size of the vessels is such that it favors the transfer of blood from one fetus to the other, one becomes the donor and hence anemic, while the other becomes the recipient and hence plethoric.

Rousen *et al.,* in a study of twins with monochorionic twin placentas, found 19 pairs with sufficient imbalance in blood transfer between the placentas to give a 5 gm hemoglobin difference and a noticeable pallor and plethora in the two twins. Littlewood recorded a hemoglobin of 27 gm% in one of his recipient twins and 5.2 gm% in its donor. A marked difference in weight is common, the plethoric twin being heavier. Unilateral hydramnios has been reported for both plethoric and anemic twins, al-

though it is probably uncommon in the latter. More often the amniotic fluid of the anemic twin is diminished and amnion nodosum has been reported.

According to Naeye, the organs of the donor twins weigh less and are morphologically similar to those of an infant with poor intrauterine nutrition secondary to poor placental function, and parenchymal cell size is reduced in many organs. Erythropoiesis in the liver is often increased (Fig. 13–11). As a result of increased blood volume the heart of the recipient twin may be enlarged and the muscle of the pulmonary arteries in the lungs increased because of the greater flow through the lungs.

Prompt postnatal relief of the cardiovascular disturbance may be necessary to maintain life in such infants. Therapy includes phlebotomy and digitalization of the plethoric twin. These twins may also develop kernicterus because of the high hemoglobin and reduced liver function. The donor twin may need replacement of fluid and blood.

SUPERFECUNDATION AND SUPERFETATION. — Conspicuous differences in size and appearance of twins have caused speculation concerning the possibility of superfecundation and superfetation. Superfecundation, the fertilization of an ovum as a result of insemination taking place after one ovum has already been fertilized, cannot be denied as a possibility but must be rare. More possible would be the more or less simultaneous fertilization of two ova by sperm cells deposited in the vagina by different men. The possibility of superfecundation has most often been suspected when a woman has given birth to infants of different skin color. However, when Negro or other colored strains are present in one or both parents, marked differences may be found among the offspring. Cases have been reported in which a woman has given birth to one albino and one normal twin. This is particularly striking if the parents are Negroes but need not indicate fertilization by sperm from different individuals (see Fig. 27–29).

Superfetation, the fertilization and development of an ovum while a living fetus is already present in the uterus, is a condition that is extremely difficult to prove. The greatest differences in size are found when one fetus dies early in pregnancy and is retained until the other reaches term, but even when both are liveborn, remarkable differences may be observed. In one case at the Chicago Lying-in Hospital there was a difference of almost 1,000 gm between liveborn twins, one weighing 1,305 gm, the other 2,300 gm. The small twin died after birth, the state of development of the lungs and kidneys, organs whose maturity can be most accu-

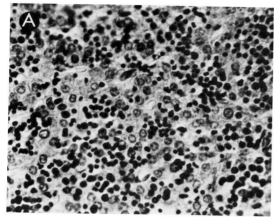 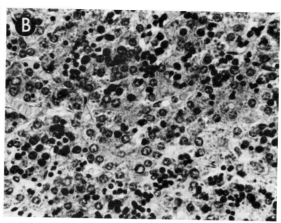

Fig. 13–11.—Twin transfusion syndrome. Fetus with a monochorionic diamniotic placenta in which the portion supplying the plethoric twin was nearly twice the size of that of the anemic twin. **A,** liver of anemic twin with an increase in erythropoiesis and reduction in liver cells. **B,** liver of plethoric twin. Gestational age 19½ weeks.

rately estimated from histologic appearance, equaling that of an infant with the weight of its twin. The formation of glomeruli, which ordinarily continues until the fetus weighs over 2,000 gm, had completely ceased in the 1,305 gm fetus. This negates the likelihood of superfetation in this case.

At the Chicago Lying-in Hospital a few twin abortuses have been observed with appearances strongly suggesting the possibility of fertilization of ova at different times. In one of these a fetus of about 16 weeks' size was associated with one of about 4 weeks' size (Fig. 13–12), the larger being slightly macerated, the smaller being normal. Although the larger fetus was dead when aborted, the state of the body did not seem compatible with death prior to the conception of the smaller fetus and it is probable that this was an example of true superfecundation.

HYDATIDIFORM MOLE.—In rare instances one blastocyst may be converted into a hydatidiform mole

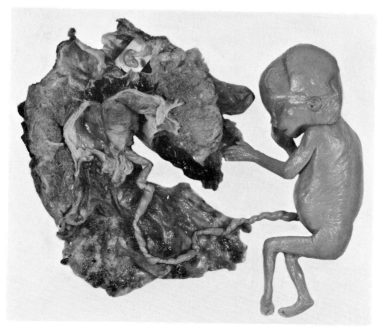

Fig. 13–12.—Superfetation. Twin pregnancy terminated 18 weeks after last menstrual period with one fetus measuring 1 cm, the other 15 cm. This is compatible with a difference of about 12 weeks' gestational age.

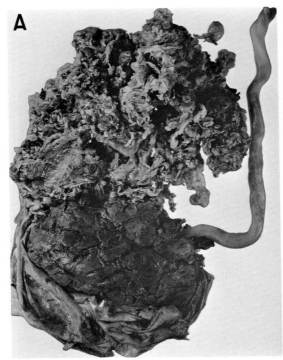

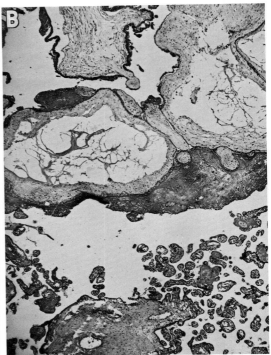

Fig. 13–13. — Twin placenta with one portion converted into a hydatidiform mole. The twin attached to the normal placenta appeared normal, weighed 650 gm and survived 2 hours. **A,** gross appearance of placenta. **B,** photomicrograph showing junction of hydatidiform mole and normal placenta. (Courtesy Dr. H. W. Hilfstein.)

while the other develops normally and contains a normal fetus. Such a case is shown in Figure 13–13. The placentas were fused and two amniotic sacs were present; the state of the chorionic membranes was unknown. Delivery was at 24 weeks and a normal premature infant weighing 650 gm who survived 2 hours was attached to the normal portion of the placenta.

Hydatidiform moles have been recognized in both dichorionic and monochorionic twin placentas. Most commonly, as in the case mentioned above, one fetus and placenta are normal. Molar changes have been observed in one of monozygotic twin pairs, but in these the molar changes have been incomplete. Chromosomal anomalies have been recognized in some hydatidiform moles (Szulman), but ordinarily in less than 50% (Carr), so that even in monozygotic twins both need not be similarly affected. Since in fully developed hydatidiform moles membranes can seldom be identified, determination of zygosity from placental structures is usually impossible.

ACARDIUS. — One of the more uncommon situations that may occur in twin pregnancies is for one twin to be normal and the other so malformed that it lacks a functioning heart. Abnormal fetuses of this variety are never found in single pregnancies, and circulation of blood is possible only by virtue of communication with the vessels supplying the normal twin. Such twins most frequently consist of a fleshy mass, often with hair on the superior surface, with two attached similarly fleshy masses representing abortive attempts at the formation of legs (Fig. 13–14, A). X-ray usually shows a fairly well-developed spine with a few ribs and surmounted by an irregular bony mass representing the base of the skull. Pelvic bones and varying portions of bones of the lower extremities are also present (Fig. 13–14, B). Viscera are seldom found although, when the legs are better developed, kidneys, portions of intestine and occasionally other organs are sometimes present.

Although this is the most common variety, many degrees of reduction of body parts have been described and names given the fetuses. Those in which some cardiac muscle is present but not formed into a functioning heart are termed hemiacardius, those with no heart holoacardius. In the

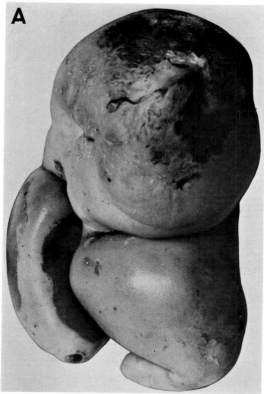

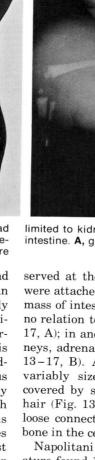

Fig. 13—14.—Acardius acephalus. Twin without head or heart. Spine, ribs and amorphous mass of bone representing base of the skull were present. Viscera were limited to kidneys, adrenal glands and small segment of intestine. **A,** gross appearance. **B,** roentgenogram.

hemiacardius, four extremities, an abnormal head and some viscera are often present although an excessive amount of myxomatous tissue usually distorts body shape to such an extent that extremities are almost hidden (Fig. 13–15). In holoacardius no cardiac muscle is present and body form is much more reduced. The latter have been subdivided into those consisting only of a head (acardius acormus), only of the lower part of the body (acardius acephalus) (Fig. 13–16) or of a mass with no distinguishable parts (acardius amorphus). It is doubtful whether an isolated head with all features distinguishable has ever been observed, and most specimens designated acardius acormus have either had a fairly well-developed trunk, sometimes even with a beating heart, or have been amorphous masses with only a semblance of some part of a face (e.g., that described by Mande Abbott with only lips, teeth and jaws). The degree to which the upper part of the body is reduced is variable but usually there is nothing above the level of the diaphragm, and one leg may be missing. In a specimen ob-

served at the Chicago Lying-in Hospital two legs were attached to a pelvis and the only viscus was a mass of intestine attached to the placenta but with no relation to the remainder of the fetus (Fig. 13–17, A); in another, one leg was absent but two kidneys, adrenal glands and testes were present (Fig. 13–17, B). Acardius amorphus fetuses consist of variably sized round, oval or indented masses covered by skin sometimes exhibiting a patch of hair (Fig. 13–18). The interior consists largely of loose connective tissue with an irregular mass of bone in the center.

Napolitani and Schreiber in a search of the literature found 149 cases described as acardiac twins. These were divided into acardius anceps (hemiacardius) (12), acardius acormus (7), acardius acephalus (93) and acardius amorphous (37). Such twins cannot be as rare as these figures indicate and it is probable that comparatively few are ever reported in the literature. Several acardius acephalus and amorphus conceptuses have been seen at the Chicago Lying-in Hospital.

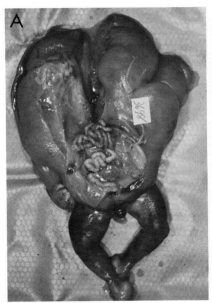 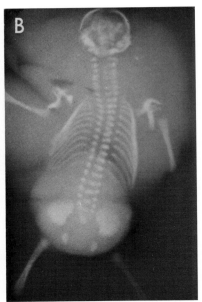

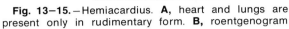

Fig. 13–15.—Hemiacardius. **A,** heart and lungs are present only in rudimentary form. **B,** roentgenogram showing a small skull with extreme edema of surrounding tissue.

Conjoined Twins

FREQUENCY.—Conjoined twins or double monsters vary widely from examples in which two well-developed individuals exist separately except for a minor superficial connection to those in which only a small part of the body is duplicated or in which amorphous masses of tissue, no more identifiable as twins than the amorphous separate twins, are found in the body or attached to the exterior of an otherwise normal individual.

Symmetrical conjoined twins are rare; only two such specimens were delivered at the Chicago Lying-in Hospital from 1931 to 1968 among over

Fig. 13–16.—Holoacardius acephalus. Monovular twin pregnancy with umbilical cord vessels of acephalic twin communicating directly with vessels of normal twin.

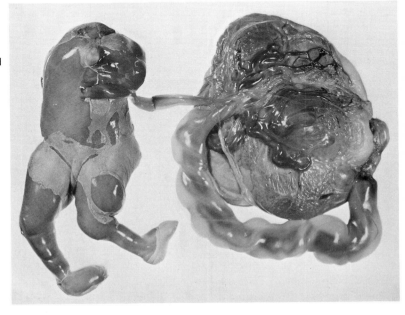

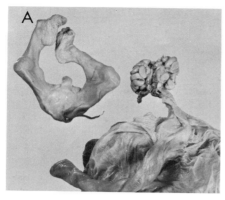

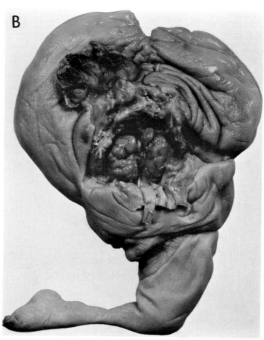

Fig. 13–17.—A, holoacardius acephalus with intestinal mass and the lower part of the fetus attached separately to the placenta. B, holoacardius acephalus with a single leg and body cavity partially surrounded by ribs and containing two kidneys, two small adrenal glands and two hypoplastic testes.

100,000 deliveries. Only one was found among the embryos and small fetuses aborted during the same time. Asymmetrical twins in whom an identifiable portion of a body is attached to a larger host are even less common, few such cases having been reported.

ETIOLOGY.—The origin of conjoined twins is probably the same as that of some normal separate monovular twins. If twinning is determined at the inner cell mass stage before the embryonic disk is differentiated, two complete separate embryos would be expected, each surrounded by an amniotic sac. If, however, twinning is not initiated until after the embryonic disk is formed, and results from the initiation on the disk of two centers of axial growth instead of one, only one amniotic sac would develop, containing both twins. If the centers of growth were not sufficiently separated, it could be anticipated that the intermediate area would be

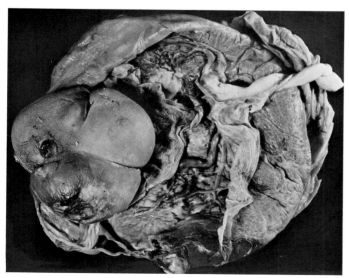

Fig. 13–18.—Acardius amorphus in separate amniotic sac on surface of placenta of its normal twin. Small irregular masses of bone and cartilage were embedded in connective tissue. Vascular connections not identified.

shared by the two embryos and that conjoined twins would result.

A more widely accepted explanation is that fission of the original embryonic area occasionally takes place and the degree and point of origin of the splitting determine the variety of conjoined twins. This might perhaps also be responsible for the origin of some of the separate twins contained in a single sac. The existence of separate or conjoined twins is ordinarily determined before the end of the second week after fertilization. It is probable that when the duplicated parts of conjoined twins are of approximately equal size, secondary fusion of two originally separate embryonic areas is rarely responsible. If secondary fusion were possible, one would expect, at times at least, to find an irregular distribution of parts instead of the bilaterally symmetrical arrangement that invariably exists. However, experimental fusion of rat blastocysts does result in normally structured chimeric embryos. Newman made the suggestion that observable differences in conjoined twins might be related to the manner of fusion.

It is difficult to differentiate between abnormalities that result from twinning and those caused by primary neoplasia or by the abnormal development of an isolated portion of the body. Duplication of parts of the face have usually been considered a phenomenon of twinning, largely because they are ordinarily bilaterally symmetrical. It has been contended that duplication of parts of the viscera such as the intestine should be considered evidence of twinning and also that extra digits have the same etiology. Carried to extremes, all tumors composed of tissues derived from three germ layers would be included in the same category.

In an excellent discussion of the causes of twinning and double and single monsters Stockard described a great variety of detailed experiments and concluded that many different types of monsters, single as well as double, could result from identical experiments and that any given variety could be produced by many different methods. He thought that all effective methods tend to decrease the rate of growth and that the type of malformation depends on the particular moment at which the developmental rate is reduced. He believed that there are many potential areas on the germinal disk that can develop into an embryonic shield but that normally the formation of one such area suppresses the development of others. If differentiation is interrupted just before differentiation of the embryonic axis, the resumption of growth could be followed by establishment of two centers of growth,

neither of which is capable of growing fast enough to inhibit development of the other. In this sense intrinsic conditions capable of giving rise to double monsters or twins exist in all eggs. Since double monsters are more common in some species than others, it is evident that the innate tendency to formation of multiple axes of growth is more prevalent in the eggs of some species than in others. This is probably due to the internal structure of the eggs and their particular manner of development. It is also true that the tendency to abnormal growth of some eggs produced by individual members of a species is greater than that of eggs produced by others.

When two embryonic axes are sufficiently close together to overlap and develop an area common to the two, or when a portion of the axis undergoes fission and parts of equal size develop, the parts formed are as strongly inclined to be normal as are single individuals; if one has an advantage over the other, however, the one suffering the disadvantage will be reduced in size and may be very abnormal in form.

In this way the smaller member of conjoined twins may show a pronounced disturbance in structure and may even be reduced to an undifferentiated mass of tissue resembling a tumor and bearing no resemblance to its twin. The same condition holds true in separate twins, and even when arising from the same zygote and enclosed by the same membranes, one may have an advantage of position and develop normally while the other becomes malformed. Consequently monozygotic twins need not be as identical as they are commonly expected to be since there are possible differences in metabolic rates related directly to placental blood supply.

Indeed, monozygotic twins may be phenotypically and genetically different. If there is a failure of proper chromosomal separation at the time the blastomeres divide, it is possible that an XO might result from an originally XY zygote. Thus one male (XY) and one phenotypic female with Turner's syndrome would result. Such occurrences have been described and if the placenta was monochorionic, would seem to belie the statement that monochorionic placentas are found only in association with identical twins. It is curious that the overwhelming majority (95%) of conjoined twins are female. It would be interesting to obtain karyotypic analyses on each member of such twin pairs.

According to Witschi, the most common cause of human conjoined twins is aging of the ovum. He thought that delayed ovulation with overripening of the ovum could be responsible for gradual decline in its ability to differentiate normally and that two centers of organization, neither able to suppress the other, would result.

When the joined twins are each fairly complete, fusion may be (1) anterior, (2) posterior, (3) cephalic or (4) caudal. Such twins are known respectively as (1) thoracopagus or xiphopagus, (2) pygopagus, (3) craniopagus or (4) ischiopagus. When doubling is less complete and only parts of the bodies are duplicated, the attachment is more often lateral. The division may extend from above downward and produce two heads and four arms, etc., or from below upward and produce three or four legs; or it may extend from both ends and produce two heads with three or four arms and three or four legs. The spine, thorax and pelvis show varying degrees of duplication directly related to the number of extremities. In all symmetrical double monsters, except the rare xiphopagus that has only the lower portions of the sternum fused, some of the viscera are shared by the two individuals and surgical separation with survival of both twins is impossible.

An excellent brief description of the various types of composite monsters was written by Wilder in 1904, and the following classification is based on his outline although it has been enlarged and rearranged.

EMBRYONIC DUPLICATIONS

I. Free monozygotic twins
   A. Symmetrical. Normal or malformed but with hearts present in each.
   B. Asymmetrical. *Acardius.*
      1. Development of the less perfect individual is reduced but the body form and various parts may still be recognized. *Hemiacardius* (see Fig. 13–15).
      2. A large part of the body, either cranial or caudal, is lacking in the less perfect individual. *Holoacardius.*
         a) Cranial part lacking. *Holoacardius acephalus* (see Figs. 13–16 and 13–17).
         b) Caudal part lacking. *Holoacardius acormus.*
      3. The general body form and various parts of the less perfect individual are wholly unrecognizable. *Holoacardius amorphus* (see Fig. 13–18).
II. Joined twins in which the components, or component parts, are equal and symmetrical. *Diplopagus.*

A. Each component is complete, or nearly so.
   1. Connection in or near the sternal region, usually median, the components face to face. *Thoracopagus* (Fig. 13–19), *sternopagus, xiphopagus, sternoxiphopagus.*
   Internal anatomy is extremely variable depending on the extent of the united area. The organs are usually disymmetrical and except for the liver are often completely duplicated. The livers are united in all but the most superficially attached twins and large anastomosing vessels extend between them. Pleural, pericardial and peritoneal cavities may be in open communication or entirely separate. The wider the zone of attachment, the more often are hearts and portions of the digestive tubes common to the two members. The portion of the intestine most often single is that from the stomach to the original attachment of the yolk sac, although it may extend from near the mouth to variable points near the anus.
   2. Connection at the sacrum, the components back to back. *Pygopagus* (Fig. 13–20).
   Although the area of fusion can be anywhere on the dorsal surface of the body, it is usually limited to the pelvic region. The internal anatomy is variable but the free portions of the vertebral columns are completely formed. Except in the most superficially united twins, the sacrum and coccyx are common to both components, the vascular trunks of the pelvis anastomose freely, the digestive tubes unite in a single common rectum and anus, and one urethra ordinarily emerges from a single bladder. The genitourinary tract varies and there may be two, three or four kidneys and one or two uteri and vaginas. There are ordinarily four adrenal glands and four gonads. The survival of several conjoined twins of this type has given it a disproportionate prominence in the series of double monsters. Actually it is one of the rarest varieties, and among almost 30 specimens and photographs of conjoined twins collected by Potter there is only one such abnormality. (Those involving older individuals published as news items were not included.)

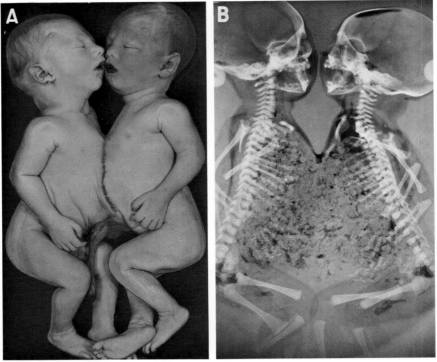

Fig. 13–19.—Thoracopagus twins. Male twins joined by thorax and upper abdomen. Umbilical cord contained four arteries and two veins. Hearts and livers were joined and only partially duplicated. Gastrointestinal tracts were separate. **A**, external view. **B**, roentgenogram. (Courtesy Drs. Bernard Mortimer and J. D. Kirshbaum.)

Fig. 13–20.—Pygopagus female twins. Infants joined by sacral areas, each of which was the site of a spina bifida. External genitalia were partially fused, and common vaginal and anal orifices were divided by septa separating the two orifices of the two twins. Bladders and all organs were duplicated except the kidneys, of which there were only three. **A**, anterior view. **B**, posterior view. (Courtesy Dr. Helen Dawson.)

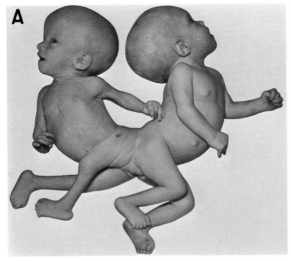
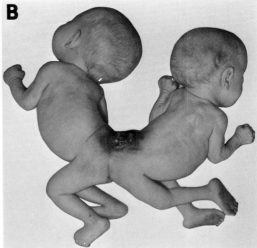

3. Connection by the heads, usually median. *Craniopagus* (Fig. 13–21).

Union may be in the region of the vertex, occiput or lateral parietal areas. The union may be slightly asymmetrical, and various combinations such as vertex to occiput or parietal area to occiput have been observed. The two components may face in the same or opposite directions. The brains are ordinarily separate or only lightly fused despite union of bones.

4. Connection in the lower pelvic region, the axes of the bodies extending in a straight line in opposite directions. *Ischiopagus* (Fig. 13–22).

The bodies are fused in the region of the pelvis as far as the level of the common umbilicus, and above this each is normally developed. The lower ends of the spines are abnormal, and sacrum and pelvis are often single and directed toward one side. Two legs extend at right angles from each lateral surface with vaginal, urethral and anal orifices opening between each pair. Those on each side are derived one from each component. If only one pelvis is present the legs on the opposite side are often fused or rudimentary, and associated genitourinary and anal orifices are absent.

B. The two components equal each other but each is less than an entire individual, usually associated with lateral fusion. These cases form a graded series illustrating almost every possible variation from normal single individuals to two normal superficially joined individuals. Duplication may affect either end and may lead to duplication of the upper part of the body while the lower part remains single; or the lower part may be duplicated while the upper remains single. Duplication may be present at both

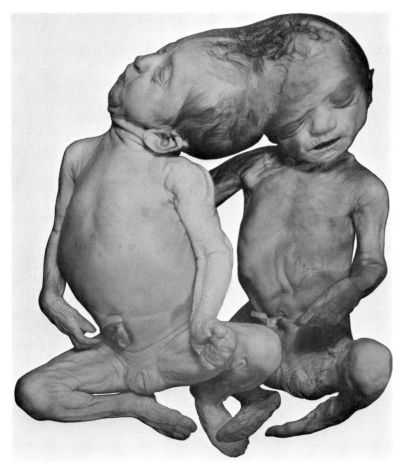

Fig. 13–21.—Craniopagus twins. Median parietal area of right twin is united with right frontoparietal area of left twin. (Courtesy Dr. Charles O. McCormick.)

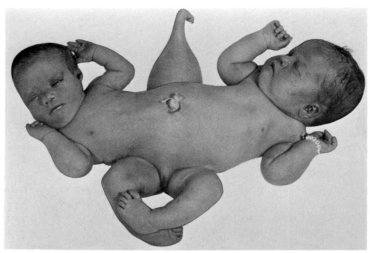

Fig. 13—22.—Ischiopagus twins. Lower abdominal areas are fused and extremities consequently displaced laterally. Only one pelvis is present, associated with single normal external genitalia, the latter located between right leg of left twin and left leg of right twin. The legs are normal except for clubfoot. Opposite legs are fused into a single composite limb. Viscera of one was in situs inversus position. Aortas were fused. The heart of one twin was hypoplastic and circulation through that twin was in reverse direction through arteries and veins. (Courtesy Dr. Hans G. Schlumberger and J. Elmer Gotwals.)

ends with only the middle area remaining single. Duplication from above downward is more common than from below upward.

1. Duplication beginning in the cranial region.
   a) Single head. *Monocephalus diprosopus.*
      (1) Partial duplication of frontal region and nose (Fig. 13–23, A and B).
      (2) Partial duplication of frontal region, nose and mouth (Fig. 13–23, C).
      (3) Duplication of the face either complete or with one eye of each face fused into a common median orbit (Figs. 13–23, D and 13–24).
   b) Two heads. *Dicephalus.*
      (1) Two arms and two legs with partial duplication of the spine and varying degrees of duplication of the median shoulder. *Dicephalus dipus dibrachius* (Fig. 13–25).
      (2) Similar to (1) but with a median third arm or arm rudiment. *Dicephalus dipus tribrachius* (Fig. 13–26).
      (3) Components united at pelvis, with varying degrees of fusion of upper parts of trunks but each component having a head and pair of arms. The pelvis is partially duplicated but only two legs are present. *Dicephalus dipus tetrabrachius* (Fig. 13–27).

2. Duplication originating in caudal region. *Dipygus.*
   a) Partial duplication of pelvis with a third median leg that may be either rudimentary or complete. *Monocephalus tripus dibrachius.*
   b) Partial or complete duplication of the pelvis with four legs, the pair belonging to one member often being fused in a sirenomelic limb. *Monocephalus tetrapus dibrachius* (Fig. 13–28).
   c) Two nearly complete components joined front to front over more or less of the trunk region, but with a single neck and with heads more or less completely fused into a single compound mass. The half-faces of the two components meet in the plane of union and form single faces of varying degrees of completeness, placed laterally with respect to the components. *Cephalothoracopagus.* In all varieties the cerebellum, brain stem

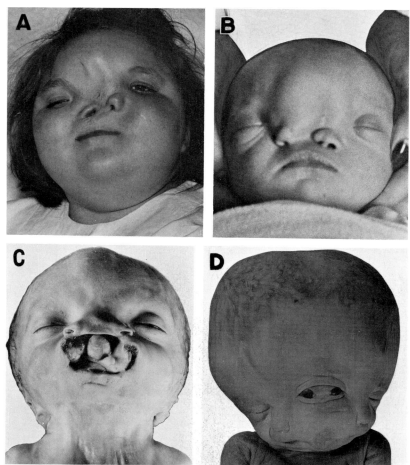

Fig. 13–23.—Monocephalus diprosopus. **A,** partial duplication of frontal region and nose. **B,** partial duplication of frontal region, nose and palate with increase in width of mouth. (Courtesy Dr. C. D. Greulich.) **C,** widening of frontal region with duplication of mouth and nose, harelip and cleft palate. **D,** duplication of face with a common median orbit. (Courtesy Dr. Henry W. Edmonds.)

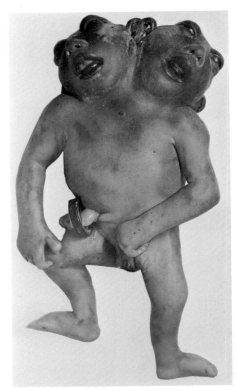

Fig. 13–24.—Monocephalus diprosopus. Anencephalus with two faces and fusion of heads. (Courtesy Dr. Raymond Mitchell.)

Fig. 13–25.—Dicephalus dipus dibrachius. **A,** external surface. **B,** roentgenogram. (Courtesy Dr. James Reaves.)

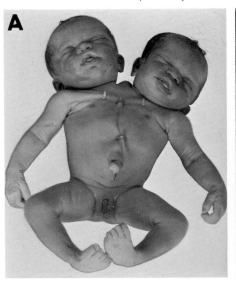
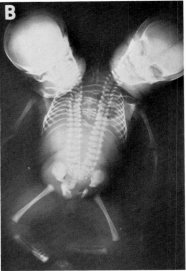

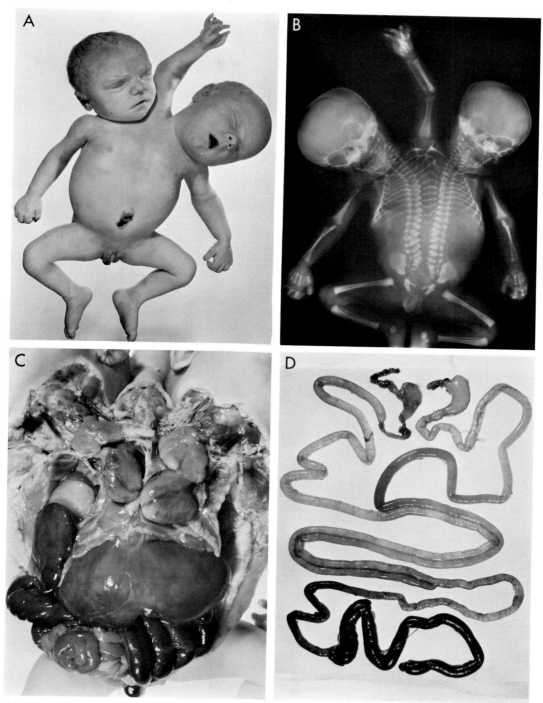

Fig. 13–26.—Dicephalus dipus tribrachius. **A,** anterior body surface. **B,** x-ray of skeleton showing common arm with fused humerus and three bones in forearm. **C,** interior of body cavity, showing two thyroids, two thymuses, two hearts in separate pericardial cavities and one liver with abnormal lobulation caused by right diaphragmatic hernia. **D,** stomachs and intestine with duplication as far as midileum. (Specimen courtesy Dr. J. B. Butler.)

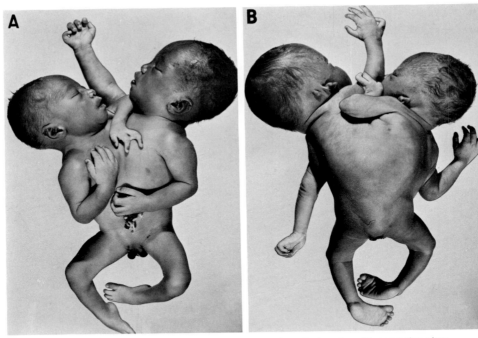

Fig. 13—27.—Dicephalus dipus tetrabrachius. **A,** anterior view. **B,** posterior view. (Courtesy Dr. B. B. Burrowes.)

Fig. 13—28.—Monocephalus tetrapus dibrachius. The two legs on one side are fused into a sirenomelic limb belonging to the left-hand component. This is to be distinguished from a median composite limb made up of components from both twin members in a tripus abnormality. **A,** exterior view. **B,** roentgenogram. (Courtesy Dr. E. C. Sage.)

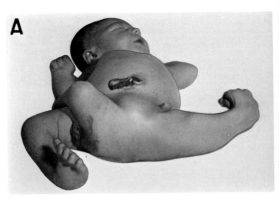

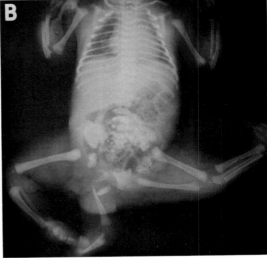

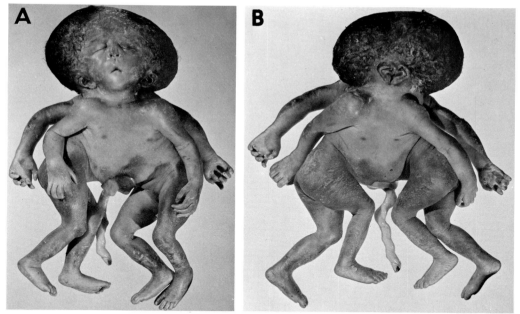

Fig. 13–29.—Cephalothoracopagus syncephalus. **A,** anterior view. **B,** posterior view.
(Courtesy Drs. Harold C. Priddle and Charles S. Stevenson.)

Fig. 13–30.—Cephalothoracopagus syncephalus. Brain from monster similar to that in Figure 13–29. Cerebrum is single, but cerebellum, brain stem and spinal cords are double. **A,** superior surface. **B,** inferior surface.

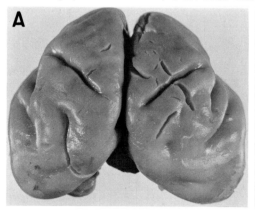
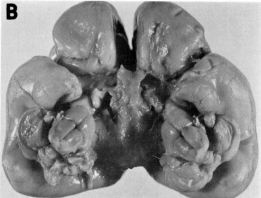

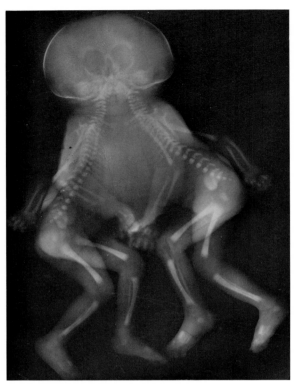

Fig. 13–31.—Cephalothoracopagus syncephalus. Roentgenogram of a fetus identical to those fetuses shown in Figures 13–29 and 13–30. (Courtesy Dr. Gordon T. Burns.)

and spinal cords are double. There are two hearts, one umbilicus and one digestive tube to the level of the stalk of the yolk sac, below which there are two.

    (1) One face with two ears and a single normally formed cerebrum. *Deradelphus.*

    (2) One face with four ears, two on the back of the head. The cerebrum may be single or partially duplicated. *Syncephalus* (Figs. 13–29 to 13–31).

    (3) Two faces on opposite sides of the head with half of each belonging to each component. *Janiceps* (Fig. 13–32).

  3. Duplication of both cranial and caudal regions. *Dicephalus dipygus.*

    a) Two members, with a common trunk but with two heads, two or three arms and three legs. The double median extremity may be rudimentary, or duplication may be so complete that fusion is only by soft tissues. *Dicephalus tripus tribrachius* (Fig. 13–33).

    b) Similar to *a)* but with either upper or lower extremities or both completely duplicated. Fusion of the trunk area may be lateral or median (Figs. 13–34 and 13–35).

    c) Complete duplication of head, arms and legs with anterior or lateral fusion of the trunk areas (see Fig. 13–19).

III. Unequal and symmetrical conjoined twins in which one component is smaller and dependent on the other. *Heteropagus.*

Two members with very unequal degrees of development, the one (autosite) being normal or nearly so and the other (parasite) being incomplete and attached to the first as a dependent growth, usually attached at some point on the ventral surface.

A. Parasite attached to the visible surface of the autosite.

  1. Parasite having arms, or a head and arms, usually attached to the autosite at or near the epigastrium.

  2. Parasite having legs and varying portions of abdomen usually attached in the same region as 1, above (Figs. 13–36 and 13–37).

  3. Parasite having arms and legs with or without a head. Attachment in the same region (Fig. 13–38).

  4. Parasite attached to the head of the autosite. This is stated to be usually only a supernumerary head attached to the parietal region, occiput or vertex of the head. An account of such a malformation was published by Home in 1790, but no other examples of this condition have been found.

  5. Parasite attached to the palate of the autosite. *Epignathus* (see Fig. 12–34).

The attachment is in the region of Rathke's pouch and may be entirely pharyngeal or may extend into the cranial cavity. The degree of development varies, but fetal parts are rarely recog-

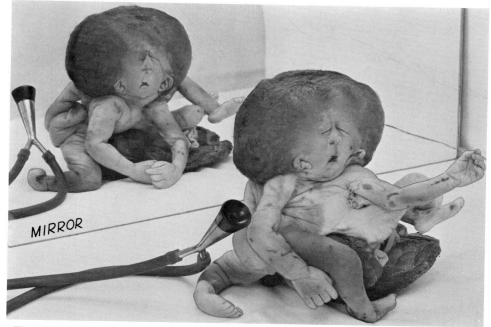

Fig. 13—32.—Cephalothoracopagus janiceps. Fetus has two faces, one of which is visible in the mirror. (Courtesy Dr. Frances Holmes.)

Fig. 13—33 (left).—Dicephalus tripus tribrachius. Upper composite limb is a result of fusion of soft tissues and bones of the two medial arms. Lower medial limb has a common femur, tibia and great toe. (Courtesy Drs. Bernard Mortimer and J. D. Kirshbaum.)

Fig. 13—34 (right).—Dicephalus tripus tetrabrachius. Medial lower extremity is rudimentary.

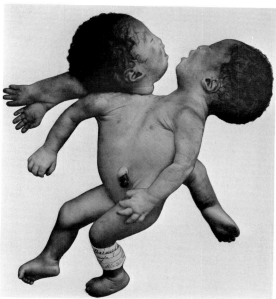

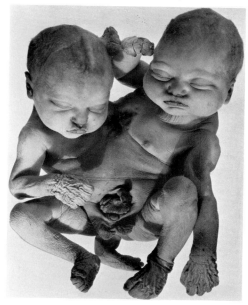

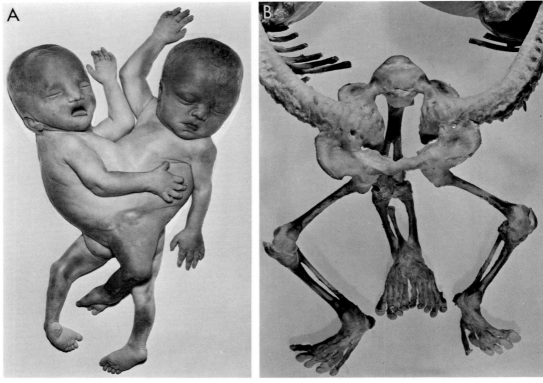

Fig. 13—35.—Dicephalus tripus tetrabrachius. This is actually a modified ischiopagus; note similarity to Fig. 13–22. **A,** anterior body surface. **B,** skeleton of lower part of the body, showing fusion of the pelvis. The common leg contains partially fused femurs, two tibias and one fibula.

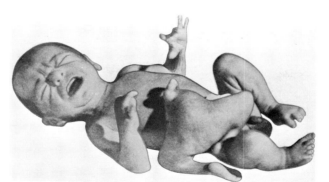

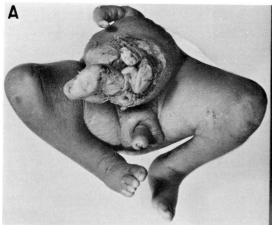
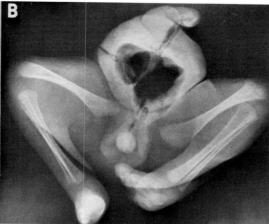

Fig. 13—36 (top).—Parasitic fetus composed of fairly well-developed legs, rudimentary pelvis and one finger attached to epigastrium of an otherwise normal male infant. (From Sarrelangue.)
Fig. 13—37 (bottom).—Parasite successfully detached.

Abdominal cavity of the parasite contains an isolated portion of intestine, urethra, bladder, one kidney with two ureters, seminal vesicles and prostate. **A,** external view. **B,** roentgenogram. (From Sarrelangue.)

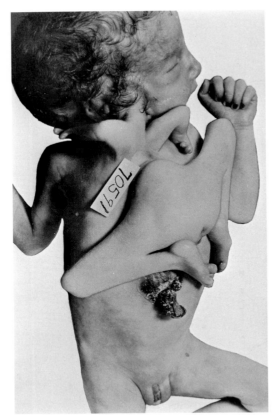

Fig. 13–38.—Parasitic fetus with abnormal arms, pelvis and legs attached to anterior thorax of autosite. (Courtesy Dr. S. A. Goldberg.)

ly well developed it is sometimes designated as "fetus in fetu." They usually show themselves in infancy, although they may not appear until adolescence or adult life. Such enclosed parasites may be found almost anywhere in the abdominal or thoracic cavity, spinal canal or scrotum (see Figs. 12–23 to 12–27). It is probable that the term "fetus in fetu" should be restricted to those growths that show some degree of internal symmetry and craniocaudal differentiation to distinguish them from the more amorphous teratomas that occur in the same areas.

REFERENCES

Aird, I.: Conjoined twins—further observations, Br. Med. J. 1:313, 1959.

Babson, S. C., *et al.*: Growth and development of twins dissimilar at birth, Pediatrics 33:327, 1964.

Benirschke, K.: Twin placenta in perinatal mortality, N. Y. J. Med. 61:1499, 1961.

Benirschke, K., and Driscoll, S.: *The Pathology of the Human Placenta* (Berlin: Springer-Verlag, 1967).

Brennenkmeijer, J. H.: Acardius acormus of het romploose hoofd, Ned. Tijdschr. Geneeskd. 81:4, 256, 1937.

Carr, D. H.: Cytogenetics of Abortion, in Benirschke, K. (ed.): *Comparative Aspects of Reproductive Failure* (New York: Springer Publishing Co., Inc., 1967), p. 96.

Dawson, H.: Pygopagus twins: Report of dissection of thorax, abdomen, and pelvis, Am. J. Dis. Child. 68:395, 1944.

Falkner, F., Banik, W. D. D., and Westland, R.: Intrauterine blood transfer between uniovular twins, Biol. Neonate 4:52, 1962.

Fogel, B. J., Nitowsky, H. M., and Gruenwald, P.: Discordant anomalies in monozygotic twins, J. Pediatr. 66:64, 1965.

Ford, G. E.: Mosaics and chimaeras, Br. Med. Bull. 25:104, 1969.

Gunter, J. U.: Cephalothoracopagus monosymmetries, Am. J. Pathol. 22:855, 1946.

Gutmacher, A. F.: Analysis of 521 cases of twin pregnancy: I. Differences in single and double ovum twinning, Am. J. Obstet. Gynecol. 34:76, 1937.

Guttmacher, A. F., and Kohl, S. G.: The fetuses of multiple gestations, Obstet. Gynecol. 12:528, 1958.

nizable and these masses are more appropriately classified as teratomas.

6. Parasite attached to the back, sacrum or pelvis of the autosite. These rarely contain recognizable parts and are often classified as teratomas (Fig. 13–39).

B. Parasite developed in the autosite, usually in the body cavity but occasionally in other regions. These are usually classified as tumors, although when the parasite is fair-

Fig. 13–39.—Amorphous parasite with single digit attached to back of an otherwise normal infant. (Courtesy Dr. Ralph V. Platou.)

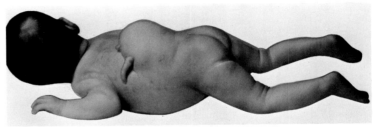

Kindred, J. E.: Twin pregnancies with one twin blighted, Am. J. Obstet. Gynecol. 48:642, 1944.

Komai, T., and Fukuoka, G.: Frequency of multiple births among Japanese and related peoples, Am. J. Phys. Anthropol. 21:433, 1936.

Littlewood, J. M.: Polycythemia and anemia in newborn monozygotic twin girls, Brit. Med. J. 1:857, 1963.

Mortimer, B., and Kirshbaum, J. D.: Human double monster (so-called Siamese twins): Anatomic presentation, Am. J. Dis. Child. 64:697, 1942.

Naeye, R. L.: Human intrauterine parabiotic syndrome and its complications, N. Engl. J. Med. 268:804, 1963.

Naeye, R. L.: Organ abnormalities in a human parabiotic syndrome, Am. J. Pathol. 46:829, 1965.

Napolitani, F. D., and Schreiber, I.: The acardiac monster, Am. J. Obstet. Gynecol. 80:582, 1960.

Newman, H. H.: Differences between conjoined twins in relation to a general theory of twinning, J. Hered. 22:201, 1931.

Newman, H. H.: Methods of diagnosing monozygotic and dizygotic twins, Biol. Bull. 55:288, 1928.

Nylander, P. P. S., and Corney, G.: Placentation and zygosity of twins in Ibadan, Nigeria, Ann. Hum. Genet. 33:31, 1969.

Potter, E. L.: Multiple pregnancies at the Chicago Lying-in Hospital, 1941–47, Am. J. Obstet. Gynecol. 58:139, 1949.

Potter, E. L.: Twin zygosity and placental form in relation to outcome of pregnancy, Am. J. Obstet. Gynecol. 87:566, 1963.

Potter, E. L., and Crunden, A. B.: Twin pregnancies in the service of the Chicago Lying-in Hospital, Am. J. Obstet. Gynecol. 48:870, 1941.

Reisner, S. H., Forbes, A. E., and Cornblath, M.: Smaller of twins and hypoglycemia, Lancet 1:524, 1965.

Rousen, A. R., Seki, M., and Strauss, L.: Twin transfusion syndrome, J. Pediatr. 66:613, 1965.

Sarrelangue, L. P.: Surgical specimen of a partially developed parasitic fetus, Arch. Surg. 52:479, 1946.

Schatz, F.: *Acardei und ihre Verwandten* (Berlin: August Hirschwald, 1898).

Schlumberger, H. G., and Gotwals, J. E.: Ischiopagus tripus: Report of two cases, Arch. Pathol. 39:142, 1945.

Stockard, C. R.: Developmental rate and structural expressivity: Experimental study of twins, double monsters, and single deformities, and interaction between embryonic organs during their origin and development, Am. J. Anat. 28:115, 1921.

Strandskov, H. H.: Plural birth frequencies in the total "white" and "colored" U. S. populations, Am. J. Phys. Anthropol. 3:49, 1945.

Strandskov, H. H., and Edelon, E. W.: Monozygotic and dizygotic birth frequencies in the total "white" and "colored" U. S. populations, Genetics 31:438, 1946.

Szulman, A. E.: Chromosomal aberrations in spontaneous human abortions, N. Engl. J. Med. 272:811, 1965.

Timmons, J. D., and de Alvarez, R. R.: Monoamniotic twin pregnancy, Am. J. Obstet. Gynecol. 86:875, 1963.

Turpin, R., *et al.*: Presomption de monozygotisme en depit d'un dimorphisme sexuel: Sujet masculine ZY and sujet neutre Haplo X, C. R. Acad. Sci. (Paris) 252:2945, 1961.

Wilder, H. H.: Duplicate twins and monsters, Am. J. Anat. 3:387, 1904.

Witschi, E.: Appearance of accessory "organizers" in over-ripe eggs of the frog, Proc. Soc. Exp. Biol. Med. 31:419, 1934.

Wyshak, G., and White, C.: Geneological study of human twinning, Am. J. Public Health 55:1586, 1965.

14

Heart and Blood Vessels

Development

DURING THE 3d week after fertilization the heart begins to develop from paired primordial vessels on the ventral surface of the embryo. These arise lateral to the foregut but gradually move toward the midline and eventually unite to form a single vessel. Fusion proceeds in a cephalocaudad direction and forms in succession the bulbus cordis, ventricle, atrium and sinus venosus. Vessels form simultaneously in other areas throughout the embryo and by the end of the 4th week contraction of the simple tubular heart is moving blood through the primitive circulatory system.

The heart is fixed at both ends but is free to grow in the middle and soon assumes an S-shaped curve, the bulbus cordis forming the upper anterior limb, the ventricle the middle central limb and the atrium and sinus venosus the lower posterior limb. The atrium expands laterally to the right and left and is connected to the ventricle, which lies above and anterior to it, by a constricted area known as the atrioventricular canal. A shift in the axis of the heart soon changes the relative position of the atrium and ventricle and, as in the definitive heart, the atrium comes to lie above and on a slightly more posterior plane than the ventricle.

Division of the heart into right and left halves begins by the more or less simultaneous ingrowth toward the atrioventricular canal of two median ridges, one extending up from the apex of the ventricle and one extending down from the area between the dilated portions of the atrium. At the same time elevations designated atrioventricular cushions appear on the dorsal and ventral walls of the atrioventricular canal and bulge into the lumen until they meet in the midline and grow together, dividing the canal into right and left halves. Shortly before the septum (septum primum) that has been growing down through the atrium toward the atrioventricular canal fuses with the atrioventricular cushions, the anterior-superior portion of the septum resorbs and reestablishes a communication between the atria. A second septum (septum secundum) then arises from the wall of the atrium to the right of the septum primum and grows down also to join the atrioventricular cushions. During growth an opening known as the foramen ovale is left in this septum. The openings in the two septa are at different levels, so that blood coming into the right atrium can push aside the septum secundum and enter the left ventricle obliquely through both openings. When the two membranes are in contact, as they are after birth, they form a complete septum.

The cephalic end of the bulbus cordis is continuous with the system of aortic arches. The central part, known as the truncus arteriosus, is divided into halves by the formation in the wall of two ridges that grow together in the midline and proceed spirally downward in such a way that at the upper margin of the ventricle they are in line with the ventricular septum, to which they immediately fuse. The lower part of the bulbus cordis, known as the conus, is gradually taken up into the wall of the right ventricle. The divided portions of the truncus arteriosus, which become the ascending aorta and main pulmonary artery, are separated from the two ventricles by small buttonlike masses of tissue that grow inward from the walls of these vessels at their junction with the ventricles. These tissue masses become hollowed out and each forms one of the semilunar cusps of the aortic and pulmonary valves.

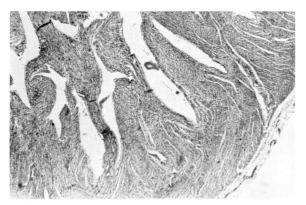

Fig. 14–1.—A cross-section of the left ventricle of a small premature infant reveals deep trabeculation in the ventricular wall. This disappears as the heart grows.

The fusion of the atrial septa with the endocardial cushions of the atrioventricular canal is completed during the 7th week; before the end of the 8th week, when the muscular portion of the ventricular septum meets the endocardial cushions of the atrioventricular canal and the conus ridges, the more complex closure of the interventricular septum is also accomplished.

While these changes are taking place, the sinus venosus shifts out of the midline and opens to the right of the interatrial septum. As the heart grows, the sinus venosus is incorporated into the wall of the right atrium, and the superior and inferior venae cavae and coronary sinus, which have arisen from it, open into the right atrium through individual ostia. The pulmonary veins at first empty through a single vessel into the left atrium, but gradually the terminal portion of this vessel is taken up into the wall of the atrium and the four pulmonary veins enter separately.

The heart assumes its definitive structure by the end of the 8th week, and any abnormality in the relationships of chambers and great vessels must arise before that time. No abnormality, however, is incompatible with intrauterine existence. Since all oxygen is derived from the placenta and none from the lungs, the manner in which blood enters and leaves the heart is of little consequence.

From the beginning of the 3d month until the end of pregnancy the only appreciable changes in the heart are in size and elaboration of muscle pattern. Early in fetal life the inner surfaces of both ventricles show prominent trabeculae (Fig. 14–1). These largely disappear from the left ventricle before birth, giving it the smooth unbroken surface that distinguishes it from the right ventricle. At

term the heart is slightly more elongated and cone-shaped than in the adult, but the general appearance is the same. The right border is made up of the right atrium. The inferior border and most of the anterior surface are made up of the right ventricle, and the left border and a narrow strip of the anterior surface are composed largely of left ventricle. The proximal portion of the common pulmonary artery where it arises from the right ventricle and a small triangular portion of the most proximal part of the aorta are visible from the front when the heart lies in its normal position. The right atrium and the auricular appendage are proportionately large and prominent in the fetus and newborn because of the important role they play in intrauterine circulation. The left atrium and auricular appendage are both small and inconspicuous (see Fig. 6–9).

Circulation of Blood Before Birth

Before birth oxygenated blood from the placenta normally passes through the umbilical vein to the umbilicus and goes to the liver in a continuation of the same vessel (Fig. 14–2). It moves through the

Fig. 14–2.—Fetal circulation.

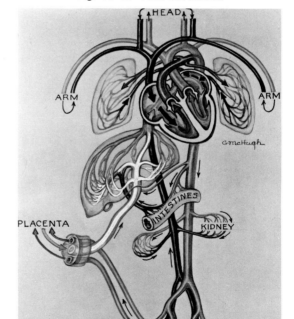

liver in a channel called the ductus venosus, which has been cut through the earlier existing anastomosing sinusoids by the stream of blood from the umbilical vein. As the ductus venosus emerges from the liver it is joined by the hepatic veins, and together they enter the inferior vena cava. Blood entering the right atrium through the inferior vena cava is a mixture of freshly oxygenated blood from the placenta and venous blood from the abdominal organs and lower extremities. It is joined in the right atrium by blood from the superior vena cava. Whether the streams from the inferior and superior venae cavae merge with a resulting intermixture of blood or whether the greater part of the blood from the inferior vena cava is shunted in an isolated stream directly through the foramen ovale into the left atrium is unsettled. Barclay *et al.* demonstrated that in sheep a definite current passes from the inferior vena cava through the foramen ovale, and in a human fetus the condition is probably the same. If this is true, the head and upper extremities receive blood somewhat more highly saturated with oxygen than the rest of the body. At any rate, a large share of the blood entering the right atrium goes through the foramen ovale into the left atrium and from there to the left ventricle and general circulation.

The rest of the blood from the right atrium passes into the right ventricle and out through the pulmonary artery. The pulmonary artery gives off branches to the right and left lungs and continues as the ductus arteriosus, which enters the aorta immediately distal to the origin of the left subclavian artery. It forms a second pathway by which oxygenated blood can be shunted past the lungs directly into the peripheral circulation. Consequently, only part of the blood entering the pulmonary artery goes into the lungs and returns through the pulmonary veins to the left atrium.

The blood in the left atrium comes largely from the right atrium through the foramen ovale and in a lesser amount from the pulmonary veins. It flows through the left ventricle into the ascending aorta and is distributed to the head, neck and arms through branches arising from the arch. Immediately distal to the subclavian artery it is joined by blood coming through the ductus arteriosus from the right ventricle; this mixture enters the descending aorta.

Blood returns to the placenta through the two umbilical arteries, which arise as branches of the right and left internal iliac arteries.

Blood pressure in the umbilical arteries at the time of birth normally averages about 80 mm Hg systolic and 45 mm Hg diastolic. It is usually about 10 mm higher in the first 24 hours, and by 10–14 days after birth the systolic pressure is 90–100 mm Hg.

Closure of the Temporary Fetal Vessels

Six structures present during fetal life disappear after birth. Four of these—the umbilical vein, ductus venosus and the paired umbilical arteries—make possible the flow of blood between the placenta and the fetus during intrauterine life. The other two—the foramen ovale and ductus arteriosus—are designed to adjust the circulation through the right and left sides of the heart before birth and to obviate the unnecessary passage of part of the blood through the lungs.

These six structures become nonfunctioning soon after birth. The umbilical arteries and vein contract, blood is forced out of them and the small lumen remaining after contraction is obliterated by proliferation of the intima. Fibrous cords persist as permanent evidence of the earlier existence of these vessels. The portion of the umbilical vein extending between the umbilicus and the liver becomes the ligamentum venosum. The proximal portions of the umbilical arteries persist as the internal iliac arteries and the more distal obliterated portions become the lateral umbilical ligaments.

Blood passes through the foramen ovale during intrauterine life only because of the greater pressure existing in the right atrium. The foramen ovale, as its name implies, is an oval foramen near the center of the interatrial septum that measures about 8 mm in diameter at term. During intrauterine life blood flows through it freely despite the fact that the curtainlike septum primum hangs down to the left and covers it. The pressure of the blood entering the right atrium from the placenta pushes the septum aside and permits easy passage into the left atrium.

After birth the volume of blood entering the right atrium is proportionately reduced and the pressure is no longer higher on the right side. When the pressure on the two sides is equalized, or is higher in the left atrium than in the right, the septum primum is held in place and covers the foramen ovale in the septum secundum. Blood normally ceases flowing through the foramen ovale as soon as the umbilical cord is cut, and the septa thereafter are in juxtaposition (Fig. 14–3). The two septa become adherent and soon are permanently fused except in a small group of individuals who retain a narrow slitlike opening throughout life.

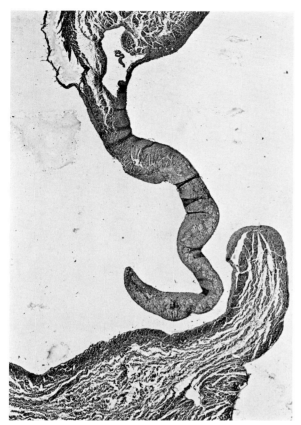

Fig. 14–3.—Foramen ovale from infant 4 days old was functionally closed although anatomically patent.

How the ductus arteriosus closes and when this is normally accomplished are not as well known as the other circulatory changes that take place after birth. Barclay *et al.* stated that the ductus arteriosus of the sheep becomes closed immediately after birth and that circulation through it is discontinued when the umbilical cord is severed. In common with many investigators, they believed the same condition to be true in human beings. Various theories offered to explain the closure of the ductus arteriosus include a change in position of the ductus with the production of a more acute angle between it and the aorta as a result of expansion of the lungs, contraction of muscle cells in the ductus wall either as a primary contraction or secondary to a nervous mechanism, obliteration of the lumen by connective tissue and so on. It has been shown in animals that increases in oxygen tension in the pulmonary artery will lead to contraction of the ductus arteriosus, and anoxic states such as the

respiratory distress syndrome may cause reopening after birth.

At autopsy it is impossible to tell from the appearance of the ductus arteriosus whether an infant was stillborn or lived for several or more hours. Before removal from the body the ductus arteriosus in a mature fetus or an infant 1–2 days old is 8–10 mm long and slightly less in diameter (see Fig. 6–9, C).

When a continuous longitudinal incision is made through the pulmonary artery, ductus arteriosus and descending aorta, the region of the ductus arteriosus is visible grossly as a circumscribed area in which the wall is thinner and more translucent than that of the permanent vessels (Fig. 14–4) and which, when unstretched, often forms fine wrinkles, a condition that is not true of the aorta or pulmonary artery. Microscopic examination reveals definite differences in the walls of the permanent vessels and the wall of the ductus arteriosus. The

Fig. 14–4.—Main pulmonary artery *(a)* gives off branches to right and left lungs and continues as the ductus arteriosus *(between arrows)* and enters aorta immediately distal to arch *(b)*. Note difference in opacity of ductus arteriosus and other vessels. Before removal from the body the ductus arteriosus appeared to be of the same caliber as pulmonary artery and aorta. Infant aged 10 hours.

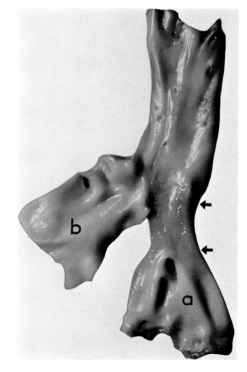

cells of the latter are much less compact and have fewer elastic fibers, slightly more muscle cells and considerably more interstitial fluid. From the appearance it might be assumed that the structure of the tissue is designed primarily to facilitate ready loss of water with condensation of cells and consequent reduction in size and eventual occlusion of the lumen.

A cross-section of the ductus arteriosus from a stillborn infant or one who dies during the 1st or 2d day of life shows a lumen about the size of the aorta and pulmonary artery. The wall is composed of loosely arranged muscle cells and elastic tissue. The internal elastic lamina is a dense compact layer except for occasional areas where slight splitting is associated with beginning intimal proliferation. Proliferation of the intima may begin before birth and resemble that ordinarily found 1–2 days after birth (Fig. 14–5). Any contraction that occurs immediately after birth must be in the nature of a spasm that disappears after death, since it is im-

Fig. 14–5.—Ductus arteriosus from infant aged 10 hours. Slight contraction shown by scalloped margin of internal elastic membrane. The small amount of intimal proliferation visible is often found in stillborn infants. Gram-Weigert stain for elastic tissue.

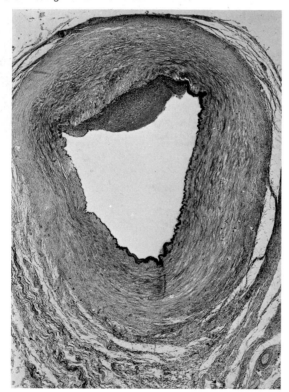

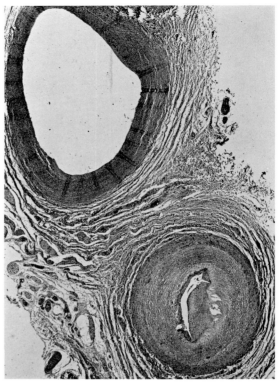

Fig. 14–6.—Ductus arteriosus *(bottom)* and aorta *(top)* from an infant 10 days old weighing 3,670 gm. Principal reduction in caliber of the ductus arteriosus is caused by contraction of the media. Hematoxylin-eosin stain.

possible to differentiate the ductus of an infant several hours or more old, which according to most investigators should have had a period of disuse, from that of a stillborn fetus in which such functional changes could not be expected to have occurred.

In infants who survive for a longer time after birth the ductus arteriosus shows a gradually increasing density of the media caused by contraction of the muscle and elastic fibers and disappearance of the intervening spaces. This is responsible for most of the reduction in the size of the vessel, and only the final obliteration of the already greatly decreased lumen is brought about by intimal proliferation (Fig. 14–6). The changes do not proceed uniformly in all parts of the ductus, and some areas may be completely closed while others retain an appreciable lumen for many weeks. Even if the ductus arteriosus becomes functionally closed immediately after birth because of the cessation of placental circulation and establishment of respiration, as contended by many investigators, the anatomic closure is only gradually brought about by the changes just described, and for at least a week or 10 days a grossly visible opening can be demonstrated in the vessel. For several months a smaller opening may be identified on microscopic examination.

The structure of the other temporary vessels is similar to that of the ductus arteriosus, and obliteration of the lumens proceeds in the same way.

Abnormalities of Cardiac Rate

During intrauterine life the only cardiac abnormalities that can ordinarily be distinguished are those of rate. The normal rate toward the end of pregnancy is 130–140 beats per minute, the belief being common that the rate is slightly higher in female than in male fetuses. The heart rate during uterine contractions often decreases 5–10 beats per minute. This has been attributed to stimulation of the sinoauricular node by overdistention of the right atrium, which may be produced when the contracting uterus forces excess blood into the heart by pressure on the placenta.

A temporary increase in cardiac rate occasionally precedes a reduction. Slowing of the fetal heart rate to fewer than 100 beats per minute, especially if not related to uterine contractions, is always a sign of fetal distress, and if delivery cannot be effected within a few minutes, the heart may stop beating. Death in such circumstances is usually attributed to anoxia, although a specific reason why oxygen failed to reach the fetus may not be demonstrable. Pathologic changes are often inconspicuous in such fetuses, although the viscera may be severely congested and a few scattered ecchymotic hemorrhages may be present on the surface of the heart and lungs.

The rate after birth is generally slightly lower than before birth, in the first few days averaging 125–130 beats per minute, although variations from 90 to 170 have been reported in seemingly normal infants. Occasionally the rate has increased to 200 or more; this increase is designated paroxysmal tachycardia and, if permitted to continue over prolonged periods, may result in heart failure and death. It is rarely associated with any demonstrable anatomic lesion. The cause is unknown but it can usually be relieved by the temporary administration of digitalis.

HEART BLOCK.—A constant fetal heart rate of 80 or less indicates heart block. Since it is possible to make electrocardiograms of the heart while the fetus is still in utero, the diagnosis of heart block can be corroborated by such a procedure. Many infants with congenital heart block die in the first few days or weeks of life, although they may survive to lead normal lives, handicapped very little by the cardiac lesion. It is ordinarily due to absence of the conduction system in the heart and is rarely, if ever, associated with absence of the interventricular septum.

At the Chicago Lying-in Hospital five infants were observed with congenital heart block before birth, of whom three died in the first few days after birth, all with intact interventricular septa. Electrocardiograms taken immediately after birth showed identical patterns in all (Fig. 14–7). The cardiac malformations consisted of cardiac hypertrophy associated with aortic isthmus stenosis in one, fibroelastosis without associated malformations in another and a large, patent interatrial septum defect in the third. The conduction system could not be identified in any of the three hearts.

In infants with major malformations of the interventricular septum evidence of heart block is rare before or after birth. Even when the interventricular septum is grossly underdeveloped or in an abnormal position, the conducting mechanism is almost always present, and differentiation of this tissue proceeds even though in an abnormal location. The bundle of His can normally be identified during the 5th week of intrauterine life and it is not until 10–14 days later that the interventricular wall is normally complete. Consequently the conducting mechanism is adequate even though the interventricular septum is grossly defective. When only a small part of the septum is present, the bundle of His traverses the posterior ventricular wall. In not more than half of the reported cases of congenital heart block have there been septal defects, and in

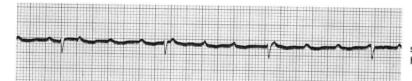

Fig. 14–7.—Electrocardiogram showing complete atrioventricular heart block in newborn infant.

these as well as in those in which the septum has been complete the fundamental defect has been an absent or abnormal conduction system.

Infections and Other Abnormalities of Valves and Muscle

HEMATOMAS OF MITRAL AND TRICUSPID VALVES. — Small, round, slightly elevated blood-filled cysts 1 – 2 mm in diameter are often found near the free margin of the mitral or tricuspid valves (Fig. 14 – 8) or, more rarely, are present as slightly larger pedunculated tumefactions attached to the free margin of a valve. They have been thought by some investigators to be evidence of endocarditis, but they actually have no relation to infection and are found most often in infants who die of anoxia shortly before or after delivery. Clefts in the walls of the valves are normal in intrauterine life, and accumulation of blood within them is responsible for the presence of the tiny blood-filled cysts. Microscopically they can be identified near the surface of the valve as accumulations of blood cells in small cavities lined by a single layer of endothelium (Fig. 14 – 9).

Fig. 14—8. — Blood cysts of tricuspid valve in heart of infant dying of intrauterine anoxia.

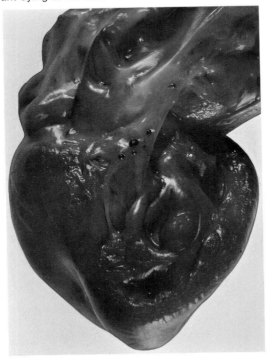

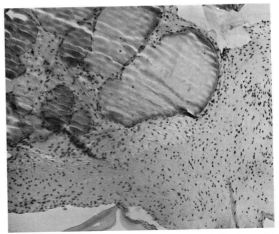

Fig. 14—9. — Microscopic view of blood-filled cavities on atrioventricular valve of a newborn infant.

VALVULAR MYXOMAS. — Several instances of myxomas or fibromyxomas have been described on the aortic or pulmonary valves of newborn infants. These are small lesions producing distortion of the valves, and although occasionally present without other disturbance, they are most often seen in association with fibroelastosis. They probably should not be considered neoplasms but rather as a persistence of tissue normal at an early embryonic stage.

ENDOCARDITIS. — Acute bacterial endocarditis is unusual in infancy and is surprisingly rare in association with congenital heart disease. When it does occur, the mitral valve is most frequently involved, with the tricuspid, aortic and pulmonary valves following in descending order. Emboli occur in about one third of the cases (MacCauley). Murmurs are rarely audible.

Acute verrucous endocarditis is even more rare. Such lesions are chiefly on the septal leaflet of the tricuspid valve with necrosis and fibrin deposition but little evidence of infection. Some have produced emboli.

ENDOCARDIAL FIBROELASTOSIS (ENDOMYOCARDIAL SCLEROSIS AND HYPERTROPHY). — Abnormalities of the heart that can be demonstrated at birth or in the first few months of life consist largely of malformations of the cardiac septa or valves or the great vessels arising from the aortic arch, all of which can be attributed to temporary inhibition of growth at a critical period in embryogenesis. Endocardial fibroelastosis is one of the few conditions that cannot be explained in this manner, although in one third to one half of the infants with this condition cardiac malformations, especially involving aortic and mitral valves, are also present. Most of the associated malformations are such that there is interference with normal movement of blood distal to the area of sclerosis; the right ventricle is affected when the pulmonary valve or artery is abnormal, the left when the aorta is involved. In most instances such malformations are not accompanied by appreciable change in the endocardium of infants who die soon after birth and why it should be severe in a few is unknown. Endocardial fibroelastosis appears to be more common in older infants with cardiac malformation; Andersen and Kelly concluded that it becomes progressive after birth as a result of increased intracardiac pressure and in locations where jets of blood impinge or cause vibration. At the Chicago Lying-in Hospital two infants who died with endocardial sclerosis soon after birth had severe changes in the left ventricle; the first was associated with mild hypoplasia of the aortic arch (Fig. 14–10) and the other with transposition of the great vessels and hypoplasia of the left ventricle (see Fig. 14–23). In Ober and Moore's series of 100 newborn infants with malformed hearts seven had endocardial sclerosis.

When fibroelastosis is not associated with other cardiac malformations, the wall of the ventricle, usually the left, is hypertrophied, and the heart is often two to four times as large as normal. The endocardium is converted into a thick fibroelastic

Fig. 14–10.—Fibroelastosis involving endocardium of left ventricle in a heart with hypoplasia of left heart and aortic outflow tract. Death at 34 hours of age.

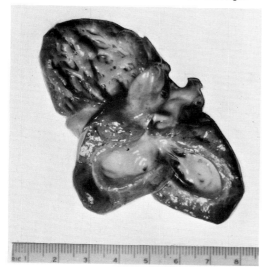

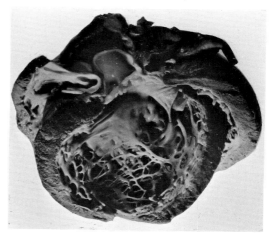

Fig. 14–11.—Endocardial fibroelastosis and verrucous thickening of aortic valve associated with left ventricular hypertrophy. Death at 3 days of age.

coat, the volume of the ventricle may be either increased or reduced and the aortic valves are often thickened and may be covered by hyalinized or myxomatous verrucous overgrowths (Fig. 14–11).

In the series reported by Keith *et al.* 98% of the infants had left ventricular involvement, with associated right ventricular enlargement in 16%. Pure right-sided involvement, although rare, has been observed (Craig). Some infants with this disturbance die soon after birth, but many develop symptoms only when they are a few months of age and do not die until the latter part of the 1st year of life. Keith *et al.* considered it the most common cause of heart failure in infants from 2 months to 1 year of age. In such infants the thickness of the myocardium and the capacity of the left ventricle are both increased (Fig. 14–12).

Kelly and Andersen, in studying their own cases and reviewing the literature, concluded that the condition is familial and suggested that it might be caused by a metabolic defect leading to myocardial weakness with secondary endocardial changes. In their study they eliminated from the group with primary fibroelastosis all infants with changes in cardiac valves. However, so many infants with this condition observed at the Chicago Lying-in Hospital have had nodular enlargement of portions of the valves that it seems questionable whether division into two groups is warranted. It is possible that the extension of the endocardial change to involve the valves indicates greater prenatal severity and is responsible for death at an earlier age.

An intraventricular viral infection has been con-

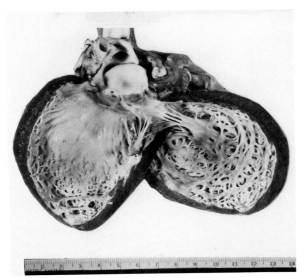

Fig. 14–12.—Fibroelastosis of endocardium of left ventricle without other malformations or abnormalities of the aortic arch. Death at 8 months.

sidered a possible cause by some investigators, but Lee found fibroelastosis in three siblings and considered this to be definite evidence against a viral infection.

Microscopic examination usually reveals a thick pale endocardium composed of an excess of fibrous and elastic tissue, with areas of calcification and irregular connective tissue septa in the muscle. Papillary muscles are often severely affected (Fig. 14–13, A). Irregularly scattered groups of large clear cells somewhat resembling Purkinje cells are often present in the deeper portion of the thickened endocardium (Fig. 14–13, B).

MYOCARDITIS.—In the newborn as well as in older individuals leukocytes may be scattered in small groups throughout the myocardium in hearts that usually are otherwise normal. The cardiac involvement is ordinarily part of a generalized infection, often viral, although it may be found without other evidence of disease.

Coxsackie B infection, especially virus types III and IV, is by far the most common cause (see Fig.

Fig. 14–13.—**A,** severe hyalinization and calcification of papillary muscles with cardiac hypertrophy and diffuse endocardial fibrosis. Associated with Turner's syndrome of ovarian agenesis. Infant aged 7 days. **B,** diffuse endo- cardial fibrosis showing prominent large vacuolated cells in the subendocardium and two masses of cartilage connected by bone in subjacent musculature. Infant aged 3 days.

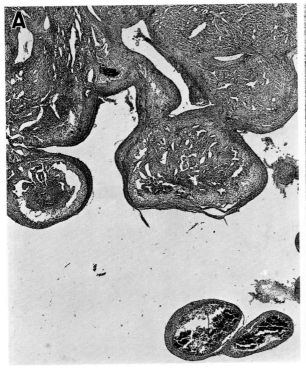
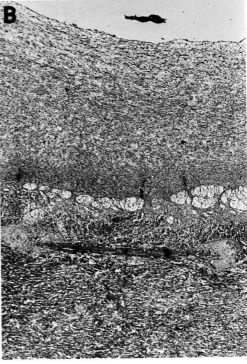

9–13,B). The heart is grossly pale and flabby and, microscopically, there are widespread focal areas of muscle destruction accompanied by infiltration of small mononuclear cells. Because the infants either die during the acute attack or survive without residual damage, only acute changes have been observed.

Cytomegalic inclusion disease may affect the heart and produce focal lesions with mononuclear cell infiltration but without the necrosis of Coxsackie virus myocarditis (Seifert).

Diphtheria, although now rare, injures cardiac muscle and may be a cause of fatal myocardial damage in the 1st year of life. Death comes from heart failure or conduction disturbances. Aside from dilatation and slight pallor of muscle, little is to be seen on gross inspection. Microscopic examination usually shows some pyknosis of nuclei with basophilic degeneration of cytoplasm and loss of cross striations. Appropriate stains often demonstrate large amounts of lipid in the heart muscle.

In congenital toxoplasmosis the heart muscle may have areas of focal inflammation (Fig. 14–14) occasionally accompanied by intracytoplasmic collections of encysted organisms.

MYOCARDIAL INFARCTION.—Gross infarction is occasionally found in the newborn or later in infancy as a result of ischemia or anoxia secondary to calcification or embolism of the coronary arteries— causes similar to those found in adults. MacMahon and Dickinson described a papillary outgrowth of muscle and elastic tissue into the lumens of coronary and renal arteries as a presumably congenital lesion responsible for infarction. In malformed

Fig. 14–14.—Focus of inflammation deep in the myocardium in a case of toxoplasmosis in the newborn.

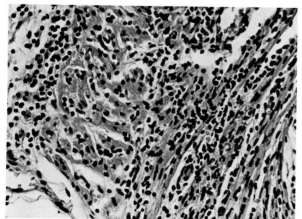

hearts, especially those associated with marked ventricular hypertrophy, Franciosi and Blanc frequently found microscopic or gross infarcts in the subendocardial myocardium and in papillary muscles of the hypertrophied ventricle. The infarcts were present in the left ventricle in aortic stenosis and in the right ventricle in pulmonic stenosis and anomalous pulmonary venous return in all cases when the infant was more than 3 months of age at death. They attributed the location to relative coronary insufficiency associated with increased myocardial mass and thought that at least half might have been diagnosed by electrocardiography.

Abnormalities of Cardiac Size

MODERATE HYPERTROPHY.—Minor changes in cardiac size may be secondary to local or systemic disturbances. At birth the right atrium is normally larger than the left and in many stillborn fetuses is excessively distended because blood from the placenta continues to enter the atrium after the heart begins to fail and can no longer maintain a normal circulation. In the liveborn infant who dies within a few days of birth the atrium is still proportionately large and may be greatly distended. This is especially true in infants with the respiratory distress syndrome.

Hypertrophy of the heart may accompany erythroblastosis. The increase is rarely more than 25% of the average weight, and the size is usually within the range of variability found in hearts believed to be normal; however, at times the enlargement is very marked (Fig. 14–15). This can be explained on the basis of increased cardiac output due to anemia. Tissue anoxia, which may also increase heart size, is also present because in severe erythroblastosis increased size of the villi makes it necessary for oxygen to travel a greater distance from maternal blood to the capillaries in the interior of the villi.

When erythroblastosis is severe before birth and many immature red blood cells are present in the circulating blood, they are often found in excessive numbers in the capillaries of the cardiac muscle (Fig. 14–16).

Moderate cardiomegaly has been observed in infants of diabetic mothers. In rare instances it is severe, but ordinarily it is less pronounced than in erythroblastosis. Infants of diabetic mothers are often unusually large and the heart weight may seem to be increased when compared with that of

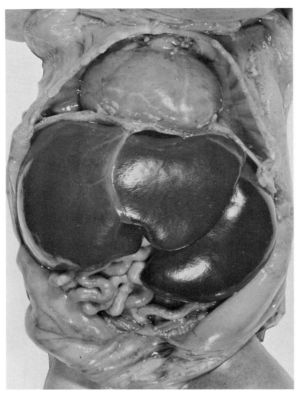

Fig. 14–15. — Marked cardiomegaly occasionally found in association with severe erythroblastosis. Spleen also greatly enlarged.

SEVERE HYPERTROPHY. — The presence at birth of severe symmetrical cardiac hypertrophy has been attributed to intrauterine infections and to other causes that cannot be proved. However, in many instances it remains "idiopathic."

The three specimens observed at the Chicago Lying-in Hospital with the greatest hypertrophy were associated with a remarkable increase in the length and tortuosity of the superficial meningeal vessels (see Fig. 24–3, A). The changes in the vessels may have produced a condition similar to an arteriovenous aneurysm in which the heart hypertrophies because of the extra work required of it. Arteriovenous shunts may have been present in these cases although none were demonstrated. In one case the shape of the heart was normal and only the size was increased. In the others the right atrium was disproportionately large and the heart had a cuboidal blocklike appearance (Fig. 14–17). The weight of each heart was about 70 gm, which is two to three times that of the normal heart of an infant at term. Similar enlargements have been described by others in congenital arteriovenous aneurysms in the brain and in infants with congenital vascular hemangiomas (Cooper and Bolande).

"CARDIAC" TYPE OF GLYCOGEN STORAGE DISEASE,

Fig. 14–16. — Erythroblastosis. Cardiac muscle showing numerous normoblasts in capillaries. Hydropic infant who died 1 hour after birth.

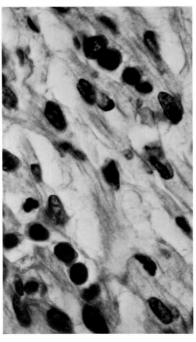

infants of normal birth weight. When compared to the average for infants with the same total weight, the seeming difference often disappears.

The enlargement of the heart of the plethoric twin in the twin transfusion syndrome and of infants with endocardial sclerosis has been noted previously. The familial idiopathic myopathy in which the heart is enlarged as a result of hypertrophy of muscle fibers and diffuse increase in fibrous tissue is usually limited to older children and not seen in the 1st year of life. However, Freundlich *et al.* described a familial myopathy, fatal in the 1st year of life, in siblings whose hearts were enlarged because of an increase in number of myocardial cells.

The heart may be enlarged as a result of malformation although the increase is usually limited to proportionate changes in size of different parts of the heart. With either aortic or pulmonic atresia the corresponding ventricle is ordinarily hypoplastic and the opposite ventricle proportionately hypertrophied.

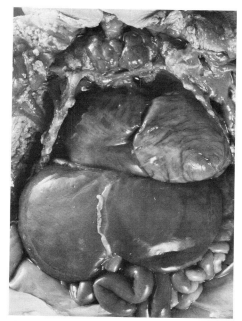

Fig. 14–17.—Severe cardiac hypertrophy associated with angiomatosis of cerebral vessels. Same infant shown in Figure 24–3, A. Weight of heart 75 gm. Death 25 hours after birth.

GLYCOGENOSIS TYPE II (POMPE'S DISEASE).—This disorder, which affects all muscles, is considered at length in Chapter 10. Symptoms begin in the first days or weeks of life with poor feeding, poor weight gain, intermittent cyanosis and dyspnea. Death occurs in a few months from cardiac failure, often precipitated by a febrile illness. At postmortem examination the heart is found to be twice or more the normal size, pale pink and of a globular shape resulting from hypertrophy of ventricular walls and septum. The atrial walls are of normal thickness. The thickened endocardium of the left ventricle may resemble that in endocardial sclerosis. The valves are normal. The muscle fibers are enlarged by deposits of glycogen. With the usual fixation and stains the muscle fibers appear vacuolated and the cytoplasm is reduced to a thin rim at the periphery of each cell. The appearance is the same as in striated muscle (see Fig. 10–3, A). When fixed in alcohol and stained with Best's carmine, the apparently empty spaces are found to be filled with glycogen.

RHABDOMYOMAS.—Single or multiple tumor nodules in the myocardium or projecting into the interior of the heart have been reported, rarely alone (see Fig. 12–36) and more often as part of the syndrome of tuberous sclerosis (see Fig. 12–37). Usu-ally designated rhabdomyomas or hamartomas because of the presence of striated myofibrils, they have sometimes been considered an overgrowth of cardiac muscle showing only mildly abnormal changes and not true neoplasia. Their most characteristic components are large round or oval cells with small central nuclei and a thin peripheral rim of cytoplasm. Connecting the nucleus with the cell wall are delicate radiating strands responsible for the designation "spider cells." Cross-striations can often be detected in these strands and at the periphery of the cells. The intervening vacuoles are filled with glycogen recognizable with appropriate staining (see Fig. 12–39). Such cells are scattered in small groups throughout the musculature as well as in masses in the grossly visible tumors. Consequently some investigators have classified such cardiac involvement under glycogen storage disease instead of rhabdomyomas. Since tuberous sclerosis in association with cardiac rhabdomyomas is a progressive disorder of the brain, the frequency with which it is found rises with the age group investigated. Kidder stated that rhabdomyomas of the heart can be found in 33% of cases of tuberous sclerosis diagnosed at 6 months and 50% at 15 years. Sixty percent of infants with rhabdomyomas die within 1 year, although not necessarily as a result of this particular lesion. The tumors do not often interfere with function of the heart unless they prevent proper closure of the heart valves or encroach on the heart chambers.

OTHER TUMORS.—True myxomas, fibromas, sarcomas, teratomas (Fig. 14–18) and angiomas have all been described in small infants.

Abnormalities of Cardiac Position

The heart is never in an abnormal location except in conjunction with malformations of some adjacent structure. Malformation of the heart itself may be associated with an alteration in shape causing an abnormal contour and exaggeration of the parts to the right or left of the midline, but the central perpendicular axis in such circumstances remains in an approximately normal location.

Ectopic hearts have been classified into cervical, thoracic and abdominal by the region in which the defect is located. According to Logan *et al.*, those in the thoracic region are by far the most common but are less amenable to surgical correction. The most severe disturbances in position are associated with a defect of the sternum and pericardium that permits extrusion of the heart to the exterior of the body. One such infant, observed by Parks and

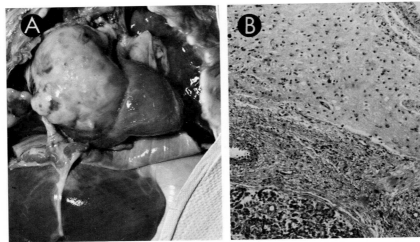

Fig. 14–18.—Teratoma of the right atrium in newborn infant. **A,** gross appearance. **B,** section showing squamous epithelium, neuroglia and glands. (Courtesy Dr. G. Vawter.)

Sweet, survived for 3 weeks despite an associated occipital meningoencephalocele. Gradually progressive epicarditis began a few days after birth and a thick layer of fibrinopurulent exudate covered the heart before death (Fig. 14–19).

Displacement downward through a defect in the diaphragm was described by Blatt and Zeldes as consistent with survival to old age.

The heart is displaced to the opposite side when one leaf of the diaphragm is incompletely developed and the abdominal viscera rise into the chest. At the same time the heart is usually forced anteriorly by herniation of displaced viscera into a saccular area produced between the esophagus and the descending aorta by pressure against this part of the mediastinum. The forward displacement of the heart stretches the aortic arch, which becomes thinned and elongated. The insertion of the ductus arteriosus may be 1 cm or more from the origin of the subclavian artery. Normally the distal margin of the subclavian artery is in an almost direct line with the proximal margin of the ductus arteriosus. This elongation of the distal part of the arch is called the fetal type of aortic coarctation (see Fig. 14–49).

Pleural effusions dating from early intrauterine

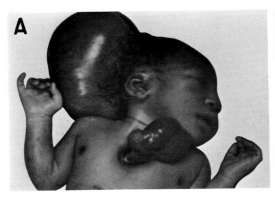

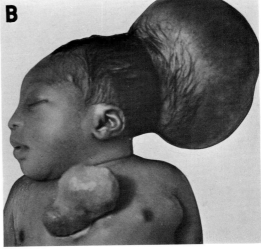

Fig. 14–19.—Ectopia cordis. **A,** infant immediately after birth. **B,** infant aged 14 days with severe epicarditis. (Courtesy Drs. Lewis K. Sweet and John L. Parks.)

life, occasionally associated with erythroblastosis fetalis and at times of unknown origin, push the heart to one side if they are unilateral, or compress it from both sides and give it an unusually vertical position if bilateral. Pneumothorax causes acute displacement of the heart toward the opposite side of the chest, and pneumomediastinum is responsible for anteroposterior compression.

Situs inversus, which is a complete lateral inversion of all viscera, resulting in a mirror image of the usual arrangement, is a rare cause of change in the relative positions of the cardiac chambers and vessels. In complete situs inversus the heart is in a normal location but the apex is pointed to the right instead of the left and the aorta descends to the right. The heart functions normally despite the reversal of its chambers and great vessels. Isolated inversion with the apex of the heart on the right side but with other organs in normal position is more rare; such malformations are often associated with severe intracardiac anomalies, abnormal venous return, abnormal lobation of the lungs and the presence of multiple spleens or splenic agenesis.

Abnormalities of the Pericardium

Abnormalities of the pericardium and pericardial cavity are uncommon except when other malformations affect the mediastinum. The pericardium is seldom either partially or completely absent in otherwise normal individuals. It has not been absent in any cases at the Chicago Lying-in Hospital except in association with defects of the anterior body wall.

Occasionally, purulent or adhesive pericarditis has been observed in very young infants, and in one stillborn fetus at the Chicago Lying-in Hospital early fibrinous pericarditis was associated with fibropurulent pleurisy.

Massive intrapericardial hemorrhage may be present even in stillborn fetuses (see Fig. 8–15). In one such case observed at the Chicago Lying-in Hospital the mother had fallen down stairs 1 week before delivery, after which no evidence of fetal life could be detected. The source of bleeding could not be established.

Hunt described a fetus with severe intrapericardial hemorrhage caused by rupture of the right atrium. The area surrounding the rupture was hyalinized but a cause could not be discovered. McInroy and Graham reported several such cases; rupture was located most often in the region of the juncture of the right atrium and inferior vena cava.

Malformations of the Heart

True malformations of the heart are extremely variable and almost no two malformed hearts are identical. Despite this, malformations do follow general patterns and in most instances a primary abnormality can be identified and distinguished from secondary disturbances produced to bring about necessary adjustments in the circulation. In certain genetic disorders such as the trisomies the type of anomaly to be expected can be predicted fairly accurately.

At postmortem examination it is essential that the external surface of the heart be examined, the various chambers identified and the vessels leaving and entering the heart recognized individually before the heart is taken from the body. If no abnormalities can be detected on external examination, usually the only malformation that will be found in the interior of the heart is a simple intra-auricular or intraventricular septal defect or a persistent atrioventricular ostium. If the viscera are removed in a single block before the great vessels are examined, it becomes more difficult to trace the path of the vessels arising from the aortic arch in the case of cardiac abnormalities being discovered subsequently. Following identification of the aortic arch vessels, removal of all of the thoracic and abdominal viscera en bloc permits an approach to the major vessels from all angles. This approach is especially fruitful if identification is to be made of such abnormalities as anomalous pulmonary drainage, anomalous subclavian vessels and the abnormal vasculature found in some cases of mitral atresia.

Since in many malformations some degree of rotation of the ventricular portion of the heart exists, it is always important to establish whether the ventricular chamber that lies to the right is the right ventricle or a displaced left ventricle. The embryologic left ventricle can best be identified by the presence of a flat smooth outflow tract lying along the interventricular septum; the embryologic right ventricle is identified by the more prominent trabeculae carneae, the papillary muscle arrangement and the presence of a conus or rounded muscular outflow tract.

Abnormal Division of the Truncus Arteriosus

A primary abnormality in the partitioning of the truncus arteriosus is responsible for a large share of the cardiac malformations that are severe enough to cause death in the early days or weeks of life. According to Patten, the partitioning starts between the fourth and sixth aortic arches and progresses through the truncus toward the ventricles. The partition begins as a pair of elevated longitudinal ridges that arise on opposite sides of the wall, grow toward each other and finally meet in the midline to form a complete partition dividing the truncus into equal parts, one of which is the aortic channel leading into the fourth aortic arches and the other the pulmonic channel leading into the sixth aortic arches. The truncus ridges grow spirally toward the ventricle; the position in which they are found at their point of origin is reversed by the time they reach the level of the ventricles. This brings the pulmonary channel into communication with the right ventricle, and the aorta into communication with the left ventricle.

Abnormalities in formation of the aorta and pulmonary artery may result from (1) failure of the truncus ridges to develop, (2) a local defect in the partition, (3) failure of the ridges to pursue a spiral course and (4) deviation from midline division with resultant decrease in the lumen of the pulmonary trunk or the ascending aorta.

Since the principal abnormality in all members of this group is due to the way the pulmonary artery and aorta are formed and united with the ventricles, no other abnormalities are necessarily present. However, since no structure without a function develops properly, in stenosis or atresia of the pulmonary artery or aorta the right or left ventricle, respectively, ordinarily fails to attain a normal size.

The atria of the heart are usually normal, as are the receiving portions of the ventricles, although the same agent causing an abnormality of truncus division may cause other disturbances in development. The truncus septum enters into the formation of the membranous portion of the interventricular septum, which is the last part of the septum to close. If the truncus septum does not form or is in an abnormal location, it cannot participate in the formation of the membranous septum. Consequently, some intercommunication between the ventricles is almost always found in association with any truncus abnormality except complete transposition of a normal-size aorta and pulmonary artery. Here a septal defect may be present or absent.

PERSISTENT TRUNCUS ARTERIOSUS. — Failure of the truncoconial ridges to divide the conus arteriosus into aorta and pulmonary artery gives rise to this anomaly. Collett and Edwards defined the minimal criterion for diagnosis of a truncus as a single arterial trunk arising from the ventricular part of the heart, supplying the coronary, pulmonary and systemic circulations. An interventricular septal defect and an overriding aorta are usually present but are not necessary for the diagnosis. According to these authors the truncus defects are classically divided into four major types and one subtype. In type I, which made up 48% of their cases, the aorta and pulmonary artery form a single trunk from which the pulmonary artery arises as a single branch; in type II (29%) the aorta and pulmonary artery arise as a single trunk, from the posterior aspect of which arise two pulmonary arteries; type III (10%) is the same as type II but with the pulmonary arteries arising laterally; in type IV (13%) the pulmonary artery, sixth aortic arches and ductus are absent and the blood supply to the lungs is by way of the bronchial arteries that originate from the descending aorta; type V, so-called persistent truncus (not included in the percentages above), has a single outflow tract, with the pulmonary trunk and aorta arising from this, the pulmonary artery then branching into the right and left pulmonary arteries rather than a single pulmonary artery arising directly from the aorta as in type I.

As would be expected, a ventricular septal defect, either alone or in combination with an atrioventricularis communis, is the most commonly associated anomaly. The semilunar cusps are often reduced in number, and in a little over half of the cases there are only three cusps in the outflow tract, although two or four cusps may be found. The prognosis is poor for infants with a truncus arteriosus; one quarter die in the first 7 days of life and over 50% within 6 months. Infants with types I and III never reach maturity, presumably because of restricted pulmonary blood flow. Four cases of truncus arteriosus found by Ober and Moore in their series of 100 malformed hearts made up 1.7% of the cases of all types of serious heart disease found in the 1st year of life by Eliot *et al.*

In a "true" truncus arteriosus there is no evidence of any partition dividing the pulmonary artery from the aorta, and the upper part of the ventricular septum is always defective (Fig. 14–20). The common trunk arises equally from both ventricles. The defect of the upper portion of the interventricular septum, which results from the failure of formation of the truncus septum, is an integral part of the malformation. The lower part of the interventricular septum may be present or absent, depending on the degree of secondary involvement of this structure. The orifice of the truncus is ordi-

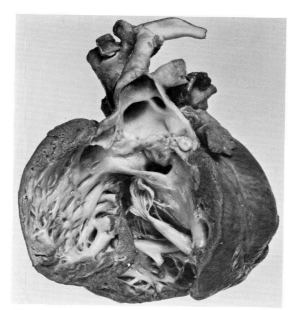

Fig. 14–20.—Truncus arteriosus. Right ventricle is open showing large defect in interventricular septum and aorticopulmonic trunk separated from ventricles by a valve composed of four cusps. Pulmonary portion of the truncus has been opened as far as the origin of the ductus arteriosus. Left pulmonary artery extends to right at base of the ductus; orifice of right pulmonary artery is visible immediately below it in interior of truncus, and the opening into the aorta is visible to the left. Arch of the aorta, ductus arteriosus and portion of the descending aorta are visible but unopened.

narily guarded by four semilunar valves formed from the four primitive endocardial cushions except, rarely, when a secondary malformation reduces the number to two or three. The ductus arteriosus may be present or absent. In its absence the two pulmonary arteries arise separately from the common trunk a short distance above the valves and proximal to the great vessels that are given off to the head and neck. If the ductus is present, the portion of the truncus that should have been separated to form the main pulmonary artery remains in open communication with the aorta, but the ductus arteriosus and the branches of the pulmonary artery to the right and left lungs arise simultaneously and form a continuation of the pulmonic portion. The atrioventricular valves and great veins are normal.

In all varieties of truncus arteriosus the heart at birth is usually of normal size and shape. The degree of cyanosis that develops after birth depends on the amount of blood reaching the lungs. In the types with pulmonary arteries arising directly from the truncus, cyanosis is minimal. When the blood going to the lungs is only the small amount supplied by the bronchial arteries as branches from the aorta, cyanosis is intense. The infant with either variety of defect rarely survives more than a few days, but if it does, the heart rapidly enlarges because both ventricles must work against the combined pulmonary and systemic circulations.

Care must be taken to differentiate these anomalies from those that result from an extreme shift in position of the truncus partition with obliteration of either the aortic or the common pulmonic trunk. Such cases have been designated pseudotruncus arteriosus. Differentiation is usually not difficult. There are ordinarily only three valve leaflets. If the shift of the septum is to the right, the pulmonary arteries receive their blood by reverse flow through the ductus arteriosus, which communicates with the aorta in its usual location distal to the origin of the three arteries to the head and upper extremities. A hypoplastic vessel or a fibrous cord representing the pulmonary artery can usually be made out, although, rarely, no vestige is present. If the shift is to the left, the ascending aorta is either hypoplastic, a fibrous cord or completely absent. In such cases the main pulmonic trunk gives rise to the right and left pulmonary arteries, and the ductus arteriosus connects the main pulmonic trunk with the descending aorta. With complete aortic atresia the innominate, left common carotid and left subclavian arteries seem to arise from a common vessel representing the aortic arch that communicates with the aorta where the latter is joined by the ductus arteriosus (see Fig. 14–27). The ductus can usually be identified by its location and by a textural difference between it and the permanent vessels. These cases are further considered among the aortic and pulmonary stenoses and atresias.

INCOMPLETE OR FENESTRATED TRUNCUS SEPTUM.— This defect is even more rare than complete absence of the septum and its actual existence has been questioned by some authors. A fenestrated septum was not included among the malformed hearts observed at the Chicago Lying-in Hospital. The defect is stated to occur a short distance above the aortic and pulmonic valves and to result from the persistence of a localized area in which the truncus ridges do not come in contact with each other. The symptoms are comparable to those of a widely patent ductus arteriosus. Since pressure is higher in the aorta than in the pulmonary artery, the work of the left ventricle is increased but cyanosis is seldom present. Gibson *et al.* reported three children with such an abnormality whose hearts were investigated surgically because of a mistaken diagnosis of patent ductus arteriosus.

TRANSPOSITION OF GREAT VESSELS. — Complete transposition of the great vessels with or without a ventricular septal defect is one of the most commonly observed complexes in the newborn period (Fig. 14–21). Ober and Moore reported this as the only lesion in 13% of their cases, and in the series of Eliot *et al.* from the 1st year of life the frequency of complete transposition was 9.8%. Eliot *et al.* found males more frequently affected than females, the ratio being 4:1. Because of the high mortality, which is over 50% in the 1st month, the incidence may be artificially reduced in any group that includes only older infants.

If the truncus ridges grow directly down in a straight line instead of pursuing a spiral course, and the development of the rest of the heart follows a normal pattern, the pulmonary artery arises from the left ventricle and the aorta from the right ventricle. Unless a secondary defect of the interventricular septum exists, or unless the ductus arteriosus or foramen ovale remains patent, oxygenated blood cannot reach the peripheral circulation. If the ventricular septum is closed and only the ductus arteriosus remains open, the head and upper extremities receive little if any oxygenated blood. The nonoxygenated blood from the peripheral circulation can reach the lungs only through a ventricular septal defect or by entering the left atrium through the foramen ovale.

Keith *et al.* found that in 60% of hearts with transposition of the main vessels examined at autopsy the ventricular septum was complete and the heart seemed normal except for the exchange of vessels at the ventricular orifices.

If two points of communication exist between the systemic and pulmonary circuits, the circulation may be fairly adequate and is compatible with moderately prolonged survival. If only one point of communication is present, the flow of blood will be in only one direction and must periodically reverse itself to equalize the amount of blood in the general and pulmonary circulations. If the interventricular septal wall is intact and the ductus arteriosus does not remain patent, death occurs soon after birth. The foramen ovale is seldom closed and atrial septal defects are rare. The coronary arteries arise from the aorta but are abnormally distributed.

In a modification of this anomaly the caliber of the pulmonary artery is reduced (Figs. 14–22 and 14–23). The artery is usually only moderately stenosed although occasionally it is completely atretic. Less frequently, the size of the aorta is reduced. In most cases the two ventricles are of approximately the same size at birth, though both soon become hypertrophied. This is usually most

Fig. 14–21.—Transposition of normal-sized aorta and pulmonary artery. **A,** intact interventricular septum. Open chamber can be identified as left ventricle by muscle pattern of septal wall. The vessel arising from the ventricle is the main pulmonary artery, which can be seen communicating directly with the branch to the left lung. Orifice visible in posterior part of lumen is opening of right pulmonary artery. Aortic arch is visible behind pulmonary artery, but ductus arteriosus is hidden by open pulmonary vessel. Infant aged 5 weeks. **B,** interventricular septal defect at base of the transposed aortic valve. Infant aged 12 weeks.

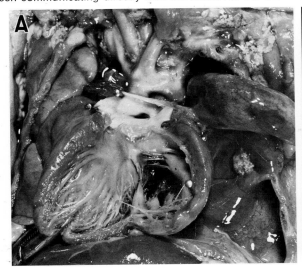
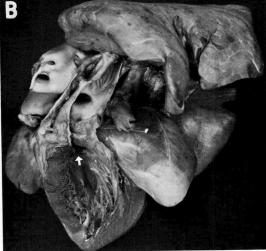

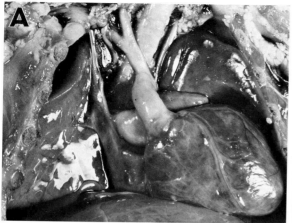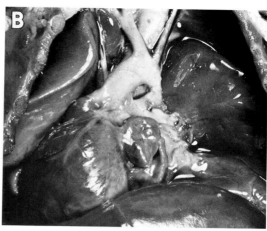

Fig. 14–22.—Transposition of the great vessels with hypoplasia of the pulmonary artery. **A,** heart in normal position showing relation of aorta to right ventricle.

B, heart drawn to the right showing hypoplasia of the pulmonary artery.

Fig. 14–23.—Transposition of the great vessels with reduction in size of the left ventricle, sclerosis of pulmonic valve and endocardium and hypoplasia of pulmonary artery. These three structures and ductus arteriosus have been opened. Aortic arch and descending aorta are unopened. Infant aged 2 days.

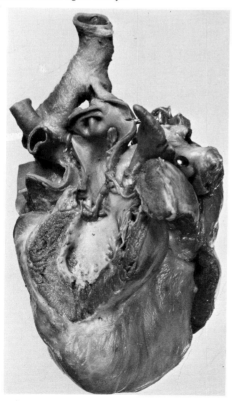

marked in the right ventricle, and the right atrium is both hypertrophied and dilated. On the other hand, if either vessel is hypoplastic, the associated ventricle is also small.

PULMONARY STENOSIS OR ATRESIA.—The extent of deviation of the truncus septum from the midline to the right determines the degree of reduction in size of the main pulmonic trunk. If the reduction is extreme, the artery is atretic and has no lumen (Fig. 14–24); if it is less severe, the vessel is stenosed but some blood is able to pass through it. Other abnormalities are always associated. Either the size of the ventricle is reduced, the upper part of the ventricular septum is defective or both disturbances are present.

If the ventricular septum is intact, the size of the right ventricle is generally greatly reduced because of failure of the bulbus cordis to develop normally, a condition secondary to the abnormal division of the truncus arteriosus. The tricuspid valve is also abnormal and often appears atretic because of the small right ventricle. If the pulmonary artery or tricuspid valve is completely atretic, blood can leave the right side of the heart only through the foramen ovale or a defect in the ventricular septum. Blood can reach the lungs only by reverse flow through the ductus arteriosus from the aorta.

If the ventricular septum is defective, the right ventricle may show any degree of development from almost complete absence to a normal size. The extent of the reduction is often proportionate to the degree of hypoplasia of the pulmonary artery, although this is not always the case and occasionally the ventricular chamber is enlarged and the wall

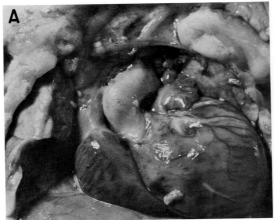

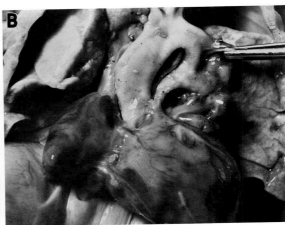

Fig. 14—24.—Atresia of pulmonary artery. **A,** actual position of heart in body, showing aorta arising from left ventricle. Dilated right atrium and proximal portion of superior vena cava are visible on reader's left. **B,** heart drawn down and to right, showing atresia of common pulmonary trunk. The lungs receive blood by reverse flow through the ductus arteriosus. Infant aged 40 hours.

hypertrophied even though the pulmonary artery is severely stenotic.

The size of the pulmonary artery determines the amount of blood going directly from the heart to the lungs. If it is greatly reduced, the lungs must receive an additional supply through the bronchial arteries or the ductus arteriosus; rarely, the ductus arteriosus also fails to develop and all blood must reach the lungs through the bronchial arteries (Fig. 14–25). If the ductus remains patent, cardiac function may be fairly adequate throughout a normal life span; if it closes soon after birth, function may be very inadequate even though bronchial arteries supply some blood to the lungs. Surgical intervention is of most value in patients with a closed ductus arteriosus because it is possible to create an artificial pathway through which the blood may reach the lungs from the aorta. If the ductus arteriosus has remained patent, no surgical treatment will improve the function of the heart.

In pulmonary atresia or hypoplasia the position of the aorta and pulmonary artery is sometimes reversed and the pulmonary artery communicates with or ends blindly in the wall of a hypoplastic left ventricle. Occasionally both vessels arise from a single chamber because of complete absence of the ventricular septum.

Rarely, the pulmonary valve is stenosed in the presence of a pulmonary artery of normal size. This malformation, which is unrelated to division of the truncus, results from abnormal development of the lower portions of the truncus ridges and their failure to differentiate into normal pulmonic cusps. In

one newborn at the Chicago Lying-in Hospital who had atresia of the pulmonic valves as an isolated cardiac malformation (Fig. 14–26) the right atrium was greatly dilated despite apparently adequate patency of the foramen ovale. An operation has

Fig. 14—25.—Extreme hypoplasia of common pulmonic trunk and branches to both lungs. Ductus arteriosus is absent and lungs are supplied almost entirely by blood from hypertrophied bronchial arteries (not visible). Infant aged 2 months.

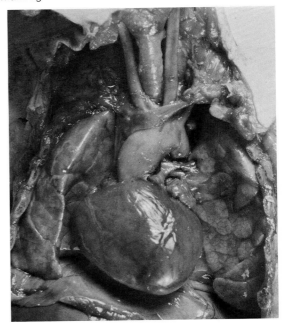

been devised by which the stenotic leaflets can be removed and blood flow through the valve established.

AORTIC STENOSIS OR ATRESIA.—This includes anomalies of the aortic valve and ascending aorta only. The caliber of the ascending aorta is variably reduced and atresia is more common in young infants than is stenosis (Fig. 14–27). According to Keith *et al.,* atresia accounts for 86% of all such anomalies, while in the remainder the valve is usually severely stenotic. With aortic valve atresia, blood reaches the coronary arteries from the ductus arteriosus by way of the aortic arch. The mitral valve is also atretic in about one half of the cases. In the latter situation the left ventricle is isolated and remains only as a slitlike potential chamber in the wall of a greatly hypertrophied and dilated right ventricle. If the mitral valve is patent, the left ventricle is ordinarily small, thick-walled and the site of marked endocardial thickening, collagenization and elastic tissue hyperplasia. The left atrium is usually enlarged and communicates with the right atrium through an open foramen secundum or abnormal ostium. The right ventricle and atrium are enlarged. Because of the circuitous route of blood flow to the coronary arteries myocardial infarction and calcification are not uncommon. Dyspnea, tachypnea and cyanosis develop soon after birth, and death usually occurs within 2

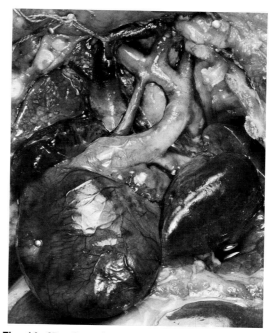

Fig. 14–27.—Complete atresia of aortic valve with marked hypoplasia of ascending aorta. Blood reaches coronary arteries and upper extremities from the ductus arteriosus by reverse flow through the aortic arch. As viewed here, the large vessel arising from the right ventricle is the common pulmonic trunk; it gives off branches to right (not visible) and left lungs and continues as the ductus arteriosus. The ascending aorta arises behind the common pulmonic trunk and joins the arch proximal to the innominate artery. Blood from the ductus arteriosus divides, part going to the descending aorta and part to the aortic arch. Ventricular septum is absent and both atria communicate with a common ventricle. Infant aged 26 hours.

weeks. Because of this high early death rate such hearts are rarely encountered after the newborn period.

ABNORMAL DEVELOPMENT OF THE INTERVENTRICULAR SEPTUM

Final closure of the ventricular septum is brought about when the endocardial cushions of the atrioventricular canal and the conus ridges meet the connective tissue crest of the muscular portion of the ventricular septum in the 15–17 mm embryo early in the 8th week of development. This final growth produces the membranous portion of the septum, which is the space that lies immediately below the aortic valve in the outlet portion of the left ventricle and behind the tricuspid valve in the inlet portion of the right ventricle. If growth of any

Fig. 14–26.—Complete stenosis of pulmonic valve with decrease in size of cavity of right ventricle but with normal lumen in pulmonary artery above valve. Infant aged 12 hours.

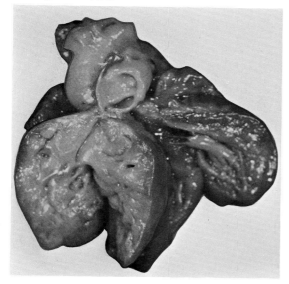

of the three structures normally bringing about the final closure is delayed, a communication between the inlet chamber of the right ventricle and the outlet chamber of the left ventricle results.

Although most interventricular septal defects are found in the fibrous septum immediately beneath the aortic valve (undefended space), especially when they are associated with other cardiac abnormalities, they may occur in any part of the septum. In Ober and Moore's series of 100 autopsies on newborn infants with cardiac anomalies a ventricular septal defect was present in 19 and was the sole cardiac defect in 10. Eliot encountered such isolated defects twice as often in the 1st year of life as at all other ages, and Keith *et al.* reported that they constitute 22% of congenital cardiac abnormalities. They are most common in infants under 1 year of age. Often, only mild physiologic disturbances are produced, and a large proportion of these infants survive the newborn period.

The size of the opening in the interventricular septum varies considerably. In small defects the upper part of the membranous septum is present and the abnormality involves only the lower part of the membranous septum and the upper part of the muscular septum. Since the defect is small and the part of the septum immediately beneath the aortic valve is present, the aortic orifice is held in its normal position and does not override the interventricular septum (Fig. 14–28). When no other abnormalities are present, this defect produces a harsh systolic murmur over the left fourth intercostal space but causes no clinical symptoms. It is known as the *maladie de Roger*.

Large defects involving the upper part of the membranous septum are always associated with some dextroposition of the aorta, so that the aorta overrides the septum. Such a condition is known as the *Eisenmenger complex* (Fig. 14–29). After birth, because the pressure is higher in the left ventricle and the aorta than in the right ventricle and pulmonary artery, blood is shunted from the left to the right ventricle through the septal defect, thus increasing the flow of blood through the lungs. Eventually, the increased flow causes pulmonary vascular sclerosis, which is responsible for increased resistance in the pulmonary circuit and for cyanosis; because this ordinarily does not occur until after the 1st year of life, the condition is not often recognized in the newborn period. However, if the septal defect is very large, heart failure may cause death in the 1st year.

Defects low in the interventricular septum are less common and, according to Keith *et al.*, make up only about 12% of total interventricular septal defects. At times a thin rim of cardiac muscle separates the defect from the membranous septum, or the defect may be far down in the septum, its contours suggesting a failure of fusion of the anlage growing in from the sides of the ventricle (Fig. 14–30). In a few cases defects low in the muscular septum have been known to close spontaneously.

TETRALOGY OF FALLOT.— The four elements of this malformation are a high interventricular septal

Fig. 14–28.—Interventricular septal defect (maladie de Roger). Two hearts with similar defects of lower part of membranous portion of interventricular septum. The aortic valve and aorta have been opened. Except for septal defects the hearts are normal. Infants aged 2 and 4 months.

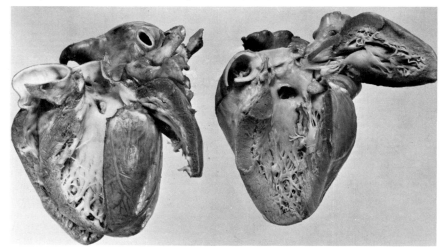

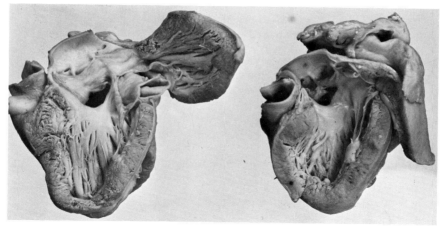

Fig. 14–29.—Interventricular septal defect (Eisenmenger complex). Two hearts each with complete absence of membranous portion of interventricular septum. The aortae show moderate dextroposition and override the edges of the septal defects so that blood from both right and left ventricles enters the aortae. Both infants aged 1 month.

defect, dextroposition of the aorta so that it overrides the septum, an obstruction to the outflow tract of the right ventricle and hypertrophy of the right ventricle. The obstruction, most commonly observed in the infundibular portion of the pulmonic outflow, was present there with tetralogy in 70% of the series of both Keith *et al.* and Eliot *et al.* It

Fig. 14–30.—Defect in lower part of interventricular septum. Infant aged 18 days.

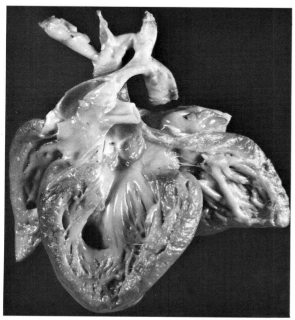

may be combined with valvular stenosis or atresia, or these anomalies may be found without infundibular involvement. The ventricular defect is usually large and always high. The crista supraventricularis is prominent. The direction of the vascular shunt and its magnitude depend on the degree of stenosis of the pulmonary outflow tract; the greater the degree of stenosis, the greater the volume of the right-to-left shunt. If the pulmonary outflow tract is atretic, the complex is sometimes termed pseudotruncus arteriosus. Cyanosis and dyspnea caused by marked right-to-left shunt and underperfusion of the lungs usually appear by 6 months of age. While Ober and Moore found that only 4% of infants with congenital heart disease who died in the 1st week of life had tetralogy of Fallot, according to Keith *et al.* and Eliot *et al.* it is the second most common diagnosis in infants with cardiac disease in the 1st year of life.

ABSENCE OF VENTRICULAR SEPTUM.—The ventricular septum is never entirely absent in a heart with otherwise normal ventricular development. Complete absence is invariably associated with such an arrest of cardiac development that only a rudimentary outlet chamber lies in the region normally occupied by the pulmonary conus of the right ventricle. This is separated from the inflow chamber—the main ventricle—by a muscular ridge, the crista terminalis. A free communication exists between the large inlet chamber, which receives blood from both atria, and the rudimentary outflow chamber, which gives rise to one or both great vessels. Ordinarily the pulmonary artery arises from the rudimentary chamber representing the conus of the right ventricle, and the aorta from the common ventricle (Fig. 14–31). However, they may be transposed (Fig. 14–32), or both may arise from the small outflow portion of the heart. Whichever vessel arises from the rudimentary chamber is usually stenosed and permits less outflow of blood than the one arising from the common ventricle. The blood in the two parts of the ventricle is completely intermixed arterial and venous blood from the two atria. If the hypoplastic vessel from the outlet chamber is the pulmonary artery, only a small amount of blood goes to the lungs and cyanosis is severe because of the small percentage of blood that is oxygenated. If the pulmonary artery arises from the main ventricle, a proportionately large amount of blood is oxygenated and cyanosis is generally absent, but the total volume of blood reaching the general circulation through the hypoplastic aorta is greatly reduced. The prognosis is

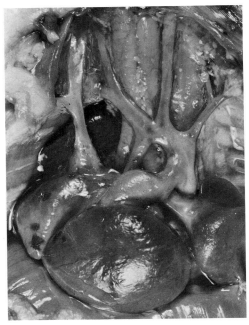

Fig. 14–32.—Common ventricle with hypoplastic aorta arising from rudimentary outflow chamber. The two atria and mitral and tricuspid valves are normal. Associated bilateral renal agenesis. Intrapartum death.

Fig. 14–31.—Common ventricle with hypoplastic pulmonary artery arising from rudimentary outflow chamber. Pulmonary artery ends in a vessel supplying the right lung. Left lung receives its blood supply directly from the aorta via a vessel that represents both ductus arteriosus and left pulmonary artery. The four vessels arising from the arch are the innominate, left common carotid, left subclavian and left vertebral arteries. Associated eventration of abdominal viscera. Respiration never established:

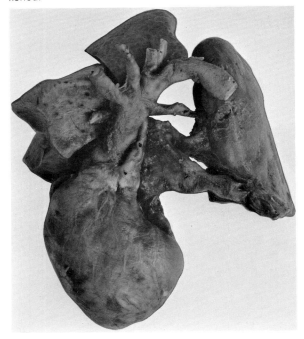

somewhat better with this type of disturbance than when the pulmonary artery is the smaller of the two vessels. With the former a child may survive for several years, whereas the latter usually results in death within a few months of birth. However, with either type the infant may die within the first few days.

Hearts with absence of the ventricular septum are sometimes designated *cor triloculare biatriatum* if the atrial septum is intact, or *cor biloculare* if the atrial septum is also absent. These are inadequate terms inasmuch as they give no indication of the state of the vessels arising from the ventricle.

Abnormal Development of the Interatrial Septum

Defects of the Septum Primum.—The septum primum arises from the upper posterior portion of the wall of the primitive atrium and grows down and forward through the center of the atrium to divide it into right and left halves by fusing with the endocardial cushions of the atrioventricular canal. The opening that exists temporarily between the septum primum and the endocardial cushions before closure is complete is called the ostium pri-

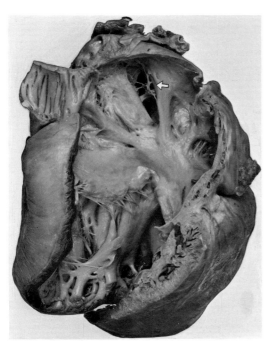

Fig. 14–33.—Defect of septum primum. Membranous covering of foramen ovale is incomplete because of fenestration of septum primum. Interventricular septum (not visible in specimen) is also defective. Infant aged 4 weeks.

mum. Shortly before this ostium closes, the upper part of the septum primum degenerates and produces a new opening between the atria. Approximately two thirds of the lower posterior portion of the septum remains intact. This becomes the membrane covering the foramen ovale when the latter develops in the septum secundum.

Defects of the septum primum consist of resorption of too much of the membrane or resorption of small secondary areas in addition to the normal one. Resorption of too great a portion, which leaves the membrane inadequate to cover the foramen ovale, is responsible for the postnatal persistence of a communication between the atria. Resorption of secondary areas causes fenestration of the membrane (Fig. 14–33), which also permits passage of blood from one side to the other if pressures in the atria are not equal. When pressure is too high in the right atrium, cyanosis results from flow of non-oxygenated blood into the general circulation.

If the rest of the heart develops normally, failure of the septum primum to fuse with the endocardial cushions of the atrioventricular canal is responsible only for an interatrial opening, the lower border of which lies at the level of the attachment of the

cusps of the atrioventricular valve. This is known as a persistent ostium primum.

DEFECTS OF THE SEPTUM SECUNDUM.—About the time that the upper part of the septum primum begins to be resorbed, a second septum starts developing in the upper anterior portion of the atrial wall immediately to the right of the first septum. This grows downward and posteriorly but during its development leaves a foramen in its wall, the foramen ovale.

During intrauterine life blood entering the right atrium passes through the foramen ovale by pushing aside the curtain formed by the septum primum. After birth, when the pressure on the left side rises, the curtain is held against the foramen ovale and the foramen functionally closes almost immediately. The septum primum gradually fuses with the margin of the foramen ovale and permanent closure results. In a small number of normal individuals fusion is never complete, but as long as the septum primum is large enough to cover it completely, patency has no clinical significance. If the opening in the foramen ovale is so large that the septum primum is unable to cover it, the functional effect is the same as if the septum primum were too small or fenestrated.

At times, in association with other malformations of the heart, the atria show little division into two chambers. The septum primum becomes largely resorbed and the septum secundum forms only a narrow rim around the periphery of the atrial wall. Such an ostium secundum always has a rim of tissue separating it from the atrioventricular ring. An

Fig. 14–34.—Lutembacher syndrome showing enlargement of foramen ovale. Pulmonary artery, right atrium and ventricle were enlarged and dilated, mitral valve was slightly stenotic. Death at 6 months from bronchopneumonia and cardiac insufficiency.

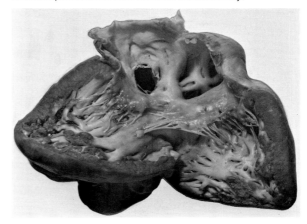

ostium secundum is more than 10 times as frequent as an ostium primum.

Any kind of septal defect that permits free communication between the atria assumes considerable importance whenever there is a significant difference in pressure on the two sides. Congenital or acquired mitral stenosis and dilatation of the pulmonary artery are sometimes associated with intra-atrial septal defects; this combination is called the Lutembacher syndrome (Fig. 14–34). The enlargement of the pulmonary artery distinguishes this condition from other atrial septal defects.

ABNORMAL DEVELOPMENT OF THE ENDOCARDIAL CUSHIONS

COMMON ATRIOVENTRICULAR CANAL. — Under normal conditions the endocardial cushions arise from the ventral and dorsal surfaces of the atrioventricular canal and grow toward each other, fusing in the midline to divide the canal into right and left channels. The interatrial septum becomes attached to the upper margin of the fused cushions, thereby closing the ostium primum, which is temporarily present in the lower part of the interatrial wall. The lower edge of the fused cushions becomes attached to the upper edge of the interventricular septum and completes the interventricular wall except for the membranous part of the septum. The leaflets of the mitral and tricuspid valves arise as ingrowths of a primitive type of connective tissue from the endocardial cushions and the outer parts of the walls of the right and left channels.

If the endocardial cushions fail to appear or do not fuse in the midline, the ventricular and atrial septa have no place to which they can attach and a common opening persists in the center of the heart that permits an intermixture of blood from all four chambers. The atrioventricular ostium thus produced is bounded above by the lower margin of the interatrial septum and below by the upper margin of the interventricular septum (Fig. 14–35). The portions of the mitral and tricuspid valves that arise from cushions formed in the outer wall of the canal are present and the opening is surrounded by five valve leaflets. Their attachments are often abnormal and they may form a continuous sheet extending through the ostium. The central portion of the sheet may be free or may be attached to the upper margin of the ventricular septum. About one fifth of such infants have associated cardiac anomalies, the most common being a patent foramen ovale (as distinct from the defect in the lower atrial septum).

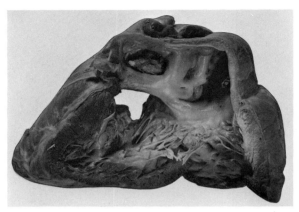

Fig. 14–35.—Persistent atrioventricular canal (atrioventricularis communis). Interatrial septum secundum is complete and the lower portion of the ventricular septum is present, but the margins of the septum primum and the interventricular septum have failed to fuse. The mitral and tricuspid valves are confluent and all four chambers are in communication. Mongolian idiot aged 15 days.

Despite the possibility of free communication in the heart the currents of blood in the two sides remain fairly separate and the heart functions better than would be expected. Cyanosis is uncommon because if there is a shift of blood flow in either direction, it is usually from left to right and at the atrial level. Comparatively little shunting occurs at the ventricular level because the ventricular septum is often nearly complete or because the valve cusps and trabeculae during systole form an effective barrier between the ventricles.

For some unexplained reason this defect is not often found except in mongolian idiots and has been called the Mongol defect. Among more than 10,000 autopsies on infants under 1 year of age at the Chicago Lying-in Hospital it was found exclusively in infants with mongolian idiocy and was present in almost all infants with mongolism. Not all investigators have observed such a constant relationship; the majority of mongoloids with this defect die in the 1st year of life. Consequently such a high incidence is to be expected only among those dying at a very early age. In Wakai and Edward's collected series of hearts with a common atrioventricular canal all but two of 17 under 1 year of age were mongoloids; of those over 1 year only two of seven were mongoloids. Rogers and Edwards and Keith *et al.* reported the incidence of mongolism as about 30%. Ober and Moore had five cases of atrioventricular communis in their series of 100 malformed hearts from newborn autopsies.

ATRESIA OF THE TRICUSPID VALVE. — This anomaly,

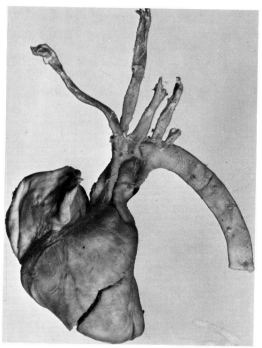

Fig. 14—36.—Mitral stenosis with hypoplasia of the left ventricle and hypertrophy and dilatation of the right ventricle and atrium. Arising from the arch are right common carotid, left external carotid, left internal carotid, left vertebral and left subclavian arteries. Infant aged 8 days.

early embryonic life effectively closes the communication between the left atrium and left ventricle. The mitral valve is represented only by a dimple of fibroelastic tissue, seen best from the left atrium. The left atrium enlarges and the septum secundum is often herniated into the right atrium, allowing passage of blood through the foramen ovale from left to right. One half of the hearts with mitral atresia have an intact interventricular septum, an isolated minute left ventricle and an atretic aortic valve. One third of the cases have an interventricular septal defect leading to a small rudimentary aortic outflow tract and a small aortic valve. The remaining one sixth have an intact interventricular septum with transposition of the aorta to the enlarged right ventricle. Mitral atresia occurs only about one third as often as tricuspid atresia. Most affected infants die in the first weeks of life with dyspnea as a prominent symptom.

STENOSIS OF MITRAL OR TRICUSPID VALVES. — As isolated lesions these are rare in the newborn period. Most often they are combined with severe stenosis or atresia of the outflow tract of the left or right ventricle, in which case the associated ventricle is reduced in size (Fig. 14–36).

HYPOPLASTIC LEFT HEART SYNDROME. — This is a combination of lesions usually causing death soon

caused by fusion of the endocardial cushions in the right heart, is always characterized by an enlarged hypertrophied right atrium, an atrial septal defect and an enlarged mitral orifice. Since the latter must carry all the blood returning both from the lungs and the peripheral circulation, the left heart is always dilated and hypertrophied. The condition of the right ventricle and its outflow tract varies and there may be (1) an intact ventricular septum with a minute isolated right ventricle and pulmonary atresia, (2) a ventricular septal defect leading from the pulmonary conus to the left ventricle and accompanied by pulmonary stenosis and (3) a single ventricle (the left) with transposition to it of a variably stenotic pulmonary artery. The most common form of tricuspid atresia is the second, in which there is an interventricular septal defect with a muscular narrowing of the pulmonary outflow tract but with the pulmonary artery in normal position. The duration of life is limited and many affected infants die in the first 3 months of life; 65% die in the 1st year.

ATRESIA OF THE MITRAL VALVE. — In this condition fusion of the atrioventricular valve cushions during

Fig. 14—37.—Hypoplastic left heart syndrome in which severe mitral stenosis is associated with hypoplasia of left ventricle, aortic stenosis and hypoplasia of the aortic arch (fetal coarctation). The superior vena cava is double with the left vena cava opening into the coronary sinus.

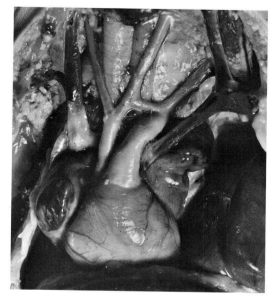

after birth. In its most distinctive form it consists of severe stenosis or atresia of the mitral valve. Because the flow of blood into the left ventricle is restricted, the left ventricle, aortic valve and aortic arch all fail to develop normally and are reduced in size. There is usually an atrial septal defect but no functional ventricular defect. From before birth the ductus arteriosus carries blood to the peripheral circulation. The aorta beyond the entrance of the ductus is of normal size, thus giving the hypoplastic arch the appearance of fetal coarctation (Fig. 14–37). (This is an integral part of this syndrome.) The restricted flow to the systemic circulation after birth results in low blood pressure and inadequate perfusion of the viscera.

ANOMALOUS ENTRANCE OF VEINS INTO THE HEART

LEFT SUPERIOR VENA CAVA. — In the young embryo the anterior and posterior cardinal veins draining the anterior and posterior parts of the body unite to form two common cardinal veins, one on each side. These empty into the sinus venosus, which communicates with the atrial portion of the heart. The sinus venosus gradually shifts out of its midline position to open into the right side of the heart. A short distance above the point at which the two cardinal veins empty into the sinus venosus, the innominate vein appears, which permits the blood from the left anterior cardinal vein to empty into the sinus venosus by way of the derivative of the terminal portion of the right anterior cardinal vein, the superior vena cava. The portion of the left common cardinal vein adjacent to the sinus venosus persists as the coronary sinus. The part between the origin of the innominate vein and the coronary sinus normally disappears.

If the innominate vein does not develop or does not attain a normal size, the portion of the left cardinal vein between the coronary sinus and the place at which the innominate vein should arise persists as a left superior vena cava (see Fig. 14–37). If the innominate vein does develop but is inade-

Fig. 14–38.—Anomalous venous drainage viewed from the front but with the heart displaced upward to show the right common pulmonary vein (*Right C.P.V.*) crossing the left behind the heart, where it joins the left pulmonary veins (*Left P. Veins*) and ascends to enter the left innominate vein. The left lung has three lobes, the right lung two lobes. The superior vena cava (*Sup. V.C.*) lies hidden by the aorta and pulmonary artery. All of the pulmonary venous drainage as well as that from the right subclavian and jugular vein is into this vessel. (From Darling, R. C., et al., Lab. Invest. 6:44, 1957).

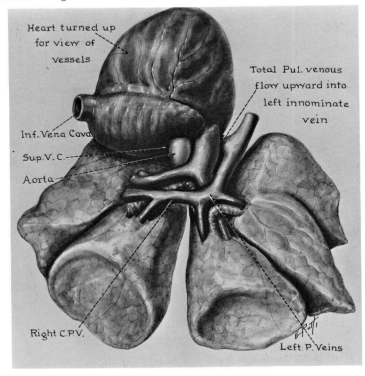

quate to carry all the blood from the left side, the left vena cava will be smaller than the right. If the heart is otherwise normal, the presence of a left superior vena cava does not interfere with function since all venous blood enters the right atrium despite the anomaly.

In the rare instances in which the left vena cava and coronary sinus open into the left atrium immediately to the left of the atrial wall moderate cyanosis results from the entrance into the left atrium of venous blood from the left side of the head and left arm.

ANOMALOUS PULMONARY VENOUS DRAINAGE. — The pulmonary veins develop as a plexus of small channels, which in the early stages of development communicate freely with the primitive cardinal

Fig. 14–39. — Anomalous venous drainage of the lungs. Pulmonary veins unite to form single vessel that passes through the diaphragm to join the portal vein. (From Darling, R. C., et al., Lab. Invest. 6:44, 1957).

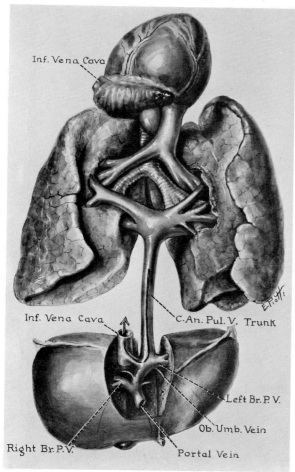

veins. As certain of these channels enlarge to form the vessels leading from the lungs to the left atrium, the communications are normally lost, but in rare instances they persist and part of the pulmonary veins empty into some vessel arising from the anterior cardinal veins. Since parts of the walls of these channels are taken up into the wall of the atrium, the pulmonary veins may enter directly into the right atrium. In the series described by Keith *et al.* of malformed hearts with anomalous pulmonary venous drainage 55% of the anomalous vessels entered above the level of the right atrium, i.e., into the superior vena cava (Fig. 14–38). In 30% they entered directly into the right atrium, in the remainder below the atrium into the portal vein (Fig. 14–39) or inferior vena cava. In a few cases the pulmonary veins communicate with both right and left atria. Discovery of drainage into the inferior vena cava is greatly aided by use of the Rokitansky method of removing the viscera, and unless the heart is carefully inspected to ensure that all vascular connections to the lungs are intact, these lesions will often be missed. The ease with which the heart may be swung anteriorly at autopsy may give a hint of the presence of the anomaly because the left atrium is not bound down to the posterior mediastinum by the pulmonary veins. Death comes early in infants with such defects; 70% of the series of Keith *et al.* died within 6 months of pulmonary congestion and hypertension. A longer life depends on establishment of an adequate communication between pulmonary venous drainage and left atrium.

ABNORMALITIES OF VESSELS DERIVED FROM THE AORTIC ARCHES

In earliest embryonic life the principal blood vessels consist of paired longitudinal dorsal and ventral arteries known as the dorsal and ventral aortae. The two ventral aortae fuse at one point to form the heart, and the two dorsal ones fuse to become the descending aorta. Anterior to these areas of fusion a series of vessels connecting the ventral and dorsal aortae, known as aortic arches, develops on each side of the body. Although six pairs develop, the first two disappear as functional vessels before the others are entirely formed. The fifth arches never become more than rudimentary structures, and only the third, fourth and sixth normally contribute to the formation of the definitive aortic arch and the vessels arising from it (Fig. 14–40).

The ascending aorta is derived from the truncus arteriosus as a result of the division of that struc-

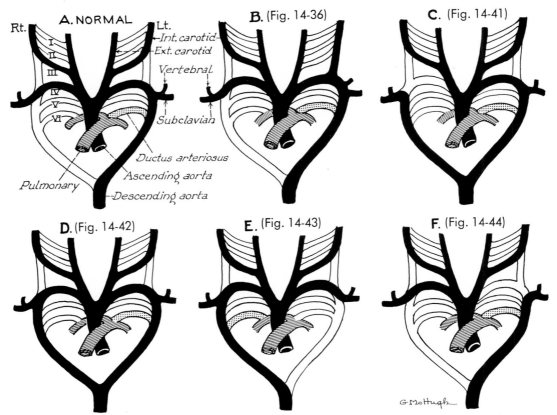

Fig. 14—40.—Diagrams showing relation of ventral and dorsal aortae and aortic arches to abnormalities of aorta and vessels to the head and upper extremities. Figure numbers refer to photographs of hearts illustrating the various anomalies. Portions that normally persist as definitive aortic vessels are black, pulmonary artery and its branches are cross-lined, ductus arteriosus stippled. **A,** schematic arrangement of ventral and dorsal aortae and six aortic arches. **B,** five vessels arising from aortic arch: innominate, external carotid, internal carotid, vertebral and subclavian arteries. **C,** right subclavian artery arises from aortic arch distal to left subclavian artery. **D,** double aortic arch with left ductus arteriosus. **E,** right aortic arch with right ductus arteriosus. **F,** absence of part of aortic arch with left subclavian artery and descending aorta receiving blood only through ductus arteriosus.

ture into the aorta and pulmonary artery. The arch of the aorta is made up of a small part of the unfused ventral aortae, the left fourth aortic arch and the portion of the left dorsal aorta extending between the origins of the fourth and sixth arches. The descending aorta arises from the fused dorsal aortae.

In the formation of the vessels that supply the head and upper extremities, the first, second and fifth arches disappear on both sides and the major part of the sixth arch disappears on the right side and persists on the left as the ductus arteriosus and the proximal part of the branch of the pulmonary artery supplying the left lung. The third arch on each side contributes to the formation of the internal carotid arteries. The fourth arch on the right becomes part of the right subclavian artery, and the arch on the left becomes part of the aortic arch. The left subclavian artery arises from the left dorsal aorta at the same level as the left fourth aortic arch.

The portions of the dorsal aortae between the origins of the third and fourth arches disappear on both sides as does the right dorsal aorta between the origin of the subclavian artery and the point at which it fuses with the left dorsal aorta to form the single trunk constituting the descending aorta.

INCREASE IN NUMBER OF VESSELS ARISING FROM THE ARCH.—The persistence or disappearance of small individual segments of the ventral and dorsal aortae and the differences in the fate of the various aortic arches make possible many divergences from the usual manner of development. Part of these have no functional significance, consisting only of variations in the way the great vessels arise directly from the arch, but not uncommonly four vessels arise from it instead of three. The fourth vessel is most often the right subclavian artery, but it may also be the right external carotid, the left internal carotid or the left vertebral artery. When the right subclavian artery arises directly from the arch, it usually comes off distal to the origin of the left subclavian artery (Fig. 14–41). It ordinarily passes behind the esophagus to reach the right side and may produce symptoms of esophageal constriction similar to those noted with persistence of both right and left aortic arches. The vertebral artery is normally a branch of the left subclavian artery, but its origin from the arch is one of the most common causes of the presence of a fourth vessel. Rarely, five or more vessels arise directly from the arch (see Fig. 14–36). At times the innominate and left common carotid arteries arise from a single trunk called the brachiocephalic artery. In this case only two vessels appear to arise from the arch—the brachiocephalic and the left subclavian.

DOUBLE AORTIC ARCH.—Severe disturbances result from persistence of the right as well as the left fourth aortic arch with the formation of a double aortic root. When both right and left arches are present, the aorta appears to divide into two large trunks near the beginning of the transverse part of the arch, and a ring of vascular tissue encircles the esophagus and trachea (Fig. 14–42). The posterior portion, which comes from the right arch, is most often the larger of the two and has the appearance of being the true arch. It gives rise to the right common carotid and subclavian arteries, while the left common carotid and subclavian arteries arise either as a single trunk or as separate vessels from the smaller anterior portion that comes from the left arch. The descending aorta is ordinarily derived from the left dorsal aorta, but since with a double aortic arch the larger branch is usually the right arch, the greater part of the blood flow to the descending aorta passes behind the esophagus. Symptoms associated with a complete aortic ring are those of tracheal compression and are aggravated during feeding. The differential diagnosis must include all conditions giving rise to chronic respiratory tract disturbances. The characteristic syndrome consists of stridorous breathing, dysphagia, chronic cough and malnutrition. Symptoms, though usually mild or absent immediately after birth, are progressive and ordinarily cause death in less than 6 months.

RIGHT AORTIC ARCH.—Persistence of the right instead of the left fourth aortic arch is rare except with some malformation of the heart, especially tetralogy of Fallot. As an isolated lesion it causes no appreciable cardiac embarrassment. It arches over the right instead of the left bronchus and gives rise successively to the left innominate, right common carotid and right subclavian arteries (Fig. 14–

Fig. 14–41 (left).—Right subclavian artery arising from arch distal to left subclavian artery. It passes behind the trachea and esophagus and is responsible for tracheal compression.

Fig. 14–42 (right).—Double aortic arch. **A,** posterior view showing two portions of the arch encircling the esophagus and trachea and uniting to form the descending aorta. **B,** anterior view showing vessels arising from the arch. (Courtesy Dr. Herman Sikl.)

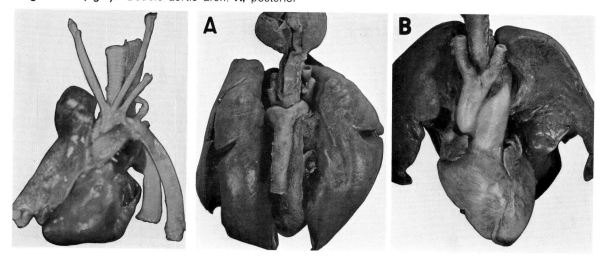

43). The right instead of the left sixth aortic arch persists to form the ductus arteriosus and consequently maintains a normal relationship to the other vessels.

STENOSIS OR ATRESIA OF THE AORTIC ARCH. — Much more serious is a localized atresia or stenosis caused by complete disappearance or reduction in caliber of portions of the arch. Any part of the aortic arch may become obliterated. The Chicago Lying-in Hospital series of autopsies included examples of (1) absence of the left ventral aorta between the fourth and sixth aortic arches, (2) bilateral absence of the fourth aortic arch and (3) absence of the dorsal aorta between the origins of the left subclavian artery and the left sixth aortic arch. In the first of these the ascending aorta terminates in the innominate artery; the left common carotid and left subclavian arteries receive blood from the ductus arteriosus by reverse flow through the distal portion of the arch. In the second the innominate and carotid arteries are supplied through the ascending aorta, while the subclavian artery and descending aorta receive blood through the ductus arteriosus (Fig. 14–44). In the third example all vessels normally arising from the arch receive arterial blood from the aorta but the descending aorta is a continuation of the pulmonary artery through the ductus arteriosus. This malformation is usually associated with other cardiac defects, especially with defects of the ventricular septum. Death usually occurs at an early age with symptoms similar to those of other severe obstructions to outflow from

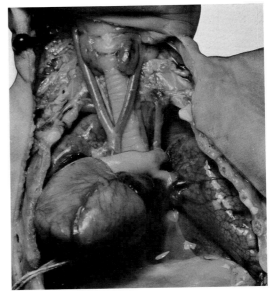

Fig. 14–44.—Absence of portion of the aortic arch between the common carotid and subclavian arteries. Ascending aorta terminates in innominate and common carotid arteries. Descending aorta is continuation of the ductus arteriosus. Left subclavian artery arises at junction of ductus arteriosus and descending aorta. Infant aged 42 hours.

the aorta, e.g., aortic valve atresia, preductal coarctation and mitral atresia.

PATENT DUCTUS ARTERIOSUS. — Functional closure of the ductus has been shown to occur quite promptly after birth under normal circumstances. From animal studies and observations in man at high altitudes and in respiratory distress it has been ascertained that contraction and closure of the ductus arteriosus ordinarily result from increase in oxygen tension in the pulmonary artery. The ductus will usually be closed anatomically by the 3d week after birth, and failure to close by 3 months indicates the probability of permanent patency. The usual patent ductus arteriosus has a lumen of such size that a pressure gradient exists between the systemic and pulmonary circuits, with a left-to-right shunt but with normal pressures in each circuit. Those patients in whom a widely patent ductus arteriosus produces a larger area of communication may develop heart failure in early infancy or, rarely, in the newborn period because of the increase in cardiac output required by the large arteriovenous shunt. Keith *et al.* suggested that in some infants under 1 month of age with cyanosis and respiratory distress a persistence of the pulmonary vascular resistance, which is normal in

Fig. 14–43.—Right aortic arch and descending aorta associated with a normal heart.

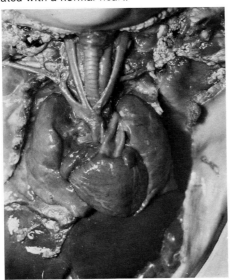

embryonic life, and a widely patent ductus may cause right ventricular hypertrophy and an increasing right-to-left shunt. This was confirmed by Kitterman *et al.* in infants weighing less than 1,750 gm at birth.

The only etiologic agent that has ever been specifically related to persistence of the ductus arteriosus is maternal rubella contracted during the 1st trimester of pregnancy. This was the most common anomaly found by the early Australian investigators as a complication of maternal rubella (Fig. 14–45), and this frequency has been confirmed by the more recent figures of Rowe *et al.* How an influence acting so early in fetal life can inhibit the closure of the ductus arteriosus many months later is unknown.

Malformation of the ductus arteriosus.—Abnormalities of the sixth aortic arch are uncommon and there are few reports of an anomalous origin or insertion of the ductus arteriosus. Such abnormalities are ordinarily found only in conjunction with other malformations of the heart. In one instance in the series at the Chicago Lying-in Hospital the ductus was a continuation of the main pulmonary artery but did not communicate with the aortic arch. It was several centimeters long and gave off small branches to the left side of the neck (Fig. 14–46). The vessels arising from the arch were also anomalous in their points of origin. In two cases the duc-

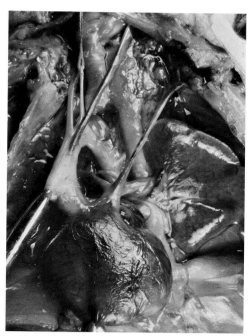

Fig. 14–46.—Ductus arteriosus ending in vessel supplying cervical muscles instead of terminating in aorta. Conus of right ventricle was hypoplastic and interventricular septum defective. Fetus stillborn at term.

Fig. 14–45.—Patent ductus arteriosus in child aged 3 years and 9 months whose mother had rubella during 2d month of pregnancy. Sudden death at beginning of anesthesia for surgical ligation of the ductus. Child was also a deaf-mute. (Courtesy Dr. Mary Heseltine.)

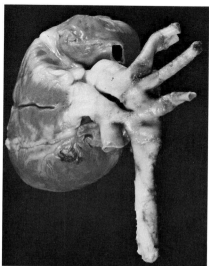

tus arteriosus was absent; in one the pulmonary arteries and arch of the aorta were otherwise normal. In another the pulmonary artery was severely stenosed.

Aneurysm of ductus arteriosus.—Such enlargement of this vessel is rare but has been observed and described as the site of thrombi that may lead to embolism and infarction of structures supplied by the aorta. Cruickshank and Marquis reviewed 60 cases, of which 51 were infants. Death was due to rupture of the aneurysm in five and thromboembolism in three. In some cases a localized disruption of the internal elastic membrane can be demonstrated (Ithuralde *et al.*).

COARCTATION OF THE AORTA.—Unusual narrowing of the distal portion of the aortic arch or upper part of the descending aorta is usually designated coarctation. A distinction is made between fetal and adult varieties because, although sometimes similar, they are usually of different etiology and may be quite different in appearance.

In the newborn infant the ascending aorta, arch, descending aorta, main pulmonary artery and ductus arteriosus are normally of about equal caliber, and the ductus arteriosus enters the aorta immedi-

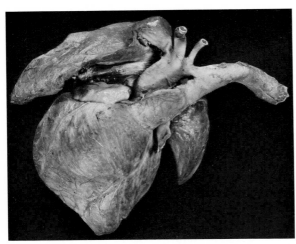

Fig. 14—47.—Coarctation of aortic arch immediately distal to origin of subclavian artery and proximal to insertion of ductus arteriosus. Associated hydrocephalus and spina bifida but no other cardiac abnormalities. Infant aged 1 hour.

ately distal to the origin of the left subclavian artery; thus, the distal margin of the subclavian artery and the proximal margin of the ductus arteriosus are in a nearly straight line.

Adult type.—This ordinarily involves the aorta immediately proximal or distal to the point where the ductus arteriosus normally enters (Fig. 14—47). It consists of an annular constriction that varies in degree, so that the aortic lumen may be only slightly affected or it may be so greatly reduced that the blood supply to the lower part of the body must be obtained entirely by means of collateral circulation. A possible etiology lies in the difference in composition of the wall of the ductus and of the permanent blood vessels. If the tissue of which the ductus arteriosus is composed extends beyond the normal limits and makes up a localized portion of the arch, this tissue can be expected to respond to the influences that cause closure of the ductus and to undergo the same cicatrizing process. This idea, first proposed by Skoda, is known as the skodaic theory. For a number of reasons, particularly because of the common association of coarctation with other congenital heart le-

Fig. 14—48 (left).—Narrowing and elongation of portion of aortic arch between origin of common carotid and subclavian arteries. Associated interventricular septal defect and rider aorta. Infant aged 36 days.
Fig. 14—49 (right).—Fetal coarctation consisting of narrowing and elongation of third part of aortic arch between origin of subclavian artery and insertion of ductus arteriosus. Associated defect of interventricular septum. Infant aged 4 days.

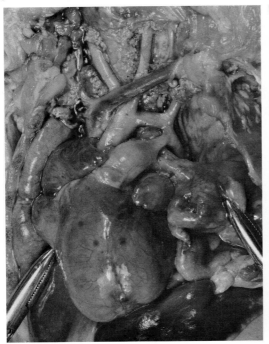

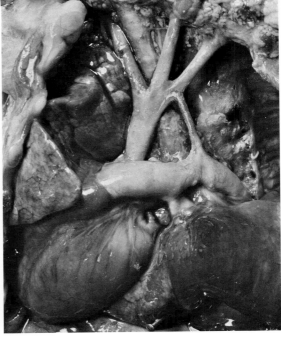

sions, Edwards considered it untenable. He found bicuspid aortic valves in over 50% of the hearts with the adult type of coarctation.

Fetal type. — In the fetal, or preductal, type of coarctation some portion of the arch is abnormally narrowed and elongated. The part involved may be between the origin of the innominate and left common carotid arteries, between the left common carotid and subclavian arteries (Fig. 14–48) or, as is most common, between the subclavian artery and insertion of the ductus arteriosus (Fig. 14–49). According to Mustard *et al.*, fetal coarctation causes death in the 1st year of life in 60% of infants so diagnosed. The adult or postductal type is recognized clinically in this age group only half as often as the fetal type.

The ductus arteriosus usually remains patent in infants with preductal coarctation and, according to Keith *et al.*, has been patent in 94% of cases. Over 80% of infants with preductal coarctation who die in the 1st year of life succumb in the first 5 weeks. The lower the defect in the arch, the more frequently it is associated with serious cardiac malformations such as transposition and ventricular septal defects. In Ober and Moore's series of 100 malformed hearts 11% had coarctations, all preductal.

ABNORMALITIES OF CORONARY ARTERIES

ANOMALOUS ORIGIN. — The anomalous origin of the right coronary artery from the pulmonary artery gives rise to no symptoms. The origin of the left coronary artery from the pulmonary artery causes cardiac hypertrophy, dilatation and electrocardiographic signs of coronary thrombosis. Symptoms are usually absent during the first few weeks after birth, not appearing for 2–3 months. Death from heart failure follows in a few weeks, the majority of infants dying in the 3rd and 4th months of life. The left ventricle is usually enlarged and its myocardium is thicker than that of the right ventricle. Both myocardium and endocardium are hyalinized and fibrotic, with myocardial changes most striking near the apex. The low pressure in the pulmonary artery with consequent low pressure in the left coronary artery is believed to be a more important cause of myocardial damage than the fact that the myocardium is supplied by venous blood. In some cases an arteriovenous shunt may be established between the high pressure branches of the right coronary and the low pressure system of the left coronary artery.

DEGENERATIVE CHANGES. — Calcification of the coronary arteries as an isolated lesion or associated

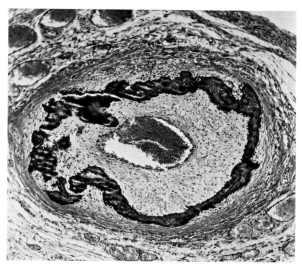

Fig. 14–50. — Coronary artery showing calcification and proliferation of the intima. Associated with endocardial sclerosis. Infant aged 3 months.

with similar changes in other parts of the body has been reported in stillborn fetuses and in infants a few days or a few months old. The cause is unknown, but the most probable explanation is an embryonically defective elastic tissue that makes the vessel unusually susceptible to any noxious agent. Deposits of calcium appear first on the surface of the internal elastic membrane adjacent to the media and spread to involve varying portions of the media (Fig. 14–50). The internal elastic membrane may remain intact or be more or less completely destroyed. Myocardial infarction, endocardial sclerosis and calcification may follow ischemia induced by narrowing of the lumens. Complete occlusion of a lumen can be responsible for sudden death.

Gruenwald reported finding isolated degenerative changes in the media of the smaller radicles of the coronary arteries in 21 infants who were stillborn or died in the first 3 days of life. Evidence of anoxia in the form of epicardial and pleural hemorrhages and excessive amniotic debris in the lungs was almost universally present.

ABNORMALITIES OF PERIPHERAL BLOOD VESSELS

Occasional reports of disturbances in the structure of blood vessels in different parts of the body are to be found in the literature. Most of these have appeared as curiosities and a cause has rarely been demonstrated. Such changes have included intimal proliferation and occlusion of small intrapulmonary arteries and widespread involvement of systemic arteries. Thromboses of the aorta and the vena cava, both with and without other vascular changes, have been observed. One infant delivered at the Chicago Lying-in Hospital, who died at 2 months with congenital heart block, had widespread endarteritis of peripheral vessels associated with aseptic necrosis of the skin (see Fig. 27–21).

PERIARTERITIS NODOSA. — According to Fetterman and Roberts, a fairly large number of cases of periarteritis nodosa have been reported in infancy. The muscle of the coronary vessels as well as the renal, cerebral, pancreatic and splenic arterial walls are infiltrated with polymorphonuclear leukocytes. The lumen of the vessels are irregularly dilated, the walls often necrotic and the site of thrombi. The myocardium is infarcted in one third of the cases, with kidney, spleen and limbs less often affected.

REFERENCES

Adams, F. H., Moss, A. J., and Emmanouilides, G. C.: Absence of Ductus Arteriosus and Foramen Ovale, in Cassels, D. F. (ed.): *Heart Disease and Circulation in Newborn and Infant* (New York: Grune and Stratton, 1966).

Andersen, D. H., and Kelly, J.: Congenital endocardial fibroelastosis: I. Endofibroelastosis associated with congenital malformations of the heart, Pediatrics 18:513, 1956.

Auld, P. M.: Delayed closure of the ductus arteriosus, J. Pediatr. 69:61, 1966.

Barclay, A. E., Franklin, K. J., and Pritchard, M. M. L.: *The Foetal Circulation and Cardiovascular System, and the Changes That They Undergo at Birth* (Oxford: Blackwell Scientific Publications, Ltd., 1944).

Batchelor, T. M., and Maun, M. E.: Congenital glycogenetic tumors of the heart, Arch. Pathol. 39:67, 1945.

Black-Schaffer, B.: Infantile endocardial elastosis, Arch. Pathol. 63:281, 1957.

Blake, H. A., Hall, R. J., and Manion, W. C.: Anomalous pulmonary venous return, Circulation 32:406, 1965.

Blatt, M., and Zeldes, M.: Ectopia cordis: Report of a case and review of the literature, Am. J. Dis. Child. 63:515, 1942.

Bleeden, L. C., Morehead, R. R., Burke, B., and Kaplan, E. L.: Bacterial endocarditis in the neonate, Am. J. Dis. Child. 124:747, 1972.

Bolande, R. P., and Tucker, A. S.: Pulmonary emphysema and other cardiorespiratory lesions as part of the Marfans abiotrophy, Pediatrics 33:356, 1964.

Calodney, M. M., and Carson, M. J.: Coarctation of the aorta in early infancy, J. Pediatr. 37:46, 1950.

Campbell, P. E.: Vascular abnormalities following maternal rubella, Br. Heart J. 27:134, 1965.

Collett, R. W., and Edwards, J. E.: Persistent truncus arteriosus; a classification, Surg. Clin. North Am. 29:1245, 1949.

Cooper, A. G., and Bolande, R. P.: Multiple hemangiomas in an infant with cardiac hypertrophy, Pediatrics 35:27, 1965.

Craig, J. M.: Congenital endocardial sclerosis, J. Tech. Methods 30:15, 1949.

Cruickshank, B., and Marquis, R. M.: Spontaneous aneurysm of the ductus arteriosus; a review and report of the tenth adult case, Am. J. Med. 25:140, 1958.

Darling, R. C., Rothney, W. B., and Craig, J. M.: Total pulmonary venous drainage into the right side of the heart, Lab. Invest. 6:44, 1957.

Edwards, J. E.: Congenital Malformations of Heart and Great Vessels, in Gould, S. E. (ed.): *Pathology of the Heart and Blood Vessels* (3d ed.; Springfield, Ill.: Charles C Thomas, 1968).

Eliot, R. S., et al.: Heart Disease in the First Year of Life, in Cassels, D. F. (ed.): *Heart Disease and Circulation in Newborn and Infant* (New York: Grune and Stratton, 1966).

Eliot, R. S., et al.: Mitral atresia: A study of 32 cases, Am. Heart J. 70:6, 1965.

Farber, S.: Congenital rhabdomyoma of the heart, Am. J. Pathol. 7:105, 1931.

Fetterman, G. H., and Roberts, F. B.: Periarteritis nodosa in infancy, J. Pediatr. 63:519, 1963.

Franciosi, R. A., and Blanc, W. A.: Myocardial infarcts in infants and children, J. Pediatr. 73:309, 1968.

Freundlich, C., et al.: Primary myocardial disease in infancy, Am. J. Cardiol. 32:721, 1964.

Gibson, S., Potts, W. J., and Langewisch, W. H.: Aortic-pulmonary communication due to localized congenital defect of the aortic septum, Pediatrics 6:357, 1950.

Gresham, G. A.: Premature obliteration of the foramen ovale, Br. Heart J. 18:296, 1956.

Gross, R. E.: Arterial embolism and thrombosis in infancy, Am. J. Dis. Child. 70:61, 1945.

Gruenwald, P.: Necrosis in coronary arteries of newborn infants, Am. Heart J. 38:889, 1949.

Hunt, W. E.: Spontaneous rupture of the heart in newborn infant, Arch. Dis. Child. 27:291, 1941.

Ithuralde, M., et al.: Dissecting aneurysm of the ductus arteriosus in the newborn infant, Am. J. Dis. Child. 122:165, 1971.

Keith, J. D., Rowe, R. D., and Vlad, P.: *Heart Disease in Infancy and Childhood* (2d ed.; New York: Macmillan Co., 1967).

Kelly, J., and Andersen, D. H.: Congenital endocardial elastosis. II. Clinical and pathological investigations of those cases without associated cardiac malformations including report of two familial instances, Pediatrics 18:539, 1956.

Kidder, L. A.: Congenital glycogenetic tumors of the heart, Arch. Pathol. 49:55, 1950.

Kirklin, J. W., and Clagett, O. T.: Vascular "rings" producing respiratory obstruction in infants, Mayo Clin. Proc. 25:360, 1950.

Kitterman, J. A., Edmunds, H. E., Jr., Gregory, G. A., Heyman, M. A., Tooley, W. H., and Rudolph, A. M.: Patent ductus arteriosus in premature infants, N. Engl. J. Med. 287:473, 1972.

Kleinerman, J., et al.: Absence of the transverse aortic arch, Arch. Pathol. 65:490, 1958.

Kunstadter, R. H., and Kaltenekker, F.: Acute verrucous endocarditis in the newborn, J. Pediatr. 61:58, 1961.

Lee, M. H.: Familial occurrence of endocardial fibroelastosis in three siblings, including identical twins, Pediatrics 52:402, 1973.

Lev, M., et al.: Premature narrowing or closure of the foramen ovale, Am. Heart J. 65:638, 1963.

Levinson, S. A., and Learner, A.: Blood cysts on the heart valves of newborn infants, Arch. Pathol. 14:810, 1932.

Logan, W. D., Jr., et al.: Ectopis cordis: Report of a case and discussion of surgical management, Surgery 57:898, 1965.

Macauley, P.: Acute endocarditis in infancy and early childhood, Am. J. Dis. Child. 88:715, 1954.

MacMahon, H. E., and Dickinson, P. C. T.: Occlusive fibroelastosis of coronary arteries in the newborn, Circulation 35:3, 1967.

McInroy, R. A., and Graham, A. L. M.: Rupture of the fetal heart during labor, Arch. Dis. Child. 30:119, 1961.

Monro-Faure, H.: Necrotizing arteritis of the coronary arteries in infancy, Pediatrics 23:914, 1959.

Mustard, W. T., et al.: Coarctation of the aorta with special reference to the first year of life, Ann. Surg. 14:429, 1955.

Ober, W. B., and Moore, T. E.: Congenital cardiac malformation in neonatal period, N. Engl. J. Med. 253:271, 1966.

Patten, B. M.: Developmental defects at the foramen ovale, Am. J. Pathol. 14:135, 1938.

Patten, B. M.: Human Embryology (3d ed.; New York: McGraw-Hill Book Co., 1968).

Rogers, H. M., and Edwards, J. E.: Incomplete division of the atrioventricular canal with patent inter-atrial foramen primum (persistent common atrioventricular ostium). Report of five cases and review of the literature, Am. Heart J. 38:28, 1948.

Ronka, E. K. F., and Tessmer, C. F.: Congenital absence of the pericardium, Am. J. Pathol. 20:137, 1944.

Rosahn, P. D.: Endocardial fibroelastosis: Old and new concepts, Bull. N. Y. Acad. Med. 31:453, 1955.

Rowe, R. B., et al.: Cardiovascular disease in rubella syndrome in heart and circulation, in Cassels, D. E. (ed.): Heart Disease and Circulation in Newborn and Infant (New York: Grune and Stratton, 1966), p. 181.

Rudolf, A. M., et al.: Patent ductus arteriosus, a clinical and hemodynamic study of 23 patients in the first year of life, Pediatrics 22:892, 1958.

Seifert, G.: Myocarditis due to cytomegaly virus, Dtsch. Med. Wochenschr. 90:149, 1965.

Stryker, W. A.: Arterial calcification in infancy with special reference to coronary arteries, Am. J. Pathol. 22:1007, 1946.

Taussig, H. B.: Congenital Malformations of the Heart (New York: Commonwealth Fund, 1947).

Wakai, C. S., and Edwards, J. E.: Pathologic study of persistent common atrioventricular canal, Am. Heart J. 56:779, 1958.

Weinberg, T., and Himmelfarb, A. J.: Endocardial fibroelastosis (so-called fetal endocarditis). Two cases in siblings, Bull. Johns Hopkins Hosp. 72:299, 1943.

Wolman, M.: Hypertrophy of branches of the pulmonary artery and its possible relationship with so-called primary pulmonary arteriosclerosis in two infants with hypertrophy of the heart, Am. J. Med. Sci. 222:133, 1950.

15

Lungs and Trachea

Development

THE PULMONARY SYSTEM begins its development as
a local expansion in the upper anterior part of the
entodermal tube. A longitudinal constriction pinch-
es off the anterior part of the expanded area and
produces a short cylindrical appendage that retains

a communication with the entodermal tube only in
its uppermost part. This appendage branches dichotomously: the left branch gives rise to two divisions,
the right to three. Further branching is less regular,
and peripheral growth proceeds throughout intrauterine life.

The first outgrowth from the entodermal tube

Fig. 15–1.—Fetal lung. **A,** branches of pulmonary tree
uniformly lined by tall columnar cells and widely separated
by primitive mesenchyme. Weight 5 gm, length 5.8 cm,
gestational age about 10 weeks. **B,** branches of pulmonary tree still lined by columnar cells but bronchi can be

differentiated from more distal portions. Condensation of
mesenchyme around groups of branches gives a lobular
appearance. Weight 98 gm, length 17 cm, gestational age
about 14 weeks.

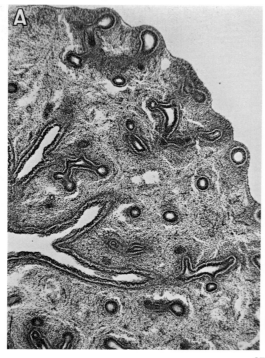
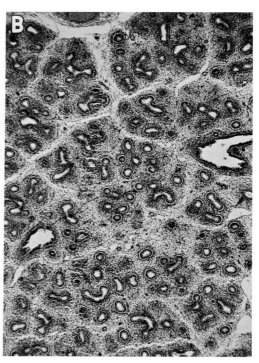

develops into the larynx and trachea; the subsequent branches become the right and left bronchi and the main bronchi of the five lobes of the lungs. The next few generations of branches develop into

smaller bronchi and bronchioles. The more distal branches become the alveolar ducts from which the alveoli arise. The bronchi and bronchioles are lined by tall columnar cells containing large, compact,

Fig. 15–2.—Fetal lung showing gradual thinning of septal walls and differentiation of alveoli. A small amount of formalin was introduced through the trachea to permit visualization of general pattern. **A,** fetal weight 670

gm. **B,** fetal weight 1,200 gm. **C,** fetal weight 3,600 gm. In C alveoli are cup-shaped structures in walls of alveolar ducts. Very few are present in A and B.

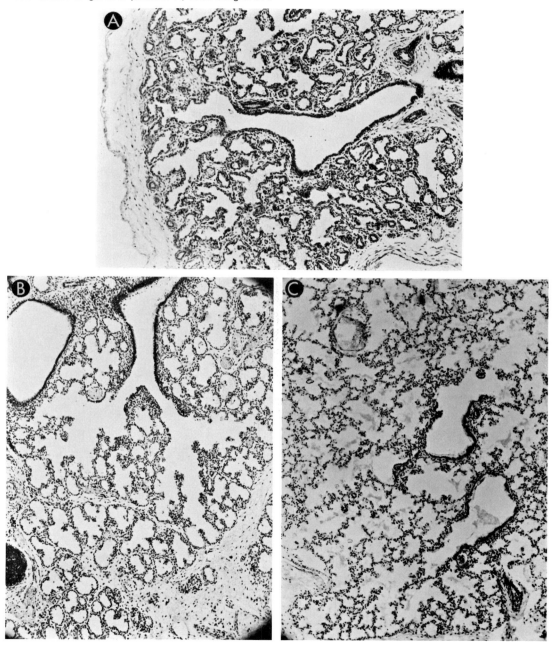

richly chromatic nuclei. The early alveolar ducts are lined by a continuous layer of large cuboidal cells with pale, poorly staining cytoplasm and prominent oval nuclei.

The original outgrowth from the entodermal tube projects into a mass of mesenchyme, which envelops it and within which further growth proceeds (Fig. 15–1, A). The proliferation of mesenchymal cells is at first more rapid than that of the entodermal cells, and the pulmonary branches are widely separated by intervening connective tissue. With further growth the cells are more concentrated in the immediate vicinity of the bronchi and a sublobular pattern is produced in the lobes of each lung (Fig. 15–1, B). Later the proportionate amount of connective tissue is gradually reduced and the lobular pattern, which is so striking in the embryo, disappears. The relative amount of connective tissue continues to decrease and by the normal time of birth only a few connective tissue cells remain in the walls of the alveolar ducts and alveoli (Fig. 15–2).

In the earliest stages of development the blood vessels lie in the mesenchyme at a considerable distance from the tubular branches. Gradually, capillaries grow out from these vessels and come to lie immediately beneath the outer surface of the single layer of cells of which the tubules are composed (Fig. 15–3, A). When the fetus is 19–20 weeks old and weighs about 400 gm, the most crucial stage in the development of the lungs begins. Capillaries penetrate the lining of the tubules for the first time (Fig. 15–3, B). The nuclei of the tubular cells are thrust aside as a capillary loop pushes its way between them to assume a position in close contact with the lumen of the tubule, the loop remaining covered only by a layer of cytoplasm so thin that it can be detected only by the electron microscope. This ingrowth of capillaries is associated with a slight local proliferation of connective tissue cells and the differentiation of elastic tissue fibers.

Once begun, capillary ingrowth progresses rapidly. The original capillaries, connective tissue and

Fig. 15–3. — Lungs from midgestation. **A,** terminal air spaces are still lined by continuous layer of cuboidal cells. No capillaries are in direct contact with a lumen and no alveoli have yet developed. Weight 400 gm; survival for 1 hour. **B,** in a few places proliferation of capillaries has brought them into contact with potential air spaces in pulmonary tree. Weight 470 gm; stillborn. Same magnification as in A.

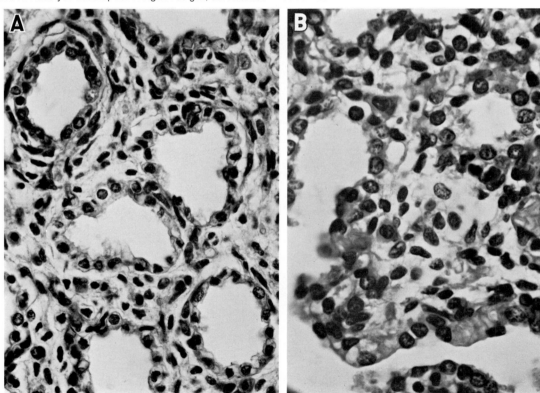

elastic tissue become definitive points in the architecture of the lung. In intervening areas the cells swell, proliferate and bulge outward to produce cuplike depressions that mark the development of new branches. Here, also, capillaries and elastic tissue invade the uniformly cellular wall and produce fixed areas between which further growth proceeds.

The first stage in the development of the lung, encompassing the first half of intrauterine life, consists of the elaboration of a system of branching tubules derived from a bud arising from the ento-

Fig. 15–4.—Lungs of stillborn fetuses from latter half of pregnancy showing gradual loss of septal cells and rise of capillaries to the surface. **A,** fetal weight 600 gm. Septa thick and young capillary loops short and thick. **B,** fetal weight 1,200 gm. Septa thinner and still largely lined by cuboidal cells; alveolar ducts present but no true alveoli yet visible. **C,** fetal weight 3,610 gm. Alveoli *(x)* now project into alveolar ducts *a* and *b.* Note absence of visible layer of cells covering the capillaries.

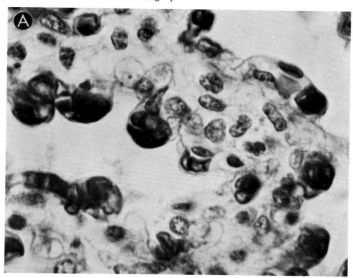

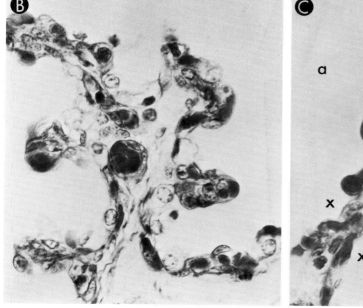

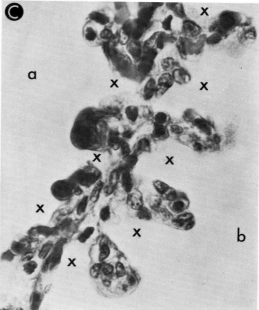

dermal tube, the branches being widely separated by the mesenchyme which proliferates simultaneously with the entodermal derivatives. The second stage begins at about mid-pregnancy and continues until after birth. It consists of vascularization of the tubular framework accompanied by progressive reduction in the intervening mesenchyme (Fig. 15–4).

About 8 weeks after the first capillaries have made contact with the tubal lumens, the capillary bed exposed to the interior of the tubules has increased sufficiently to allow transfer of enough oxygen to support life if air is permitted to enter. The ingrowth of capillaries marks the gradual differentiation of alveolar ducts and alveoli, and by the end of the 28th week, when the fetus weighs about 1,000 gm, the vascular development of the lung is such that it can supply enough oxygen to permit conversion of the fetus from a parasite entirely dependent on the maternal circulation into a viable human being capable of independent existence. Because the capillary bed exposed to the potential air spaces in the lungs continues to proliferate throughout fetal life, each succeeding week of intrauterine life increases the efficacy with which pulmonary ventilation can be maintained when the infant must oxygenate its blood through the lungs instead of the placenta.

Since ultra-structural studies with the electron microscope have shown that there is a continuous layer of attenuated epithelium covering the entire alveolar surface, much of the former speculation as to whether or not such a covering exists is no longer pertinent. Two types of cells are recognized among those covering the alveolar surfaces. Type I cells have greatly attenuated cytoplasm that covers the greater part of all capillaries. Type II cells have a prominent endoplasmic reticulum and contain large numbers of mitochondria, lipid bodies and myelin figures. They are thought to be the source of a lipoprotein complex, surfactant, which acts to lower surface tension. The two types of cells are intermixed over the alveolar surfaces. Type I cells, although usually cuboidal before birth in small premature infants, are capable of undergoing great stretching and consequently may lose their cuboidal appearance very rapidly after the onset of breathing. As term approaches, the continuous growth of the capillary net stretches and attenuates the cytoplasm of these cells; thus, in a mature newborn infant, even one that has never breathed, the cytoplasm of the cells over the capillary loops cannot be seen at magnifications possible with the light microscope.

Respiration before Birth

As long as the fetus is in the uterus, fluid is present in the lumens of all portions of the growing lung. At no time after a lumen is established are the walls normally in coaptation. While experiments on rabbits and sheep seem to show that in utero the lungs produce fluid, the quantities produced are still under investigation (Towers; Goodlin and Rudolph). Due to muscular contraction at the laryngeal level this flow is intermittently obstructed and pressure builds up in the lung parenchyma, causing distention of the alveoli. It has been reported that if the trachea is kept occluded in experimental animals until the lungs are excised, the lungs will remain distended until the tracheal ligature is removed, after which they will collapse.

In the embryo there seems to be no doubt that the fluid is a transudate from surrounding tissues, but as the fetus develops, the possibility that it is derived at least in part from the amniotic fluid cannot be denied. Windle and his followers maintained that the fetus does not normally inspire amniotic fluid and that debris from it found in the alveoli and alveolar ducts indicates that the respiratory center was abnormally stimulated by anoxia resulting from interference with intrauterine circulation. Snyder and his co-workers, on the other hand, presented evidence to show that the animals with which they worked normally drew amniotic fluid into the lungs before birth by active inspiratory movements, and Farber and Sweet found squamous epithelial cells in 88% of autopsies on newborn infants, indicating that respiratory movements are common.

Davis and Potter were able to show that human respiratory activity begins early in fetal life. In a group of women who required therapeutic abortion a radiopaque substance (Thorotrast) was introduced into the amniotic sac from 15 minutes to 48 hours before the fetus was surgically removed from the uterus. Roentgenograms of the fetuses were made immediately after their removal and the lungs examined microscopically. The lungs of all of those that had been exposed to Thorotrast for 18 hours or more contained this material in greater concentration than did the amniotic fluid (Fig. 15–5, A). The longer the exposure to Thorotrast, the greater the concentration in the lungs. When Thorotrast had been injected 12 hours or less before operation, the lungs showed a lower concentration, although whenever it had been present in the amniotic fluid for more than 1 hour before removal of the fetus, some could be demonstrated in the lungs.

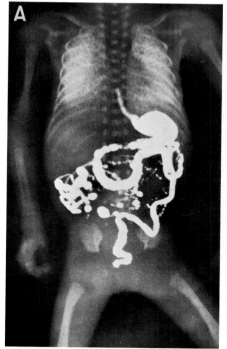 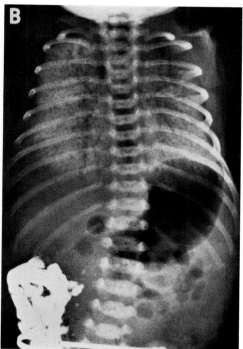

Fig. 15–5.—Thorotrast in lungs and gastrointestinal tract. **A,** Thorotrast had been introduced into amniotic cavity 26 hours before fetus was removed by hysterotomy. Weight 115 gm, gestational age about 16 weeks. **B,** Thoro-trast had been introduced into amniotic fluid 24 hours before delivery by cesarean section. Weight 3,250 gm, gestational age about 38 weeks.

To prove that the operative procedure itself did not induce respiration, in several instances Thorotrast was injected into the amniotic sac immediately before the operation was begun and consequently was present for only 15–20 minutes before the fetus was removed. In these cases no Thorotrast could be demonstrated in the lungs by x-ray and was identified on microscopic examination in only one.

The evidence leaves no doubt that these fetuses inspired amniotic fluid before the beginning of the operative procedures by which they were removed. Snyder found respiration in fetal rabbits intermittent, and it is probable that the same intermittent pattern is characteristic of the human fetus. When fluid is aspirated, much of it is absorbed through the wall of the pulmonary tree and any nonabsorbable substance such as Thorotrast becomes concentrated in the potential air spaces. The use of water-soluble materials such as Renograffin for such a purpose is unsatisfactory since such material appears to be absorbed from the lungs immediately even if aspirated.

Thorotrast was also injected by Davis and Potter into the amniotic sacs of several infants at term prior to cesarean operations. These infants were entirely normal and breathed immediately after birth; x-ray examination revealed Thorotrast in the lungs of all (Fig. 15–5, B).

One objection voiced to the belief that all fetuses normally make respiratory movements that draw amniotic fluid into all parts of the lungs before birth is that the presence of amniotic fluid would interfere with the establishment of respiration after birth. However, respiration before birth is normally very shallow; the lumens of the alveolar ducts are small and the area occupied by fluid is only a fraction of the potential air space. Moreover, the fluid that is present can be absorbed rapidly through the rich capillary bed of the alveoli. Abnormal stimulation of respiratory activity before birth may distend the potential air spaces, in which case much more fluid may be present than if the fetus had not been stimulated to inspire more deeply than is normal. Even then, absorption through alveolar walls can rapidly remove it.

The fact that fluid can be absorbed rapidly from the alveoli has been demonstrated by several investigators in different animals, but two particularly striking examples have been seen. A cannula was placed in the trachea of a full-grown rabbit and 130 ml of amniotic fluid was introduced slowly. At the end of 35 minutes the animal was killed. The combined weight of both lungs was 30 gm, indicating almost complete absorption of the fluid in this short period. In a second experiment, fluid was introduced by a tracheal catheter into the lungs of a 2-day-old infant with extreme hydrocephalus and spina bifida; 70 ml of fluid was allowed to flow in slowly over a period of 15 minutes with no apparent ill effect. When the child died 3 days later, permission to perform autopsy could not be obtained but there was no reason to believe that the death was in any way related to this introduction of fluid.

As the fetus approaches term, the glands of the skin become more active, an increasing amount of sebaceous material is excreted and epithelial desquamation is accelerated. The increasing concentration of these substances in the amniotic fluid makes it increasingly probable that they will be present in the lungs of normal infants. Some investigators have stated that the more frequent presence of such debris in the lungs of infants at term is evidence that the younger fetus does not breathe; however, another reason may be that the amniotic fluid in younger fetuses contains no epithelial cells and sebaceous material.

The question still exists as to whether the fluid in the alveolar spaces of the normal mature fetus is of local origin and is produced in such amounts that it normally flows out of the lung and contributes to the volume of the amniotic fluid, or whether it comes from the fluid in the amniotic sac and is inspired in such amounts as to remove part of the amniotic fluid. A review of data presented by many investigators shows that definitive experiments have not yet been devised and it is impossible to reach a final conclusion concerning the source and fate of the fluid present in the fetal lung at birth.

Appearance of Lungs before Birth

By the time a fetus is mature the lungs have a characteristic pattern that is invariably present unless altered by the effects of intrauterine anoxia, external compression, malformation or infection. This normal picture is not often observed because death during labor frequently follows a period of anoxia, or if death occurs before the onset of labor, degenerative changes are usually sufficient to obscure the normal appearance. Almost all infants who are alive at birth and who do not breathe spontaneously are subjected to artificial resuscitation, and this too alters the normal appearance.

In those rare instances in which the normal pattern still exists it is possible to detect uniform lumens in all portions of the pulmonary tree (Fig. 15–6, A). The irregular shape of the alveolar ducts is largely responsible for the "crumpled sac" appearance of the parenchyma. These potential air spaces are normally small and contain only a little fluid.

If the fetus is stimulated to increased respiratory activity because of anoxia, it aspirates more fluid than is normal and the potential air spaces become dilated (Fig. 15–6, B). The intratracheal introduction of fixing under low pressure similarly distends the alveolar ducts and alveoli and produces an appearance identical to that found in the lungs of infants who have died of anoxia before birth, except that when the distending fluid is artificially introduced, little or no debris is present. Such intratracheal instillation dilates the potential air spaces and permits visualization of the normal structure of the lung in a way not otherwise possible (see Fig. 15–2). It allows observation of the extent of alveolar development, thickness of alveolar septa, location of abnormal infiltrations of cells, etc., which is often impossible in a lung handled by the usual methods. It often seems desirable to inject one lung, leaving the other in its natural state.

Fluid entering the lungs as a result of active intrauterine respiration may expand them to a greater extent than that normally produced when air enters in the first few hours of extrauterine life. If the fetus that is stimulated to respire excessively survives and continues to breathe in utero, a constant absorption of fluid permits concentration of the solid material, and the alveolar ducts may become distended by epithelial cells and vernix caseosa (Fig. 15–6, C). In this event the debris may seriously interfere with the breathing of air after birth.

Infants who die 6 or 8 weeks postnatally may reveal histiocytes and aspirated epithelial squames still filling scattered groups of alveoli (Fig. 15–7). In some cases there are enough to give a "snowflake" appearance on x-ray examination.

Normally there is little debris in the amniotic fluid and respiration appears to be very shallow. This accounts for the fact that epithelial cells are not invariably present in the lungs of mature infants. The fetal activity attendant on anoxia increases the amount of particulate material in the amniotic fluid by freeing more cells and vernix from the surface of the body and agitating whatever may have already accumulated.

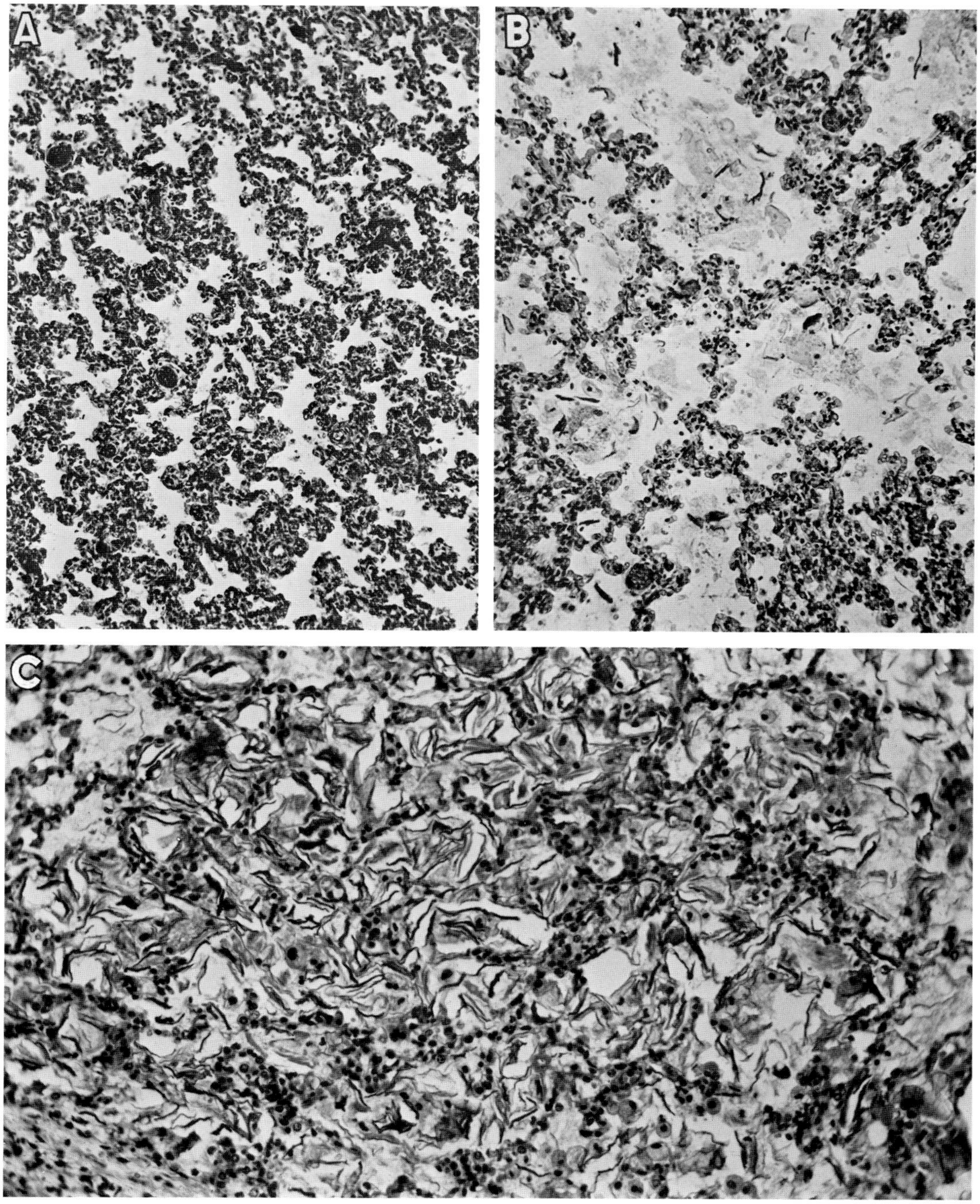

Fig. 15–6.—Lungs of mature stillborn fetuses. **A,** pattern of alveolar ducts associated with normal intrauterine respiratory movements. Nonexpansion of ducts obscures alveoli and few can be individually distinguished. **B,** lung following increased respiratory activity associated with anoxia. Capillaries are distended with blood and individual alveoli can be distinguished in walls of alveolar ducts. A few epithelial cells and a little debris inspired with amniotic fluid are visible. **C,** alveolar ducts distended by squamous epithelial cells concentrated as result of prolonged increase in respiratory activity and constant absorption of fluid.

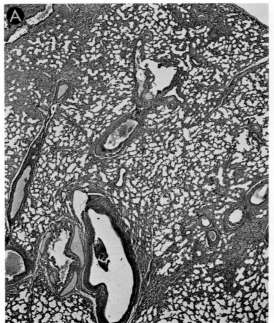
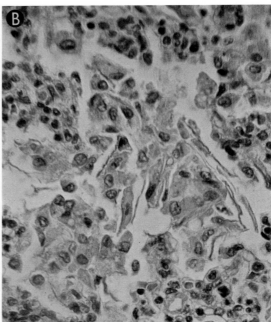

Fig. 15—7.—Lung of infant who died at 6 weeks of age showing persistence of large numbers of epithelial cells from amniotic fluid. **A,** solid-appearing areas are filled with epithelial cells and macrophages. **B,** high magnification of a solid area showing macrophages in the process of removing cornified epithelial cells.

It is a curious phenomenon that at postmortem examination lungs that are filled with amniotic sac contents as a result of massive aspiration can be easily and completely inflated with air under controlled pressures.

Respiration after Birth

All infants whose central nervous systems have not been depressed before birth will breathe air immediately after delivery. It is doubtful that immaturity of the respiratory center is ever responsible for failure to breathe after birth. Fetuses weighing only a few ounces that are removed surgically from the uterus will inflate their lungs and may continue to breathe a considerable length of time if they are kept in a warm moist atmosphere. We learned long ago that it was necessary to ligate the trachea in order to be able to study the intrauterine pattern of the lungs of any fetus of more than a few weeks' gestation. When small fetuses whose pulmonary tree is still completely lined by tall columnar epithelium inspire air, the lumens become dilated and the cells are somewhat flattened but they remain easily identifiable as a complete layer (Fig. 15–8). By 20–22 weeks, when a fetus weighs about 400 gm, breathing may continue in an ordinary atmosphere for more than an hour. At this time alveolar development is in its initial stages and a few capillary loops are in contact with the air spaces although most of the lung is still lined by a continuous layer of cuboidal cells. Figure 15–9 shows a well-expanded lung from a fetus weighing 450 gm who breathed for approximately 1 hour after delivery. The pattern of terminal air spaces is visible on the surface of the lungs as is also the large amount of interductal mesenchyme.

The stage of development at which a fetus will be able to survive outside the uterus depends largely on the maturity of the lungs. The average fetus weighs about 1,000 gm at the end of the 28th week (counting from the 1st day of the last menstrual period)—the approximate age at which alveolar development is sufficient to provide adequate oxygenation of the blood. In a 10-year period 350 infants weighing 400–1,000 gm were born at the Chicago Lying-in Hospital. Only nine survived, all of whom weighed over 800 gm.

An infant with a very low birth weight who does

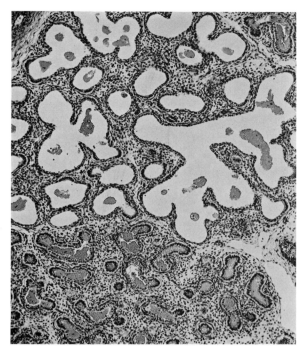

Fig. 15—8.—Lung of 115 gm fetus who breathed after removal from uterus, showing difference in size of lumens of pulmonary tree in expanded and unexpanded states. All spaces are lined by a continuous layer of columnar cells which have become somewhat flattened in areas containing air. Same fetus as in Fig. 15−5, A.

survive must gradually develop a normal number of alveoli arranged normally around alveolar ducts. We have seen a few very small infants, however, surviving a few weeks whose lungs were still extremely immature. Few alveoli had developed and the alveolar ducts had an almost cystic appearance. The septa were thick, and cuboidal cells still covered much of the surface (Fig. 15−10). In a set of twins of similar birth weight who were observed at the Boston Lying-in Hospital one died after a few hours, the other after 1 week. There was a marked difference in the appearance of the lining cells; they were largely cuboidal in the younger infant and completely flattened in the second.

Alveolar development continues throughout intrauterine life and the probability of survival increases in proportion to advancing pulmonary maturity. At the normal time of birth no portion of the lung distal to the bronchi possesses an epithelial lining distinguishable with light microscopy even though electron microscopy shows an extremely thin layer of cytoplasm covering all of the capillar-

ies. The connective tissue septa separating the outer surfaces of the alveolar ducts have disappeared and the alveolar ducts are visible only as the central spaces around whose periphery the alveoli are located (see Fig. 15−2).

The vital capacity increases progressively during the 1st week of life. The expansion of the lung after birth has been described as a gradual process and likened to the opening of a fan. From observations on the manner in which the lungs expand in young fetuses and from experiments in artificial insufflation of the lungs of infants soon after death we have concluded that probably the entire lung expands more or less uniformly under normal conditions and that the increase in vital capacity is a result of a progressive increase in size of each alveolus rather than the expansion of an increasing number of alveoli.

Radiologic studies of normal newborn infants immediately after birth show an almost immediate aeration of the lungs with the first breaths. Further increase in alveolar size and change in lining cells and septa probably continue for some time.

Fig. 15—9.—Lung of a fetus of 21 weeks' gestation weighing 450 gm who breathed for 1 hour after delivery. Lung surface shows the pattern of the expanded air spaces and the large amount of interstitial connective tissue still present.

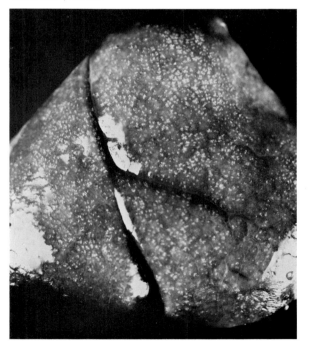

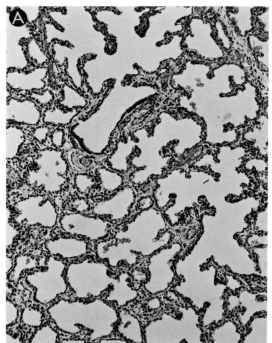
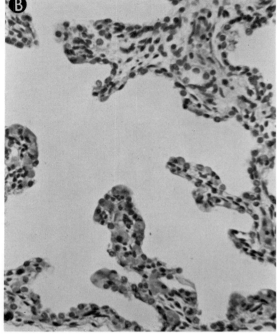

Fig. 15–10.—Lung of an infant with birth weight of 790 gm; survival for 26 days. No true alveoli have developed; open spaces are alveolar ducts. **A,** low magnification showing general pattern. **B,** high magnification showing alveolar ducts largely lined with slightly flattened cuboidal epithelium.

Evidence of Live Birth

To establish the time of death in relation to birth may be impossible from evidence obtained by postmortem examination. An infant is considered to be born when it is entirely outside the mother's body, even before the cord is cut. If the heart is beating, it is liveborn even though it never breathes. (See Chapter 5 for further discussion.)

If air does not enter the infant's lungs after birth, there is no way of determining at autopsy whether the heart stopped beating before or after delivery. We have seen two infants who were delivered in intact amniotic sacs and who were stated to have been active immediately after birth but who stopped moving before a medical attendant arrived and opened the sac. Neither showed petechiae, pulmonary hemorrhage or other abnormality. The lungs were distended with fluid, but similar distention is found following intrauterine death from anoxia.

The dilatation of alveolar ducts and alveoli resulting from breathing air can generally be easily distinguished from the uniform dilatation produced by inhalation of fluid. If an infant, especially one that is premature, has breathed air for only a few minutes or even a few hours, the proximal air spaces after death are proportionately more distended than the more distal ones, and many of the more distal ones may be collapsed and the walls approximated. Because of the surface tension at an air-fluid interface, the air-containing alveoli, even though not fully expanded, tend to assume a rounded outline due to the natural tendency to form the smallest possible surface area. This rounded appearance is not seen in alveoli expanded by fluid, and alveoli that have never contained air do not show collapsed lumens except as a result of postmortem degeneration.

Since air in the lungs will cause the lungs to float, this has generally been considered evidence of live birth, but it may be present either as a result of artificial resuscitation or the infant's own efforts. Failure to float is not necessarily a sign of absence of breathing, for when death is preceded by the formation of pulmonary hyaline membranes, resorption of air is often sufficient to cause complete collapse of alveoli, and the lungs immediately sink when placed in water even though the child has survived for many hours. In rare instances gas-forming organisms invading the tissues after death may produce enough gas to cause the lungs to float in water. Such lungs contain irregularly distributed gas bubbles, the position of which bears no relation to the bronchial tree. Moreover, large organisms are easily recognized within the gas-filled spaces.

If an infant has been willfully prevented from breathing after birth, as in some cases of infanticide, hemorrhage rarely occurs and the viscera are normal unless pathologic changes resulting from other causes are present. In the absence of air in the lungs there is ordinarily no conclusive evidence that an infant was alive at birth and then died of intentional suffocation.

The Role of Pulmonary Surfactant in the Maintenance of Alveolar Expansion

A lipoprotein complex can be extracted from the lungs of mature infants and healthy adults, and a similar substance can be shown to line the alveolar spaces in animals. On lateral compression this material reduces the surface tension of an air-water interface. Known as surfactant, it contains dipalmitoyl lecithin, which can reduce the surface tension of the alveolar-air interface from 20 to 5 dynes/cm^2. According to Laplace's law, the pressure (P) needed at an air-liquid interface to keep a bubble open is equal to twice the surface tension (T) divided by the radius (R) of the bubble (P = 2T/R). Consequently, the pressure needed to keep an individual alveolus open will increase with the reduction in its radius during expiration. If no surface-active material is present, the value for T remains constant, the pressure needed to keep an alveolus open increases and the alveolus tends to collapse. When it is present, a reduction in the value of T takes place with deflation, so the pressure required to keep the alveolus open is little changed.

This material, which in animals has been shown to originate in type II alveolar lining cells, does not appear in the extracts of lungs of human fetuses until 34–36 weeks of gestation; its appearance is heralded by the presence of lipid inclusions demonstrable by the electron microscope in the type II cells. Severe atelectasis causes surfactant material to disappear and extracts of affected lungs, even in adult life, fail to show its presence.

Because this substance is not yet being formed in the lungs of very premature infants, their lungs tend to collapse at the end of respiration. This tendency is increased in infants breathing 100% oxygen since the oxygen tends to be absorbed from nonaerated lung. Air is also absorbed from any lung in which the circulation continues after respiration has ceased. Consequently, atelectasis alone gives little indication of the state of the air spaces before death.

Other factors adding to the difficulty experienced by the premature infant in expanding its lungs, include the increased thickness of the alveolar walls and the cuboidal epithelium covering the walls of the air spaces.

Interstitial Emphysema and Pneumothorax

Air is found not infrequently in the interstitial, interlobular and subpleural portions of the lungs and in the thorax or mediastinum. In a living infant pneumothorax should always be considered in the differential diagnosis of dyspnea. With a large amount of free air in the chest the diaphragm may be depressed, the viscera pushed down and the abdomen made unusually prominent (Fig. 15–11). If the diaphragm on the right side is abnormally low, the liver may seem enlarged because downward displacement makes it more easily palpable.

Air may be found in any part of the mediastinum. An air bubble may elevate the thymus several centimeters above the pericardium, and on rare occasions the pericardium may be distended by air. More often the air is present between the sternum and the anterior mediastinum. Subcutaneous emphysema is most common in the neck and under the scalp, although it may be present over any part of the body. During investigation of the history of an infant with mediastinal and generalized subcutaneous emphysema the statement was obtained that during attempted resuscitation by the intratracheal introduction of oxygen "something seemed suddenly to give way" and the subcutaneous tissues over the entire body became crepitant. Radiographically, recognition of interstitial emphysema limited to the lungs is difficult unless air outlines a large interstitial vessel lying outside the alveolar space (Ovenfors). As a result mediastinal air is much more frequently recognized radiologically than air in the lung proper (Chasler; Morrow et al.).

Pneumothorax may produce severe dyspnea and can even cause death. If the condition is recognized and the air removed, recovery is usually dramatically prompt. Mild pneumothorax is often symptomless.

Air in the anterior mediastinum has been reported to produce symptoms of cardiac embarrassment, but it probably does so infrequently and may be

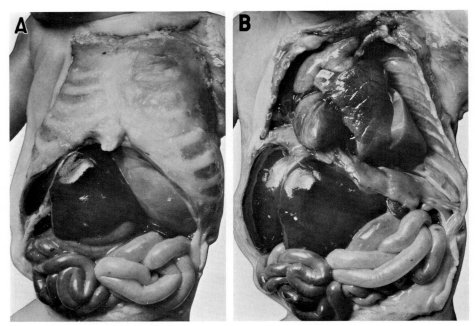

Fig. 15–11.—Extreme tension pneumothorax involving left thoracic cavity. Death at 5 hours. **A,** diaphragm presents a convex surface toward abdomen; liver and in-testine are displaced downward. **B,** chest opened showing left lung and mediastinum displaced into right side.

discovered accidentally in newborn infants without symptoms. The retrosternal introduction of air for the purpose of delineating the thymus in an attempt to determine the etiology of an increase in mediastinal width has been reported as an innocuous procedure producing no symptoms.

The means by which air escapes into the mediastinum and subcutaneous tissues has never been entirely understood but it seems probable, as stressed by the Macklins, that the accumulation of air in the mediastinum ordinarily follows interstitial emphysema (Fig. 15–12, A) with the transfer of air along the sheaths of the pulmonary arteries, the air coming from alveoli that have ruptured and permitted escape of air into the adventitia of the adjacent vessels (Fig. 15–12, B). Local compression of the blood vessels may follow and further aggravate the symptoms by interfering with the circulation in the pulmonary vessels. Air moving along the vessel sheaths may accumulate in the mediastinum or follow the adventitia of the aorta and other blood vessels to produce intraperitoneal, retroperitoneal or subcutaneous emphysema. From the mediastinum it may also break through around the hilar vessels into the pleura and produce secondary pneumothorax. With unilateral pneumothorax air is usually present in the interstitial tissues of the lung on the opposite side.

According to the Macklins, air enters the sheaths of the blood vessels as a result of the establishment of an abnormal pressure gradient caused by (1) overinflation of alveoli without corresponding expansion of the vascular lumens with which the alveolar walls are in contact or (2) reduction of vascular lumens without a corresponding decrease in the lumens of the alveoli to which they are attached. The second factor rarely if ever operates in the newborn.

In all but rare cases of interstitial emphysema and pneumothorax in the newborn a history of artificial resuscitation can be obtained. When respiration is claimed to have been spontaneous and unaided by mechanical means, it can only be supposed that the infant's attempts to overcome an obstruction in its bronchi or trachea raised the intraalveolar pressure sufficiently to cause rupture of the walls. Spontaneous interstitial emphysema and spontaneous pneumothorax occasionally occur in the respiratory distress syndrome. Chasler, and Chernick and Avery, found that a large proportion of infants who suffered a spontaneous pneumothorax while still in the delivery room were postmature and meconium-stained. Massive aspiration of amniotic sac contents was implicated as a cause. In excised lungs obtained at autopsy we found that, when unsupported by the thoracic cage, interstitial em-

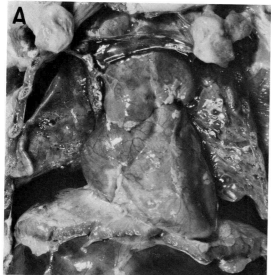

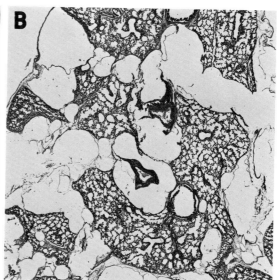

Fig. 15—12.—Interstitial emphysema in infant weighing 2,000 gm who survived 2 hours. **A,** air-filled bullae in interlobular and subpleural spaces were caused by hyperdistention of alveoli with rupture into perivascular connective tissue. **B,** nonexpanded portion of lung with large amounts of air around major blood vessels and in interlobular connective tissue.

physema would develop on expansion by air with as little as 20 cm of water pressure. Air may enter the thoracic cavity on the involved side if the rupture extends through the pleura, or it may escape into the opposite side via the sheaths of the blood vessels and the mediastinum. The pneumothorax that results from rupture of alveoli directly into the pleural space, or from rupture of an air cyst, which has been postulated as a possible congenital malformation responsible for pneumothorax, is no greater than that which can be produced by the elimination of negative pressure in the pleural cavity. Then air enters the pleura under atmospheric pressure, and unless complicating factors are pres-

Fig. 15—13.—Air in abnormal locations in the chest. **A,** pneumomediastinum with substernal accumulation of air. **B,** extreme pneumothorax with displacement of left lung and mediastinum into right side of chest.

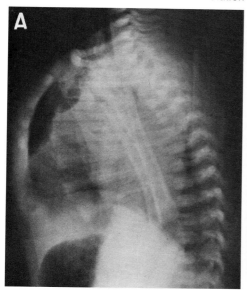

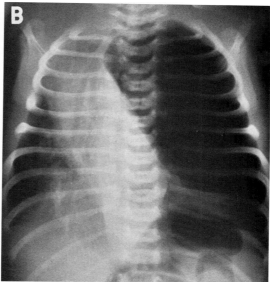

ent, the air in the pleural space remains at that pressure.

In tension pneumothorax the pressure is greater and rises more rapidly at the end of inspiration than does the pressure within the alveolus. This can only result from the forceful introduction of air or the development of a valvelike opening in the pleura. Consequently, if air is under sufficient tension to balloon out the diaphragm and produce a flat or convex surface, artificial introduction of air is by far the most probable cause. However, Chernick and Avery reported that three of 11 survivors of spontaneous pneumothorax required intrathoracic catheters for control and thus no doubt had a tension pneumothorax.

In the living infant pneumomediastinum is best diagnosed from lateral x-ray projections of the chest (Fig. 15–13, A). Pneumothorax is best diagnosed from an anteroposterior view (Fig. 15–13, B).

Atelectasis

Atelectasis may result either from nonexpansion of the lungs after birth or the subsequent collapse of alveoli. The former is primary and the latter secondary atelectasis. Primary atelectasis is found in all stillborn infants and in liveborn infants who die before normal respiration is established. It is almost never present in infants after even a brief period of normal breathing and crying.

Secondary atelectasis is found on postmortem examination of almost all infants who die in the first weeks of life and, except for the variety associated with a hyaline membrane, is never a primary cause of death and should not be used on a death certificate. The newborn lung is highly elastic and, because of the small size of the alveoli, contains little residual air. Consequently, a large share of the air is resorbed during the agonal period and may be completely absorbed if the infant has been exposed terminally to 100% oxygen, as is so often the case. Then all of the gas may be absorbed if respiration stops before the circulation ceases. Thus the absence of gas or "air" in the alveolar spaces of the dead infant ordinarily has little clinical significance.

The Respiratory Distress Syndrome

(Atelectasis with Hyaline Membrane Formation, Bronchopulmonary Dysplasia or Oxygen Toxicity)

This condition has been recognized for many years and has been described under a variety of names such as resorption atelectasis, hyaline membrane and vernix membrane.

The clinical and pathologic findings are characteristic and when recognized are rarely confused with those of any other disease. It is more frequent in premature than in full-term infants. The infants often breathe spontaneously at birth, and for the first hour or two often seem normal; after that, progressive cyanosis and dyspnea gradually develop. Breathing becomes extremely labored, the sternum and lower ribs retract with each inspiration (Fig. 15–14) and breath sounds become gradually less audible. Death usually takes place in 8–30 hours as a result of exhaustion and inability to obtain enough oxygen to maintain life.

The pathologic findings in such an infant can be foretold before the chest is opened. The lungs have a striking appearance. They are the size of well-expanded lungs but have the consistency of liver. Instead of having the yellow-pink color of lungs containing air or the light violet of the nonexpanded fetal lungs they are a uniform dark red-purple. If the infant has continuing symptoms and survives more than 24 hours, a reactive process is usually superimposed. In such instances the lungs may seem slightly granular on palpation; ordinarily, however, they are of uniform consistency. The whole lung or individual portions sink when placed in water despite the fact that a little air always remains in the proximal portions of the pulmonary tree.

Histologic examination reveals widespread resorption of air, and the walls of many alveolar ducts and most of the alveoli are collapsed, giving a solid appearance to the lung tissue between the few alveoli that remain open (Fig. 15–15). This picture is so different from normal unexpanded lung that it has sometimes led to the mistaken conclusion that it is a result of primary maldevelopment of pulmonary tissue. If an attempt is made to expand such lungs with air after removal from the body, the proximal spaces ordinarily become greatly hyperdistended and the distal ones even more completely

Fig. 15–14.—Infant in incubator showing the extreme retraction of lower sternum often associated with hyaline membranes and atelectasis.

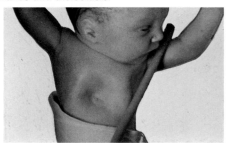

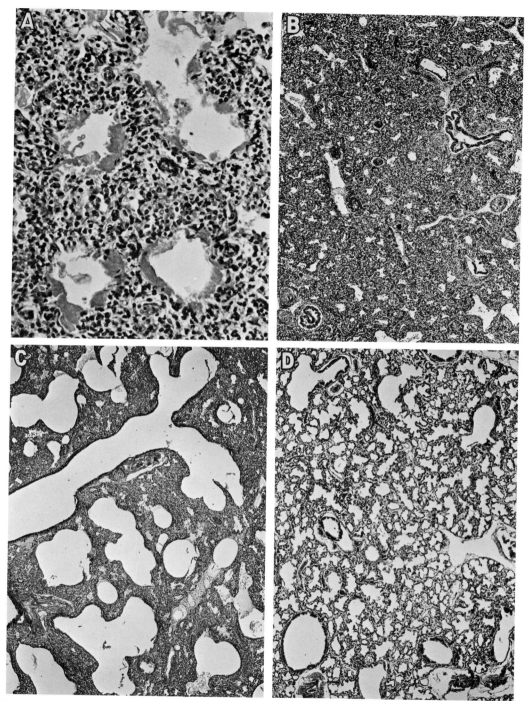

Fig. 15–15.—Lungs in respiratory distress syndrome showing hyalinelike membrane and atelectasis. **A,** the few air spaces that have remained open are lined by an irregular layer of homogeneous, finely granular eosinophilic material. Distal alveoli are collapsed and, as a result, the intervening areas appear solid. **B,** low power view showing generalized absence of air. **C,** attempted insufflation by air. Bronchi and proximal alveolar ducts are greatly hyperdistended; alveoli remain collapsed. **D,** intratracheal injection of fluid resulting in reopening of alveoli, proving that they are of normal anatomic structure. B, C and D from same infant at same magnification. Weight 1,970 gm, age 30 hours.

collapsed (Fig. 15 – 15, C). If saline instead of air is injected via the bronchi, the alveolar spaces will gradually open, but they may leak fluid into interstitial tissue. Though on microscopic examination the alveoli are partially expanded, the lymphatics and interlobar spaces are often distended, indicating that fluid has passed through the alveolar walls at random (Fig. 15 – 16, A). On deflation only a small portion of the fluid can be recovered from the bronchi. If fluid with a high oncotic pressure, such as 5% gelatin solution, is used instead of saline, this does not pass the alveolar barrier (Fig. 15 – 16, B). Then a marked restriction in the distribution of the expanding fluid is found in lungs with hyaline membranes. As by expansion with air, the proximal alveoli are well filled but the distal alveoli only sparingly (Craig *et al.*, unpublished). In immature lungs without membranes no such filling defect is found.

Intense capillary engorgement, which is responsible for the color and increased weight of lungs with hyaline membranes, is one of the most striking findings on histologic examination. In the first few hours of life the infant with severe respiratory distress has masses of necrotic material containing much nuclear debris in the terminal bronchioles and alveolar ducts, but there is no inflammation. At first debris does not line the spaces but is present as irregular masses (Fig. 15 – 17). The nuclear chromatin gradually fades, the necrotic material becomes uniformly homogeneous and eosinophilic and covers the inner surfaces of the alveolar ducts that remain open. A few polymorphonuclear leukocytes may be present, especially in infants who survive more than 36 hours, but in the majority there is no evidence of infection.

The membranes stain for lipid and are periodic acid-Schiff (PAS)- and Feulgen-positive. The latter reaction indicates the presence of degenerated nuclear material in the membrane. Immunofluorescent studies have demonstrated the presence of fibrin and other proteins (Gitlin and Craig). When the arteries of excised lungs are injected with a mixture of gelatin and india ink to demonstrate the patency and distribution of the capillary nets, a decrease in local filling beneath the areas covered by membranes is revealed (Craig, unpublished). The membranes apparently thus form a barrier to normal respiratory exchange by blocking off some portions of the pulmonary tissue, obstructing the capillary nets, presumably by thrombi beneath the membrane, and coating other capillaries so that they are deprived of contact with an oxygen-rich atmosphere.

A picture characteristic of hyaline membrane disease is never seen in stillborn infants, in those who die within 1 hour of birth or in those who survive more than 10 days. It is uncommon in infants

Fig. 15 – 16. – A, lung of newborn after saline injection of trachea. The alveoli are moderately expanded; the interlobular space is markedly widened due to the leakage of fluid from the alveoli into the interstitium.

B, lung of newborn after dextran injection of the trachea. The alveoli are distended; only a small amount of dextran is present in the interstitium of the interlobular space.

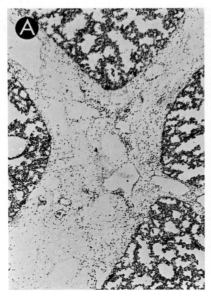
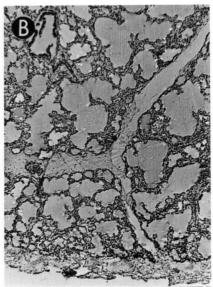

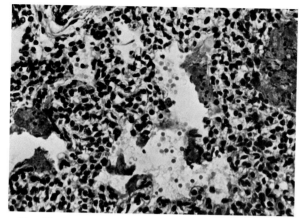

Fig. 15–17.—Lung of infant 2 hours old with respiratory distress syndrome. Masses of necrotic cells lie in the lumen of the alveolar ducts. Pyknotic nuclei are still present within the masses.

over 2,500 gm and seems to be directly related to the stage of development at birth and to extrauterine age. The lungs of stillborn fetuses may contain evenly distributed, finely granular material that stains light pink with eosin, but it does not resemble that found in infants with this disorder.

This clinical picture occurs disproportionately often among infants of all weights delivered by cesarean section. It seems to be fairly well agreed, however, that cesarean section alone does not cause the respiratory distress syndrome but that the gestational age at which section is performed is the most important factor (Usher *et al.*). The indication for cesarean section is also an important determinant for the predilection to respiratory distress: fetal distress, obstructed labor, abruptio placentae, placenta previa and maternal diabetes all increase the hazard. Infants of diabetic mothers, because of their large size, may fall into weight categories ordinarily regarded as mature yet have gestational ages associated with a higher risk. Although repeat elective cesarean sections at term in patients with previous sections for placenta previa or dystocia carry little risk of neonatal mortality, the incidence of the respiratory distress syndrome in infants of such mothers is higher than that found in those of a comparable group of women delivered vaginally (Potter).

An associated finding in many infants dying after cesarean section has been an increase in subarachnoid fluid (see Fig. 24–1). The normal amount of subarachnoid fluid varies with age, the premature infant of 1,500–2,000 gm normally having more fluid both actually and proportionately than

the infant of any other weight. The normal amount of fluid at this weight is about 15 ml. At term there is normally so little that it cannot be measured. In infants who die of progressive respiratory distress following cesarean section, 40–60 ml or even more may be obtained (Potter and Rosenbaum). Whether cerebral compression in these infants may contribute to the abnormal pulmonary function is unknown.

We have been struck by the infrequency with which hyaline membranes are found in autopsy material in areas outside the United States and Europe—areas where the use of supplemental oxygen is negligible. Several years ago at the Chicago Lying-in Hospital a reduction in frequency of hyaline membranes followed a reduction in the use of oxygen in premature infants pursuant to the discovery of the relationship of oxygen therapy to retrolental fibroplasia. In the 4 years from 1956 to 1959 the frequency was only 25% of the average for the preceding 10 years. It seemed difficult to ascribe this difference to reduction in the use of oxygen for at no prior time had concentrations greater than 50% been used, but no other changes were discovered in conduct of labor, delivery or postnatal care of the infant that might have accounted for this change. In subsequent years even in those infants whose deaths were ascribed to the respiratory distress syndrome the amount of hyaline material in most instances was minimal and atelectasis was the principal finding.

At the Chicago Lying-in Hospital mortality attributed to hyaline membranes from 1961 to 1966 was 2.5/1,000 live births divided between 0.3 for infants over 2,500 gm at birth and 2.2 for those under 2,500 gm. At the Boston Hospital for Women in 1968 the mortality was 5.2/1,000 live births with 0.2 for infants over 2,500 gm and 5/1,000 for those under 2,500 gm. Premature infants made up 10% of births at the Boston Hospital for Women and 8% of those at the Chicago Lying-in Hospital (Potter and Davis), a fact that accounts for part of the difference in frequency of deaths from the respiratory distress syndrome in the two hospitals.

The etiology and pathogenesis of hyaline membranes in the newborn lung are still uncertain but a few facts appear incontrovertible at the present time. First, no lesion that can be identified as a precursor of atelectasis and hyaline membranes can be demonstrated in the lungs of infants who are stillborn or die in the first moments of life. Second, in premature infants dying between half an hour and 2 hours after birth with respiratory distress necrobiotic or necrotic epithelial masses can be identified lying in the alveolar ducts and proximal alveoli. Third, the first identifiable membranes, which can be seen after 2 hours of life, contain remnants of epithelium as well as fibrin and other elements. If damage to the alveolar wall occurs, enough thromboplastin of tissue origin will be released to preclude the presence of an inhaled thromboplastin-like material from the amniotic sac, which has been postulated as playing a role. Fourth, after 24 hours of life, evidence of proliferation and repair of the damaged epithelium, together with a macrophage response, begins to appear. Fifth, in the infants requiring oxygen levels over 50% for survival, and especially those placed on artificial respiration, the process of necrosis, new membrane formation and repair continue with ever-increasing thickening of the alveolar walls and distortion of the normal lung architecture.

In infants who survive more than 24 hours there may be evidence of resolution of the membranes, infiltration of macrophages and presence of large immature cells lining the alveolar spaces, all of which suggest a repair process (Boss and Craig). When respiratory distress continues for several days, the alveolar walls may become thickened and the alveolar lumens filled with desquamated cells. Evidence of continued degenerative and regenerative processes can be identified in infants given oxygen in high concentration and maintained with

artificial respiration (Fig. 15–18, A) (Northway *et al.*). There may also be squamous metaplasia of bronchial epithelium (Fig. 15–18, B). Radiologically, the lungs of a few infants who recover from the respiratory distress syndrome may have irregular streaking, and lung biopsy may show such histologic abnormalities as distention of the alveolar ducts and thickening of the peribronchial tissue and alveolar walls (Shepard *et al.*). A high oxygen concentration similar to that administered to severely ill infants is capable of producing the same lesion in adults when given for prolonged periods (Nash *et al.*). Attempts at experimental production of this process in newborn animals exposed to similar high oxygen levels have not been successful.

Effective vascular perfusion of the lung may be greatly reduced in the respiratory distress syndrome; anoxia may cause the ductus arteriosus to reopen and shunt the blood away from the lungs, and much of the blood that does pass through the lungs goes to collapsed and unaerated alveoli; also, injection studies show that many of the capillaries beneath the membrane do not fill (Craig). For these reasons the effective gas exchange and particularly the elimination of carbon dioxide from the blood are diminished. Severe respiratory acidosis results even though a high ambient oxygen level may produce a normal oxygen tension in the blood.

It may be concluded that infants dying with hya-

Fig. 15–18.—Lung of infant 9 days old with severe respiratory distress who required oxygen at high concentration throughout life. **A,** the lung parenchyma contains almost no open alveoli. The epithelium of the bronchioles is metaplastic and debris fills the lumens. **B,** bronchus showing squamous metaplasia of the epithelium. **C,** pulmonary artery injected with gelatin and india ink. Only a few of the alveolar capillaries are filled.

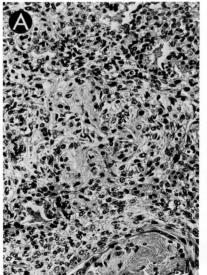
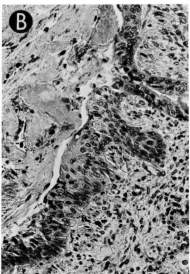
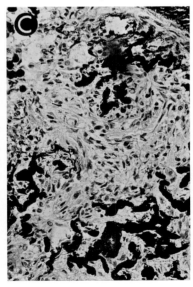

line membranes and respiratory distress are faced with two separate problems. Because of prematurity and/or other factors such as anoxia surrounding birth the lungs lack the surface active material needed to maintain the lung in expansion; therefore atelectasis and anoxia become progressive. To remedy this anoxic state oxygen is given, which induces the necrosis, membrane formation and repair associated with this condition. These changes further impair the ability of the lungs to expand and function normally.

Pneumonia

In the perinatal period.—Bacteria enter the lungs in inspired fluid and are more widely and evenly distributed than when they are carried in by air. Consequently when pneumonia develops before birth, the potential air spaces in the lungs are often diffusely infiltrated by polymorphonuclear leukocytes (Fig. 15–19). The leukocytes, usually intermixed with debris from the amniotic fluid, are distributed throughout the lungs, although they may be more numerous in some areas than in others. Polymorphonuclear cells can also enter the amniot-

ic fluid from the maternal or fetal circulation. As noted in the section on the placenta, inflammation in the chorion and amnion is not necessarily caused by bacterial infection of these structures, although Bernstein and Wong found histologic or cultural evidence of the presence of bacteria in the lungs of 55 infants with amniotic fluid aspiration and infection. The more immature the infant, the less commonly can bacteria be cultured from the placenta and the less often does the infant show evidence of infection by culture or histology, even when the placenta does have histologic evidence of inflammation. While the amniotic fluid may be sterile, it may contain many polymorphonuclear leukocytes. These cells may be aspirated and fill the alveolar spaces without producing interstitial, bronchial or nodal inflammation. Consequently, aspirated polymorphonuclear cells cannot be considered definitive evidence of pneumonia although, when accompanied by interstitial or peribronchial infiltrates, the process is generally known as "congenital aspiration pneumonia," as distinct from ordinary bronchopneumonia, which is less diffuse and extends more directly from bronchi to the surrounding parenchyma.

Fig. 15–19.—Intrauterine pneumonia in stillborn fetus. All potential air spaces are uniformly filled with poly- morphonuclear leukocytes. No fibrin is present. **A,** low magnification. **B,** high magnification.

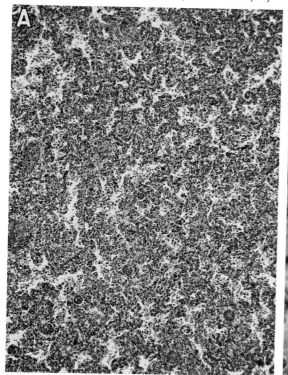
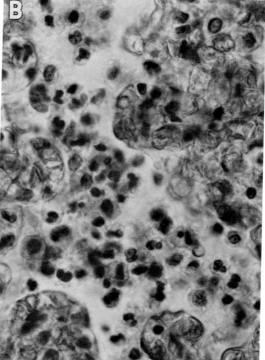

A positive diagnosis of pneumonia can almost never be made on gross examination of the lungs of a stillborn fetus or a young infant. A diffuse increase in density indistinguishable from that produced by inflammatory cells may result from the presence of large numbers of epithelial cells inspired with amniotic fluid. If the concentration of leukocytes varies in different portions of a lobe, a granular sensation suggestive of pneumonia may be obtained on palpation, but it is never possible to determine positively whether or not inflammation exists except by microscopic examination. On rare occasions a severe infection may extend to the pleura, and exudative pleuritis or actual empyema may develop (Fig. 15–20). Evidence of a more chronic or resolving pneumonia can be identified by lymphocytic infiltration of the interstitium accompanied by a macrophage response.

Despite the fact that sterile inflammation without bacterial contamination may occur, almost all true pneumonias originating before birth are caused by aspiration of amniotic fluid containing bacteria. Enteric pathogens such as fecal streptococci, colon bacilli, and *Aerobacter aerogenes* are most often found as causative organisms, with Beta streptococci or staphylococci less common. The high incidence of staphylococci in congenital aspiration pneumonias reported by Anderson *et al.* has not been found at the Boston Lying-in Hospital, nor was it the experience of Bernstein and Wong. A few cases of hematogenous pneumococcic infections have been reported, but such a source of infection is rare. It has been shown that bacteria are present in the amniotic fluid within a few hours after the onset of labor even though the membranes are still intact and that they are present almost immediately after rupture of membranes. In view of the fact that within a few hours after rupture of membranes the amnion and chorion are often infiltrated by leukocytes, it is somewhat surprising that the fetal lungs are not affected more commonly. Although most cases of intrauterine pneumonia follow early rupture of membranes, long labors or complicated deliveries, in all of which there are both increased likelihood of bacteria in the fetal environment and increased respiratory activity from attendant anoxia, the actual frequency with which such conditions are complicated by pneumonia is low.

Clinical diagnosis in the newborn is often difficult. The temperature is of little help for it may be normal in pneumonia or temporarily elevated in infants whose subsequent course is uneventful. Changes in breath sounds and rales are difficult to detect and may be duplicated by mild irregularity in pulmonary expansion. Even x-ray examination is ordinarily of little help because of the diffuseness of the pneumonic involvement and the fact that vascular markings in the lungs are normally unusually prominent for a few days after birth. Infants who die unexpectedly without previous evidence of illness more often have pneumonia than any other pathologic condition.

However, infants with pneumonia usually seem ill and occasionally have positive blood cultures. They may be hyperirritable with irregular twitching or actual convulsions, or they may be lethargic and unresponsive. A differentiation between pneumonia and cerebral injury resulting from trauma or anoxia may be impossible.

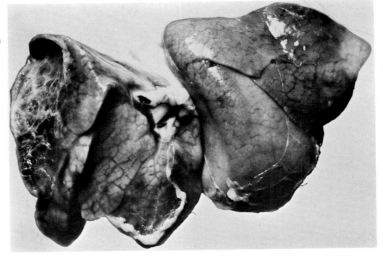

Fig. 15–20. — Exudative pleuritis with pneumonia. Weight 2,560 gm, age 4 hours.

The gross appearance of the lungs on postmortem examination may be misleading and microscopic examination is essential before a diagnosis can be established. The granular sensation mentioned previously is often even more pronounced than in the lungs of stillborn infants owing to the presence of air in the unaffected areas. If large portions of lung tissue are involved, it may be impossible to differentiate pneumonia from areas of alveolar collapse.

Microscopic examination usually reveals a diffuse infiltration of cells similar to that found in the pneumonia of stillborn infants. Debris from the amniotic fluid is usually intermixed with the leukocytes. The presence of air in some parts of the lungs accentuates the affected areas and makes them somewhat more prominent than they are in the lungs of infants who have never breathed. Red cells are occasionally present. Fibrin is rarely present in pneumonia of intrauterine origin although it is common in pneumonia originating after birth.

IN OLDER INFANTS.—Pneumonia becomes responsible for an increasing share of the total number of deaths in each succeeding month of the 1st year of life, although in actual numbers of cases it constantly decreases. By the end of the 1st month, when prematurity, malformations, birth trauma and the other causes of high postnatal mortality have claimed most of their victims, infections then become the principal cause of death with pneumonia far outranking any other. Pneumonias caused by pneumococci are rare, but bronchopneumonia may become confluent and involve large portions of the lungs, giving a gross appearance of lobar pneumonia.

In the immediate postnatal period gram-negative organisms are the most common etiologic agents, but in the remainder of the 1st year of life staphylococci play a disproportionately large role.

Of 24 cases of staphylococcal pneumonia in childhood collected by Huxtable et al. 20 occurred during the first 3 months of life with 12 being of the aggressive 80/81 strain. Perhaps because of the virulence of the organisms or because of the relative lack of collagen in the interstitium of the lung at this early age partial obstruction of an airway associated with some necrosis of distal alveolar walls may produce cysts of entrapped gas in the interlobar septa. These cysts have thin walls, show some evidence of tissue necrosis on their inner aspect and are surrounded by an acute inflammatory exudate.

In a child who is more than a few days old the leukocytic infiltration begins in the peribronchial

areas and extends outward into the surrounding air spaces. Destruction of tissue seems to occur more readily than in older individuals and abscesses are more common. Fibrin, which is seldom found with pneumonias originating before birth, becomes a prominent component of the alveolar exudate (Fig. 15–21). Pleural exudates composed of fibrin and leukocytes may also be present. Bronchopneumonia can be diagnosed on gross examination more readily in these older infants than in those only a few days old. The normal portions are well filled with air, and if irregularly distributed firm areas can be palpated, the microscopic findings will usually confirm a diagnosis of pneumonia. Neither at this nor at any other age, however, should a positive diagnosis be made without corroboration by microscopic examination.

The severity of the pneumonia as shown by the outcome of the disease often seems to bear little relation to the pathologic appearance of the lungs. Some infants who die with pulmonary symptoms show remarkably little evidence of pneumonia. Varying amounts of edema with a few scattered inflammatory cells that seem worthy only of a diag-

Fig. 15—21.—Pneumonia in infant aged 2 weeks. Fibrin, leukocytes and bacteria are present. Fibrin is not present in pneumonia of intrauterine origin.

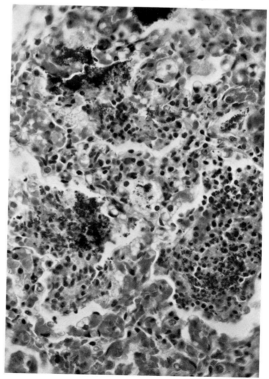

nosis of inflammatory edema may be all that is visible. The term interstitial pneumonia has occasionally been applied when no exudate is visible but the alveolar walls seem abnormally thick. In some instances when occasional leukocytes can be seen, such a diagnosis may be warranted, but in most cases the apparent thickening of the walls is due to contraction of tissues brought about by the presence of a diminished amount of air and is a mechanical rather than a pathologic state.

On the other hand, in infants with few or no clinical symptoms of pulmonary infection postmortem examination may reveal definite evidence of pneumonia. In the few cases of sudden death in the 1st year of life in which a definite pathologic process can be identified pulmonary infection is the most common.

LIPID PNEUMONIA. — This type, characterized by the presence of numerous fat-filled histiocytes in the alveolar spaces, may follow the regurgitation and aspiration of milk or the frequent use of nose drops. It more often occurs in small infants fed by gavage than in older ones who can nurse successfully. It is also found in infants who are doing poorly and nurse with difficulty and in those with severe neurologic defects whose deglutitory function is impaired.

VIRUS PNEUMONITIS. — A pulmonary infection principally affecting young infants was described by Adams and his co-workers in epidemic and sporadic form. It was characterized clinically by coughing, sneezing, dyspnea, cyanosis and variable elevation of temperature. Throat smears showed characteristic cytoplasmic inclusion bodies in epithelial cells, and throat smears of the mother often had similar inclusions. In one epidemic described by Adams mortality was 83% among affected premature infants and 8% among mature infants. Pathologic changes in the lungs consisted largely of proliferation and sloughing of bronchial epithelium associated with mild peribronchial or interstitial infiltration by mononuclear cells. Atelectasis, edema and hemorrhage were common. Diseased epithelial structures in the lung at times contained acidophilic cytoplasmic inclusion bodies measuring $3-6\ \mu$ in diameter similar to those seen in throat smears. The etiologic factor was presumed to be a virus because of the association of inclusion bodies, but no virus was identified.

Goodpasture also described a virus pneumonia in infants characterized by intranuclear inclusion bodies (see Fig. 9–15).

Cytomegalic inclusion disease is responsible for the presence of characteristic large mononuclear cells with prominent round intranuclear inclusions. Such cells may be free in the alveoli or, less frequently, in bronchial or septal cells (see Fig. 9–9, C). They are most common when the infection is acquired prenatally but are occasionally found in older infants.

Becroft described adenovirus pneumonia in young children. He found that affected lungs are often voluminous, with necrosis and repair in the alveolar walls and intranuclear inclusions in the alveolar lining cells. Pleural effusions were present in some of his patients.

Fatal herpes virus infection of the newborn may be associated with extensive coagulation necrosis of alveolar walls often accompanied by hemorrhage and edema. These changes have been found only in the acute stages of the disease and the lungs have lacked evidence of repair. Intranuclear inclusions may be difficult to find despite the severity of the disease process.

GIANT CELL PNEUMONIA. — Pneumonia characterized by the presence of giant cells arising from bronchial or alveolar epithelium has been found in infants as an accompaniment of various systemic diseases and occasionally as a primary infection. In all cases in which a virus has been isolated it has been that causing measles. Such infection has been recognized as a complication of tuberculosis, cystic fibrosis of the pancreas, Letterer-Siwe's disease and treated leukemia (Enders et al.).

The giant cells are syncytial masses of varying size (Fig. 15–22) that may be present in bronchi or alveoli or sometimes form a pseudolining over localized portions of alveolar walls. Inclusions are sometimes visible in nuclei or cytoplasm. The accompanying exudate is variable but often consists largely of mononuclear cells. In such cases giant cells with inclusions may also be found in other organs such as lymph nodes, stomach, intestine, bone marrow and heart.

Pneumocystis carinii PNEUMONITIS (INTERSTITIAL PLASMA CELL PNEUMONIA). — A particular variety of pneumonia characterized by moderate thickening of alveolar septa with plasma cell infiltration was first described in Switzerland, Germany, Italy and other European countries as occurring most often in infants a few months of age who were born extremely prematurely. More recently, attention has been focused particularly on the exudate in the lumens of the alveolar ducts and alveoli, which with hemotoxylin-eosin staining is visible as a characteristic acidophilic foamy-granular material. Only with silver impregnation or certain other stains can oval bodies be identified as responsible for the foamy

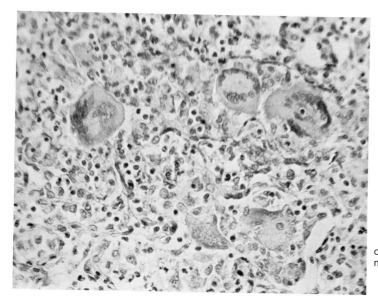

Fig. 15—22.—Giant cell pneumonia complicating measles in child aged 11 months.

appearance since they stain with neither hematoxylin nor eosin (Fig. 15—23). Whether this is a protozoan parasite or a fungus has not been definitely settled. Robbins pointed out that the organism is a slowly growing one causing no necrosis and little reactivity on the part of the host. Both lungs are usually involved.

A few cases have been reported in the United States in which the lungs have exhibited a similar exudate although the plasma cell infiltration described by the European investigators has not been a prominent feature. Most of the United States cases have been in infants slightly older than the majority of those reported from Europe and have

not been premature. The disease has been characterized by a protracted respiratory illness, and at death the lungs often have had a uniformly wooden consistency. In some instances all alveoli and alveolar ducts have been distended by typical exudate but the walls have been relatively unaffected. Gradually, over a prolonged period, focal emphysema and thickening of the alveolar walls occur. The posterior portions of the lung are most often affected. In advanced late cases emphysema is both interstitial and interlobular. Organisms are difficult to find and identify in the sputum. An open lung biopsy is usually necessary for diagnosis since the stiffness of the lungs leads to pneumothorax if nee-

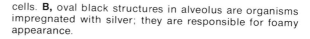

Fig. 15—23.—*Pneumocystis carinii* pneumonia. **A,** alveoli distended by uniformly granular foamy-appearing material; septa infiltrated with lymphocytes and plasma cells. **B,** oval black structures in alveolus are organisms impregnated with silver; they are responsible for foamy appearance.

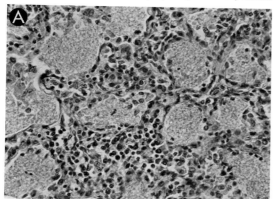

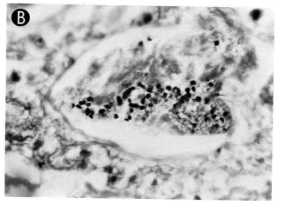

dle biopsy is attempted. Hamperl reported several cases in which alveoli contained large cells with inclusions typical of those caused by cytomegalic inclusion disease virus intermixed with exudate characteristic of that produced by *Pneumocystis carinii*. Robbins believed that, like other infections, cytomegalic inclusion disease may predispose to pneumocystis infections and that immunosuppressive drugs, disseminated tuberculosis and corticoids may alter defenses sufficiently to permit growth of the organism. On ultramicroscopic examination Barton and Campbell described the pneumocystis organism as complex, with five outer layers, nuclei, endoplasmic reticulum and mitochondria.

PNEUMONIA ALBA: SYPHILIS. — Infants of untreated syphilitic mothers who are delivered near term are often severely affected by the disease and either are stillborn or die immediately after birth. Their lungs are frequently enlarged, heavy, uniformly firm and yellow-pink. The increased weight and density result from distention of the alveolar ducts

and alveoli by macrophages and from an increase in connective tissue in the interalveolar septa (Fig. 15–24). Alveoli may have failed to develop and may be absent even in an infant at term. The pulmonary tree is then composed only of bronchi and alveolar ducts, the latter widely separated by connective tissue heavily infiltrated by different kinds of mononuclear cells. Polymorphonuclear leukocytes may also be present, but in syphilis the predominant cells in the exudate are always mononuclear. It is of interest that in a review by Oppenheimer and Hardy of recent cases of congenital syphilis in infants, most of whose mothers had had some treatment with penicillin, the lungs were involved in only 25% and none had classic pneumonia alba.

CANDIDIASIS (THRUSH). — The frequency of thrush varies in different hospitals and has been reported as occurring in 15–20% of newborn infants. Since vaginal candidiasis is present in a large proportion of women during pregnancy, most infections in infants appear to be acquired during passage through

Fig. 15–24. — Pneumonia alba due to syphilis in mature stillborn fetus. **A**, low power photomicrograph showing wide masses of connective tissue densely infiltrated by mononuclear leukocytes separating alveolar ducts. No alveoli can be identified. **B**, high power view showing macrophages filling alveolar ducts.

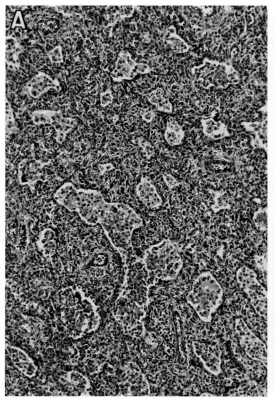
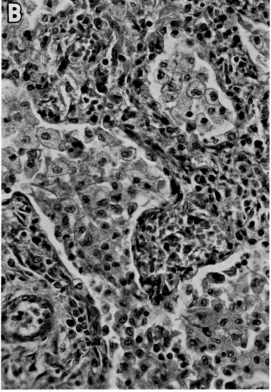

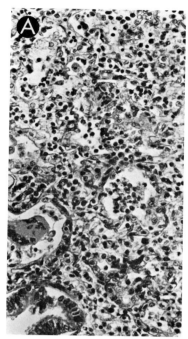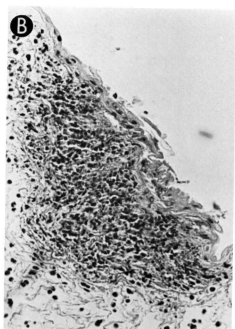

Fig. 15–25.—Congenital candidiasis of the lung in newborn infant. **A,** lung diffusely infiltrated with mononuclear cells and giant cells containing yeast forms (PAS stain). **B,** umbilical cord of same infant showing inflammation and necrosis.

the birth canal, although occasionally Candida infection of the amniotic sac is followed by aspiration pneumonia (Fig. 15–25) and organisms are often present in the bowel. The lungs are infiltrated with mononuclear and giant cells but pseudohyphae are usually rare despite a marked histiocytic response. Such lung involvement may cause death in the newborn period; Emanuel recorded 15 cases, 6 of which were in premature infants. Convulsions, apnea, cyanosis and jaundice are among the symptoms.

Pulmonary Hemorrhage

Pulmonary hemorrhage is observed not infrequently on postmortem examination of stillborn fetuses and infants who died during the 1st week of life. It may be subpleural, intra-alveolar, interstitial or perivascular and at times may involve all sites.

A few small ecchymotic hemorrhages, sometimes called "flame" hemorrhages, are often visible on the surface or deep in the substance. They are probably agonal, are presumably caused by terminal anoxia and do not differ from similar hemorrhages at other ages.

Sharply circumscribed petechiae 2–3 mm in diameter are present in great numbers beneath the visceral pleura in association with anoxia caused by premature separation of the placenta. A few similar hemorrhages may be found when anoxia results from other causes, but when present in large numbers, such petechiae are pathognomonic of separation of the placenta from the uterine wall before the infant's birth (see Fig. 7–1). Parietal pleura, epicardium and mediastinal connective tissue are usually similarly affected. The alveolar capillaries are ordinarily greatly distended with blood.

Perivascular and interstitial pulmonary hemorrhage (Fig. 15–26, A), which most often appears to be secondary to anoxia, is found more frequently in fetuses dying in utero than in liveborn infants. Hemorrhage is particularly striking in the tissues surrounding the larger bronchi and major blood vessels but may extend into the interlobular connective tissues and under the pleura. The alveoli often remain free of blood cells. The lungs of anencephalic monsters often have a severe form of this variety of hemorrhage.

Diffuse intra-alveolar hemorrhage (Fig. 15–26, B) may be observed in infants a few hours to a few days of age and is the most difficult form to inter-

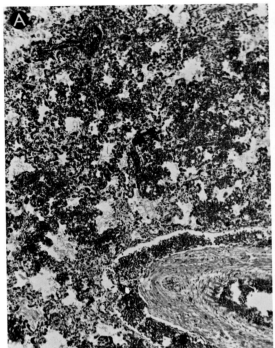

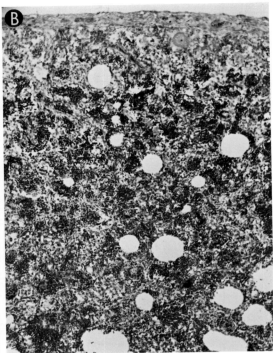

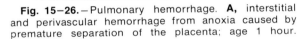

Fig. 15–26.—Pulmonary hemorrhage. **A,** interstitial and perivascular hemorrhage from anoxia caused by premature separation of the placenta; age 1 hour.

B, intra-alveolar hemorrhage of unknown cause; age 3 days.

pret. Except in erythroblastosis it is usually limited to infants with a birth weight of less than 2,000 gm. The appearance suggests that the infant drowns in its own blood but the cause of the bleeding is generally unknown. When present in infants who have not breathed independently after birth or who have breathed poorly for only a short time, there is always the possibility that the blood was of maternal origin and was aspirated during labor and delivery. It may also be a result of capillary injury produced by anoxia sustained before birth. It is found more commonly, however, in infants 3–5 days old in whom there seems less probability of anoxia being the causative agent, and under such circumstances it has been variously interpreted. A few associated conditions that have been accepted as possible causes are increased intracranial pressure, erythroblastosis with or without kernicterus, and anoxic changes in the brain (Esterly and Oppenheimer; McAdams). More doubt is expressed over the role of respiratory distress and hyaline membranes. While certain gram-negative organisms predispose to hemorrhagic pneumonia, this accounts for only a small percentage of cases of

pulmonary hemorrhage in the newborn period. Esterly and Oppenheimer reported that 40% of such hemorrhage in newborn infants occurs in the first 24 hours and two thirds within the first 48 hours after birth, but at the Chicago Lying-in Hospital such hemorrhage as a probable cause of death usually occurred somewhat later. Those who believe that hemorrhagic disease is a specific entity caused by hypoprothrombinemia due to deficiency of vitamin K consider pulmonary hemorrhage one form of this disease. Its occurrence on the 2d or 3d day coincides with the period during which prothrombin time is generally most greatly prolonged. Massive bleeding in other locations, which would be expected to occur at times at least in conjunction with pulmonary hemorrhage if it were caused by lack of vitamin K, is almost never present. Infants with erythroblastosis occasionally die suddenly of pulmonary hemorrhage on the 2d or 3d day of life even though vitamin K has been administered and hemoglobin and erythrocyte levels in the blood are adequate. The reason for this is also unexplained. Until more definite information is available concerning the etiology of the intra-alveolar hemorrhage that occurs after extrauterine existence has been well established, it seems wisest to list such cases only under intra-alveolar hemorrhage rather than to obscure them under such titles as hemorrhagic disease, hemorrhagic pneumonia and so on.

Erythroblastosis

The lungs are important organs from which to obtain contributory evidence of the existence of erythroblastosis in the infant and stillborn fetus. In the liveborn infant they are less important than in the fetus because the degree of abnormal erythropoiesis can also be estimated from other organs. In stillborn fetuses whose tissues have become partially autolyzed the pulmonary tissue retains its affinity for nuclear stains long after it is lost by the spleen, liver and most other organs. In such instances the lung may be the only tissue to yield evidence of an increased number of immature red cells (Fig. 15–27, A). Blood cells are almost never formed locally in the lungs, but the small caliber of the pulmonary capillaries seems to impede the circulation of large primitive erythroblasts, and these cells, if present in the circulating blood, stand out prominently in the capillaries of the alveolar walls (Fig. 15–27, B). Increased numbers of nucleated cells can also be observed in the larger blood vessels.

Erythroblasts and normoblasts in the pulmonary capillaries and larger blood vessels, however, are not specific evidence of erythroblastosis as they will be found whenever there is an increase in immature erythrocytes in the circulation. Such an increase may be observed in congenital syphilis, cytomegalic inclusion disease, rare anemias of unknown origin and other conditions. In our material, which includes little syphilis, the presence of erythroblasts in pulmonary capillaries has been largely limited to erythroblastosis due to maternal immunization to the Rh factor.

Tuberculosis

Lesions of tuberculosis in the lungs of stillborn infants or those who die in the early neonatal period are extremely uncommon. Tubercle bacilli are rarely present in the maternal circulation except in association with miliary tuberculosis or an acute fulminating infection, and women with such lesions seldom become pregnant. They are not present in amniotic fluid, and the few cases of tuberculosis that have been reported in infants at birth have been of hematogenous origin. The involvement of the lungs has been only incidental to miliary tuberculosis. Active tubercles, often showing large caseous centers and associated with diffuse pneumonia, have been reported. Epithelioid cells, giant cells and lymphocytes make up the tubercles of the newborn as they do of the adult.

The newborn infant is extremely susceptible to tuberculosis and, if exposed to the disease in early

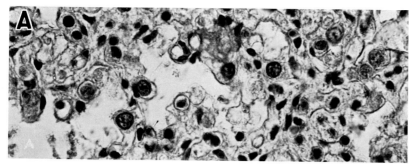

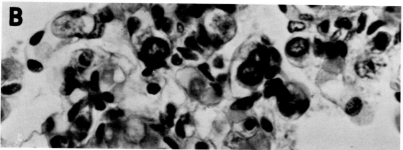

Fig. 15–27.—Erythroblastosis. A, lung from moderately macerated fetus. Largest nuclei visible are primitive erythroblasts in the pulmonary capillaries. These establish the presence of erythroblasts in the circulation and are indicative of severe extramedullary erythropoiesis. B, lung of infant 6 hours old showing erythroblasts in alveolar capillaries.

infancy, will often die in a few months. Tubercles are widespread throughout the body, but the lungs are usually more severely involved than other organs. They are often the site of abscesses and caseous, necrotizing lesions. Tuberculous pneumonia and meningitis are common complications.

Toxoplasmosis

Organisms have been reported in cells in the alveoli of a few young infants with a generalized Toxoplasma infection. Their appearance is similar to that in other locations (see Fig. 9–22).

Malformations

Malformations of the lungs are common if included under this title are minor anomalies such as incomplete separation of lobes and the reductions in size that are caused not by an abnormality of the lungs themselves but by encroachment of other organs on the space normally allotted to them. Primary malformations of the lungs sufficiently important to interfere seriously with function are rare in relation to the frequency with which malformations are observed in other major organs.

ABNORMAL SIZE

SECONDARY HYPOPLASIA.—Any condition that reduces the capacity of the thoracic cage early in fetal life will cause hypoplasia of lung tissue. To develop normally the lung must have adequate room for growth, which will be inhibited in proportion to lack of space. It has been contended that intrauterine respiration is also necessary for normal development and that absence of respiratory activity is the main cause of hypoplasia.

The three conditions most characteristically associated with pulmonary hypoplasia are diaphragmatic hernias, craniospinorachischisis and renal agenesis. Less often, idiopathic cardiac hypertrophy, large pleural effusions and polycystic kidneys have been observed. In one case observed at the Boston Hospital for Women there were no accompanying abnormalities except for absence of amniotic fluid.

Almost all of these conditions excluding renal agenesis limit the space in the chest available for growth of the lungs; with renal agenesis there is a lack of amniotic fluid. Opinions differ as to whether the diminished growth and maturation are a direct result of inadequate space or whether the primary

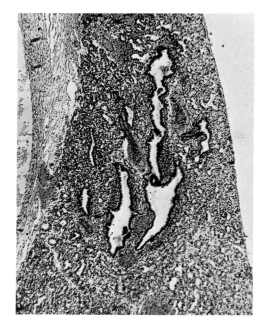

Fig. 15–28.—Hypoplastic lung of infant with eventration of the diaphragm. The bronchi are unusually prominent and lack of alveolar development causes them to be closer to the lung surface than normal.

cause is lack of intrauterine respiratory activity caused in some cases by lack of space and in others by lack of amniotic fluid. It is possible, however, that the cause may be different when hypoplasia accompanies a reduction in available space from that acting when it occurs with absence of amniotic fluid. In the former the bronchi and bronchioles are well developed and the abnormality is largely a reduction in number of alveolar ducts and alveoli. The bronchi consequently appear disproportionately numerous and close to the surface (Fig. 15–28). With renal agenesis the degree of differentiation is more variable; at times growth appears arrested at midpregnancy at about the time that alveolar development normally begins (Fig. 15–29) and at other times is moderately more advanced. The two conditions are ordinarily easily distinguishable and may result from two different causes, or the primary cause may be inhibition of respiratory activity.

PRIMARY HYPOPLASIA OR AGENESIS.—Complete agenesis of pulmonary tissue is extremely rare except in acephalous monsters who also lack a heart and upper gastrointestinal tract. In 1958, when Claireaux and Ferreira reported an otherwise normal infant with such an abnormality, they were able to find only three cases previously described. The trachea is usually also absent. (One such case

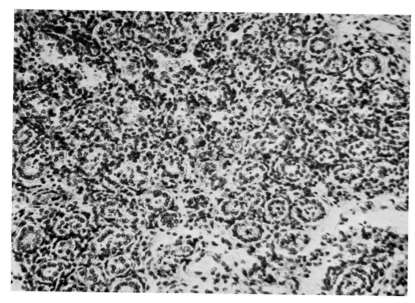

Fig. 15–29. – Lung. Extreme hypoplasia associated with renal agenesis in infant at 38 weeks' gestation. Almost no semblance of alveolar ducts or alveoli.

was observed at the Boston Hospital for Women.) Both lungs may be extremely hypoplastic and weigh only a few grams at birth (Fig. 15–30), but this too is usually found only with other severe malformations.

Fig. 15–30. – Pulmonary hypoplasia in infant with many other malformations.

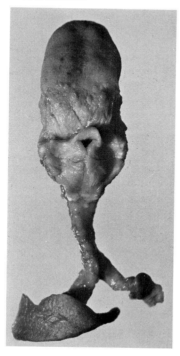

Unilateral hypoplasia is slightly more common, and in a few instances complete absence of one lung and the bronchus leading to it has been reported in otherwise normal individuals. The heart and mediastinum are pushed toward the affected side, and the existing lung becomes enlarged. Unilateral absence or hypoplasia is compatible with a normal existence in the absence of other malformations. The left lung is involved in 70% of cases and males are twice as frequently affected as females. Higher mortality is associated with absence of the left lung than with absence of the right. Tracheoesophageal fistulas or cardiac malformations were present in 13 of 17 cases collected by Booth and Berry.

HYPERPLASIA. – We have not observed this rare condition except in association with pulmonary cystic disease (see page 305).

ABNORMAL POSITION

This is always secondary to some other abnormality. A defect in the diaphragm permits the abdominal viscera to enter the thorax and displace the lungs and mediastinum into the opposite side of the chest. Unilateral pneumothorax or hydrothorax may cause a similar displacement. Situs inversus, either limited to the chest or involving all viscera, causes a reversal in position of the right and the left lungs.

Abnormalities of the parietal pleura may be responsible for abnormal position and associated hypoplasia of the lungs. Either a part or all of one lung may fail to be enclosed by pleura and may develop in an extrapleural space. Rarely, part or all of one lung is enclosed in the pericardium.

ABNORMAL LOBATION

Incomplete separation of the lobes of either lung is sufficiently common to be classed as a normal variant instead of a malformation. Partial fusion of the right upper and middle lobes is most common. Complete lack of separation into lobes is unusual, although, rarely, each lung is an undivided unit.

Division into more than the conventional number of lobes may occur. The so-called azygos lobe is an additional lobe found at the apex of either lung. The relation to bronchi is normal and the separation into an individual lobe does not interfere with function.

Infrequently, the number of lobes is reversed so that there are two on the right and three on the left.

SEQUESTERED LOBES. — Masses of pulmonary tissue sequestered from the normal lung and having no communication with the bronchial tree have been described as intralobar, extralobar or completely sequestered, depending on whether they are part of the lobe of a lung, a separate lobe but still attached to the main pulmonary mass or entirely independent of the lungs. In a few reported cases tissues believed to be respiratory in character have been found outside the pleural cavity, usually in the wall of the esophagus, stomach or intestine; rarely, the principal bronchus of this mass communicates with or is attached to the esophagus although it ends blindly in the wall. Various theories to account for the sequestration include (1) fortuitous separation of a tip of the embryonic bronchial tree with acquisition of a new blood supply by secondary attachment to some other area; (2) separation of a bronchial tip as a result of the traction of an adventitious blood supply, usually an abnormal pulmonary artery; and (3) an independent outgrowth from the entodermal tube having no connection with the normal pulmonary anlage. The intralobar sequestrations are somewhat different from the extralobar varieties and consequently have been thought by some, especially Boyden, to have a different pathogenesis. Boyden considers the presence of a systemic pulmonary artery and an intralobar area of sequestration to be coincidental and not necessarily causally related. In the intralobar variety the involvement of right and left sides is of fairly equal frequency, whereas the extralobar and complete types are largely limited to the left side and most often occur with a defect of the left leaf of the diaphragm. The arterial supply of both varieties is usually a vessel arising directly from the thoracic or abdominal aorta: the venous return of the intralobar variety is generally the normal pulmonary vein; of the extralobar variety it is the hemiazygos vein. The artery supplying an intralobar area is usually interpreted as an abnormal pulmonary artery, not as a bronchial artery. It may supply only the sequestered lobe or may also send branches into normal lung tissue. Although the intralobar masses on the right contain air and fluid, the extralobar masses on the left are usually radio-opaque. Intralobar masses may contain tissues resembling pancreas (Beskin). Infections develop commonly in the intralobar but not in the extralobar variety.

The sequestered lobe, whether in the lung or separate from it, is ordinarily composed of fairly normal-appearing pulmonary tissue showing bronchi and structures that have been interpreted as alveolar ducts and alveoli. According to Jordan, however, there are no true alveoli, and capillaries should be considered nutritive only.

Only one case belonging to this group was observed at the Chicago Lying-in Hospital. An infant with a left diaphragmatic hernia had a completely separate lobe of pulmonary tissue in the left thoracic cavity attached only by an artery arising from the aorta and a vein emptying into the inferior vena cava (Fig. 15–31, A). The lobe lay behind the heart in a hernial sac produced in the posterior mediastinum by pressure from abdominal viscera in the left side of the chest secondary to a diaphragmatic hernia. It was composed of bronchi and structures that were interpreted to be alveolar ducts. The lumens of alveolar ducts were larger than in normal lung and few alveoli could be identified (Fig. 15–31, B). It is interesting that in this case, in which there were both reduced space and complete inability of fluid to enter the pulmonary tissue, the appearance was entirely different from that associated with renal agenesis or diaphragmatic hernias. Although this was once used to support the contention that intrauterine respiration is not necessary for normal development of the lung (Potter and Bohlander), further knowledge of lung structure indicates that this tissue is not normal. Alveolar ducts are distended, and few if any normal alveoli are present. It might be concluded that lack of an escape route for fluid secreted by pulmonary tissue is responsible for hyperdistention and that this fact could be used to support the idea that the lung is a source of amniotic fluid.

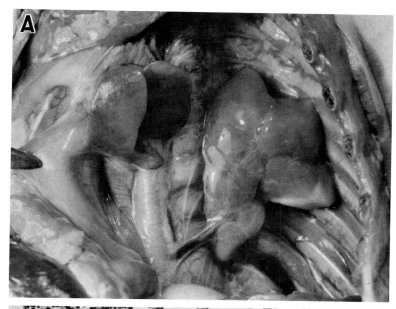

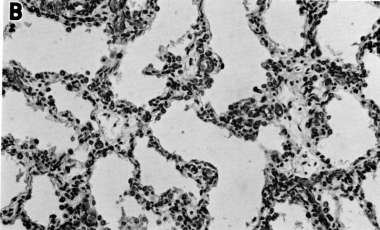

Fig. 15–31.—Sequestered portion of lung attached only by a blood vessel arising from the aorta. Hypoplasia of left lung is due to a diaphragmatic hernia. **A,** gross appearance. **B,** histologic structure showing large alveolar ducts and a few alveoli in the sequestered lobe.

ABNORMAL COMPOSITION

ADENOMATOID CYSTIC MALFORMATION OF THE LUNG.—This term is used to indicate the existence of multiple cysts of congenital origin. The lesions are more typical in fetuses who are dead at birth or infants who live only a short time than they are in older individuals in whom infection and fibrosis alter the appearance. In two cases observed at the Chicago Lying-in Hospital there was involvement of all of one or more lobes in stillborn infants. One was a severely macerated fetus with no demonstrable abnormalities except for diffuse cystic hyperplasia of the upper lobe of the right lung (Fig. 15–32).

The other was an iniencephalic fetus with tracheal atresia and involvement of all lobes of both lungs (Fig. 15–33). The cysts, which in both cases were too small to be visible to the naked eye, were composed of innumerable small cavities lined by epithelium similar to that lining the bronchi. Only a few scattered areas seemed to be alveolar ducts. The appearance resembled a great overgrowth of bronchi occurring at the expense of the portions of lung tissue that normally develop distal to the bronchi. Ch'in and Tang described this condition as a congenital adenomatoid malformation; in reviewing the literature they could find only 10 reported cases with involvement of an entire lobe and only one

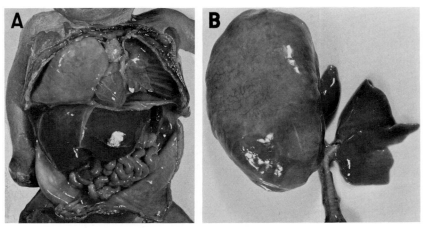

Fig. 15–32.—Cystic disease involving entire upper lobe of right lung.
A, thoracic viscera in situ. **B,** lungs removed from body.

with involvement of all lobes. In all of the reported cases generalized anasarca was also present. This was not true of the cases at the Chicago Lying-in Hospital.

Cystic changes are not always so extensive, being limited at times to a single part of one lobe (Fig. 15–34) or, less often, to several parts of a lobe. They may be isolated abnormalities or may be accompanied by abnormalities in other parts of the body. They occasionally accompany cystic disease of the

Fig. 15–33.—Cystic disease involving all lobes of both lungs in infant with iniencephaly. **A,** large submandibular masses are pulmonary tissue. **B,** viscera removed from body showing size of lungs in relation to liver, spleen and

intestine. Upper portions of the lungs that are separated by a groove from the rest of the lung tissue were present above the clavicle in the submandibular region.

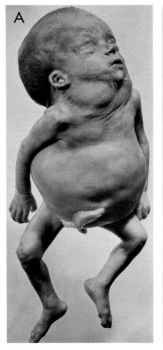
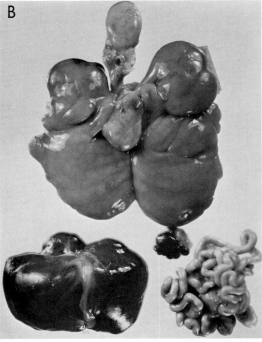

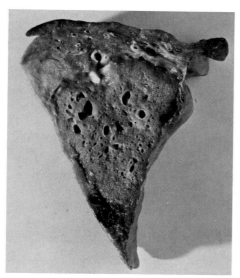

Fig. 15–34.—Cross-section of a lung removed for adenocystic disease showing sharply circumscribed area of malformation.

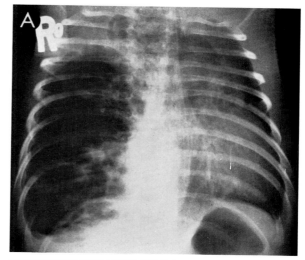

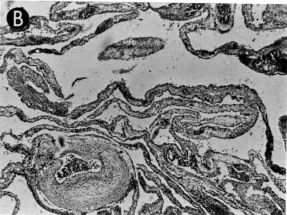

Fig. 15–35.—Unusual malformation in which the lung consists of large irregular air spaces that caused a shift in the mediastinum. **A,** roentgenogram of chest. **B,** photomicrograph of lung showing absence of normal air spaces; the walls of the cystic space contain large veins and arteries. (Courtesy Dr. A. Kashkula.)

kidneys when involving only part of the lobe. They are seldom discovered until the cysts become infected or, as sometimes happens, greatly distended with air (Fig. 15–35). A diagnosis can sometimes be made in the first hours of life because of respiratory distress and a radiographically demonstrable enlarging mass that gradually becomes more radiolucent as air enters the area. Although respiratory epithelium may be present in the larger air passages of some of these masses, a deficiency of cartilage leads to obstruction and focal emphysema.

The histologic appearance of these masses shows considerable variation. At times all cavities are lined by a bronchial type of epithelium (Fig. 15–36, A); at other times the pattern is that of the normal lung before the time of vascularization and consists of structures resembling bronchi, intermediate zones and terminal pneumomeres (Fig. 15–36, B and C). These were described by Stowens as cystic bronchiectatic type and embryonal type. Tufts of tall, columnar mucus-secreting epithelium with the appearance of gastric mucosa, when present, are diagnostic of this malformation.

Dyspnea and cyanosis are common symptoms of cystic disease and if the cysts communicate with bronchi, there may be an excessive amount of bronchial secretion. However, when the involved areas are composed only of small cavities lined by bronchial epithelium, the cysts rarely communicate with bronchi and may remain undiscovered for many years.

In a review of 46 cases Merenstein found anasarca in one third and maternal hydramnios in one fourth. It has been suggested by those who believe that the lungs actively secrete fluid before birth that this hyperplasia of lung tissue causes maternal hydramnios by overproduction of fluid.

SOLITARY CYSTS.—These are rarely found in the newborn although symptoms may be present within a few weeks of birth. Most of the solitary cysts described have contained mucus glands, smooth muscle and cartilage in the wall and have appeared to be greatly dilated bronchi. They may become distended with air if they communicate with a bron-

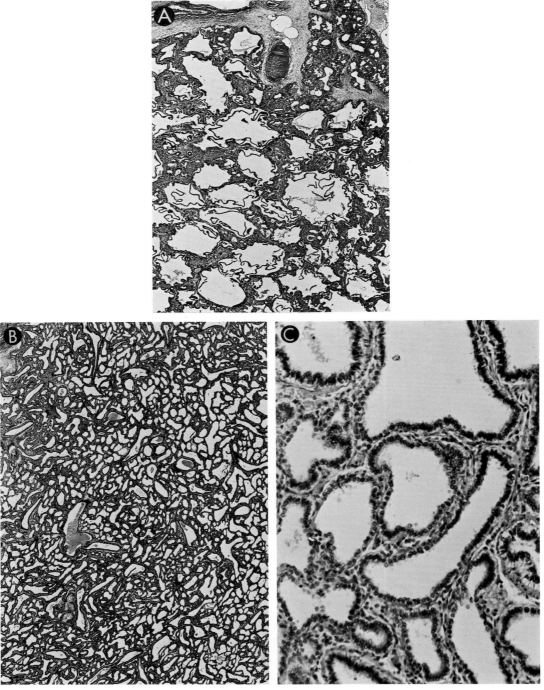

Fig. 15—36.—Cystic disease of the lungs. **A,** low power view of part of a lung in which all cavities are lined by a bronchial type of epithelium. **B** and **C,** lung from another infant showing cysts lined by three varieties of cells re-sembling those normally present in early fetal lung before the beginning of the vascularization responsible for alveolar development.

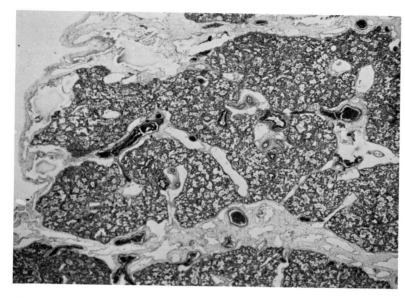

Fig. 15—37.—Lung showing enlarged, proliferated lymphatic channels in subpleural and interlobar areas. (Courtesy Dr. K. M. Laurence.)

chus and may reach such a size that compression of pulmonary tissue leads to a diagnosis of pneumothorax. On the other hand, a cyst may become filled with thick mucoid fluid and be confused with a pleural effusion. Dyspnea and cyanosis, the most common symptoms, are caused by compression of the remaining pulmonary tissue.

CONGENITAL PULMONARY LYMPHANGIECTASIA.—

Fig. 15—38.—Lobe of lung containing large amounts of striated muscle from stillborn fetus weighing 780 gm. **A,** view showing excessive numbers of large blood vessels with intervening tissue composed of striated muscle and groups of capillaries representing a rudimentary attempt at alveolar formation. **B,** view showing striations in muscle cells.

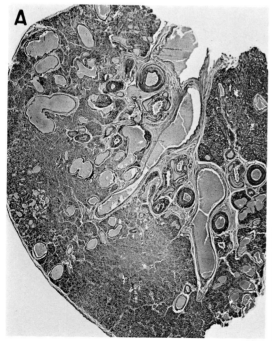

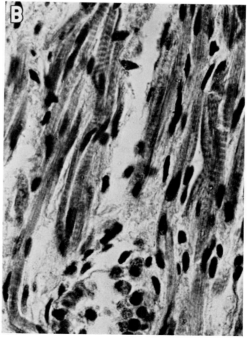

An increase in number and size of lymphatic channels in the lungs was described in 13 stillborn and newborn infants by Laurence. Ekelund *et al.* pointed out that one half of these infants are stillborn and most of the remainder die within the first few weeks of life. An occasional infant may survive for several months. In the first minutes of life the liveborn infants may breathe normally, but soon coughing, cyanosis, dyspnea and gasping supervene. Radiographically, a finely granular pattern is present throughout the lung. Grossly, the lungs have a characteristic appearance; they are large, firm and honeycombed with small smooth-walled fluid-filled cysts. These channels have a normal distribution under the pleura, in interlobar tissue and in the immediate vicinity of blood vessels but are unusually large and variably increased in number (Fig. 15–37). Microscopically, they are lined by endothelium, the adjacent connective tissue is normal and they seem to be continuous with normal lymphatics. Such areas are to be distinguished from both cystic disease of the lung, in which the cysts are lined by tissue characteristic of some part of the pulmonary tree, and from neoplastic lymphangiomas. Laurence believed that lymphatic channels are much more prominent between 14 and 20 weeks of fetal life than at term and that lymphangiectasia is a malformation in which the lymphatics maintain their early relationship to the pulmonary parenchyma.

TISSUE OF EXTRAPULMONIC ORIGIN. — Although few cases have been reported in which tissues other than those derived from the tracheobronchial anlage are present in the lungs, several such cases have been observed at the Chicago Lying-in Hospital. One of the most spectacular was discovered only on microscopic examination, and whether it involved more than the two lobes through which the sections were taken is unknown. Both lobes showed a great increase in the size and the number of blood vessels, and although the bronchi seemed fairly normal, the more distal parts of the pulmonary tree were hypoplastic and no normal alveoli could be found. In regions where blood vessels were largest and most numerous there were large interlacing masses of striated muscle cells (Fig. 15–38). This might actually be called a hemangiorhabdomyoma.

A few cases have been reported including two from the Chicago Lying-in Hospital in which small

Fig. 15–39. — Lung of anencephalic monster containing brain tissue. **A,** lung showing solid areas, the structure of which resembles brain tissue. **B,** high power view from one of the solid areas containing cells that resemble those found in the brain.

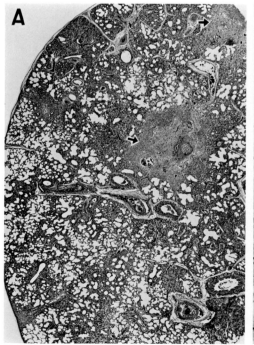
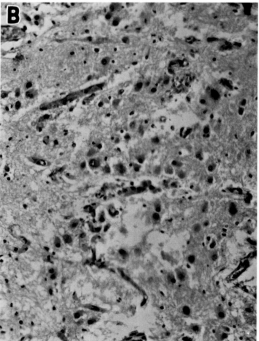

masses of brain tissue were found growing in the lungs of anencephalic monsters (Fig. 15–39). Since such changes have never been described except in anencephalic monsters, this finding suggests that destruction of the brain may have been responsible for the presence of these cells in the amniotic fluid and that the fluid may have been aspirated into the lungs with subsequent implantation and growth of the cells.

Embolism of brain tissue to the pulmonary arteries was found by Fobes and Hirst in a newborn infant after breech extraction and application of forceps to the after-coming head. There was a tear in the great vein of Galen but no evidence of cranial bleeding.

Small masses of tissue resembling fetal adrenal cortex have also been observed in the lungs. In one stillborn fetus with a widespread neuroblastoma, masses of tumor cells were present.

Other Pulmonary Disorders

INFANTILE CONGENITAL LOBAR EMPHYSEMA. — Leope and Longino described a condition of focal overexpansion of part of the lung with compression of the surrounding parenchyma (Fig. 15–40). Such tension emphysema arises from a unidirectional valvular obstruction of the air spaces. The etiology—in cases in which one could be identified—was deficient cartilage, redundant bronchial mucosa, alveolar fibrosis from previous infection, aberrant blood vessels or bronchial stenosis.

Onset of symptoms is ordinarily within the first 4 months of life; when the onset is very early, the symptoms are usually severe and operation may be necessary. Because only the emphysematous area is ordinarily removed, the causative abnormality is seldom defined. In fatal cases the affected lobar segment may show alveolar walls thickened by an increased amount of immature collagen. Jones et al. pointed out that congenital heart disease is frequently associated (8 of 14 patients). Some mild restriction of pulmonary function may be expected even in patients treated surgically (Demuth and Sloan).

THE PULMONARY SYNDROME OF MIKITY-WILSON. — This process is even less well defined than is the more localized condition of lobar emphysema. Mikity and Wilson described a diffuse lung lesion in small premature infants (1,123 gm mean weight) who, soon after birth, developed progressive dyspnea, tachypnea and cyanosis leading to chronic pulmonary insufficiency and right heart failure. Failure to thrive and recurrent pulmonary infec-

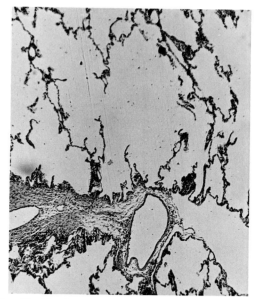

Fig. 15–40.—Surgical specimen from an infant with congenital lobar emphysema. The alveoli and alveolar ducts are greatly distended.

tions completed the picture. The lungs of such infants are voluminous and hyperaerated, with a reticular pattern and multiple small cysts demonstrable by x-ray (Baghaassarian). Physiologically, the lungs have reduced compliance and increased resistance to inspiratory and expiratory flow. After death they have a hobnail appearance when hyperinflated; microscopically, there may be many small cysts, and alveoli may be emphysematous and have thickened walls. Smooth muscle cells about the bronchioles are hypertrophied. Suspected cases examined at the Boston Hospital for Women have not been identifiable by pathologic means. In the collected series of Swyer et al. 10 of 22 infants died. This syndrome is believed to be distinct from the sequelae of the respiratory distress syndrome, cystic fibrosis of the pancreas and familial fibrocystic pulmonary dysplasia.

FAMILIAL FIBROCYSTIC PULMONARY DYSPLASIA. — In 1959 Donahue et al. described a familial form of pulmonary disease having many features of the adult Hamman-Rich syndrome. Dyspnea, fever or feeding problems may occur as early as 3 days. The course is remittent but progressive, with increasing respiratory distress requiring oxygen administration for relief. The course is more rapidly fatal in infants with onset of symptoms before 6 months than after 2 years of age (Hooft et al.).

At autopsy the lungs are heavy, with cystic em-

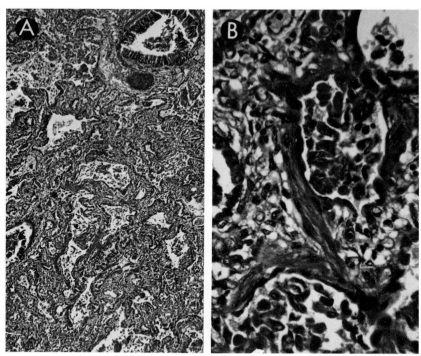

Fig. 15–41.—Lung of infant who died at 2 months of fibrocystic pulmonary dysplasia. The alveolar ducts are lined by metaplastic epithelium that is partially desquamated into the lumens. Some ducts are irregularly dilated. No normal alveoli are visible. **A,** low magnification show-ing diffuse involvement. **B,** high magnification showing fibrous tissue beneath capillaries with diffuse increase in interstitial connective tissue. Hyperplastic duct epithelium largely desquamated.

physematous areas intermixed with rubbery, firm white areas. The alveolar walls are thickened by bands of fibrous tissue or smooth muscle that lie beneath the capillaries. Many alveoli are lined by cuboidal metaplastic epithelium. Macrophages and desquamated cells are present in the alveolar lumens (Fig. 15–41), and occasionally there are microabscesses or chronic inflammation in the interstitium. Death may be caused by congestive heart failure.

The familial distribution of cases suggests a genetic metabolic disorder. In some families inheritance appears to be by an autosomal dominant gene (Kack).

PULMONARY ALVEOLAR PROTEINOSIS.— This is usually considered a disease of adults but was diagnosed in two infants at the age of 3 months by Wilkinson *et al.* Both had progressed normally for about 1 month, then began to vomit and cough and stopped gaining weight. Respiratory rate was increased; pulmonary roentgenograms showed evidence of hyperaeration with a reticular pattern of infiltration and numerous rounded lucent areas in one infant and a diffuse increase in density in the other. Cardiac rate increased, dyspnea developed and one had fever. Following a gradual progression of symptoms one died at the age of 13 weeks and the other at 18 weeks. At autopsy the lungs of both weighed more than twice the normal, and in both the cells lining the alveoli were unusually prominent and alveolar spaces were distended with a granular, eosinophilic, PAS-positive substance containing acicular spaces and infiltrated with numerous macrophages. In one, inclusion bodies characteristic of cytomegalic inclusion disease were found in the lungs, kidneys and salivary glands. A third case of an infant who died at 30 months with a similar although more protracted illness was reported by the same authors. Autopsy findings were similar to those of the younger infants except that intranuclear inclusions characteristic of herpes simplex virus infection were present in the lungs, liver and adrenal glands. The cause of the pulmonary changes is unknown.

Trachea and Larynx

The larynx and trachea are rarely the site of pathologic changes demonstrable after death. Passage of a tracheal catheter for resuscitation may infrequently cause mild congestion of the larynx, but there is seldom evidence of actual trauma.

Noisy respiration (stridor) may be caused by unusual flaccidity of the epiglottis or by abnormality of the vocal cords. Temporary paralysis of one or both vocal cords has been observed on several occasions in association with such symptoms. A laryngeal web or a stenosing diaphragm that obstructs breathing most often lies at the level of the vocal cords, less commonly above or below.

Tracheal tumors are rare but, when present, are found most often in the upper third of the trachea and are principally papillomas, fibromas or angiomas. They are usually associated with a brassy cough and respiratory difficulty.

Compression of the trachea by mediastinal cysts (see Fig. 12–42) may cause respiratory embarrassment with or without stridor. Such cysts, most often present near the bifurcation of the trachea, are usually thin-walled structures lined by mucus-secreting cells. An enlarged thymus rarely if ever causes compression of the trachea.

The trachea may be occluded by cartilage immediately below the level of the vocal cords. Such a malformation was observed at the Chicago Lying-in Hospital in three infants, all of whom had a solid mass of cartilage approximately 3 mm thick ex-

tending across the entire larynx at this level. Upper and lower surfaces were covered by normal tracheal epithelium. In two cases a hairlike canal connecting the upper and lower segments was present posteriorly in the midline (Fig. 15–42, A); pulmonary development was normal except that the alveolar duct lumens were slightly larger than usual (Fig. 15–42, B). The other case was that of the infant with pulmonary cystic disease mentioned earlier.

Sudden Death in Infancy

The occurrence of sudden death in infancy is all too frequent. In material from the city of Copenhagen, Geertinger found that the syndrome was present in one third of all infants dying between 2 and 4 months of age, which period covers the peak incidence of the phenomenon. As infant deaths due to diarrhea and pneumonia decrease, this syndrome becomes more significant.

The history of such infants is usually unremarkable; either they are without symptoms (33% in Adelson's series) or have only mild symptoms such as fussiness or coryza. The usual history is that the infants are found lifeless in bed in the morning with no recognized acute events such as struggling or crying. They are usually found on the back or side; in the latter case blood-stained fluid may be found about the nose and mouth.

At autopsy the lungs have some abnormality in over 70% of cases, but changes are usually of doubt-

Fig. 15–42.—Cartilaginous obstruction of trachea in infant weighing 1,130 gm. **A,** cartilage has been split through the center. A channel less than 1 mm wide connects pharynx and trachea. **B,** lung showing pulmonary development. Material in the lumens has been precipitated by fixative in which lungs were immersed.

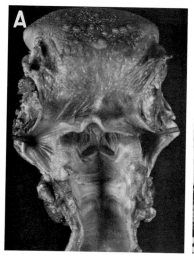
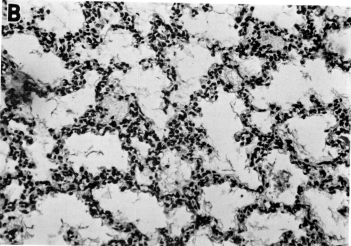

ful significance and are rarely considered sufficient in themselves to have caused death. The lungs may be hyperemic and have focal intra-alveolar hemorrhages and edema or changes that may suggest asphyxia, with petechiae in the thymus and pleura. Occasionally there may be subepiglottic edema. Interstitial pneumonia with thickening of the alveolar walls and a mononuclear cell infiltrate may be found; more rarely the infiltrate is peribronchial in distribution. In a few cases evidence of undiagnosed Coxsackie virus infection or endocardial sclerosis has been found in the heart. In some series undiagnosed congenital heart or central nervous system diseases have been the cause of the unexpected death, but the "sudden death syndrome," as now defined, includes only those cases with the minimal findings listed above (Bergman *et al.*). The etiology is unknown; many causes such as mild allergy, virus infections, vasovagal syndrome and laryngospasm have been suggested but none is widely accepted.

There are a few epidemiologic facts that may be important in the eventual identification of a cause. At times there seems to be a strong familial incidence. The syndrome occurs more frequently among twins and a few instances of simultaneous death of both members of a twin pair have been reported. It is most common in the lowest socioeconomic groups and is more common among infants of low birth weight than in the general population at risk; this tendency may account for its greater frequency among twins.

REFERENCES

Adair, F. L., and Potter, E. L.: Evidence of intrauterine death of the fetus, Am. J. Med. Jurisprudence 2:252, 1939.

Adams, F. H., Desilets, D. T., and Towers, B.: Control of flow of fetal lung fluid at the laryngeal outlet, Respir. Physiol. 2:302, 1967.

Adams, J. M.: Sudden death in infants due to pneumonia, J. Pediatr. 23:189, 1943.

Adams, J. M.: Third epidemic of primary virus pneumonitis among infants in Minnesota, Lancet 65:192, 1945.

Adelson, L.: Specific Studies of Infant Victims of Sudden Death, in Wedgewood, R. J., and Benditt, E. P. (eds.): *Sudden Death in Infants* (Seattle: University of Washington Press, 1963), p. 11.

Anderson, G. J., *et al.:* Congenital bacterial pneumonia, Lancet 2:585, 1962.

Anderson, W. R., and Strickland, M.: Pulmonary complication of oxygen therapy in the neonate, Arch. Pathol. 91:506, 1971.

Avery, M. E.: *Lung and Its Disorders in the Newborn Infant* (2d ed.; Philadelphia: W. B. Saunders Co., 1968).

Baghaassarian, O. M., Avery, M. E., and Neuhauser, E. B. D.: Form of pulmonary insufficiency in premature infants. Pulmonary dysmaturity, Am. J. Roentgenol. 89: 1021, 1963.

Barnard, W. G., and Day, T. D.: Development of the terminal air passages of the human lung, J. Pathol. Bacteriol. 45:67, 1937.

Barton, E. G., Jr., and Campbell, W. G.: Further observation on the ultrasource of pneumocystis, Arch. Pathol. 83:527, 1967.

Becroft, D. M. D.: Histopathology of fatal adenovirus infection of respiratory tract in young children, J. Clin. Pathol. 20:561, 1967.

Bergman, A. B., Beckwith, J. B., and Ray, C. G.: *Sudden Infant Death Syndrome* (Seattle: University of Washington Press, 1970).

Bernstein, J., and Wong, J.: The pathology of neonatal pneumonia, Am. J. Dis. Child. 101:350, 1961.

Beskin, C. A.: Intralobar enteric sequestration of the lung containing aberrant pancreas, J. Thorac. Cardiovasc. Surg. 41:314, 1961.

Booth, J. B., and Berry, C. L.: Unilateral pulmonary agenesis, Arch. Dis. Child. 42:361, 1967.

Boss, J., and Craig, J. M.: Reparative phenomena in lungs of neonates with hyaline membranes, Pediatrics 29:891, 1962.

Boyden, E. A.: Bronchogenic cysts and the theory of intralobular sequestration: New embryologic data, J. Thorac. Surg. 35:604, 1958.

Burger, R. A.: Agenesis of the lung, Am. J. Dis. Child. 73: 48, 1947.

Chasler, C. N.: Pneumothorax and pneumomediastinum in the newborn, Am. J. Roentgenol. 91:550, 1964.

Chernick, V., and Avery, M. E.: Spontaneous alveolar rupture at birth, Pediatrics 32:816, 1963.

Ch'in, K. Y., and Tang, M. Y.: Congenital adenomatoid malformation of one lobe of a lung with general anasarca, Arch. Pathol. 48:221, 1949.

Claireaux, A. E., and Ferreira, H. P.: Bilateral pulmonary agenesis, Arch. Dis. Child. 33:364, 1958.

Corbett, D. P., and Washington, J. E.: Respiratory obstruction in newborn and excess pulmonary fluid, Am. J. Roentgenol. 112:18, 1971.

Craig, J. M.: Distensibility curves and expansion patterns of newborn lungs, Am. J. Dis. Child. 106:174, 1963.

Craig, J. M., Fenton, K., and Gitlin, D.: Obstructive factors in pulmonary hyaline membrane syndrome in asphyxia of the newborn, Pediatrics 22:847, 1958.

Davies, P. A.: Congenital pneumonia, Arch. Dis. Child. 37:598, 1962.

Davis, M. E., and Potter, E. L.: Intrauterine respiration of the human fetus, J.A.M.A. 131:1194, 1946.

Demuth, G. R., and Sloan, H.: Congenital lobar emphysema: Long-term effects and sequelae in treated cases, Surgery 59:601, 1966.

Devi, B., and More, J. R. S.: Total tracheopulmonary agenesis, Acta Paediatr. Scand. 55:107, 1966.

Donahue, W. L., *et al.:* Familial fibrocystic dysplasia and its relation to Hamman-Rich syndrome, Pediatrics 24:786, 1959.

Ekelund, H., Palmstierna, S., and Ostberg, G.: Congenital pulmonary lymphangiectasia, Acta Paediatr. Scand. 55: 171, 1961.

Emanuel, B.: Pulmonary candidiasis in the neonatal period, J. Pediatr. 61:44, 1962.

Enders, J. F., McCarthy, K., Mitus, A., and Cheathem, W. J.: Isolation of measles virus at autopsy in cases of giant cell pneumonia without rash, N. Engl. J. Med. 261:875, 1959.

Esterly, J. R., and Oppenheimer, E. H.: Massive pulmonary hemorrhage in the newborn. Pathologic considerations, J. Pediatr. 69:3, 1966.

Esterly, J. R., and Oppenheimer, E. H.: Primary pulmonary hemorrhage in the newborn. Clinical considerations, J. Pediatr. 69:11, 1966.

Farber, S., and Sweet, L. K.: Amniotic sac contents in lungs of infants, Am. J. Dis. Child. 42:1372, 1931.

Fobes, C. D., and Hirst, A. E.: Brain embolism to the lung, J.A.M.A. 218:735, 1971.

Gajdusek, D. C.: *Pneumocystis carinii:* Etiologic agent of interstitial plasma cell pneumonia of premature and young infants, Pediatrics 19:543, 1957.

Geertinger, P.: *Sudden Death in Infancy* (Springfield, Ill.: Charles C Thomas, 1968).

Giammalvo, J. T.: Congenital lymphangiomatosis of the lung: A form of cystic disease, Lab. Invest. 4:456, 1955.

Gitlin, D., and Craig, J. M.: Nature of the hyaline membrane in asphyxia of the newborn, Pediatrics 17:64, 1956.

Glaser, J., and Epstein, J.: Empyema of the newborn, Am. J. Dis. Child. 41:110, 1931.

Glaser, J., Landau, D. E., and Heatley, C. A.: Subglottic laryngeal stenosis in infancy, Am. J. Dis. Child. 50: 1203, 1935.

Gleissner, P., Asante, F., and Schubert, G. E.: Congenital pulmonary lymphangiectasias, Dtsch. Med. Wochenschr. 94:1987, 1969.

Goodlin, R. C., and Rudolph, A. M.: Tracheal fluid flow and function in fetuses in utero, Am. J. Obstet. Gynecol. 106:597, 1970.

Goodpasture, E. W., *et al.*: Virus pneumonia of infants secondary to epidemic infections, Am. J. Dis. Child. 57:997, 1939.

Gregg, R. H., and Bernstein, J.: Pulmonary hyaline membranes and respiratory distress syndrome, Am. J. Dis. Child. 102:871, 1961.

Gruenwald, P.: Course of respiratory distress syndrome of newborn infants as indicated by poor stability of pulmonary expansion, Acta Paediatr. Scand. 53:470, 1964.

Gruenwald, P.: Exaggerated atelectasis of prematurity, Arch. Pathol. 86:81, 1968.

Hamperl, H.: Pneumocystis infection and cytomegaly of the lungs of newborn and adult, Am. J. Pathol. 32:1, 1956.

Hanna, E.: Bronchoesophageal fistula with total sequestration of the right lung, Ann. Surg. 159:599, 1964.

Hooft, C., *et al.*: Le syndrome d'Hamman-Rich dans l'enfance, Arch. Fr. Pediatr. 21:413, 1964.

Horowitz, R. N.: Extra-lobar sequestration of lung in newborn infant, Am. J. Dis. Child. 110:195, 1965.

Howard, R. M., and Sheldon, W. H.: Pneumocystic pneumonia, Am. J. Dis. Child. 95:18, 1958.

Huxtable, K. A., Tucker, A. S., and Wedgewood, R. J.: Staphylococcal pneumonia in childhood, Am. J. Dis. Child. 108:262, 1964.

Jones, J. L., *et al.*: Lobar emphysema and congenital heart disease in infancy, J. Thorac. Cardiovasc. Surg. 49:1, 1965.

Jordan, H.: Respiratory malformations, Am. Rev. Tuberc. 53:57, 1946.

Kack, B.: Familial fibrocystic pulmonary dysplasia, Can. Med. Assoc. J. 92:801, 1965.

Landing, B. H.: Anomalies of the respiratory tract, Pe-

diatr. Clin. North Am. 4:73, 1957.

Laufe, L. E., and Stevenson, S. S.: Pulmonary hyaline membrane syndrome: Some effects of O_2 and amniotic fluid pathogenesis, Obstet. Gynecol. 8:451, 1956.

Laurence, K. M.: Congenital pulmonary lymphangiectasis, J. Clin. Pathol. 12:62, 1959.

Le Tan-Vinh, Couchard, A. M., and Vu Trieu Dong: Lymphangiectasies pulmonaires congenitales et lymphangite pleuro-pulmonaire cancereuse metastatique de l'enfant, Arch. Fr. Pediatr. 21:165, 1964.

Leope, L. L., and Longino, L. A.: Infantile lobar emphysema, Pediatrics 34:246, 1964.

Loosli, C. G., and Potter, E. L.: Pre- and postnatal development of the respiratory portion of the human lung, Am. Rev. Respir. Dis. 80:5, 1959.

MacGregor, A. R.: Pneumonia in the newborn, Arch. Dis. Child. 14:323, 1939.

Macklin, C. C., and Macklin, M. J.: Pulmonic Interstitial Emphysema and Its Sequelae: An Anatomical Interpretation, in *Essays in Biology* (Berkeley: University of California Press, 1943).

McAdams, A. J.: Pulmonary hemorrhage in the newborn, Am. J. Dis. Child. 113:255, 1967.

Merenstein, G.: Congenital cystic adenomatoid malformation of lung. Report of a case and review of literature, Am. J. Dis. Child. 118:772, 1969.

Morgan, T. E.: Pulmonary surfactant, N. Engl. J. Med. 284:1185, 1971.

Morrow, G., III, Hope, J. W., and Boggs, T. R., Jr.: Pneumomediastinum, a silent lesion of newborn, J. Pediatr. 70:554, 1967.

Naeye, R. L.: Children at high altitude; pulmonary and renal abnormalities, Circ. Res. 16:33, 1965.

Naeye, R. L.: Pulmonary arterial abnormalities associated with hyaline membrane disease, Am. J. Pathol. 48:867, 1966.

Nash, G., Blennerhassett, J. B., and Pantoppidan, H.: Pulmonary lesions associated with oxygen therapy and artificial respiration, N. Engl. J. Med. 276:368, 1967.

Nelson, N. M.: On the etiology of hyaline membrane disease, Pediatr. Clin. North Am. 17:943, 1970.

Northway, W. H., Jr., Rosan, R. G., and Porter, D. Y.: Pulmonary disease following respiratory therapy of hyaline membrane disease, N. Engl. J. Med. 276:357, 1967.

Oppenheimer, E. H., and Hardy, J. B.: Congenital syphilis in newborn infant: Clinical and pathological observations in recent cases, Johns Hopkins Med. J. 129:63, 1971.

Outerbridge, E. W., Nogrady, M. B., Beaudry, P. H., and Stern, L.: Idiopathic respiratory distress syndrome. Recurrent respiratory illness in survivors, J.A.M.A. 123: 99, 1972.

Ovenfors, C. O.: Pulmonary interstitial emphysema, Acta Radiol. [Diag.] [Suppl.] (Stockh.) 224:1, 1964.

Potter, E. L.: Respiratory disturbances in the newly born infant, Ill. Med. J. 83:100, 1943.

Potter, E. L., and Bohlender, G.: Intrauterine respiration in relation to the development of the fetal lung, Am. J. Obstet. Gynecol. 42:14, 1941.

Potter, E. L., and Davis, M. E.: Perinatal mortality: The Chicago Lying-in Hospital, 1931–1966, Am. J. Obstet. Gynecol. 105:335, 1969.

Potter, E. L., and Rosenbaum, W.: The association of mild external hydrocephalus with death in the early days of life, Am. J. Obstet. Gynecol. 45:822, 1943.

Potter, E. L., and Young, R.: Heterotopic brain substance found in the lung, Arch. Pathol. 34:1009, 1942.

Robbins, J. B.: *Pneumocystis carinii* pneumonitis — a review, Pediatr. Res. 1:131, 1967.

Robertson, R., and James, E. S.: Congenital lobar emphysema, Pediatrics 8:795, 1951.

Rudolf, A. M., *et al.:* Patent ductus arteriosus. A clinical and hemodynamic study of 23 cases in the first year of life, Pediatrics 22:892, 1958.

Shepard, E. M., *et al.:* Residual pulmonary findings in clinical hyaline membrane disease, N. Engl. J. Med. 279:1063, 1968.

Smith, C. A.: Intrapulmonary pressures in the newborn infant, J. Pediatr. 20:338, 1952.

Smith, R. A.: Theory of origin of intralobar sequestration of the lung, Thorax 11:10, 1956.

Snyder, F. A., and Rosenfeld, M.: Intrauterine respiratory movement of the human fetus, J.A.M.A. 108:1946, 1937.

Snyder, F. F.: *Obstetric Analgesia and Anesthesia* (Philadelphia: W. B. Saunders Co., 1949).

Soergel, K. H., and Sommers, S. C.: Idiopathic pulmonary hemosiderosis and related syndromes, Am. J. Med. 17:25, 1962.

Spencer, H.: *Pathology of the Lung* (Oxford: Pergamon Press, 1968).

Spock, A., Schneider, S., and Bayler, G. J.: Mediastinal gastric cysts: A case report and review of the literature, Am. Rev. Respir. Dis. 94:97, 1968.

Stein, J.: Hamartoma of lung, Am. J. Surg. 89:439, 1955.

Stowens, D.: *Pediatric Pathology* (2d ed.; Baltimore: Williams & Wilkins Co., 1966).

Stowens, D.: Sudden unexpected death; a major problem in infancy and early childhood, Arch. Pathol. 61:341, 1956.

Strang, L. B.: Uptake of Fluid from the Lung at Start of Breathing, in *Development of Lung, Ciba Foundation Symposium* (New York: Longman, 1967), p. 348.

Swyer, P. B., *et al.:* The pulmonary syndrome of Mikity-Wilson. Pediatrics 36:374, 1965.

Tannenberg, J.: Fetal and postnatal atelectasis, Am. J. Clin. Pathol. 32:305, 1959.

Thomson, J., and Forfar, J.: Regional obstructive emphysema in infancy, Arch. Dis. Child. 33:97, 1956.

Towers, B.: The Fetal and Neonatal Lung, in Assali, N. (ed.): *Biology of Gestation* (New York: Academic Press, 1968).

Usher, R., *et al.:* Respiratory distress syndrome in infants delivered by caesarean section, Am. J. Obstet. Gynecol. 88:806, 1964.

Wessel, M. A.: Chylothorax in a 2-week-old infant with spontaneous recovery, J. Pediatr. 25:201, 1944.

Wilkinson, R. H., Blanc, W. A., and Hagstrom, J. W. C.: Pulmonary alveolar proteinosis in three infants, Pediatrics 41:510, 1968.

Wilson, M. G., and Mikity, V. G.: A new form of respiratory disease in premature infants, Am. J. Dis. Child. 99:489, 1960.

16

Thymus and Glands of Internal Secretion

Thymus

THE THYMIC PRIMORDIA originate during the latter part of the 6th gestational week as hollow pear-shaped outgrowths from the entoderm of the third pharyngeal pouches. As they migrate down into the neck they lose their lumens and become solid masses of small cells. Gradually the cells lose their compact arrangement, take on a reticulum-like structure and are slowly invaded by lymphocytes. The thymus grows by sending out branches in all directions and soon assumes a lobulated pattern. The peripheral portions of the lobules become more densely infiltrated by lymphocytes, and the inner medullary portions, which make up the central cores holding the lobules together, show a proportionately greater growth of reticulum.

In the young fetus the lobules are small and are separated by loose connective tissue, permitting the branching character of the gland to be easily visualized (Fig. 16–1, A). As the fetus approaches term, the lobules become larger due especially to a proportionate increase in the lymphocyte mass (Fig. 16–1, B). Hassall's corpuscles, made up of small groups of acidophilic cells arranged in a whorl-like pattern around small central areas of hyalinization or necrosis, appear in the medulla in small numbers early in intrauterine life but are not conspicuous until some time after birth. Myeloid cells, especially eosinophilic myelocytes, are often present in interstitial tissues during the latter part of fetal life. They disappear soon after birth, as they do from other areas such as the portal triads in the liver, where they are a temporary source of leukocytes.

The primitive gland migrates down to a position in the midline of the upper part of the chest between the sternum and the heart. The two parts of the gland, which arise from the right and left pharyngeal pouches, are held together by loose connective tissue but usually are easily separated. Each consists of an upper lingual portion that passes behind the sternal notch and ends 1 cm or so below the thyroid isthmus, and a broader triangular mass covering the great vessels and base of the heart (see Fig. 6–8). The thymus is closely adherent to both the sternum and the pericardium and ordinarily encircles the innominate vein. By careful dissection it can be separated from these structures leaving it and the parts to which it was attached both intact.

The gland is soft and its shape is largely a result of its position. The thickest part, found just below the junction of the lingual portions with the lower triangular parts, lies over the area where the great vessels arise from the heart. The size is extremely variable; it normally increases gradually throughout intrauterine life, the average weight being 11 gm in newborn infants weighing 3,500 gm. Almost any disturbance, however, may cause a decrease in size. In infants who die during labor or immediately after birth it is ordinarily of maximum size and always heavier than the average. It is smaller in macerated fetuses of comparable weight and in infants who die of any cause a few days after birth.

Until recently no function had been found for the thymus, but it is now believed to play two roles in immunity. In the first, it acts as a "way station" for lymphoid cells thought to arise in the bone marrow and reticular tissue that proliferate here and then

317

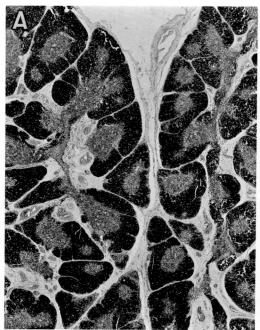
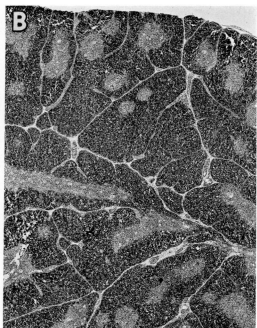
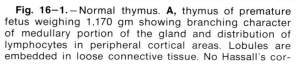

Fig. 16—1.—Normal thymus. **A,** thymus of premature fetus weighing 1,170 gm showing branching character of medullary portion of the gland and distribution of lymphocytes in peripheral cortical areas. Lobules are embedded in loose connective tissue. No Hassall's cor-puscles. Weight of thymus 5 gm. **B,** thymus of mature fetus weighing 3,365 gm showing relative increase in volume of cortical portions and decrease in interlobular connective tissue. The few Hassall's corpuscles are very small. Weight of thymus 17 gm. Same magnification.

pass on to the lymph nodes and spleen. The cells are small "T" lymphocytes that are involved in tuberculin and delayed hypersensitivity reactions and transplant rejection. They populate the paracortical regions of the lymph nodes after passing through the thymus; there they show a marked lymphoblastic response to foreign tissues when previously sensitized to the appropriate antigen. The second role is less certainly defined, but the thymus is thought to be responsible for a humoral influence that acts on the peripheral lymphoid tissues to stimulate the development of preplasma and plasma cells. These in turn supply the humoral antibody of the globulin system. The cells that are under this thymic influence are found in the germinal centers and medulla of the lymph nodes.

Absence of all or specific anatomic elements, or a deficiency of either function, gives rise to various syndromes related to immunologic deficiency (Good).

HYPOPLASIA AND INVOLUTION

The thymus, like nearly every other organ in the body, may fail to form, partially or completely.

Such alterations are to be distinguished from involutionary changes, which may occur before or after birth at a slow or rapid rate.

The most obvious failure of thymic formation is found in *DiGeorge's syndrome,* in which other derivatives of the third and fourth pharyngeal pouches such as the parathyroids may also be absent. Other malformations are frequently present in the same region as well as elsewhere in the body. They include esophageal atresia, a right or absent arch, tetralogy of Fallot, interventricular septal defects, shortened upper lip, micrognathia and narrowed palatal arch (Kretschmer; Gilmour). As a result of the lack of a thymus affected infants have an abnormal immunologic apparatus. Their lymph nodes and spleen contain germinal centers and plasma cells but the deep cortical and perivascular peripennicilar cell concentrations are deficient in adult lymphocytes. Although serum immunoglobulin levels are normal, the humoral responses to antigen stimulation are variably deficient. The cellular responses involved in the delayed hypersensitivity reaction, such as the tuberculin reaction, are absent. Absence of parathyroids is responsible for hypocalcemic tetany, and even though this may be satisfactorily treated, death usually results from some type of infection. This constellation of anatomic and functional deficiencies does not appear to be genetically determined.

In partial failure of thymic differentiation, such as that seen in the genetically determined autosomal *Swiss or sex-linked agammaglobulinemias,* the thymus is small and lacks lymphoid cells (small thymocytes) and Hassall's corpuscles (Fig. 16–2) (Hitzig; Gitlin and Craig). Lymphoid cells are depleted or absent in the circulation and peripheral lymphoid organs (Fig. 16–3). The circulating gamma globulins are either absent or markedly deficient. Humoral responses to antigen are generally lacking, and delayed hypersensitivity reactions do not occur. The thymus is made up of large thymocytes, large cells with vesicular nuclei that are capable of a macrophage response and that remain after small thymocytes are lost during involution of the thymus. In a related form of disease, *Netzeloff's syndrome,* general findings are similar but circulating immunoglobulins may be normal.

In the syndrome of *ataxia-telangiectasia* (Louis-Bar syndrome), which is an autosomal recessive genetic disorder, immunologic defects develop in three fourths of all affected individuals during the 1st year; these are manifested by repeated respiratory infections involving sinuses, bronchi and lungs (Peterson *et al.*). Immunoglobulin A, secreted by the mucous cells of the affected organs, is decreased. Both humoral and cellular responses to antigens may be abnormal. The thymus is reported to be small, absent or lacking in normal corticomedullary division and Hassall's corpuscles. The lymphoid tissues are variably deficient in plasma cells, germinal centers and lymphocytes. The dilatation of blood vessels, which gives the disorder its name, may eventually become widespread, with skin, conjunctivae and cerebellum most often involved. However, vascular changes rarely begin the 1st year of life. Symptoms attributable to the central nervous system also usually do not become apparent until after the 1st year. The cerebellar lesion consists primarily of an absence of Purkinje cells in the telangiectatic areas with associated atrophy of the adjacent internal granular layer (Thieffry *et al.*).

The above disorder with absent, hypoplastic or dysontogenic thymic structure and lack of peripheral lymphocytes is associated with severe humoral (agammaglobulinemia) and cellular delayed hypersensitivity immune deficiencies. They are in contrast to the *Bruton type of agammaglobulinemia* in which the thymus and circulating lymphocytes are normal but germinal centers and plasma cells in the lymph nodes, intestine and spleen are decreased.

INVOLUTION. — In a healthy person the thymus does not ordinarily involute until puberty. With disease, infection, malnutrition or states associated with excessive adrenal glucocorticoid discharge, involution may occur at any time following the development of well-defined cortical and medullary layers and Hassall's corpuscles.

Fig. 16–2. — Thymus of infant with lymphopenic form of agammaglobulinemia. **A,** the lobules of the thymus are small and lack small lymphocytes and Hassall's corpuscles. **B,** high power view. (Courtesy Dr. David Gitlin.)

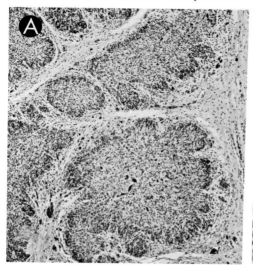
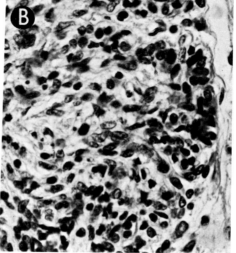

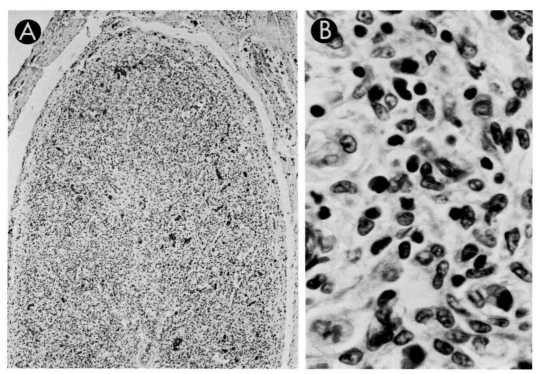

Fig. 16–3.—Lymph node of infant with lymphopenic form of agammaglobulinemia. **A,** the cortex and medulla are poorly differentiated and contain few lymphocytes and no germinal centers. **B,** high power view. A few plasmacytoid cells are present. (Courtesy Dr. David Gitlin.)

The earliest evidence of mild involution can be recognized in the medulla by pyknosis and beading of the nuclei of the small thymocytes. In more rapidly progressing involution the small cortical thymocytes undergo the same changes, and if involution is protracted, macrophages appear among the large thymocytes. Because of the loss of thymocytes Hassall's bodies seem more numerous (Fig. 16–4). In very chronic states of malnutrition Hassall's corpuscles may become cystic. In rare instances massive destruction of small thymocytes produces large masses of disintegrated nuclear material that later calcifies because of the high phosphate content of the nuclear elements (Fig. 16–5). In more active states of involution Hassall's corpuscles swell and become infiltrated with polymorphonuclear leukocytes. As the process advances, the loss of small thymocytes leads to encroachment of the medulla on the cortex until the dense layer of cortical cells completely disappears. During the most active involutionary periods similar pyknosis of lymphocytes can be recognized in the spleen and lymph nodes, particularly in young infants.

Involutionary changes, when recognized, may give a clue to the presence of a chronic state of stress such as intrauterine anoxia or malnutrition. Since involution is largely mediated by glucocorticoid secretion from the adrenal glands, conditions in the newborn in which the adrenal glands are enlarged, such as erythroblastosis or maternal diabetes, are characteristically associated with smaller than normal thymuses.

SYPHILIS.—Syphilis ordinarily produces a characteristic form of atrophy. The connective tissue is very dense and seems to replace the peripheral portions of the lobules so that only sharply marginated areas made up largely of medullary tissue remain (Fig. 16–6, A). Very rarely, nonspecific lesions called Dubois' abscesses are present. Located in the medulla and usually multiple, they consist of cavities lined by an irregular layer of squamous epithelial cells and filled with polymorphonuclear leukocytes (Fig. 16–6, B). They are Hassall's corpuscles that have become cystic and heavily infiltrated with leukocytes in the process of involution. The necrotic cavities may be visible on gross inspection.

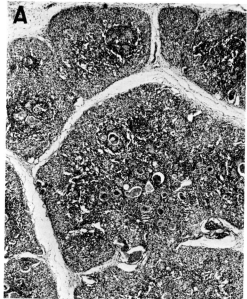

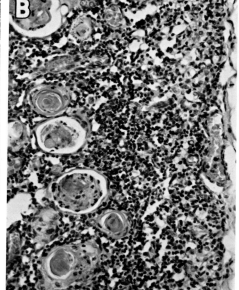

Fig. 16–4.—Involuted thymus from infant aged 5 days weighing 2,850 gm who died of pneumonia. Gland is small and weighs only 4 gm as a result of loss of lymphocytes due to acute involution. Hassall's corpuscles are increased in size and prominence. No increase in connective tissue. **A,** low power view showing lack of demarcation between cortex and medulla. **B,** high power view showing structure of Hassall's corpuscles and proportionate decrease in lymphocytes.

Not infrequently, small areas of liquefaction are found in an otherwise normal thymus as a result of postmortem degeneration. These may be erroneously diagnosed as Dubois' abscesses on gross examination but are easily distinguished microscopically by the absence of squamous epithelial cells and polymorphonuclear leukocytes.

HYPERPLASIA

Hyperplasia of the thymus in times past was often considered a cause of sudden death in the neonatal period either by compressing the trachea or by inducing some occult disturbance generally designated status thymicolymphaticus. The fact that the function of the gland was unknown was probably responsible for its frequent indictment as the cause of sudden infant deaths. Years ago, when the small thymus of the sick infant was believed to be the normal size, the discovery of a nonatrophic (and normal) thymus in any infant who had not been ill led to the assumption that the gland was hypertrophied. Large-scale x-raying of the chest to determine thymic size led to many diagnoses of enlarged thymus, and since lymphoid tissue shrinks under x-ray therapy, it was usually recommended that the gland be so treated. In some communities the diagnosis is still made and x-ray therapy still given. However, recent studies have indicated that little benefit results from this procedure and that more infants who receive x-ray therapy for an enlarged thymus develop carcinoma of the thyroid in adolescence and die of leukemia than those who have not been so treated.

Most infants with so-diagnosed enlargement of the thymus show spontaneous regression in the size of the gland if left untreated (Fig. 16–7).

When the chest of a newborn infant is examined by x-ray, it is extremely important that the roentgenograms be taken in the true anteroposterior diameter. Even slight rotation may show an apparent enlargement of mediastinal structures, leading to an erroneous diagnosis of thymic or cardiac enlargement (Fig. 16–8). Whether the infant is quiet or crying also affects the apparent width of the upper mediastinum, and two successive films may show a striking difference in the size of what is interpreted as the thymus.

Among the 12,000 autopsies on infants under 1 year of age at the Chicago Lying-in Hospital the

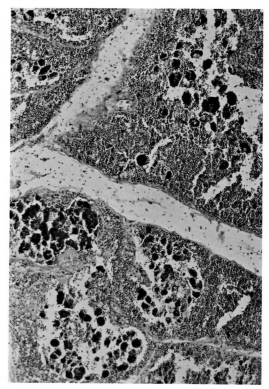

Fig. 16–5.—Thymus showing complete involution with calcium encrusting degenerated nuclear material in the medulla. Infant aged 8 months.

thymus has never shown enlargement that might have led to death.

ANENCEPHALY.—Moderate hyperplasia of the thymus is common in anencephalic monsters. The anteroposterior diameter is ordinarily increased, and although the gland often weighs less than that of a normal infant, it is large in relation to total body weight. An increase in size of individual lobules from unusually wide cortical zones is histologically characteristic. Because of the close approximation of the margins of the individual lobules the branching character of the gland is never visible. This change in the thymus appears to be related to the lack of adrenocorticotropic hormone (ACTH) discharge by the pituitary and the small adrenal glands of such infants.

TUMORS

Lymphoblastomas of the thymus gland have been reported in older individuals and in rare instances in infants. The majority have been composed principally of immature lymphocytes, and symptoms have usually been limited to those caused by pressure on adjacent organs.

ANOXIA

The thymus, since it lies in a protected retrosternal position, is almost never a site of direct mechanical injury and does not show diffuse confluent hemorrhage or other signs of trauma. However, petechial hemorrhages in the cortex are invariably associated with the anoxia resulting from abruptio placentae and occasionally, although in smaller numbers, with anoxia from other causes. They are small, sharply circumscribed hemorrhages visible grossly on the surface and in the substance of the gland (see Fig. 7–2). Similar hemorrhages are ordinarily present simultaneously under the visceral and parietal pleura and epicardium.

Hypophysis

The hypophysis is composed of two portions, each arising from an independent source and each developing its own specific functions. The two parts are in no way related except by anatomic proximity.

The primordium of the anterior lobe (pars distalis) is an ectodermal projection arising as an extension of the stomodeal depression anterior to the oral membrane known as Rathke's pouch. It grows upward in the midline toward the infundibular process of the floor of the diencephalon.

The primordium of the posterior lobe (pars neuralis) is a downward projection of the floor of the diencephalon known as the infundibular process. The upward growth of Rathke's pouch and the downward growth of the infundibular process bring the terminal portions of the growing structures in close apposition, one immediately behind the other. The posterior lobe, like the anterior lobe, is of ectodermal origin, but its derivation from cells already differentiated into nervous tissue gives it a structure similar to that of other portions of the nervous system. The two parts of the gland lie one behind the other in the sella turcica at the base of the skull.

The anterior wall of Rathke's pouch becomes markedly thickened and makes up the greater part of the gland. The posterior wall fuses with the anterior surface of the infundibular process and develops into the intermediate lobe (pars intermedia). The lumen of Rathke's pouch may persist as a narrow slit called the residual lumen, which separates

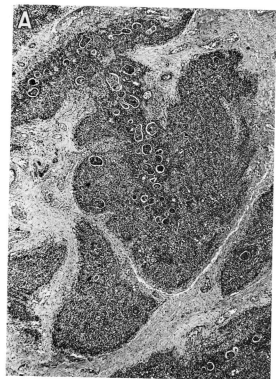
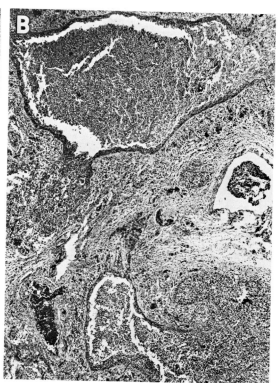

Fig. 16–6.—Syphilis involving thymus of two mature stillborn fetuses. **A,** lobules are small, distinction between cortex and medulla is lost and the interlobular connective tissue is increased in extent and density. Involution is nearly complete. **B,** Dubois' abscesses. The central portions of Hassall's corpuscles have become cystic and are filled with leukocytes and granular debris.

the anterior lobe from the fused intermediate and posterior lobes.

The anterior lobe gradually differentiates during intrauterine life into a structure quite similar to that found in the adult (Fig. 16–9). It is composed of many large, closely packed polyhedral cells separated by a richly anastomosing network of capillarylike vessels. At birth acidophilic cells are fairly

Fig. 16–7.—Wide shadow with rounded margins in upper mediastinum usually diagnosed as hypertrophy of thymus. **A,** normal newborn infant who received no therapy. X-ray 6 months later showed normal thymus. **B,** infant of 2 months with noisy respirations and slight wheezing cough. No therapy. Chest x-ray 3 months later showed normal mediastinum; no change in symptoms.

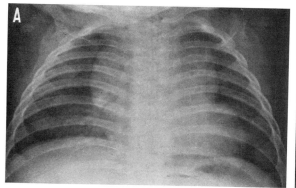
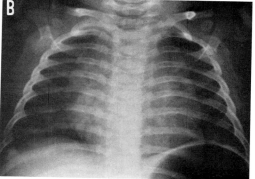

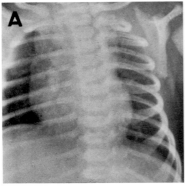 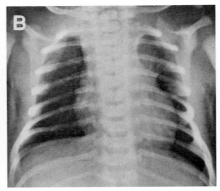 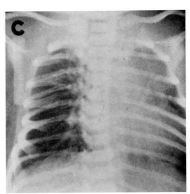

Fig. 16–8.—Three views of chest of newborn infant showing apparent change in contour of mediastinum as a result of rotation. **A,** rotation to right. **B,** direct anteroposterior view. **C,** rotation to left.

Fig. 16–9.—Normal hypophysis in mature newborn infant. Anterior lobe is composed largely of eosinophilic and chromophobe cells separated by connective tissue containing numerous sinusoidal blood vessels. The vessels cannot be distinguished because of the small amount of blood they contain. The intermediate lobe contains several small glandlike structures lined by cuboidal cells and is separated from the anterior lobe by a cleft (residual lumen). Posterior lobe is attached to intermediate lobe and is composed of neurosecretory cells.

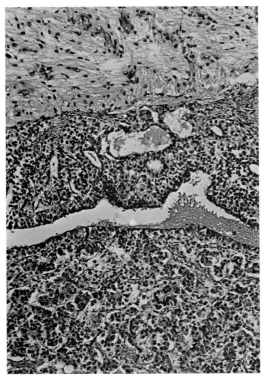

numerous but there are few basophilic cells. The remaining cells are not typically chromophobic, although they contain no specific granules, but appear instead to be undifferentiated; most can be expected to develop along specific lines later. The anterior lobe has many functions, two of the most important being its regulatory effect on the growth and maturation of bones and its stimulating effect on the gonads. The hormones responsible for these effects appear to be elaborated before birth, and the newborn hypophysis actually contains more growth hormone than does the adult. However, acidophilic cells, which are thought to produce this hormone, are not increased (Russfield).

At birth the anterior surface of the intermediate lobe is covered by a single layer of prominent cuboidal cells. Several small cavities lined by similar cells are present in the adjacent tissue. It is a relatively narrow portion of the gland and its posterior surface is attached to the posterior lobe.

The posterior lobe is composed of cells and fibers resembling neuroglia. Blood vessels are small and inconspicuous. This lobe secretes hormones capable of causing an elevation of blood pressure and contraction of uterine muscle.

Few pathologic changes are known to occur in the hypophysis before or immediately after birth. The principal abnormalities are associated with anoxia or anencephalus. With anoxia the vessels in the anterior lobe become engorged with blood, and at times the distention is so great that the cells seem to be compressed into small groups as a result of diffuse hemorrhage. Actually the blood is contained in the endothelial-lined channels, and only a simulated, not a real, hemorrhage is seen. Similar changes may be found at the same time in the thyroid and adrenal glands.

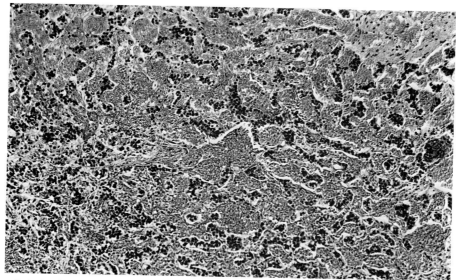

Fig. 16–10.—Anterior lobe of hypophysis of an anencephalic monster showing compression of cellular elements (small groups of dark cells) by greatly distended sinusoids.

In anencephalic monsters the hypophysis frequently cannot be identified grossly but can sometimes be found in microscopic sections of the usual site or within the occipital bone (Fig. 16–10). The vascular channels are ordinarily greatly distended and the cells compressed into small cords. The appearance is an exaggeration of that sometimes found after death from anoxia.

Absence of the hypophysis has also been observed in newborn infants without anencephalus. Whenever the hypophysis is absent the adrenal glands are abnormal: they are extremely small, lack fetal cortex and resemble miniature adult glands. Most infants with normal brains do poorly and die without specific symptoms at a few days of age. Accompanying malformations are seldom present.

Duplication of the hypophysis, sella turcica and stomatodeal structures has been described as a minimal attempt at twinning.

Thyroid Gland

The thyroid gland originates during the 3d gestational week as a diverticulum from the floor of the pharynx. It rapidly becomes bilobed and descends in the neck by elongation of the tissue attaching it to the pharynx. This stalk is known as the thyroglossal duct. The gland soon loses its connection with the pharynx but the point of origin may remain visible as the foramen caecum, which is a depression in the posterior portion of the tongue. The thyroglossal duct normally resorbs but, rarely, remains patent entirely or in part and may be responsible for cysts or a fistulous tract in the midline of the neck anterior to the hyoid bone.

In its early development the thyroid is immediately adjacent to the heart and great vessels. With further growth the heart descends and becomes removed from the region of the thyroid. Occasionally, portions of thyroid tissue are carried down with the heart and small masses consequently may be found in the thoracic cavity. Rarely, the whole gland is substernal. The close association of the primordia of the parathyroid glands, thymus and thyroid is responsible for the location of the parathyroid glands on the surface or in the substance of the thyroid and also for the occasional presence of nodules of thymic tissue in the thyroid or on its surface.

Initially the gland consists of solid cords of cells whose branching is responsible for the lobular structure of the fully developed organ. These cords are gradually hollowed out to form small follicles that become filled with acidophilic material known as colloid (Fig. 16–11). At birth the cells lining the follicles are composed of a moderate amount of colorless cytoplasm surrounding small central nuclei. The cytoplasm often bulges into the lumens of the follicles, giving the colloid a scalloped margin. The follicles at the periphery of the lobules usu-

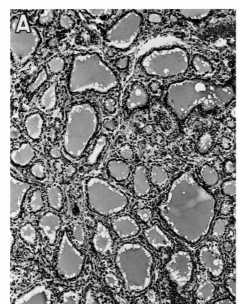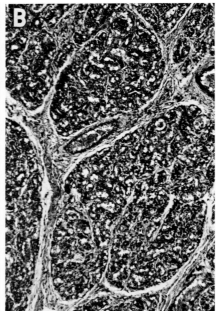

Fig. 16–11.—Thyroid gland at birth. **A,** normal gland weighing 2 gm. Acini are lined by secretory cuboidal cells and filled with colloid. Rich vascular bed is normally present between the acini, but here the vessels are col-lapsed and cannot be individually distinguished. **B,** gland weighing 14 gm. No colloid is present and acini are reduced in size and increased in number.

ally contain more colloid than those in the center.

The gland is highly vascular, and large numbers of small vessels are present between the follicles. Usually they contain only a moderate amount of blood and are relatively inconspicuous. At times, however, they become intensely engorged and the intervening follicles are so compressed that identification of the gland is difficult. This is especially true if postmortem degeneration is also present.

The size of the thyroid gland seems to vary in different localities. In areas with a high incidence of thyroid disease the weight of the thyroid at birth is often increased. For example, weights of 5–7 gm with an average well over 3 gm were found in the mid twenties in Minneapolis by Adair (unpublished data) in contrast to a maximum weight of 3 gm at the Chicago Lying-in Hospital in later years.

Occasionally, thyroid glands of normal weight in normal infants fail to contain colloid and the lumens are filled with loosely arranged, large cuboidal cells. These have been variously interpreted, but it seems probable that they result from postmortem degeneration. One suggestion that this is a change due to a sudden thyrotropic hormone discharge seems untenable because the change is also found in infants with anencephalus and little or no hypophyseal tissue.

Inadequacy of thyroid function may be due to many causes but all produce the same changes in affected infants. During intrauterine life sufficient thyroid secretion reaches the fetus through the placenta to permit normal development, and even though the thyroid gland itself may be enlarged, the infant's appearance at birth is usually normal. Within a few weeks characteristic changes begin to appear and become progressive unless replacement therapy is instituted. An infant with manifestations of an absence of thyroid secretion is known as a cretin. The retarded bone growth is associated with myxedema, thickened dry skin, coarse hair, constipation and a reduced basal metabolic rate. Myelinization of major neural pathways in the brain is delayed and mental retardation becomes evident (Fig. 16–12, A). Replacement therapy often produces dramatic results, and if treatment is started early enough, development usually proceeds normally (Fig. 16–12, B).

ABSENCE OF THYROID GLAND.—This is the most common cause of lack of thyroid secretion in cases of "sporadic" cretinism. It is not genetically determined and consequently is not repeated in subsequent pregnancies. Radioscanning technics demonstrate the absence of the gland. According to Little *et al.*, thyroid tissue is commonly present (23 of 39

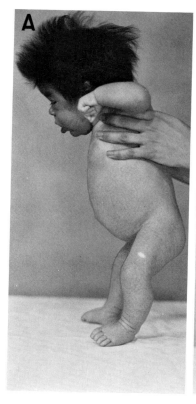 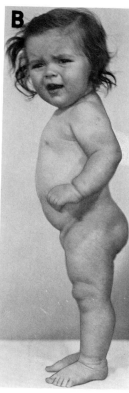

Fig. 16–12.—Absence of thyroid gland. **A,** infant aged 1 month showing characteristics of cretinism: hair coarse and bushy, skin thick and dry, mouth held open and expression dull and apathetic. **B,** normal appearance at age 13 months following thyroid therapy. (Courtesy Dr. Rustin MacIntosh.)

cases studied) at the base of the tongue or above the level of the cricoid bone. Unfortunately, the amount is insufficient to prevent cretinism.

ENLARGEMENT OF THE THYROID GLAND (GOITER)

FAMILIAL GOITER.—Thyroid enlargement is found at birth or in the 1st year of life in two forms of genetically determined metabolic block to the uptake of iodine, thyroxin formation or release. In *Pendred's syndrome* of familial goiter with deafness the defect may be present at birth but is not associated with myxedema or local symptoms other than the thyroid enlargement. The gland is hyperplastic, has little colloid and is composed of many small follicles lined by columnar epithelium having some infolding into the lumen. Malignant degeneration may occur. The metabolic defect is associated with a slowed release of hormone (Stanbury).

A second familial metabolic defect is caused by lack of iodotyrosineiodenase. A goiter develops in the 1st year and the infant becomes cretinous. The glands are multinodular and intensely hyperplastic but have some areas containing colloid (Stanbury).

In other forms of familial goiter the patients may be cretins and although the glands are probably hyperplastic at birth, they do not become significantly enlarged until later.

CONGENITAL GOITER DUE TO EXOGENOUS INFLUENCES.—Such enlargements are usually mild but may be great enough to interfere with breathing and necessitate surgical intervention. They arise from three general causes: (1) Administration of large amounts of iodine to the mother, as for an expectorant, may cause a block in iodine uptake in the fetus and produce thyroid enlargement. Such thyroids either have large colloid-filled acini or small acini with hyperplasia of the columnar lining epithelium (Fig. 16–13). The infants are euthyroid. (2) In maternal Graves' disease, when antithyroid drugs are given, the newborn may have a large hyperplastic goiter and show some retardation of bone development (Burrow). Infrequently, it may be cretinous. Samuels *et al.* reported a euthyroid mother with previous thyroidectomy and the persistent exophthalmos of severe Graves' disease who gave birth to an infant with an enlarged and hyperplastic thyroid gland. They speculated that this resulted from passage of thyroid-stimulating hor-

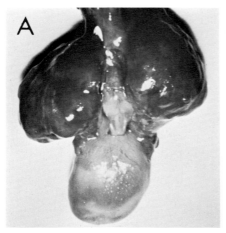

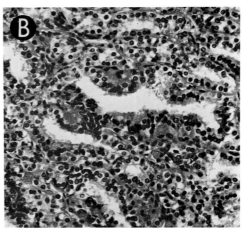

Fig. 16–13.—Marked hyperplasia of the thyroid gland in a newborn infant whose mother received iodides in pregnancy. **A,** gross appearance showing great enlarge- ment of both lobes. **B,** microscopic section composed of cellular acini that contain almost no colloid.

mone or thyroid-stimulating hormone-releasing factor across the placenta. (3) Para-aminosalicylic acid given to the mother for tuberculosis, or cobalt such as the hematinic Roncovite given for anemia, may cause marked microfollicular hyperplasia with sufficient enlargement and encroachment on the airway to threaten life. The latter drug may also impose a metabolic block on the conversion of iodine to thyroxin (Sommers). Probably any drugs given to the mother in doses large enough to cause goiter in the fetus will cause some hypofunction. All such goiters disappear in the first months after birth. The thyroid gland of one infant born at the Chicago Lying-in Hospital whose mother had received propylthiouracil for hyperthyroidism was considerably enlarged at birth, but the size gradually diminished and was normal at 3 months. It was not associated with any abnormality in development.

ENDEMIC GOITER.—Hypothyroidism, usually attributed to a lack of iodine in the water, is endemic in some parts of the world and in such areas is often also associated with enlargement of the thyroid (Schamaun). It has been stated that in certain parts of Switzerland the first generation of children born in an endemic area are mildly affected and are considered myxedematous, while the second generation—delivered by myxedematous women—are often cretins.

In cases of nutritional goiter in the mother the goitrous infant, if euthyroid, will have a hyperplastic gland with small follicles; if he is hypothyroid, follicles will be large and colloid storage marked (Louw).

Parathyroid Glands

The four parathyroid glands arise as bilateral outgrowths of the third and fourth pharyngeal pouches and migrate downward to lie on the surface of the thyroid gland near the upper and lower

Fig. 16–14.—Normal parathyroid gland from newborn infant composed of interlacing cords of cells (chief cells) separated by interstitial blood vessels and connective tissue.

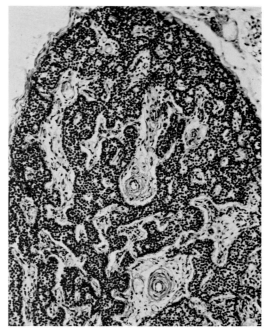

poles. They are frequently embedded in the thyroid, and since at birth they measure only 1–2 mm in diameter, are difficult to distinguish on gross examination. Nodules attached to the thyroid that can be detected grossly often prove to be small masses of thymic tissue. In the newborn the glands are composed of large, pale and polyhedral cells with small compact central nuclei known as "chief" cells. They are arranged in solid masses that have numerous small lacunae containing sinusoidal blood vessels Fig. 16–14. In the adult, acidophilic "oxyphil" cells are also present but do not appear until about the 10th year of life. The glands produce the hormone parathormone, which is important in calcium and phosphorus metabolism. It influences the liberation of calcium into the blood and controls phosphorus excretion in the urine by action on tubular resorption.

Disturbances in the action of these glands is rare in infancy, with the exception of temporary hypofunction leading to tetany. Only a few abnormal conditions have been described.

HYPERPLASIA

Primary hyperplasia most often results from tumor formation but is virtually unknown in infants. Secondary hyperplasia most commonly results from chronic renal disease, rickets or bone tumors, and this too is rare inasmuch as these conditions seldom exist in infants. The osteitis fibrosa cystica that may be found in older individuals as a result of the excessive activity of the glands in association with chronic renal disease also does not occur because renal disease in infants usually results from maldevelopment and causes death before secondary changes take place.

HYPOPLASIA

The parathyroid glands are almost never absent except in DiGeorge's syndrome (see section on thymus) in which the derivatives of the third and fourth branchial pouches fail to develop. Since the difficulties arising from the immunologic defects caused by the failure of thymic development are more difficult to treat than is the absence of parathyroid secretion, these infants die from infection more often than from tetany.

Hypoparathyroidism is seen in childhood in certain auto-immune glandular deficiency syndromes which include the thyroid, adrenal and ovary, but such syndromes are rarely found in the 1st year of life, perhaps because of the incompletely developed function of the immunologic apparatus. When present, the parathyroid glands are infiltrated with lymphocytes, and glandular parenchymal cells are gradually lost.

TETANY OF THE NEWBORN

This results from a lowered level of ionized calcium in the body fluids and hypofunction of the parathyroid glands, except in DiGeorge's syndrome, and is rarely associated with observable pathology in the gland structure.

Bakwin, who found the serum calcium content of infants on the 2d or 3d day of life to be lower than at birth, concluded that this was caused by a physiologic hypofunction of parathyroid glands. Saville and Kretchmer found the frequency greater following traumatic than normal delivery and suggested that stress at birth could cause increased adrenal gland secretion that might be a contributing factor. It is also said to occur most often in infants born by cesarean section, those of diabetic mothers and in premature babies. If infants with unstable calcium metabolism receive excessive amounts of phosphates from an endogenous source either as a result of liberation during the physiologic starvation of the newborn or by the ingestion of cow's milk, which contains six times as much phosphorus as human milk, hypocalcemia may result.

In older infants lack of vitamin D has the same sensitizing effect as parathyroid deficiency in the newborn, and in vitamin-D-deficient states excessive ingestion of phosphates may also cause hypocalcemia. Lack of vitamin D does not appear to be associated with tetany in the newborn, for the administration of this vitamin is not followed by a return of serum calcium to a normal level as it is later in infancy.

Another cause of tetany in infants is alkalosis resulting from hyperventilation, loss of chloride ions through vomiting and ingestion of large amounts of bicarbonate.

The clinical picture of tetany is not specific, but the diagnosis should be suspected and the serum calcium content estimated whenever abnormal irritability, exaggerated facial and peroneal reflexes, twitchings or convulsions appear. Projectile vomiting, laryngospasm, carpopedal spasm and edema have also been reported as characteristic of tetany. According to Shannon, edema of the brain may be caused by hypocalcemia; it causes symptoms identical to those of intracranial hemorrhage and is possibly responsible for symptoms of intracranial hemorrhage in infants who recover without residual damage.

The normal level of blood calcium is usually stated to be between 9 and 11 mg/100 ml. Symptoms are not invariably present with a serum calcium content of less than 8 mg/100 ml, nor is a low serum calcium value always associated with hyperirritability. It is possible that the amount of ionizable or usable calcium is reduced even though the total calcium content is normal and that this may explain apparently normal calcium levels in infants with symptoms of tetany.

Adrenal Glands

DEVELOPMENT

The adrenal glands are derived from two sources and, like the hypophysis and pancreas, are actually two glands combined in a single capsule. The outer, cortical layer is derived from mesodermal cells situated near the cephalic pole of the mesonephros. These cells are first visible at about the 8 mm stage; slightly later, at about the 12 mm stage, other smaller cells are formed that gradually spread out over the surface of the original mass. The smaller cells develop into the definitive cortex; the larger, more central cells become the fetal or provisional cortex, which rapidly disappears after birth. The inner, medullary portion of the gland arises from ectodermal cells that migrate down from the neural crest and are first visible at about the 14 mm stage. They originally form a mass on the medial aspect of the cortical portion of the gland but gradually become completely surrounded by the cortex. They are part of a widespread system of cells of similar origin located in close proximity to the sympathetic ganglions and along the lower portion of the aorta. The early cells have deeply staining nuclei with little cytoplasm and poorly defined walls that are similar to the immature neuroblasts found in neuroblastomas arising in the adrenal gland. The more mature cells are larger, are stained brown by chromic acid salts and consequently are called chromaffin cells. They secrete epinephrine, norepinephrine and other catecholamines, and although these substances have been demonstrated early in fetal life, the amount secreted is very limited until after birth. The total mass of chromaffin tissue in the adrenal gland is proportionately much less in the fetus and newborn than it is later in life.

The inner part of the cortical portion of the gland is known as the provisional or fetal cortex. It develops rapidly and is relatively more advanced during the first half of pregnancy than are the other abdominal and thoracic organs. Before birth it is made up of a thick layer of anastomosing cords of large polyhedral acidophilic cells that merge with the more basophilic cuboidal cells that form a thin outer zone under the capsule and will become the definitive cortex. The provisional cortex has a rich sinusoidal blood supply, and endothelium-lined channels separate the cells into cords that usually are only one cell thick (Fig. 16–15). In conjunction with the placenta, it is capable of producing a wide variety of steroids including mineral and glucocorticoids. The provisional cortex has no recognized homologue in any other species and is not equivalent to the x-zone that appears near maturity in the mouse and rat.

The peripheral part of the cortex maintains a fairly uniform thickness during the last few months of pregnancy. The several layers are not well differentiated and the glomerular, fascicular and reticular portions cannot be specifically identified. The inner, provisional cortex continues to grow as long as the fetus remains in the uterus, but immediately after delivery it begins to retrogress. No other organs in the body except the uterus and the mammary gland grow in this manner. The interstitial cells of the testis hypertrophy and become active in the 2d and early 3d trimester of pregnancy, but unlike the adrenal fetal cortex, which involutes only after birth, the interstitial cells become inactive before birth. The growth of the uterus and mammary glands is attributable to maternal estrogen secretion; the trophic hormones supporting the provisional adrenal cortex must include fetal pituitary ACTH as well as maternal luteinizing hormone.

The function of the provisional cortex has not been established but it seems probable that it produces a precursor steroid that passes to the placenta for conversion to estriol. This is suggested by the fact that maternal estriol excretion is greatly reduced when the fetus is anencephalic, inasmuch as such fetuses lack a normal fetal zone. Some increase in estriol excretion may be seen with maternal diabetes and severe erythroblastosis, in both of which the fetal zone of the adrenal is generally enlarged if the fetus is in good condition. Bolande called attention to the presence of hemorrhage and vacuolar degeneration in the adrenal cortex of postmature and small-for-date neonates. The mothers of such infants excrete less estriol than the normal for the period of gestation but this may result in part from depression of steroidogenesis in the placenta as well as from depressed function of the fetal adrenal.

The average weight of the adrenal glands at birth in the 3,400 gm infant is about 5 gm each. They grow in proportion to body size, however, and in two infants at the Chicago Lying-in Hospital weighing about 6,500 and 6,800 gm at birth the combined weight of the adrenals in each was 20 gm.

In small premature infants who weigh only 1,200–1,500 gm, and whose adrenal glands weigh about 2 gm, the inner zone shows progressive degeneration beginning immediately after birth, as it does in those weighing a great deal more. This zone behaves as if it has a definite function before birth that ceases immediately after delivery, and since it no longer has a purpose to serve, promptly disappears.

By the 2d or 3d day after birth the outer portion of the cortex, which will persist and become the definitive cortex of the older individual, is often fairly well set off from the inner fetal zone. The inner cells become pale and vacuolated and gradually disappear, causing a general shrinkage of the gland. For a time some of the stroma remains and for several months makes up a gradually diminishing mass of connective tissue filling the space between the medulla and the definitive cortex.

In infants with fatal infections or severe shock the fetal cortex may be infiltrated with polymorphonuclear cells, and necrosis of the parenchymal cells may produce a more rapidly progressive change than is seen in normal involution. Inflammation does not occur during the normal involutionary processes.

By the end of the 1st month the greatest part of the reduction in size has occurred. From then until the 2d or 3d year the combined weight of the adrenal glands is about 4 gm.

Normally there is little lipoid material in the adrenal cortex at birth. The small amount present is limited to the peripheral part of the definitive cortex and to a few cells scattered through the central part of the provisional cortex. Ordinarily, within a few days after birth considerably more lipoid material is present, and after a few weeks the definitive cortex is well delineated and appears to be as rich in lipoid as the adult cortex. The one exception is in the adrenal glands of anencephalic monsters. These are miniature at birth and contain almost no provisional cortex, but the definitive cortex is rich in lipoid.

HEMORRHAGE

The cortex of the adrenal glands of the mature fetus is extremely vascular and the cords of cells are covered by endothelium forming the lining of sinusoids that separate the cords of cells. These sinusoids may become extremely distended with blood as a result of anoxia or any condition causing visceral congestion. Consequently, in many fetuses and young infants the interior of the gland is red or red-brown and is softer than the outer portion. This appearance has led to the statement that hemorrhage into the adrenal gland is a universal phenomenon in the young infant. This is untrue for in most instances the blood is limited to the endothelium-lined spaces.

Bleeding does occur occasionally but is uncommon and always pathologic. Small hemorrhages presumably may be completely absorbed, but the blood may also remain in the central portion of the gland and become calcified or even ossified. Massive hemorrhage may destroy the entire substance and distend the capsule to a size several times that of the normal gland. If the capsule ruptures, blood usually extends into the retroperitoneal space and causes perirenal hemorrhage (see Fig. 8–17). Hemorrhage in this area is most common in infants dying after breech extraction and is thought to be caused by the pressure of the obstetrician's hands.

Hemorrhages having no relation to trauma may occur in infants who are somewhat beyond the newborn period. Commonly called the *Waterhouse-Friderichsen syndrome,* this is a rapidly fatal condition characterized by hemorrhage into both adrenal glands and accompanied by purpura of the skin. The symptoms, usually acute in onset, consist of malaise, vomiting, diarrhea, fever, rapid pulse, cyanosis, lethargy and coma. Death often occurs within 24–48 hours. At postmortem examination the adrenal glands are ordinarily not enlarged but are intensely congested and hemorrhagic. Microscopic examination often shows evidence of peripheral sinus thrombosis. Even though destruction is extensive, function of such adrenals seems adequate in the acute stage of the disease. Death is believed to result from an endotoxin or bacterial shock, not from hypoadrenocorticism. Most such lesions are sequelae of meningococcemia but other gram-negative organisms may sometimes be the cause. A sequela of this process may be the bilateral calcification of the adrenals that is seen by x-ray in some young children. Most such children have no recognizable abnormality of adrenal function but a few have addisonian symptoms (Williams and Robinson). Marked enlargement of the adrenals with cyst formation and adrenal insufficiency was reported by Moore and Cermak. The cysts, which

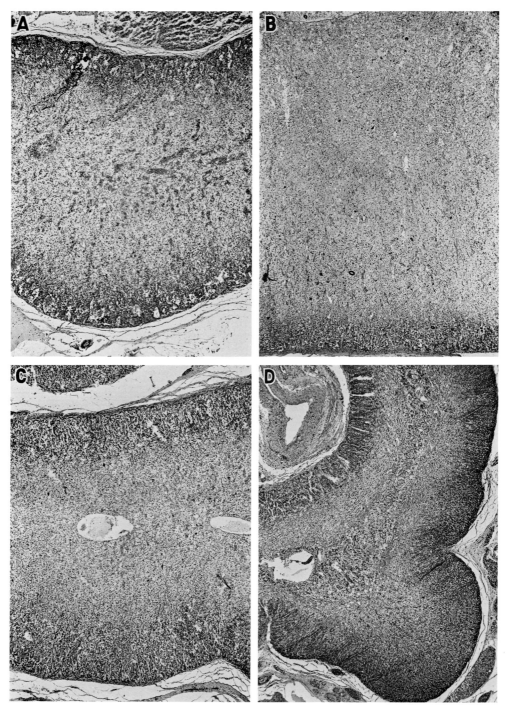

Fig. 16–15.—Appearance and relative thickness of normal adrenal glands at different ages. Each photograph includes entire thickness of the gland except B, which is only half the width of the others and extends from central vein to capsule. No medullary tissue in any section. All magnifications the same. **A,** stillborn fetus weighing 440 gm, about 22 weeks' gestation. **B,** stillborn fetus weighing 3,600 gm. **C,** infant aged 3 days weighing 3,200 gm. **D,** infant aged 3 weeks. *(Continued.)*

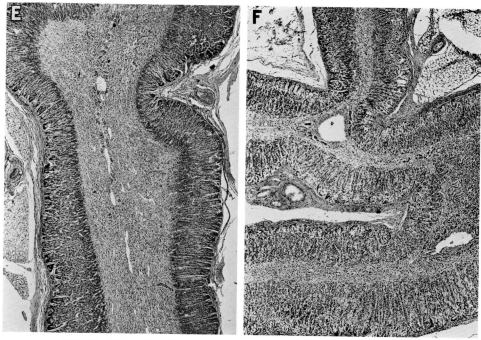

Fig. 16–15 (cont.). — **E**, infant aged 10 weeks. **F**, infant aged 8 months.

were filled with brown fluid, may have resulted from destructive adrenal hemorrhage.

Small cystic spaces are common in the outer portion of the adrenal glands of small premature infants (Fig. 16–16). Oppenheimer considered them to be similar to the tubular transformation described in adults by Rich, which he believed to be the result of stress. In infants anoxia often appears to be the cause of the stress.

Erythroblastosis

In severe erythroblastosis the adrenals are larger than those of normal infants of the same gestational age, and the cells of the fetal cortex often show marked vacuolation (Bartman and Driscoll). The etiology of these changes is not known; stress, ACTH discharge and anoxia have all been invoked. The increased size of such adrenals (Fig. 16–17) appears closely associated with the fatty infiltration and vacuolation (Fig. 16–18).

Syphilis

Severe syphilitic infection may produce fibrosis of the adrenal glands. The connective tissue increase is most pronounced immediately beneath the cap-

sule, and irregular tonguelike projections extend inward between the cords of cells of the permanent cortex (Fig. 16–19). Organisms can be demonstrated more often in the adrenal glands than in any other organ except the liver.

Cytomegaly

The fetal portion of the cortex, especially the central part, occasionally shows a widespread change in the size, shape and nuclear pattern of its constituent cells. Craig and Landing described 37 cases from the Children's Hospital in Boston, and over 20 cases were seen at the Chicago Lying-in Hospital. In only one was any disturbance suspected on gross examination and this was because of a difference in size of the two glands. In most instances when both adrenal glands have been examined, only one has been affected, although in some cases both glands are involved, and in one case of previable triplets observed at the Chicago Lying-in Hospital typical cells were present in the glands of all three infants.

This condition has been known as adrenal cytomegaly because some of the cells in the fetal zone of the cortex become irregularly larger and greatly altered in appearance (Fig. 16–20, A). The cells are polyhedral, measure up to 50 μ in diameter and the

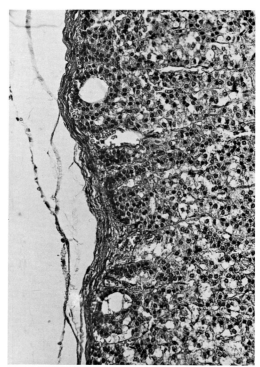

Fig. 16–16.—Adrenal gland with vacuolated spaces beneath the capsule giving the appearance of cysts. They were believed to have been due to stress resulting from anoxia caused by respiratory insufficiency. Infant of 37 weeks' gestation weighing 1,940 gm. Death at 2 days.

volume of both cytoplasm and nuclei is increased. The nuclear chromatin is generally arranged in large irregular clumps, and vacuoles may be present or absent. The latter single or multiple, clearly outlined, spherical acidophilic bodies sharply contrasted with the basophilic chromatin (Fig. 16–20, B). Borit and Kosek believed these to be invaginations of the cytoplasm into the nucleus. The cytoplasm is often occupied by circumscribed masses of finely granular acidophilic material (Fig. 16–20, C), and the periphery of the cell may be composed of a rim of small vacuoles giving a characteristic foamy appearance. Occasionally, the acidophilic granules seem to enlarge and become basophilic. In some cells the entire cytoplasm is filled with fine vacuoles.

Such changes in the adrenal glands have been observed in white and Negro fetuses and infants weighing 400–4,500 gm. There has been no recognized similarity in maternal conditions or in causes of infant death although some authors have postulated an increased frequency in erythroblastosis. Recently these changes have been described in association with pancreatic hyperplasia and hypoglycemia, bilateral renal hyperplasia, omphalocele and macroglossia, a condition known as Beckwith's or Beckwith-Wiedemann's syndrome. The adrenal abnormality may involve the fetal zone of adrenal rests in other parts of the body. In one case in which cells were present in the fetal adrenal cortex there was intravascular spread to the lung (Sherman *et al.*). Craig and Landing noted the similarity of such cells to those making up adrenal tumors in this age group, and the suggestion that these tumors originate from such cells was made because of the known increased frequency with which such tumors occur in the 1st year of life and their relative infrequency in the next few years. Accompanying cellular changes of the same variety have been found in no other organs of affected pa-

Fig. 16–17.—Enlarged adrenal gland with peripheral zones of erythropoiesis from full-term infant with hydropic form of erythroblastosis. **Inset,** hypoplastic adrenal gland of infant with pituitary agenesis; this is identical to the appearance ordinarily associated with anencephalus. Same magnification.

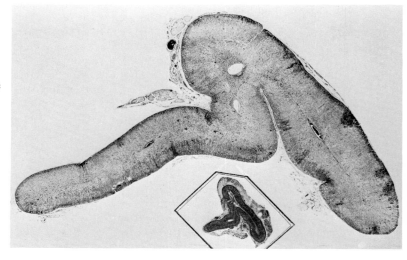

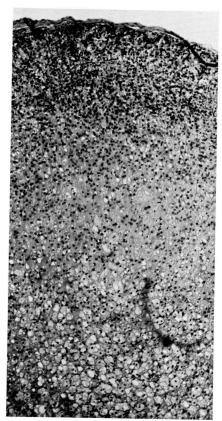

Fig. 16–18.—Section from the cortex of an infant who died with hydropic form of erythroblastosis. The fetal cortex is increased in width and contains an increased amount of fat in the inner portion.

tients, except for one of Craig and Landing's series in whom enlarged cells and nuclei were seen in the islet cells of the pancreas of the infant of a diabetic mother.

ABNORMALITIES OF SHAPE AND POSITION

The shape of the adrenal glands is largely a result of their proximity to the kidneys. If a kidney is not present to push the lower pole of the adrenal gland upward and give it a characteristic triangular shape, it remains a round flat disk against the posterior abdominal wall. Position varies in relation to the size and location of the kidneys; with polycystic or hydronephrotic kidneys the adrenal glands lie higher and often more anterior than is usual.

The adrenal glands are fused behind the aorta, in some cases with other midline abnormalities (see Fig. 22–18, A). The microscopic appearance is not altered.

Small nodules of cortical tissue, often designated accessory adrenal glands, are so common that they are ordinarily considered an anatomic variant rather than a malformation. They may be attached to an adrenal gland, embedded in the peripheral portion of the cortex or separated from the main portion of the gland and present in or attached to other organs at a considerable distance from their normal position. Frequent locations are the testes or spermatic cord in the male, less often the ovary or broad ligament in the female. These may be the source of tumors of the ovary or testis in the adult.

HYPOPLASIA

By far the most common of the several structural abnormalities of the adrenal glands of the newborn is hypoplasia secondary to absence or hypoplasia of the hypophysis or the diencephalic centers control-

Fig. 16–19.—Syphilis of the adrenal gland. Connective tissue is growing inward from the capsule in fingerlike processes. Infant aged 38 days. Same magnification as in Figure 16–15.

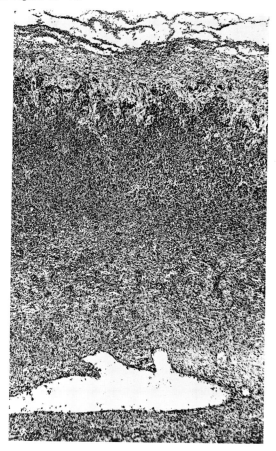

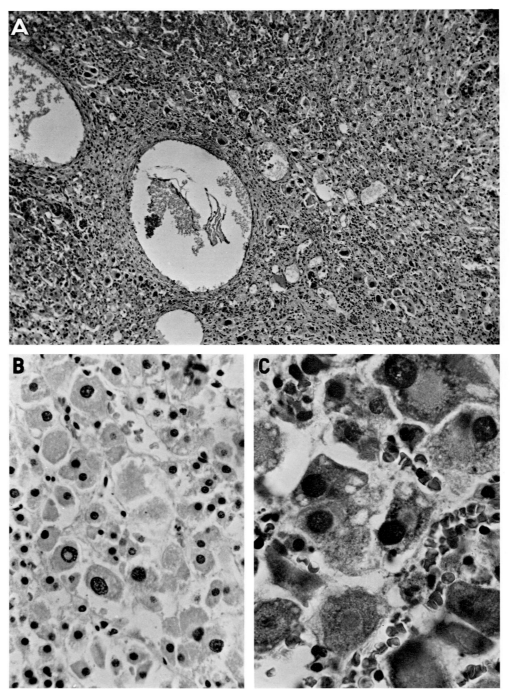

Fig. 16–20.—Adrenal glands of newborn infants with cytomegaly of central portion of the fetal zone. **A,** low power view showing general distribution. **B,** cells with giant nuclei and one area of cytoplasmic invagination into the nucleus. **C,** typical cells with cytoplasmic inclusions and vacuolation.

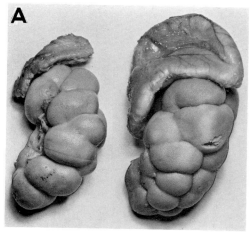
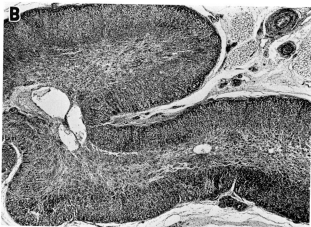

Fig. 16–21.—A, adrenal gland and kidney of an anencephalic monster *(left)* with adrenal gland and kidney of a normal infant *(right)*. Both were born at term as calculated from the mother's last menstrual period. **B,** hypoplastic adrenal gland of an anencephalic monster at term showing remarkable histologic similarity to that of an infant several months old. The definitive cortex is more completely differentiated, the provisional cortex much narrower, and the medullary tissue proportionately more abundant than in a normal newborn infant. Same magnification as in Figure 16–15.

ling the release of ACTH. Infants with anencephaly are predominantly affected.

In anencephaly, hypophyseal tissue can almost never be identified grossly, and although it has been said that some can always be found on microscopic examination, this has not been our experience.

In most anencephalic infants no brain tissue exists except for small groups of glial cells distributed between large vascular channels intimately associated with masses of meningeal tissue. Since the combined weight of the adrenals is often less than 1 gm, without care they may be completely overlooked on postmortem examination (Fig. 16–21). A few infants without cerebral hemispheres have a fairly well-developed cerebellum and spinal cord; in these cases the glands, although hypoplastic, are larger than those completely lacking brain tissue. About one quarter of infants born with severe hydrocephalus have some reduction in the size of the adrenal glands, though not as severe as in the anencephalics.

It is interesting that up to about 20 weeks' gestation the adrenal glands in anencephalics are of normal size and structure (Fig. 16–22). Although the reason for the change after this time is not definitely known, it may possibly be due to premature involution of the fetal zone and failure of subsequent growth coupled with precocious maturation of the definitive cortex; or perhaps the growth until 20 weeks is autonomous and after this time further

Fig. 16–22.—Anencephalic fetus of 12 weeks, 5 cm total length, with adrenal glands of normal size. Legs detached.

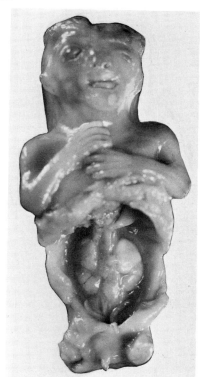

development requires an intact diencephalic-hypophyseal system. The adrenal glands are miniature replicas of the glands of infants several months old. The definitive cortex is well differentiated, the provisional cortex almost entirely absent and the medullary tissue present in a somewhat larger amount than is normal.

The hypophysis may also be absent or hypoplastic in infants without anencephaly, and the adrenal glands are the same as in that condition.

Three such infants—two male and one female—were delivered at the Chicago Lying-in Hospital. All weighed between 2,500 and 3,000 gm, survived 10–19 hours and had cyanosis and poor respiratory activity. One had two convulsions. No definite clinical diagnosis was made, although cardiac malformations were considered possible in two and meningitis in the one with convulsions. One infant had several malformations including harelip, cleft palate and multiple digital abnormalities. Both adrenal glands were extremely small in each infant and closely resembled those found in anencephalus; the pituitary was absent in one and hypoplastic in the others. The pregnancies of all mothers were uneventful and the cause is unknown.

Congenital hypoplasia of the adrenal glands has been reported as a rare cause of Addison's disease in small children. One of the youngest infants with bronzing of the skin and other evidence of adrenal insufficiency was reported by Sikl. Death occurred from pneumonia at 33 days of age and the adrenal glands were estimated to have only one hundredth of the normal volume. The small amount of tissue present appeared to be definitive cortex. Few medullary cells could be identified.

A form of adrenal hypoplasia thought to be a genetic defect since it has appeared in siblings was reported by Roselli and Barbosa. The volume of both adult and fetal cortices is reduced and cortical cells are small and devoid of lipid. Death occurs from adrenal insufficiency in the first days of life unless the condition is recognized and replacement therapy given.

In another form the adrenal hypoplasia appears to be progressive. Although symptoms are usually present by 1 month of age, death often does not occur until months or years later (Baker *et al.*). The adrenal glands are severely hypoplastic and have a narrow cortex in which the cords of cells are disorganized and without the usual stratification into the three adult zones. The individual cells are large and eosinophilic with pyknotic nuclei. The condition bears some resemblance to the cytotoxic atrophy found in adults except that in infants no in-

flammation is present. The nature of the process is not known.

Iatrogenic adrenal hypoplasia was observed at the Boston Lying-in Hospital in a newborn whose mother had received prednisone constantly during pregnancy for control of symptoms of adrenal virilism. All zones of the cortex were narrower than usual, but within each zone the cellular distribution was normal.

HYPERPLASIA

All of the recognized forms of adrenal hyperplasia in the infant except that associated with Cushing's syndrome are secondary to specific metabolic blocks in the production of the normal end-products of the adrenal gland. Because of a deficiency in the normal end-product the diencephalon and pituitary react by increasing ACTH secretion; this causes hypertrophy of the gland and excessive production of the precursors of the end-metabolite. These precursors then produce an excess of abnormal androgen- and aldosterone-like substances, which leads to virilism and hypertension.

The most common form of secondary adrenal hyperplasia is that associated with virilism—sometimes accompanied by a loss of salt—due to a decrease but not complete absence of the enzyme 21 hydroxylase. In both the pure masculinizing form and the salt-losing form with masculinization, varying degrees of masculinization appear in the female; in the male, only increased pigmentation of the scrotum and slight enlargement of the phallus may be evident at birth. In the most severe form of virilization the female has a phalluslike clitoris (Fig. 16–23, A) with some degree of hypospadias, complete fusion of the labia and a vagina that opens into the posterior urethra (Fig. 16–23, B). Only areas that are susceptible to androgen stimulation are affected. The internal female genitalia—uterus, tubes and ovaries—either because of their insusceptibility or their exposure to elevated levels of androgen only late in pregnancy, are anatomically normal. In the less severe forms only partial fusion of the labia or enlargement of the clitoris are present, the degree of alteration depending on the amount of abnormal steroid and the time it is first produced. Other features of the disease include hyperpigmentation of the areola and labia or scrotum, increased wrinkling of the labial surface and advanced bone age.

In the series of Collip *et al.* of 74 cases of adrenal hyperplasia due to 21 hydroxylase deficiency, 36 had the simple virilizing form and 38 the salt-los-

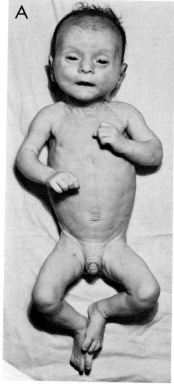
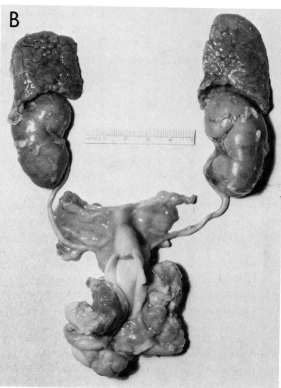

Fig. 16–23.—Newborn female who died with the severe form of adrenal virilism. **A,** the clitoris is greatly enlarged. **B,** the adrenal glands are nearly as large as the kidneys, and surfaces have many microadenomas. The vagina opens into the posterior urethra.

ing form. Of the 36 with the simple virilizing form twice as many females were affected as males, probably because of the ease with which it can be recognized in females early in life. Males may come to attention only later in life because of sexual precocity or late growth failure due to premature closure of the epiphyses. Sixteen of the total group of 74 had other major anomalies, 8 cardiovascular and 8 genitourinary.

In the salt-losing form the hydroxylase block is complete rather than partial, as it is in the simple virilizing form, so that no salt-retaining hormone is produced. Unless exogenous hormone is supplied, an adrenal crisis due to salt loss causes death in half of the affected infants in the 1st week and in the remainder in the 1st 7 weeks of life. Among the salt losers the sexes are equally affected, probably because of more complete case finding among the males in this group.

In both forms of this condition the adrenals are large and may weigh as much as twice the normal amount (Fig. 16–23, B). They have a normal outline but the surface is marked by numerous folds, which has aptly been called "cerebration." The depth of the cortical layer is not ordinarily increased in young infants, but in older individuals the reticularis becomes more prominent and the demarcation from the fasciculi is obscured. The fetal cortex is not involved in the process and the increase in weight is largely due to the increased length of the infolded cortical ribbon. The cortical cells may have less lipid than is normal; in older patients the normal pigmentation of the reticularis is much increased. Older patients, if untreated, of necessity have the simple virilizing form since without therapy the salt losers die in infancy; with therapy the adrenal regains its normal appearance or even becomes atrophic.

Both forms are autosomal recessive in inheritance. There is no cross-over in families between the simple virilizing and salt-losing varieties.

An uncommon form of adrenal cortical hyperplasia due to an 11-hydroxylation defect is associated with hypertension. Here desoxycorticosterone is produced, which causes salt retention and hypertension. The heart enlarges and may fail because of an expanded blood volume even before hypertension is obvious. The adrenal glands in these first three forms of congenital adrenal hyperplasia are not histologically separable one from another.

In another form of adrenal hyperplasia complete failure of steroid synthesis leads to lipoid adrenal hyperplasia, or the *Prader-Willi syndrome* (O'Doherty). In this disorder the defect is an absence of the 3 beta-O1 (R 20–22 desmolase) dehydrogenase enzyme system (Visser). Because of the absence of androgen production, along with the failure of other steroid synthesis, affected individuals who are chromosomal males have no stimulation of their androgen-sensitive end-organs and consequently appear to be females because of absence of a penis and failure of fusion of the two portions of the scrotum. Hence, without careful study all might be considered female. Because of the complete absence of steroid synthesis, affected infants rarely survive the first few days of life and die with acute adrenal insufficiency. The adrenals are enlarged but the cortex lacks the cerebration of the other forms just discussed. The glands are thicker than normal and the cut surface is bright yellow. Microscopically the cortical cells are filled with fat. Small eosinophilic cells close to the capsule enlarge and become foam cells filled with finely distributed fat.

A deficiency in 18-dehydrogenase, which converts 18-dehydroxycorticosterone to aldosterone, is accompanied by adrenal hypertrophy. Symptoms are relieved by administration of desoxycorticosterone and salt. No virilization is present.

In the Wolman syndrome adrenal enlargement is associated with calcification and increased amounts of fat in the adrenal cortex (Wolman *et al.*; Crocker *et al.*), but adrenal function is normal and no enzymatic defect has been identified. The disorder is generalized and involves the intracellular metabolism of cholesterol. The principal symptoms are failure to gain weight, recurrent diarrhea and marked hepatosplenomegaly with anemia. The serum lipids are not elevated and serum cholesterol is low. The tissue cholesterol level is 7–10 times normal in the liver, 15–20 times normal in the spleen, but brain lipids are not increased. The liver, spleen, mesenteric lymph nodes, lamina propria of the small intestine and bone marrow all contain large numbers of cholesterol-containing foam cells (Fig. 16–24, A). In the liver these fill the sinusoids and distort the portal triads; severe periportal fibrosis may result. The bone marrow may contain up to 14% foam cells. The adrenal glands may be twice the normal size and have a bright yellow outer and a gray inner cortex, the latter being gritty owing to deposits of calcium (Fig. 16–24, B). The enlargement appears to be caused by the massive lipid content of the cells rather than true hyperplasia. The fetal cortex may contain fatty cysts. The central calcification is easily demonstrable by x-ray during life. It has been suggested that since cholesterol is found in the liver only in macrophages and not in parenchymal cells, abnormal synthesis rather than a lysozymal defect is most probably responsible.

Cushing's disease resulting from simple adrenal enlargement must be distinguished from Cushing's syndrome in which symptoms like those of Cush-

Fig. 16–24.—Wolman's disease. **A,** small intestine stained with Sudan black for lipid. The lamina propria is massively infiltrated with lipid-laden macrophages. **B,** adrenal gland showing enlarged fat-filled cells in the fasciculi and local calcification. (Courtesy Dr. A. C. Crocker.)

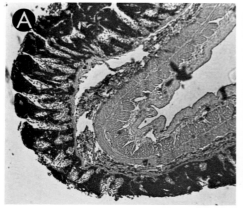
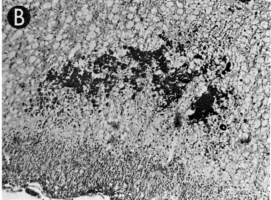

ing's disease may result from other causes. Either may be found in the 1st year of life. Of 27 cases of Cushing's syndrome occurring in the 1st year described by Gilmour, 11 were caused by adrenal cortical carcinomas, 10 by benign adenomas and 6 by simple hyperplasia. The last six were true Cushing's disease. In this condition the symptoms are thought to result from a disturbance in the level of ACTH-releasing factor from the diencephalon and not from intrinsic adrenal or pituitary abnormalities. However, the adrenal glands are enlarged and have many irregularities (microadenomas) on the surface. The cell columns, especially in the fasciculi, are disrupted and irregular as a result of variation in cell size and degree of lipidization. These changes result from varying degrees of cellular activity and look quite different from the rather monotonous pattern of the adrenal hyperplasia that occurs with enzymatic defects. The symptoms found in association with adrenal cortical hyperplasia as well as with tumors result from an excess of adrenal glucocortical hormone. They include obesity, especially of the face and arms, thinning of the skin, abdominal striae, hypertension and osteoporosis.

TUMORS

Adrenal cortical tumors often produce symptoms in the 1st year of life, particularly virilizing adrenal cortical carcinomas; in the series of Goldstein *et al.*, of 54 such cases 57% developed symptoms in the 1st year of life and 87% in the 1st 4 years. Carcinomas outnumber adenomas 3:1 from birth to 3 years of age (Hayles *et al.*). Most of the primary tumors are encapsulated even though malignant. Both adenomas and carcinomas may contain large cells with polyploid hyperchromatic nuclei. A disorganization of the linear configuration of the cortex is most obvious in the malignant tumors, and mitoses and necrosis are more evident than in the adenomas (Figs. 16–25 and 16–26). The decision as to whether the tumors are benign or malignant must often rest on whether they invade and metastasize. Hormonally active adrenal tumors are rare in the 1st year of life, although virilizing and glucocorticoid-secreting tumors producing Cushing's syndrome have been described (Goldstein *et al.*; Gilbert and Cleveland).

NEUROBLASTOMA. — One of the most common tumors found in the newborn infant, this arises from neural crest cells that normally migrate into the adrenal gland and differentiate into chromaffin tissue. In some instances these cells reach the adre-

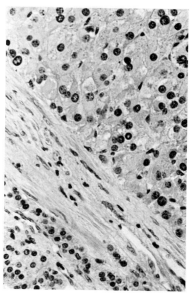

Fig. 16–25. — Adrenal adenoma. The large cells of the adenoma *(top)* have distorted and compressed the adrenal cortical cells *(bottom)*.

nal gland but retain their primitive character and proliferate, forming masses that vary in size from a few millimeters to several centimeters with or without a central cavity. Cortical tissue frequently

Fig. 16–26. — Adrenal cortical carcinoma; the size and staining qualities of the tumor cells show marked variation in comparison to the cortical adenoma shown in Fig. 16–25.

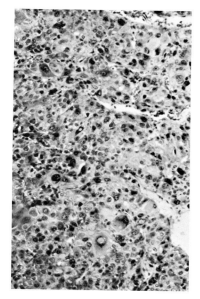

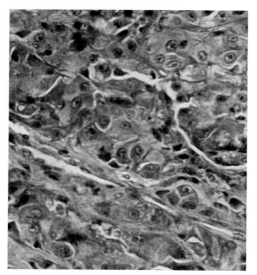

Fig. 16–27.—Pheochromocytoma in a newborn infant. The tumor lay outside the adrenal gland above the left kidney.

surrounds part or all of the tumor. Tumors may be bilateral or unilateral and may be limited to the adrenal gland or widespread throughout the body.

PHEOCHROMOCYTOMAS.—These are rare but one histologically typical tumor of the adult type without metastases was seen in a newborn infant at the Boston Hospital for Women (Fig. 16–27).

REFERENCES

Angevine, D. M.: Pathological anatomy of hypophysis and adrenals in anencephaly, Arch. Pathol. 26:507, 1938.

Aterman, K. Kerenyi, N., and Lee, M.: Adrenal cytomegaly, Virchows Arch. Pathol. Anat. 355:105, 1972.

Baker, W. De C., Wise, G., and Mezger, M. L.: Cytomegalic adrenal hypoplasia in a 4½ year old boy. Am. J. Dis. Child. 114:180, 1967.

Bakwin, H.: Tetany in newborn infants, J. Pediatr. 14:1, 1939.

Bartman, J., and Driscoll, S. G.: Fetal adrenal cortex in erythroblastosis, Arch. Pathol. 87:393, 1969.

Baulieu, E. D., Peillon, F., and Migeon, C. J.: Congenital Adrenal Hyperplasia, in Eisenstein, A. B. (ed.): *The Adrenal Cortex* (Boston: Little, Brown and Co., 1967), p. 579.

Beck, K., Tygstrup, J., and Nerup, J.: The involution of the fetal adrenal cortex, Acta Pathol. Microbiol. 76:391, 1969.

Beckwith, J. B.: *Macroglossia, Omphalocele, Adrenal Cytomegaly, Gigantism, and Hyperplastic Visceromegaly,* Birth Defects Original Article Series, No. 5 (New York: The National Foundation-March of Dimes, 1969), p. 188.

Beckwith, J. B., *et al.*: Hyperplastic fetal visceromegaly with macroglossia, omphalocoele, cytomegaly of adrenal fetal cortex, postnatal somatic gigantism and other abnormalities, Abs. Am. Pediatr. Soc. p. 56, 1964.

Bolande, R. P.: Adrenal changes in post-term infant and the placental dysfunction syndrome, Am. J. Pathol. 34:137, 1957.

Bongiovanni, A. M., and Root, A. W.: The adrenal genital syndrome, N. Engl. J. Med. 268:1283, 1342, 1391, 1963.

Borit, A., and Kosek, J.: Cytomegaly of the adrenal cortex, Arch. Pathol. 88:58, 1969.

Boyd, E.: Weight of the thymus gland in health and disease, Am. J. Dis. Child. 43:1162, 1932.

Burrow, G. N.: Neonatal goiter after maternal propylthiouracil therapy, J. Clin. Endocrinol. 25:403, 1965.

Cohen, M. M., Jr., Gorlin, R. J., Feingold, M., and Bensel, R. W.: The Beckwith-Wiedemann syndrome, Am. J. Dis. Child. 122:515, 1971.

Collip, P. J., Irani, N. G., and Plachte, F.: Congenital anomalies and congenital adrenal hyperplasia, Calif. Med. 104:278, 1966.

Craig, J. M., and Landing, B. H.: Anaplastic cells of the fetal adrenal cortex, Am. J. Clin. Pathol. 21:940, 1951.

Crocker, A. C., *et al.*: Wolman's disease, Pediatrics 35:637, 1964.

David, R., Golan, S., and Drucker, W.: Familial aldosterone deficiency: Enzyme defect, diagnosis, and clinical course, Pediatrics 41:403, 1968.

deLorimer, A. A., Bragg, K. U., and Linden, G.: Neuroblastoma in childhood, Am. J. Dis. Child. 118:441, 1969.

DiGeorge, A. M.: Congenital Absence of the Thymus and Its Immunological Consequences; Concurrence with Congenital Hypoparathyroidism, in Good, R. A. (ed.): *Immunologic Deficiency Diseases in Man,* Birth Defects Original Article Series, No. 4 (New York: The National Foundation-March of Dimes, 1968), p. 116.

French, F. S., and Van Wyck, J. J.: Fetal hypothyroidsim, J. Pediatr. 64:589, 1964.

Gilbert, M. G., and Cleveland, W. W.: Cushing's syndrome in infancy, Pediatrics 46:217, 1970.

Gilmour, J. R.: Some developmental abnormalities of the thymus and parathyroids, J. Pathol. Bacteriol. 52:213, 1941.

Gitlin, D., and Craig, J. M.: Thymus and other lymphoid tissues in congenital agammaglobulinemia: Thymic alymphoplasia and lymphocytic hypoplasia and their relation to infection, Pediatrics 32:517, 1963.

Goldstein, A. E., Rubin, S. W., and Oskin, J. A.: Carcinoma of adrenal cortex with adreno-genital syndrome in children, Am. J. Dis. Child. 72:563, 1946.

Good, R. A. (ed.): *Immunologic Deficiency Diseases in Man,* Birth Defects Original Article Series, No. 4 (New York: The National Foundation-March of Dimes, 1968).

Hayles, A. B., *et al.*: Hormone secreting tumors of the adrenal cortex in children, Pediatrics. 37:19, 1966.

Hitzig, W.: The Swiss Type of Agammaglobulinemia, in Good, R. A. (ed.): *Immunologic Deficiency Diseases in Man,* Birth Defects Original Article Series, No. 4 (New York: The National Foundation-March of Dimes, 1968), p. 82.

Johannisson, E.: The foetal adrenal cortex in the human, Acta Endocrinol. (supp. 130) (Kbh.) 58:7, 1968.

Kaplan, E.: Parathyroid gland in infancy, Arch. Pathol. 34:1042, 1942.

Kretschmer, R., *et al.*: Congenital aplasia of the thymus (DiGeorge's syndrome), N. Engl. J. Med. 279:1295, 1968.

Little, G., *et al.*: Crypto-thyroidism, the major cause of

sporadic athyrotic cretinism, J. Clin. Endocrinol. 25: 1529, 1965.

Louw, J. H.: Congenital goitre, S. Afr. Med. J. 37:976, 1963.

Moore, F. P., and Cermak, E. G.: Adrenal cysts and adrenal insufficiency in infant with fatal termination, J. Pediatr. 36:91, 1950.

More, G. H.: Thyroid in sporadic goitrous cretinism, Arch. Pathol. 74:35, 1962.

Morton, W. R. M.: Duplicaton of the pituitary and stomatodeal structures in 38-week male infant, Arch. Dis. Child. 32:135, 1957.

O'Doherty, N. S.: Lipoid adrenal hyperplasia, Guys Hosp. Rep. 113:368, 1964.

O'Donahue, N. V., and Holland, P. D. J.: Familial congenital adrenal hyperplasia, Arch. Dis. Child. 43:717, 1968.

Oppenheimer, E. A.: Cyst formation in the outer adrenal cortex, Arch. Pathol. 87:653, 1969.

Perlmutter, M., *et al.:* Cushing's syndrome in infancy, Metabolism 11:946, 1963.

Peterson, R. D. A., Kelley, W. D., and Good, R. A.: Ataxia-telangiectasia: Its association with defective thymus, immunologic deficiency and malignancy, Lancet 1:184, 1964.

Powell, L. W., Newman, S., and Hooker, J. W.: Cushing's syndrome, Am. J. Dis. Child. 90:417, 1955.

Prader, A.: The Adrenal Cortex in Childhood and Adolescence, in *The Human Adrenal Cortex* (Ciba Foundation Study Group no. 27) (Boston: Little, Brown and Co., 1967).

Provenzano, R. W.: Adrenocortical hypolasia in newborn infant, N. Engl. J. Med. 242:87, 1950.

Reid, J. W.: Congenital absence of the pituitary gland, J. Pediatr. 56:568, 1960.

Rich, A. R.: A peculiar type of adrenal cortical damage associated with acute infections and its possible relation to circulatory collapse, Bull. J. Hop. Hosp. 74:1, 1944.

Roselli, A., and Barbosa, I. T.: Congenital hypoplasia of the adrenal glands, Pediatrics 37:70, 1964.

Russfield, A. B.: Adenohypophysis, in Bloodworth, J. M. B. (ed.): *Endocrine Pathology* (Baltimore: Williams & Wilkins Co., 1968).

Samuels, S., *et al.:* Neonatal hyperthyroidism in an infant born of a euthyroid mother (A case report with 4 from the literature), Am. J. Dis. Child. 121:440, 1971.

Saville, P. D., and Kretchmer, N.: Neonatal tetany; report of 125 cases and review of the literature, Biol. Neonate 2:1, 1960.

Schamaun, H. M.: Pathologische-anatomische Unter-

suchungen uber die Struma congenita im Kanton Aargau 1940-1951, Helv. Paediatr. Acta 9:455, 1954.

Seligman, M., Fudenberg, H. N., and Good, R. A.: A proposed classification of primary immunologic deficiencies, Am. J. Med. 45:817, 1968.

Shannon, W. R.: Tetany, generalized edema and cerebral compression in the new-born, Arch. Pediatr. 48:153, 1931.

Sherman, F. E., Bass, L. W., and Fetterman, G. H.: Congenital metastasizing adrenal cortical carcinoma associated with cytomegaly of the fetal adrenal, Am. J. Clin. Pathol. 30:439, 1958.

Sikl, H.: Addison's disease due to congenital hypoplasia of adrenals in infant aged 33 days, J. Pathol. Bacteriol. 60: 323, 1948.

Smith, D. W., Blizzard, R. M., and Wilkins, L.: Mental prognosis in hypothyroidism of infancy and childhood: Review of 128 cases, Pediatrics 19:1011, 1957.

Sommers, S. C.: Thyroid Gland, in Bloodworth, J. M. B. (ed.): *Endocrine Pathology* (Baltimore: Williams & Wilkins Co., 1968), p. 131.

Stanbury, J. B.: Familial Goiter, in Stanbury, J. B. (ed.): *Inherited Basis of Metabolic Diseases* (New York: McGraw-Hill Book Co., 1966), p. 125.

Stemfel, R. S., and Tompkins, G. M.: Congenital Virilizing Adrenal Cortical Hyperplasia (The Adreno-Genital Syndrome), in Stanbury, J. B. (ed.): *Inherited Basis of Metabolic Disease* (New York: McGraw-Hill Book Co., 1966), p. 635.

Stevenson, J., MacGregor, A. M., and Connelly, P.: Calcification of the adrenal glands in young children, Arch. Dis. Child. 36:316, 1961.

Stowens, D.: Neuroblastoma and related tumors, Arch. Pathol. 63:454, 1957.

Theiffry, S. T., *et al.:* L'ataxie-telangiectasie, Rev. Neurol. (Paris) 105:390, 1961.

Visser, H. K. A.: The adrenal cortex in childhood, Arch. Dis. Child. 41:113, 1966.

Williams, A., and Robinson, M. J.: Addison's disease in infancy, Arch. Dis. Child. 31:265, 1956.

Wolman, M., *et al.:* Primary familial xanthomatosis with involvement and calcification of the adrenals, Pediatrics 28:742, 1961.

Yonis, Z., *et al.:* Primary hypoparathyroidism in an infant, Am. J. Dis. Child. 104:307, 1962.

Young, M., and Turnbull, H. M.: Analysis of data collected by the Status Lymphaticus Investigation Committee, J. Pathol. Bacteriol. 35:344, 1949.

17

Pancreas

Development

THE PANCREAS grows by repeated branching of cell cords that come from two portions of the duodenum. They develop central lumens and give rise to two additional varieties of cells, one with exocrine and one with endocrine function. The original cell cords become pancreatic ducts; the cells to which they give rise become acini and islands of Langerhans.

The early pancreatic buds are surrounded by mesenchymal tissue within which they grow. In the young fetus the branching ducts are widely separated by connective tissue. As the pancreas matures, the amount of connective tissue is proportionately decreased, and at term the organ is almost entirely glandular with little connective tissue remaining (Fig. 17–1).

The acini first appear early in the 3d month as small cap-shaped groups of cells along the sides and tips of the ducts (Fig. 17–2, A). They are penetrated by other duct cells, some of which come to lie in the center of the acini and are known as centroacinar cells (Fig. 17–2, B) and some of which elongate to form the connections between acini and main ducts and are known as intercalated duct cells (Fig. 17–2, C). Proliferation of the acini continues after birth.

The first appearance of acini is slightly preceded by the appearance of a primitive generation of islands of Langerhans. These are seen first as small clusters of cells on the outer surfaces of the ducts. They detach themselves from the ducts, enlarge to reach a maximum size by the 5th to the 6th month, degenerate and disappear. A second generation, the definitive islands, is first seen early in the 4th month as individual or small aggregates of angular cells from which they arise (Fig. 17–3, A). These islands gradually increase in size throughout intrauterine life by proliferation and fusion of adjacent groups of cells (Fig. 17–3, B). The two types of islands are composed of the same three varieties of

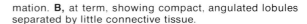

Fig. 17–1.—Pancreas. **A,** at 3d month of gestation, showing proliferation of ducts with beginning lobule for- | mation. **B,** at term, showing compact, angulated lobules separated by little connective tissue.

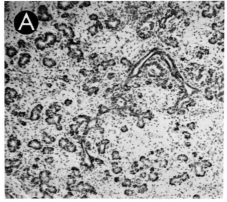
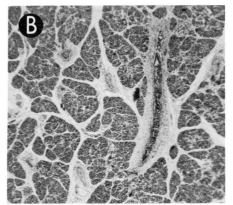

344

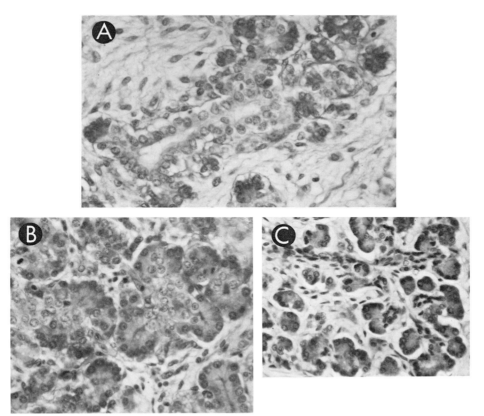

Fig. 17–2. — Pancreas. **A,** at 3d month of gestation, with groups of acinar cells differentiating from terminal portions of ducts. Nuclei of acinar cells darker than duct cells. **B,** at 6th month of gestation, with acinar cells larger, more numerous and often enclosing centroacinar (duct) cells. **C,** at term, showing relation of intercalated ducts and acini.

Fig. 17–3. — Pancreas. **A,** at 10 weeks, showing a small group of secondary island cells *(arrow)* differentiating from a primitive duct. **B,** at term, with isolated beta cells and secondary islands of varying size identified by specific granules. Gomori stain.

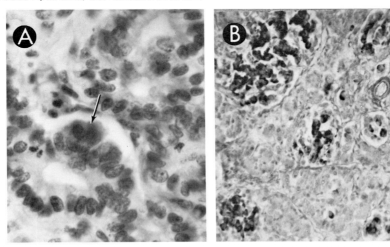

cells: alpha cells, which produce glucagon; beta cells, which produce insulin; and delta cells, whose function has not been definitely established. They are distinguishable principally by the findings that the primitive islands appear earlier, are larger, are located in the interlobular connective tissue close to the main ducts and show degenerative changes, while the second generation, or definitive, islands appear later, are located in the center of the lobules at some distance from the main ducts and are surrounded by acini (Liu and Potter).

The pancreas is commonly the site of early erythropoiesis, and small groups of immature red blood cells may be found even at term. Groups of lymphocytes are common throughout the organ but are especially numerous in the head near the principal duct.

Hypertrophy and Hyperplasia of Islands of Langerhans

The most common cause of an increase in size or number of islands of Langerhans is *maternal diabetes,* and infants of diabetic mothers who die in the latter weeks of pregnancy or in the first few days after birth almost always have a striking increase in size, and sometimes in number, of islands. This seems to be true regardless of the severity of the diabetes and the degree to which it has been controlled during pregnancy. The islands are composed largely of beta cells, and the structure is often normal except for increase in size (Fig. 17–4). How-

ever, single cells of the islands are occasionally enlarged (Fig. 17–5). The centers of the islands may have irregular areas of degeneration in which cells appear to be replaced by connective tissue. The islands are sometimes infiltrated and surrounded by leukocytes, chiefly lymphocytes, mononuclear cells and eosinophils. In some cases in which the eosinophilia is striking, Charcot-Leyden crystals, a proteinaceous deposit, can also be found in the periacinar connective tissue. The pancreas contains more insulin than normal.

Infants of diabetic mothers frequently have an excessive accumulation of subcutaneous adipose tissue, which is thought to be related to an excessive production of insulin by the fetus and a greater availability of carbohydrate in maternal blood. Not only are infants of diabetic mothers unusually heavy as a result of excessive fat deposit, but they are longer than normal for the length of gestation, and organ size is proportionately increased. Histologic differentiation fails to keep pace with organ size, however, and histologic structure is often disproportionately immature. Normally, new glomeruli are rarely being differentiated in the kidneys of infants weighing over 2,300 gm, but they are often being formed in infants weighing over 3,000 gm whose mothers are diabetic. Only the brains are smaller in size than normal. Driscoll *et al.* found no significant change in adrenal weight but the thymus tended to be small and show evidence of chronic involution.

Infants of diabetic mothers have been described

Fig. 17–4.—Marked hypertrophy and hyperplasia of islands of Langerhans in pancreas of newborn infant of a diabetic mother.

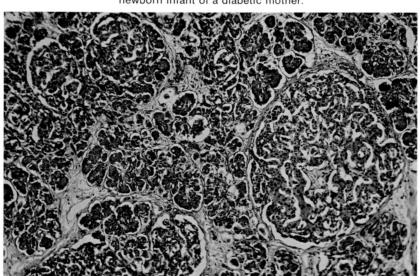

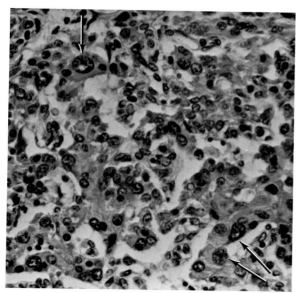

Fig. 17–5.—High power view of hyperplastic island from pancreas of an infant of a diabetic mother to show mild infiltration of mononuclear cells and cytomegaly of individual island cells *(arrows).*

as resembling those with Cushing's syndrome. However, in any unusually heavy newborn the adipose tissue is an important component of the total body weight, and infants with the same appearance may be delivered by normal women. Some women whose babies are abnormally large develop symptoms of diabetes at a later time, but this is by no means universally true.

In the preinsulin era it was commonly believed that diabetic women improved during the latter half of pregnancy. This was attributed to activity of the fetal pancreas, which was thought to produce enough insulin to compensate for the inadequacy of the maternal pancreas. Later studies have failed to corroborate this contention, and there seems to be little evidence to support the belief that the fetal pancreas contributes in any way toward regulating maternal carbohydrate metabolism.

Despite the increase of island tissue in children of diabetic women it seems probable that hypoglycemia from this cause rarely occurs. The blood sugar of the newborn is normally lower than that of the adult, the range generally being from 40–80 mg%. Priscilla White, who has had more experience in treating diabetic women and their children than any other person, thought that the blood sugar of the offspring of diabetic women is no lower after birth than that of other children and that it is not necessary to give them sugar solutions to prevent

hypoglycemia. Premature infants in general tend to have lower glucose values in the early postnatal period, and premature diabetic infants may suffer from the same difficulty. The infant of a severely diabetic mother with renal difficulties, like the offspring of any woman with renal disease, may be small in relation to the length of pregnancy; such infants have hypoglycemia because of low glycogen and protein stores.

Although islands of Langerhans are more greatly and more constantly enlarged in infants of diabetic women than in those of any other group, they are sometimes enlarged in infants with severe erythroblastosis and rarely in infants who have died of birth injury or some such unrelated cause whose mothers show no evidence of deranged carbohydrate metabolism. Potter *et al.* reported several infants, none of whose mothers were diabetic, who had striking increases in size and number of islands of Langerhans (Fig. 17–6). Miller subsequently described similar changes in the islands of infants of prediabetic women, and whether the cases reported by Potter *et al.* should be placed in the same category is not known. One of the women in that group had abnormal glucose tolerance but no evidence of hyperglycemia, and it is quite possible that she might have developed diabetes subsequently. In the years since publication of that paper very few infants with definite enlargement of the islands whose mothers were not diabetic have been observed, and it seems probable that island hyperplasia in children of normal women is rare.

Miller's investigation showed that unusually large infants with a presumed increase in island secretion were sometimes born to prediabetic women and that at times the subsequent development of diabetes in the mothers could be prognosticated from the infant's appearance. Such infants, as he described them, were large, often weighing over 4,500 gm, the organs including the heart were enlarged (although usually not out of proportion to total body weight) and an abnormal number of nucleated red blood cells were present in the circulation. If these infants died, island hyperplasia was usually found.

Infants of diabetic mothers appear to be unusually susceptible to respiratory distress compared with other infants of the same birth weight. This increase is less marked if gestational ages are used for comparison, but there still appears to be an excess of respiratory distress among infants of diabetic mothers. Driscoll *et al.* found that among 95 infants of diabetic mothers 32 had some variety of intracranial hemorrhage, in six of whom it was massive. Four had massive pulmonary hemor-

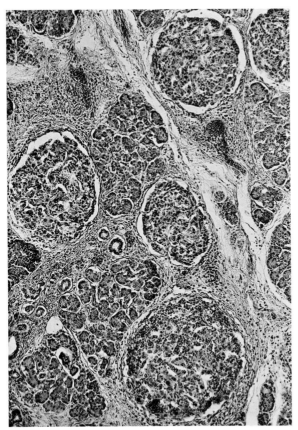

Fig. 17−6 −Pancreas with hypertrophy and hyperplasia of islands of Langerhans of unknown origin (probably from a prediabetic mother). There is severe infiltration of eosinophilic leukocytes and immature red blood cells. Death at 2 days of pneumonia of intrauterine origin.

rhage, and in 49 infants diffusely spread hyaline membranes were the only significant lesion. An additional 22 infants had less extensive membranes, bringing the total with respiratory distress to 78%. Offspring of diabetic women have also been described as having a high incidence of malformations, although this has not been true at the Chicago Lying-in Hospital. Driscoll *et al.* reported a two- to threefold increase and found malformations in 23 to 95 autopsied infants. They were most frequent among infants of mothers with severe diabetes, especially those in Joslin classes C and D. The varieties of malformations are variable, the most frequent being an interventricular septal defect. Kucera, who reviewed reports on 7,101 fetuses and infants of diabetic mothers, found a number of malformations with a high specificity. The most striking was agenesis of the lumbar vertebrae and sa-

crum (syndrome of caudal regression) (Fig. 17−7). Others with a high but less striking degree of specificity included situs inversus of the viscera, arthrogryposis, double ureter and pseudohermaphroditism. An unusual lesion and one we have not seen in infants born to nondiabetic mothers is spontaneous thrombosis of the renal vessels and inferior vena cava. No clue to the origin of the thrombosis is evident, but fetal renal glycosuria and hemoconcentration have been suggested as predisposing factors.

True *diabetes mellitus in the newborn period* is almost unknown but there are a few reports of infants with temporary hyperglycemia. Such infants are usually in the small-for-date group and, according to Gentz and Cornblath, the increased blood glucose level, which may be as high as 600 mg%, usually is normal by 6 weeks of age. Mental retardation appears to occur with increased frequency in such infants, but this may be related to the cause of the low birth weight rather than to the hyperglycemia. At times hyperglycemia is intermittent and may alternate with periods of hypoglycemia.

Fig. 17−7. −Roentgenogram showing absence of the lower lumbar and sacral vertebrae in infant of diabetic mother. This is known as the caudal regression syndrome, a condition significantly increased in frequency among infants of diabetic mothers. (See also Fig. 25−57 for infants whose mothers were not diabetic.)

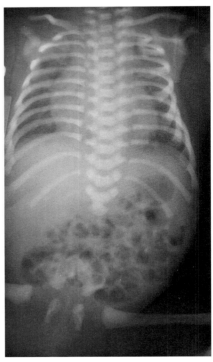

Most cases of infantile hypoglycemia, according to Warren *et al.,* have no organic pathology, although Haworth and Coodin found hypertrophy and/or hyperplasia of the pancreatic islands in 9 of 29 cases. In the hypoglycemia of infants induced by protein intake, especially by the amino acid leucine, no pathologic change in the pancreas has been described.

Island hyperplasia is also found in Beckwith's syndrome (p. 174).

Erythroblastosis

In severe erythroblastosis the pancreas may be the site of marked erythropoiesis. Immature cells, which are diffusely distributed throughout the connective tissue, are especially prominent in the perivascular regions. This is never to be considered diagnostic of erythroblastosis, however, because similar, although usually less extensive, erythro-

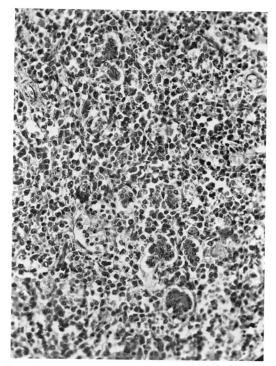

Fig. 17–9. — Leukemic involvement of pancreas of mature infant surviving 2 days. Islands and acini are largely obscured by immature myeloid cells.

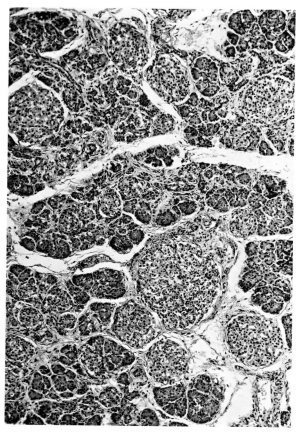

Fig. 17–8. — Moderate increase in size and number of islands of Langerhans in pancreas of an infant with erythroblastosis.

poiesis may be observed without known cause. Miller pointed out a few similarities between infants of diabetic mothers and those with erythroblastosis. They consist principally of an increased number of nucleated red blood cells in the circulation and varying degrees of cardiomegaly. We have also observed a moderate increase in the amount of island tissue in erythroblastosis (Fig. 17–8). This increase has been attributed to a decrease in reactive insulin as a result of its being bound by the free hemoglobin in the blood, which is increased as a result of blood destruction. The pancreas in the erythroblastotic infant, like that of the infant of a diabetic mother, has more than a normal amount of insulin.

Leukemia in the newborn ordinarily profoundly affects the pancreas, and all of the connective tissue is flooded with immature leukocytes (Fig. 17–9).

Syphilis

The pancreas is one of the principal organs involved in congenital syphilis. The characteristic change results in hypertrophy from an increase in

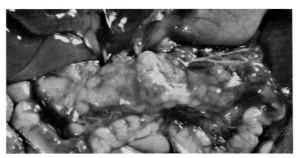

Fig. 17–10.—Great hypertrophy of the pancreas in newborn infant with congenital syphilis.

interacinar connective tissue (Fig. 17–10). It is distributed throughout the organ and causes wide separation of individual acini, ducts and islands (Fig. 17–11). The increase may be so pronounced as almost to mask the identity of the organ, and gland structures may be visible only as isolated groups of cells in a dense connective tissue matrix. The proliferation of connective tissue increases the density

Fig. 17–11.—Syphilitic pancreatitis. Islands of Langerhans and acini are reduced, and interstitial connective tissue is greatly increased and infiltrated with lymphocytes, plasma cells and macrophages. Infant weighed 3,100 gm and survived 20 minutes.

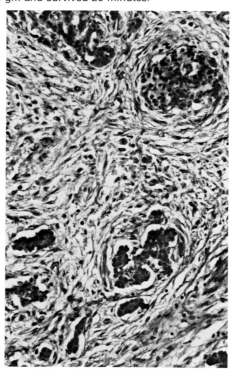

of the pancreas, which becomes almost cartilaginous in consistency.

Cytomegalic Inclusion Disease

The virus responsible for cytomegalic inclusion disease most often produces changes in the kidneys and lungs, but lesions have also been described in the pancreas. Any epithelial or glandular tissue appears to be a possible site for intranuclear inclusions in this disease, and they are occasionally found in the cells of the pancreatic acini (see Fig. 9–9) or islands of Langerhans.

Nonspecific Pancreatitis

Among 17 cases of inflammation of the pancreas, excluding those attributable to congenital syphilis, gathered by Frey and Redo, 8 patients were under 1 year of age. Most of these inflammations appeared to be extensions from peritoneal, bowel or mesenteric lesions or were associated with generalized sepsis or toxoplasmosis. This is in accord with our experience in a few cases in which nonspecific pancreatitis was never a primary or isolated lesion. The inflammation is acute and spreads diffusely through the stroma, with secondary involvement of acini and islands.

Fibrocystic Disease

Fibrocystic disease is a generalized metabolic disturbance affecting all mucus-secreting cells in the body but producing the most severe changes in the pancreas and lungs. Symptoms may be present at birth in the form of meconium ileus or may not develop until later in the form of chronic pulmonary infection.

The secretions normally produced by the exocrine pancreas are largely or entirely absent. Their absence during intrauterine life causes a change in the consistency of the meconium, which becomes hard and gray and resembles putty. It accumulates in the distal part of the ileum, seemingly unable to pass the ileocecal valve, and produces the condition known as meconium ileus. Proximal to the hardened mass the ileum is often distended by a large amount of more normal-appearing meconium. Farber, who demonstrated that the dry meconium can be softened by exposure to pancreatic substance, was one of the first to attribute the abnormal consistency to absence of pancreatic digestion. This observation has led to the treatment of meconium ileus by irrigation of the ileum with pancreatic enzymes. However, infants may have hypoplasia of the exocrine pancreas and no pancreatic secretions in the intestine and yet have normal meconium. Holsclaw *et al.* found protein increased in the meconium in pancreatic fibrosis; this may be an additional factor required for the production of abnormal meconium.

In the newborn the symptoms of fibrocystic disease are primarily those of intestinal obstruction. Unless the inspissated meconium is softened so that it can pass through the intestine or is removed surgically, the infant will die. Meconium ileus may be responsible for volvulus or overdistention, and ulceration may cause perforation of the ileum, leading to dense adhesive meconium peritonitis. The exudate in the peritoneal cavity contains many squamous cells, foreign body giant cells and calcium. The caliber of the colon is reduced because of disuse even though it is anatomically and functionally normal.

If death occurs in the first few days after birth, the lesions in the pancreas may be inconspicuous. The increase of connective tissue is usually mild and localized. Only the larger ducts are obstructed and they contain granular or amorphous material instead of the concretions found in older children (Fig. 17–12).

The bronchial mucosa of newborn infants with fibrocystic disease is normal, and before 5–7 weeks of age it is usually not possible to identify affected lungs from the pathologic changes. When the condition does not become evident until later, bronchial infection may be one of the first noticeable symptoms. Bronchial secretion is increased in amount and viscosity and causes a severe, persistent cough. *Staphylococcus aureus hemolyticus* almost always can be isolated early in the course of bronchial symptoms. In untreated infants the chronic bronchial infection usually leads to death from bronchopneumonia, bronchogenic abscesses, pyopneumothorax, focal emphysema or atelectasis from plug-

Fig. 17–12.—Cystic fibrosis of the pancreas. **A,** infant who died at age 3 months with chronic respiratory symptoms. Lumens of the acini are dilated and filled with acidophilic hyalinelike material arranged in concentric layers. Interstitial connective tissue is conspicuously increased. **B,** infant who died at 2 days of age after laparo-

tomy for meconium ileus. The larger ducts are dilated and filled with finely granular debris. A few of the small ducts are dilated but not to the extent commonly seen in infants who survive for a longer period. Connective tissue moderately increased.

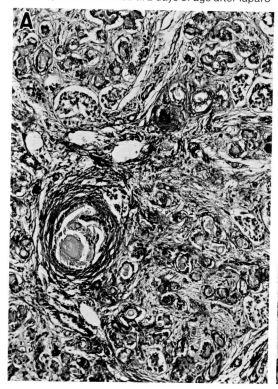
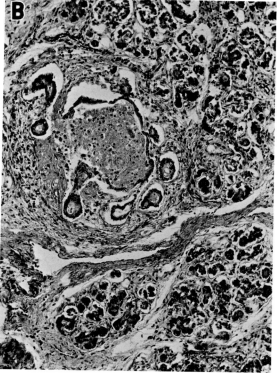

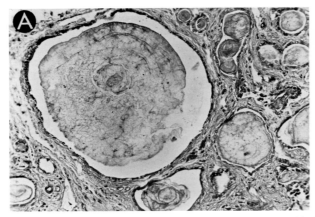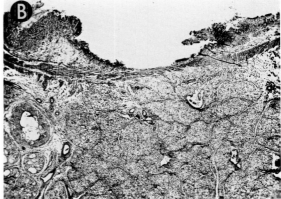

Fig. 17—13.—Cystic fibrosis of the pancreas, with death due to hemorrhage from duodenal ulcer. **A**, pancreas. **B**, duodenal ulcer. (Courtesy Dr. K. Aterman.)

ging of a bronchus. The bronchial secretions are not inspissated or massive enough to make these lungs distinguishable from those affected by other pneumonic processes. An interesting exception is the case of Claireaux, whose patient had abnormal bronchial and biliary secretions recognized at the time of birth but lacked evidence of meconium ileus. The liver is usually less fatty in very young infants than in older children. The gallbladder may be small and empty or may contain inspissated bile. Periportal fibrosis and fatty infiltration increase as survival time increases. In infants dying in the latter part of the 1st year of life both Craig *et al.* and Claireaux described focal biliary cirrhosis with inspissated secretions in the proliferated bile ducts. Squamous metaplasia of the bronchial epithelium is often present owing to lack of vitamin A.

Aterman observed five infants with fibrocystic disease of the pancreas who also had duodenal ulcers (Fig. 17–13). Hemorrhage from such an ulcer occasionally causes death.

In older children the inspissated secretions in the ducts and acini of the pancreas are deeply eosinophilic and arranged in concentric rings in dilated gland lumens. As the deposits become large, the ducts become cystic and the acini atrophy and are replaced by connective tissue or fat. The main ducts often remain patent, although they may become atretic or obstructed by secretion. Since all of the mucus-secreting cells in the body are affected by the metabolic abnormality, increased amounts of mucus may be detectable in the salivary glands, duodenum, large intestine (Fig. 17–14) and uterine cervix. In these areas, however, aside from the increased mucus in the cells and adjacent gland lumens, no pathologic alterations are found.

The assessment of sweat electrolytes, obtained by elution from sweat gathered into an absorbent gauze attached to the skin, is an important diagnostic aid. Concentrations of sodium and chloride are significantly greater in the sweat of patients with cystic fibrosis than in that similarly collected from normal individuals. Despite repeated investigation no histologic abnormality has been detected in the sweat glands. Until the development of the sweat electrolyte test the most reliable laboratory means of confirming the diagnosis of fibrocystic disease during life was the assay of duodenal juice for pancreatic enzymes. Trypsin and lipase are normally present at birth, whereas amylase does not appear for 2–3 months. Consequently, trypsin is the best enzyme to investigate in attempting to establish the diagnosis in early age groups.

Fig. 17—14.—Colon of a newborn infant who died with meconium ileus. The glands are dilated and filled with concentrated mucus. (Courtesy Dr. G. Vawter.)

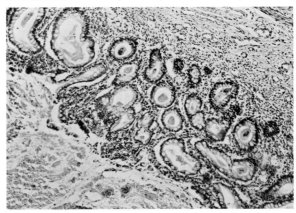

Cystic fibrosis of the pancreas is a genetic disorder produced by the homozygous state of an autosomal recessive gene. Heterozygotes do not have the disease and are not identifiable. DiSant'Agnese found the frequency of the homozygous state to be 1:2,000.

Mantle and Norman's life table for cystic fibrosis showed a high mortality. Three quarters of those with meconium ileus died before the 3d month of life; one seventh of those without this early symptom died by the end of the 1st year and three quarters by their 15th year.

Hypoplasia of the Exocrine Tissue of the Pancreas

Another disorder in which trypsin is absent from the pancreatic secretions is congenital hypoplasia of the acinar tissue of the pancreas. Nineteen such cases were gathered by Burke et al; 11 of these infants showed absence of both trypsin and lipase associated with chronic thrombocytopenia, and all but two had neutropenia. A few infants develop symptoms in the first weeks of life but most are not seen until they are several months old. The first symptoms are steatorrhea and failure to thrive. The sweat test is normal. Because of the frequency of neutropenia respiratory infection is common, but the characteristic obstructive emphysema and bronchiectasis of cystic fibrosis do not develop. Pathologically, the acinar tissue is largely or completely absent and is replaced by fat, and secretion is not inspissated in the ducts. The islands are normal. In a few cases the metaphyses are irregularly calcified. Biopsies of the small intestine may show blunting of the villi and mild inflammation of the lamina propria. Periportal fatty infiltration of the liver may result from lack of adequate intestinal absorption. The bone marrow is hypoplastic, and myeloid cells and megakaryocytes are decreased in infants with neutropenia. Although two patients reported by Lumb and Beautyman died in the 1st year of life, death usually comes much later.

Cysts of the Major Ducts

Cystic hyperplasia of major ducts of the pancreas has been found in conjunction with cysts in the kidneys on rare occasions. It was present only twice among 370 cases of renal cysts in infants in the Chicago Lying-in Hospital autopsy series, a frequency lower than that of cysts of the lung or liver.

Tumors of the Pancreas

Moynan et al., in an incomplete list of carcinomas of the pancreas in childhood, included three cases occurring in the 1st year of life. Such tumors, like those in adults, are either limited to the head of the pancreas or are multifocal and present throughout the pancreatic body. There is histologic evidence that the tumors arise from both ductal and acinar elements. Metastases are found primarily in the liver and regional lymph nodes.

One round, circumscribed tumor measuring 1.5 cm was present in the head of the pancreas in a newborn infant born at the Chicago Lying-in Hospital. Appearing histologically benign, it was composed of uniform cells, none of which contained specific granules. They were arranged in irregular sheets penetrated by blood vessels and small amounts of connective tissue.

Several cases of diffuse proliferation of the islands designated nesidioblastosis (Gr. *nesidion* is-

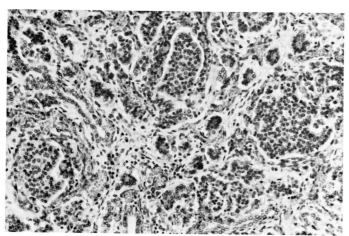

Fig. 17–15.—Nesidioblastosis. Diffuse hyperplasia of the islands in the pancreas associated with hypoglycemia in a newborn infant. The island cells are diffusely distributed and not limited to circumscribed masses.

lands, *blastos* germ) have been seen. In these cases the island cells proliferate individually or in small groups throughout the pancreas (Fig. 17–15). True tumors composed exclusively of islands have not been recognized. In one or two instances nesidioblastosis has been associated with infantile hypoglycemia (Yakovac and Baker).

REFERENCES

Andersen, D. H.: Cystic fibrosis of the pancreas and its relation to celiac disease, Am. J. Dis. Child. 56:344, 1938.

Assemany, S. R., Muzzo, S., and Gardner, L. I.: Syndrome of phocomelic diabetic embryopathy (caudal dysplasia), J.A.M.A. 123:489, 1972.

Aterman, K.: Duodenal ulceration and fibrocystic pancreatic disease, Am. J. Dis. Child. 101:210, 1961.

Bodian, M.: *Fibrocystic Disease of the Pancreas* (New York: Grune & Stratton, 1953).

Burke, V., *et al.*: Association of pancreatic insufficiency and chronic neutropenia, Arch. Dis. Child. 42:147, 1967.

Claireaux, A. E.: Fibrocystic disease of pancreas in newborn, Arch. Dis. Child. 31:22, 1956.

Craig, J. M., Haddad, H., and Schwachman, H.: The pathological changes in the liver in cystic fibrosis of the pancreas, Am. J. Dis. Child. 93:357, 1957.

DiSant'Agnese, P.: The Pancreas, in *Nelson's Pediatrics* (9th ed.; Philadelphia: W. B. Saunders Co., 1968), p. 857.

Driscoll, S. G., Benirschke, K., and Curtis, G. W.: Neonatal deaths among infants of diabetic mothers, Am. J. Dis. Child. 100:818, 1960.

Engleson, G., and Zetterqvist, P.: Congenital diabetes mellitus and neonatal pseudodiabetes mellitus, Arch. Dis. Child. 32:193, 1957.

Farber, S.: Pancreatic function and disease in early life: V. Pathologic changes associated with pancreatic insufficiency in early life, Arch. Pathol. 27:238, 1944.

Frey, C., and Redo, S. F.: Inflammatory lesions of the pancreas in infancy and childhood, Pediatrics 32:93, 1963.

Gentz, J. C. H., and Cornblath, M.: Transient diabetes in newborn, Adv. Pediatr. 16:345, 1969.

Haworth, J. C., and Coodin, F. J.: Idiopathic spontaneous hypoglycemia in children: Report of seven cases and review of the literature, Pediatrics 25:748, 1960.

Holsclaw, D. S., Eckstein, H. B., and Nixon, H. H.: Meconium ileus—20 year review of 109 cases, Am. J. Dis. Child. 109:101, 1965.

Kucera, J.: Rate and type of congenital anomalies among offspring of diabetic women, J. Reprod. Med. 7:61, 1971.

Kyle, G. C.: Diabetes and pregnancy, Ann. Intern. Med. (supp. no. 3) 59:1, 1963.

Liu, H. M., and Potter, E. L.: Development of the human pancreas, Arch. Pathol. 74:439, 1962.

Lumb, G., and Beautyman, W.: Hypoplasia of the exocrine tissue of the pancreas, J. Pathol. Bacteriol. 64:679, 1952.

Mantle, D. J., and Norman, A.: Life table for cystic fibrosis, Pediatrics 25:748, 1960.

McKay, D. G., Benirschke, K. and Curtis, G. W.: Infants of diabetic mothers, Obstet. Gynecol. 2:133, 1953.

Miller, H. C.: Effect of diabetic and prediabetic pregnancies on fetus and infant, J. Pediatr. 29:455, 1946.

Moynan, R. W., Neerhaut, R. C., and Jackson, T. S.: Pancreatic carcinoma in childhood, J. Pediatr. 65:711, 1964.

Norris, R. F., and Tyson, R. M.: Pathogenesis of polycystic pancreas: Reconstruction of cystic elements in one case, Am. J. Pathol. 23:485, 1947.

Potter, E. L., Seckel, H. P., and Stryker, W. A.: Hypertrophy and hyperplasia of the islets of Langerhans of fetus and newborn, Arch. Pathol. 31:467, 1941.

Spicer, S.: Histochemistry of Cystic Fibrosis, in *Research on the Pathogenesis of Cystic Fibrosis* (Washington, D.C.: National Institutes of Health and Cystic Fibrosis Foundation, 1964).

Warren, S. LeCompte, P. E., and Legg, M.: *Pathology of Diabetes Mellitus* (Philadelphia: Lea & Febiger, 1966).

Yakovac, W. C., and Baker, L.: Beta cell nesidioblastosis in idiopathic hypoglycemia in infancy, J. Pediatr. 79:226, 1971.

Zuelzer, W. W., and Newton, W. A.: Pathogenesis of fibrocystic disease of the pancreas, Pediatrics 4:53, 1949.

18

Mouth, Esophagus, Stomach and Intestine

DURING THE EARLY STAGES of fetal development the entodermal tube, from which the gastrointestinal tract arises, lies in the midsagittal plane adjacent to the neural tube. It is at first confluent with the yolk sac but the gradual infolding of the splanchnopleure forms the foregut and hindgut and finally the midgut. At the end of the 1st month the entodermal tube is closed and the area in communication with the yolk sac is greatly reduced. During the same time the length has increased more rapidly than that of the neural tube and the close association of the two structures has disappeared.

During the 4th week a slight local dilatation appears, which marks the location of the stomach. This is at first high and the esophageal area is short, but the stomach, as it enlarges and assumes a more definitive form, moves downward, causing a considerable elongation of the esophagus.

The midportion of the intestine begins to elongate rapidly during the 5th week. The point at which the yolk sac is attached forms the apex of a hairpin-shaped loop that is herniated outward into the body stalk. The intestine continues to elongate, and for the next 4 or 5 weeks the midgut remains outside the body in the umbilical cord (see Fig. 3–50). The yolk sac is attached slightly above the region that develops into the ileocecal valve, and consequently all of the large intestine and about 3 ft. of the adult ileum come from the portion distal to the attachment of the yolk sac. The rest of the gastrointestinal tract comes from the proximal portion.

When first formed, the primitive intestinal tract is closed at both ends. Small depressions appear in the regions of the future oral and anal orifices. The anterior end of the entodermal tube comes in contact with the oral depression and breaks through to form a communication with the exterior during the 4th week. The point of rupture marks the approximate junction of buccal cavity and pharynx. The lower end does not establish a communication with the exterior until early in the 8th week. At that time the cloacal membrane ruptures and the urogenital sinus and intestine open to the exterior.

During the latter part of the 2d month the epithelial lining of the intestinal tract appears to grow faster than the outer wall. Proliferation is stated to be especially rapid in the esophagus, the upper part of the small intestine and the rectum. The epithelium is described as temporarily occluding these areas but the lumens soon reappear, the channels widen and the definitive mucosa begins to develop. Some atresias, stenoses and reduplications of the intestine are thought to be related to a failure of normal recanalization.

Buccal Cavity

Malformations of the buccal cavity occur principally with abnormal development of the branchial arches and are discussed in Chapter 25.

Rarely, the tongue is held too close to the floor of the mouth by a short thick frenulum, a so-called tongue-tie (Fig. 18–1, A), or the frenulum may be absent (Fig. 18–1, B).

Often in mongolian or microcephalic idiots the tongue is mildly enlarged and the tip protrudes from the mouth, or at times it protrudes without any demonstrable increase in size. In infants who

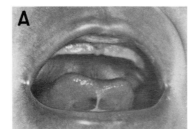

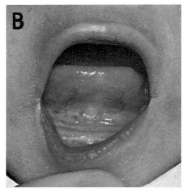

Fig. 18–1.—Abnormal frenulum. **A,** short frenulum extending to tip of tongue, generally called tongue-tie. **B,** absence of frenulum.

are stillborn or die soon after birth of *erythroblastosis,* edema is largely responsible for the almost constant protrusion of the tongue. Edema of other parts of the body is often associated, although at

Fig. 18–2.—Macroglossia. Spontaneous recovery without treatment. Normal at age 4 months.

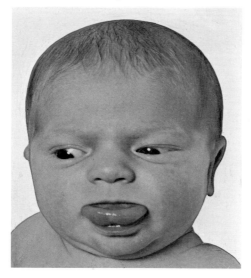

times the tongue and eyelids seem to be the only regions involved. With severe erythroblastosis perivascular foci of erythropoiesis may be found in the muscle or connective tissue of the tongue. A somewhat greater increase in size is often associated with *glycogenosis, type II* as a result of abnormal deposits of glycogen in the muscles. Macroglossia is part of *Beckwith's syndrome,* which also includes visceromegaly, omphalocele, cytomegaly of the adrenal cortex and micrognathia (see Fig. 11–4). Severe macroglossia with protrusion may be caused by lymphangiectasia or by an actual increase in muscle and connective tissue. Its cause is unknown. Occasionally it regresses spontaneously (Fig. 18–2).

A *lingual thyroid* occurring as a result of nondescent of the thyroid anlage may be found as an obstructing mass in the posterior one third of the midline of the tongue.

Fig. 18–3.—Teeth erupted before birth. **A,** lower central incisors. **B,** upper lateral incisors.

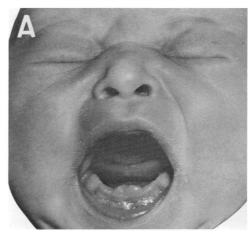

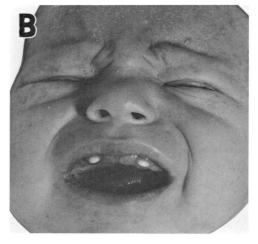

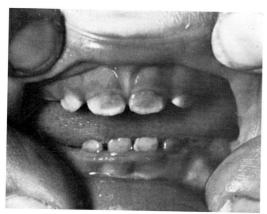

Fig. 18—4.—Deciduous teeth with blue discoloration resulting from deposit of bilirubin between dentine and enamel during period of severe jaundice associated with erythroblastosis. Permanent teeth are normal.

Teeth, especially the two lower central incisors, may be present at birth (Fig. 18–3, A). They are rarely of normal form and generally have little enamel and no roots. Because of the possibility of suffocation if they become detached and lodge in the larynx they are often removed. One infant born at the Chicago Lying-in Hospital had two normal-appearing upper incisors partially erupted at birth (Fig. 18–3, B). The enamel was well developed and they grew and remained in the jaw for several years.

In some cases of erythroblastosis associated with severe prolonged hemolytic icterus those teeth in which the enamel and dentine have developed by the time the icterus is at its height show a deposit of bile pigment between these layers. The teeth, when erupted, may have portions that are either bright blue-green or brown. All of the surfaces of the upper and lower incisors are discolored (Fig. 18–4). The extent of discoloration of the cuspids and bicuspids is variable, being dependent upon the stage to which the teeth are developed at birth since the deposit of bile is limited to the areas in which enamel is present. The permanent teeth are normal.

Tetracycline taken by the mother over a long period of time will stain the developing teeth of the fetus; if given to the infant after birth it will have a similar effect.

TUMORS

Ranula is a term applied to a retention cyst of the sublingual or submaxillary gland (Fig. 18–5). The cysts, located beneath the tongue, are round or oval, usually unilocular and lined by large, mucus-secreting cells. They sometimes disappear spontaneously or may persist until surgically removed.

Bohn's nodules are small white or yellow nodules 1–2 mm in diameter arising as retention cysts in mucous glands. They are found soon after birth in the roof of the mouth near the midline and disappear spontaneously in a few days.

Cystic enlargement of the enamel organ may be responsible for cysts on the gum margin (Fig. 18–6).

Epulis (on the gum) is a nonspecific term for a localized mass. Willis distinguished three kinds, all of which may be found in the 1st year of life. The first, which is non-neoplastic, is a reactive, often cystic, lesion containing fibroblasts and osteoclastic giant cells; it is related to the remodeling of the jaw that occurs during tooth formation and replacement. The second has the appearance of a benign, granular cell myoblastoma but comes from para-dental epithelial residues. The third is melanotic and consists of a mixture of pigmented epithelium and connective tissue (Fig. 18–7); although often associated with widespread destruction and distor-

Fig. 18—5.—Ranulas—sublingual cysts of salivary glands. **A,** large elongated cyst to right of frenulum. Infant aged 3 days. **B,** small round cysts to left of frenulum. Stillborn fetus.

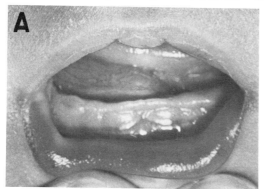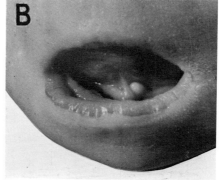

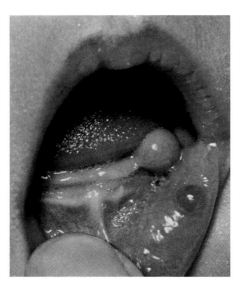

Fig. 18—6.—Cyst of the enamel organ with area of irritation on apposed surface of the lip.

tion of the jaw, it is benign. The tissue of origin of the third variety of epulis is in dispute. Halpert and Patzer called them retinal anlage tumors, and Stowens suggested an origin from phylogenetic cells analogous to the lateral line organ of teleost fish. Willis believed them to be of paradontal origin. Similar tumors have been described in other parts of the body.

Large tumors arising in the mouth are rare and an exact point of origin may be impossible to determine. The majority appear to come from the region of Rathke's pouch and most of them are teratomas (see Fig. 12–34). Occasionally they are composed of a mixture of cell types with no specifically identifiable tissues (Fig. 18–8).

THRUSH

Caused by the yeast organism *Candida albicans*, this infection is almost never found in the infant unless it was present in the mother's vagina. The disease may be contracted rarely in utero from infected amnion and chorion or more often during delivery from organisms in the vagina. Infection from other sources is rare, and even in the presence of a vaginal infection prophylactic treatment of the infant's tongue and buccal mucosa will ordinarily prevent the disease. It is characterized by slightly elevated white areas of irregular size and shape on the tongue or buccal mucosa. The lesions spread rapidly and the entire buccal mucosa may become involved (Fig. 18–9). When the patches are wiped off, a red denuded area remains. The lesions usually heal readily if properly treated, but in infants who are in poor condition from other causes they may spread, and involvement of the esophagus, pharynx, lung and intestine may lead to severe disease with fatal outcome. The diagnosis is confirmed by the finding of mycelial threads and small oval

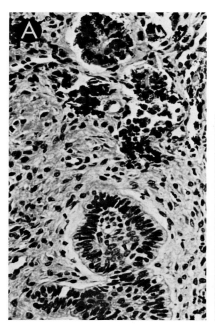

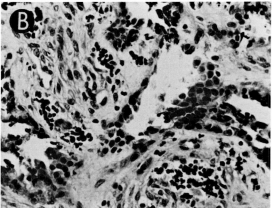

Fig. 18—7.—Melanotic epulis. **A,** characteristic plump stroma cells are intermixed with a pigmented epithelium above and primitive tooth anlage below. **B,** irregular spaces of highly vascular connective tissue lined by pigmented epithelium.

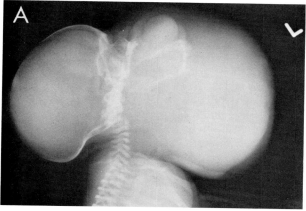

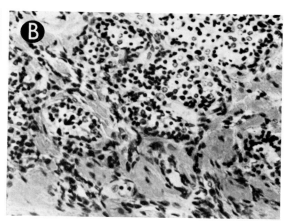

Fig. 18–8. – **A,** roentgenogram of an enormous tumor of the lower jaw of uncertain origin. **B,** photomicrograph of the same tumor made up of large pale cells with vesic- ular nuclei and small dark pyknotic cells with scant cyto- plasm.

spores in stained smears. Histologic examination of the involved areas may reveal masses of mycelia and spores replacing the squamous epithelium (see Fig. 9–25).

Esophagus

The esophagus may share in the generalized congestion of tissues found in anoxia. Ulceration and esophageal varices, the existence of which was

Fig. 18–9. – Thrush caused by *Candida albicans.* Infant aged 5 days.

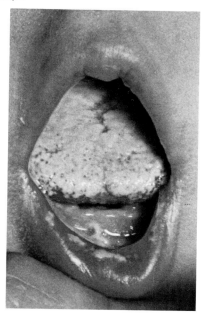

not suspected clinically, have been reported as inci- dental findings on postmortem examination. In a few instances they have been thought to have caused bloody emesis but usually they are symp- tomless. The etiology is unknown, although capil- lary injury associated with anoxia may predispose to their formation.

Gruenwald and Marsh reported finding acute esophagitis often accompanied by ulceration in one of every six infants under 6 months of age exam- ined at autopsy. The abnormality was suspected when the esophageal surface was hyperemic, lus- terlous or ulcerated, although occasionally cellular infiltration was found when the gross appearance was normal. The most common location was just above the cardia but it never extended beyond the edge of the gastric mucosa. At times the entire length of the esophagus was involved. Bacteria could be demonstrated in about half of the cases. The disorder was sometimes asymptomatic and probably unrelated to death but at other times was associated with vomiting and hematemesis and even caused death from perforation. It can be a source of infection in other parts of the body. The diagnosis should be suspected in any infant with blood in the stools or vomitus. The etiology is un- known but the authors felt that it might be a "shock lesion" and that other evidence of shock should be sought whenever esophagitis is sus- pected.

An even more common lesion, although very rarely giving rise to symptoms, is erosion of the esophagus at the level of the thyroid gland. Mer- riam and Benirschke found a 30% incidence of such lesions in 190 consecutive autopsies on newborns.

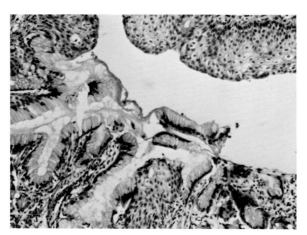

Fig. 18—10.—Ectopic gastric epithelium in the mid-portion of the esophagus.

These ulcerations were most common after intubation.

Ectopic gastric epithelium (Fig. 18–10) may be found in the esophagus in about 8% of autopsies on newborn infants, according to Rector and Connerly, and ciliated respiratory epithelium in about 4%. The latter is more common in very premature infants and disappears as term is reached. The gastric epithelium is found most often in the upper one third of the esophagus and the ciliated epithelium in the lower one third. Such aberrant epithelium almost never produces symptoms.

The esophagus may rupture spontaneously in very young infants, usually after violent vomiting. It most often ruptures into the right pleural space and causes pneumothorax.

The position of the esophagus is altered by any condition causing a shift in the location of the mediastinal structures. A defective diaphragm that permits the abdominal viscera to enter the thoracic cavity is the most common cause of lateral displacement. The esophagus may be displaced anteriorly by herniation of bowel into the posterior mediastinum. Air in the displaced esophagus may be visible in a chest roentgenogram (see Fig. 19–5) before enough is swallowed to be visible in the loops of intestine lying in the chest cavity.

TRACHEOESOPHAGEAL FISTULA

Tracheoesophageal fistula is the condition of outstanding interest in the esophagus. Several varieties have been described but in the majority the esophagus is separated into two noncommunicating parts with the lower part opening into the trachea and the upper part ending blindly in a sacculated pouch 2–4 cm below the epiglottis (Fig. 18–11). The lower portion has a considerably smaller lumen than the upper portion and generally arises in the midline of the posterior wall of the trachea about 1 cm above the bifurcation (Fig. 18–12). The esophagus widens as it descends and is of normal caliber when it reaches the stomach. In other less frequently encountered varieties the upper end of the esophagus communicates with the trachea, both ends communicate with it or stenosis or atresia of the esophagus exists without a tracheal communication. The sacculation of the upper segment is probably the result of distention caused by swallowed amniotic fluid. According to Holinger et al., the frequency with which the four types are encountered is 87%, 1%, 4% and 8%, respectively.

In the classic form of fistula, material taken into the mouth quickly fills the esophageal pouch, is regurgitated into the pharynx and aspirated into the lungs. Even if the infant is not fed, large amounts of mucus accumulate in the pouch, and any baby who brings forth an unusually large amount of mucus should be suspected of having esophageal atresia. Pneumonia develops early because of aspiration into the lungs, and the child's life can be saved only if a diagnosis is made and the defect repaired within a few hours of birth. Barium should never be used as the opaque medium for a diagnostic roentgen study because of its almost certain aspiration into the lungs. In the presence of esophageal obstruction the demonstration of air in the stomach and intestines on x-ray examination is evidence of a fistulous opening into the trachea (Fig. 18–13, A); its absence indicates a lack of communication between trachea and esophagus (Fig. 18–13, B).

Microscopic examination of the trachea and esophagus reveals normal mucosa and muscularis. The esophageal mucosa ends abruptly at its junction with the trachea (Fig. 18–14).

If no other anomalies exist, prompt diagnosis and skilled operative intervention may permit survival in as many as 78% of infants with the most common form of tracheoesophageal fistula (Holinger et al.). However, in the approximately 50% of such infants who have other major anomalies the chance of survival is greatly reduced. According to Haight, cardiovascular or gastrointestinal malformations each occur in about 22% of cases and genitourinary and bony anomalies about half as often. The central nervous system is infrequently involved.

Absence of the trachea, with the lungs individ-

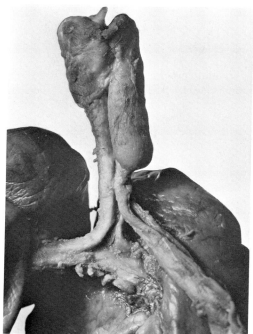

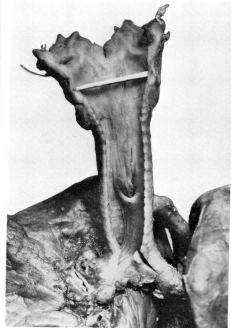

Fig. 18–11 (left).—Tracheoesophageal fistula. External surface showing sacculated blind upper esophageal pouch with fibrous cord connecting it to lower segment arising from trachea.

Fig. 18–12 (right).—Tracheoesophageal fistula. Interior of trachea showing communication with esophagus 1 cm above the bifurcation. Same case as Fig. 18–11.

ually attached to the lower esophagus by the main bronchi, was reported by Witzleben from the Boston Lying-in Hospital.

Duplication of the esophagus or cysts derived from gastric tissues may be found in the posterior mediastinum. Some of the latter contain pancreatic tissue (Fig. 18–15). Such cysts must be distinguished from mediastinal teratomas, neurenteric

Fig. 18–13.—Roentgenograms of infants with esophageal fistulas. **A,** air in stomach and intestine indicates presence of fistulous opening between trachea and lower end of esophagus. **B,** absence of air in stomach and intestine indicates absence of communication between trachea and esophagus.

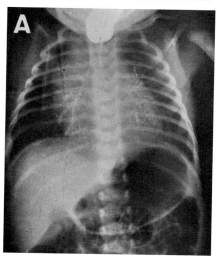

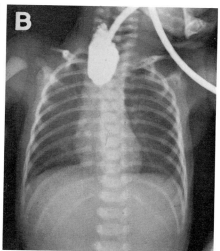

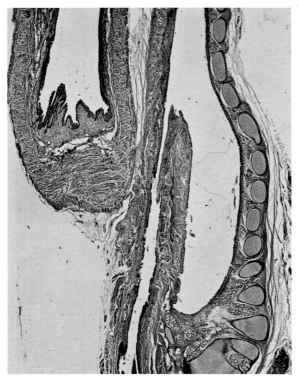

Fig. 18−14.−Photomicrograph showing blind esophageal pouch and origin of lower portion of the esophagus from the trachea.

canals associated with diastomyelia and defects in the upper thoracic vertebrae.

Stomach

During fetal life the stomach is filled with a gray-white mucoid material composed of secretions from the gastric mucosa, desquamated gastric cells and fluid and debris derived from swallowed amniotic fluid. Maternal blood swallowed during delivery may also be present and is probably the most frequent source of occult blood in the stools in the first few days of life. Experiments at the Chicago Lying-in Hospital indicated that 4 ml of blood is sufficient to produce a tarry stool.

Occasional regurgitation, which is most often a result of overdistention or too rapid filling of the stomach, is common in the newborn and usually is of no pathologic significance. It may be associated with an excessive amount of mucus in the stomach and relief may be obtained from lavage. Air swallowed during feeding, if not expelled before the child is returned to its crib, often carries food material with it when it escapes. Vomiting may be

observed in any infant who is not doing well, especially those with signs of intracranial injury. If it occurs soon after birth and continues, obstructive lesions in the gastrointestinal tract must be considered. When it occurs first at 2 or 3 weeks of age and becomes projectile, it is almost always a result of pyloric stenosis.

Ulcerations of the stomach and duodenum have been described in the newborn and have been considered a possible source of hematemesis as well as a cause of perforation and obstruction. The mucosa may be injured by passage of a stomach tube, and subsequent action by gastric juice may produce necrosis and inflammation. Multiple ulcerations have been reported as embolic phenomena caused by sepsis originating from infection of the umbilicus. Leix and Greaney reported that nearly one half of all peptic ulcerations in infants and children occur in the 1st year and that half of these are found in infants who are otherwise well. Care must be taken not to confuse the punctate areas of necrosis caused by postmortem digestion of the mucosa with actual ulceration.

Bloody emesis, designated clinically as hemorrhagic disease, is stated to result from capillary hemorrhage of the gastric mucosa. No lesions have been described as characteristic of this disease, and whether hemorrhage occurs from an intact gastric

Fig. 18−15.−Wall of a cyst in the posterior mediastinum. The lumen is at the upper right without specific lining. Below to the left is ectopic pancreatic tissue. (Courtesy Dr. W. D. Bradford.)

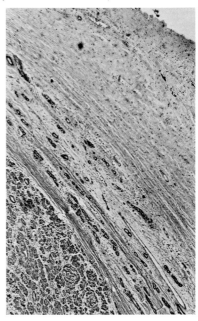

mucosa because of a prothrombin deficiency is questionable. Blood in vomitus may have its origin in the lungs or nasopharynx, in a fissured maternal nipple or, rarely, in blood dyscrasias such as purpura and leukemia.

Rupture of the stomach is limited largely to the first few days of life. It is most often observed in infants who have been fed by gavage and the site is frequently the greater curvature of the stomach in the region most susceptible to damage from introduction of a gavage tube. Accidental introduction of a tracheal catheter into the esophagus and stomach during attempts at resuscitation may also produce injury. It seems probable that in most instances the mucosa is traumatized, infection sets in and perforation follows. The escape of gastric contents into the abdomen leads to peritonitis. The stomach wall in the vicinity of the perforation becomes progressively necrotic and by the time of death a large defect is usually visible.

Rarely, defective formation of the musculature of the stomach is responsible for areas that give way under the postnatal distention occasioned by early feedings. In one infant observed at the Chicago Lying-in Hospital who died of peritonitis following gastric rupture, the muscle coats became gradually thinner and disappeared at the margin of the tear in the stomach wall (Fig. 18–16). This appeared to be a congenital defect of the musculature.

Shaw *et al.,* after studying sections of the stom-

ach following experimental rupture, noted marked retraction of the muscle away from the edge of the rupture and a gradual thinning of the muscle as the point of rupture was approached. They concluded that rupture of a stomach with normal musculature would produce an appearance identical to that attributed to malformation and that the latter diagnosis was generally due to misinterpretation of findings.

The stomach ordinarily varies in size and shape only in relation to the amount of material within it. Its position is remarkably constant except as it is altered by malformation of other structures in the abdominal or thoracic cavities. When the left leaf of the diaphragm is defective the stomach usually lies partially or entirely within the chest along with most of the abdominal viscera (see Fig. 19–3). Hiatus hernias produce less extensive displacement and usually only a few centimeters of stomach appear above the diaphragm. Filler *et al.* found 30 cases of hiatus hernia among 142 cases of diaphragmatic defects; in the majority vomiting and malnutrition occurred in the first 3 weeks of life.

Intrinsic malformations are less common in the stomach than in the intestinal tract and diverticuli; stenosis or other malformations are almost unknown. Most so-called hourglass stomachs in infants are not abnormalities of the stomach but are the result of distention of the proximal portion of the duodenum secondary to atresia or stenosis of

Fig. 18–16 (left).—Ruptured stomach. Photomicrograph of margin of the rupture showing a defect in the muscular layer.

Fig. 18–17 (right).—Section through the pyloric end of the stomach showing a small cyst lined by gastric mucosa. The muscle lies exterior to the cyst. This is one form of duplication of the stomach.

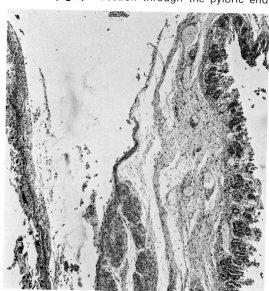

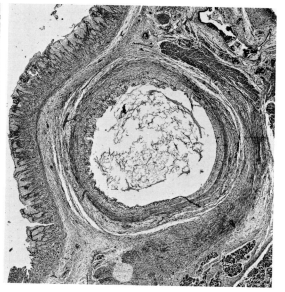

the distal portion. The distended duodenum is mistaken for part of the stomach (see Fig. 18–26, A).

Partial duplication of the stomach is rare but has been reported. One case was observed at the Chicago Lying-in Hospital in which a small closed cavity lined by gastric mucosa was present in the wall of the pyloric end of the stomach (Fig. 18–17). Only two of 67 gastrointestinal duplications reported by Gross *et al.* involved the stomach. Absence of the stomach is unknown except in grossly malformed fetuses such as acardiac acephalic monsters.

Pyloric Stenosis

Congenital hypertrophic pyloric stenosis is the most common gastric lesion found in infancy. It is much more common in boys than in girls, the ratio being 4:1; according to Burmeister and Hamilton, it is found most often in firstborn infants and frequently in siblings. Inheritance has been described as polygenic and sex-modified, with the process transmitted more frequently from an affected mother than a father. The hypertrophy of the pylorus is believed to exist before birth and to be responsible for a narrowing of the pyloric lumen. Vomiting occurs only when the mucosa becomes edematous and infiltrated by inflammatory cells because of mechanical irritation produced by passage of milk curds through the narrowed sphincter. Usually occurring at 2 or 3 weeks of age, this is an important point in differentiating pyloric stenosis from stenosis or atresia of other parts of the gastrointestinal tract. In the latter, vomiting occurs in the first few days of life; in pyloric stenosis it begins as ordinary emesis but soon assumes a characteristic projectile pattern. The enlarged pylorus can often be palpated through a relaxed abdominal wall, and peristaltic waves may be visible.

The lesion consists of hypertrophy of the circular layer and, to a lesser degree, of the longitudinal layer of muscle in the wall of the pyloric sphincter. The pylorus is increased in length and width and has a gray-white gristly appearance. At the gastric end the thickened muscle tapers off gradually but at the duodenal side it ends abruptly. The mucosa is often edematous and mildly infiltrated by inflammatory cells. The muscle is increased in amount but is otherwise normal. In one case observed at the Children's Hospital Medical Center in Boston benign mucosal glands were abnormally distributed throughout the thickened pyloric muscle. It was designated adenomyosis of the pylorus.

Milder degrees of vomiting that are suggestive of pyloric stenosis may respond to treatment with drugs such as atropine or barbiturates that tend to relax the pyloric sphincter. In affected infants there is no actual increase in the volume of sphincteric muscle and the condition seems to be a disturbance of the nervous mechanism responsible for relaxation rather than an anatomic reduction of the lumen.

Because of the partial response to sympathetic blocking agents among certain patients with pyloric stenosis attempts have been made to demonstrate an abnormality of the nerve cells in order to explain the muscular hypertrophy. Belding and Kernohan described degenerated nerve cells in the duodenal wall but no decreases in ganglion cells. Friesen and Pearse, because they found a reduced histochemical reaction for esterase, suggested that maturation of the nerve cells was delayed.

Intestine

Meconium

The fetus normally swallows large amounts of amniotic fluid during intrauterine life, and it seems probable that this helps to regulate the amount of fluid in the amniotic sac since the existence of high intestinal obstruction is usually associated with polyhydramnios. The ingested fluid normally leaves the stomach rapidly and passes into the intestine where most of the water is absorbed and only the nondigestible elements such as lanugo hairs and cornified epithelial cells remain. This detritus, together with desquamated cells and secretions from the gastrointestinal mucosa, liver and pancreas, make up meconium.

Normal meconium is a green-black viscid substance that fills the colon at birth. The anal sphincter normally remains closed and no meconium is evacuated during intrauterine life except occasionally when delivery is from a breech position. If the oxygen supply is reduced, the anal sphincter relaxes and the intestine may be more or less completely emptied. Consequently meconium in the amniotic fluid with a cephalic presentation is ordinarily a sign of fetal distress.

Much of the meconium in the intestine may be passed before birth by fetuses that are stillborn or before death by infants who fail to survive after birth. When the total amount of meconium has been retained until the time of autopsy, the large intestine in infants at term is often 2–3 cm in diameter. Since the intestine of the newborn is more redundant than that of an older individual, especially in the region of the sigmoid flexure, and the total amount of meconium is rarely seen, an erroneous diagnosis of megacolon may be made if no meconium has been passed before autopsy is performed. Partial evacuation may leave distended portions interspersed between sharply contracted empty portions. The extreme difference in diameter of the lumens in the contracted and noncontracted areas may lead to an incorrect diagnosis of multiple areas of intestinal stenosis.

The consistency of normal meconium is fairly constant. The terminal part of the rectum may be filled with a plug composed of dense meconium that has become abnormally firm because of excessive absorption of water. This plug may interfere temporarily with defecation and cause symptoms of intestinal obstruction but is usually passed before severe symptoms develop. Rarely, the meconium filling part or all of the colon and lower ileum is abnormally firm and dry and so impacted that intestinal obstruction is diagnosed from x-ray examination because radiopaque material does not penetrate the meconium mass.

Although deficiency of biliary or pancreatic secretions is the most common cause of a lack of normal fluidity of the intestinal contents, diminution of the volume of amniotic fluid swallowed during intrauterine life could be responsible for a less than normal amount of fluid in the intestinal tract and this in turn for abnormal consistency of meconium. In some infants this is an isolated phenomenon of unknown cause and the subsequent course of the infant is normal.

If the hepatic or common bile ducts are obstructed or if the intestine is atretic at a point distal to the papilla of Vater, the meconium is gray instead of green-black. It is also firmer and less viscid than normal meconium. With high intestinal obstruction the amount of meconium is decreased because of the absence of fluid and of debris from the swallowed amniotic fluid.

MECONIUM ILEUS. — With rare exceptions true meconium ileus is associated with deficient pancreatic secretions, a result of the hereditary disorder *cystic fibrosis of the pancreas*. In that disease the meconium has an abnormally high protein content, which may be due in part to a deficiency of trypsin and in part to the abnormal mucoprotein secretion of the pancreas and intestinal glands.

In some cases the intestinal obstruction may be relieved by irrigation of the intestine with "pancreatin," which causes liquefaction of the meconium. More often resection of the impacted area is necessary to relieve the obstruction. Although the distal portion of the large bowel may have a very small diameter, a so-called "microcolon," it is func-

tionally normal and assumes a normal size once the obstruction is relieved.

INFECTION

Epidemic diarrhea of the newborn is a condition dreaded in any nursery. The discovery of diarrhea necessitates prompt isolation of the affected infant for cross-infections are common and if diarrhea becomes established in a nursery, its spread may not stop until the nursery is closed and all of the affected infants have been discharged.

In different epidemics different bacteria and viruses have been found in the stools. However, it is now generally accepted that most such epidemics are caused by a small group of *Escherichia coli*, which can be identified by serologic typing. Before their immunologic specificity was recognized, these organisms were thought to be part of the normal bowel flora. They are now designated "pathogenic *E. coli*." This term has meaning only as related to their behavior in the intestine and the fact that they give rise to serious disease in the very young; in the kidney or peritoneal cavity "nonpathogenic *E. coli*" strains are equally disease-producing at any age. The pathologic changes in infantile epidemic diarrhea are minimal and often no bowel lesions can be demonstrated. Such a diagnosis can be accepted only during an epidemic and when specific *E. coli* strains are isolated. If death occurs, it is usually the result of toxicity, electrolyte imbalance or secondary pneumonia. The severity of symptoms in reported epidemics has varied, but in some the infants have been greatly prostrated and the mortality has been more than 50% of affected infants.

Enteritis may also occur in a nonepidemic form in individual infants. The young infant, especially when premature, may develop diarrhea in association with severe para-enteric infections, and pneumonia or pyelonephritis, for instance, may be found at autopsy in an infant whose chief difficulty appeared to be diarrhea.

Autopsy findings following death from infectious diarrhea are often meager. The intestinal mucosa may be congested and reddened but there is ordinarily little evidence of local infection, and unless a history is available the cause of death may be unsuspected at postmortem examination. Infection by dysentery organisms in older infants may produce widespread ulcers that involve much of the mucosa of the large and small intestines.

A specific form of *acute necrotizing enteritis* was described by Berdon *et al.* and Mizrahi *et al.* in young premature infants usually weighing less than 1,500 gm. Loss of the mucosa in large portions of the ileum, appendix and colon was accompanied by an acute inflammatory reaction and often by pneumo-intestinalis. The latter appeared in the bowel submucosa and muscularis as large bubbles with occasional giant cells in large, otherwise empty interstitial spaces. Some of these infants were born following early rupture of the membranes, and cultures of the bowel showed the same variety of enteric organisms usually found in the amniotic sac after prolonged rupture. Bell *et al.* often found such lesions in the respiratory distress syndrome, and Hardy *et al.* stated that they are strikingly frequent in infants receiving exchange transfusions for erythroblastosis. Such infections may lead to perforation of the bowel and peritonitis.

PERITONITIS

This condition most often follows the rupture of a viscus, but rarely it may be found with an intact gastrointestinal tract. In several instances we have observed fibrin containing a few leukocytes forming delicate adhesions holding loops of bowel together in stillborn infants or those dying in the immediate postnatal period. Bacteria are rarely demonstrable and there has been no other evidence of infection in any infant except one in whom the chorionic surface of the placenta was densely infiltrated by leukocytes. It is generally presumed that such peritonitis arises from placental transmission of bacteria, although this has never been proved. It has also been suggested that the ingestion of amniotic fluid containing bacteria might give rise to enteritis, which in turn might lead to peritonitis; this idea, too, is largely conjectural. Peritonitis that develops several days after birth may be a direct extension of an infection arising in the umbilicus. This is uncommon and even with severe omphalitis the peritoneum is not ordinarily involved.

Meconium peritonitis is the name given peritoneal involvement secondary to meconium ileus, peritoneal bands, mesenteric herniation or volvulus. The peritonitis is due to the irritation produced by bile and other material in the meconium and is originally sterile. If an infant is born alive and food is ingested, bacteria soon appear in the intestine and continued leakage through the rupture rapidly leads to bacterial peritonitis and death.

If rupture occurs before birth, the material in the abdominal cavity may become calcified when it can be seen outlining the loops of intestine on roentgen examination (Fig. 18–18).

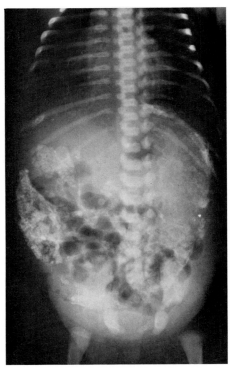

Fig. 18–18. — Roentgenogram showing widespread calcification throughout the abdomen in meconium peritonitis secondary to intrauterine rupture of the intestine. (Courtesy Dr. Sidney Farber.)

Mucus, epithelial cells from the amniotic fluid, calcium and other debris may be identified histologically on the surface of the liver, spleen, intestine and other organs (Fig. 18–19, A). Foreign body giant cells are also often visible (Fig. 18–19, B).

In one infant observed at the Chicago Lying-in Hospital a peculiar form of calcification was widespread over the abdominal surface of the diaphragm and present in small areas over the kidneys, adrenal glands and parts of the posterior abdominal wall. The calcium was present in small wormlike masses 1–2 mm in diameter (Fig. 18–20, A) and on microscopic examination was found as flakelike material filling the lumens of small muscular tubes resembling blood vessels. Intervening tissue also contained many small vascular channels (Fig. 18–20, B) and the appearance was that of multiple small, unusually well-differentiated angiomas that had become partially obstructed and undergone secondary calcification. Other blood vessels in the body showed no abnormalities.

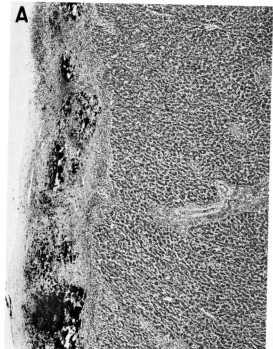

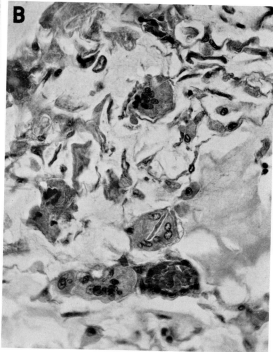

Fig. 18–19.—Calcification of surface of the liver secondary to meconium peritonitis. **A,** low power view. **B,** high power view of the abdominal exudate from another patient showing keratinized epithelial cells derived from ingested amniotic fluid and foreign body reaction to these cells. (B, courtesy Dr. Sidney Farber.)

RUPTURE OF INTESTINE AFTER BIRTH

Spontaneous rupture of the intestine after birth is rare and usually without known cause. We have observed only one case. This infant appeared normal for the first 24 hours of life, then suddenly became pale and dyspneic and appeared acutely ill. Moderate abdominal distention led to roentgen examination, which revealed free air in the peritoneal cavity (Fig. 18–21, A). The infant died in a short time and at autopsy two areas of rupture were found, with a third area almost on the point of rupture. One perforation was at the base of the appendix and the other was close to a Meckel's diverticulum, with the unruptured area adjacent to it (Fig. 18–21, B). Meconium was present in the abdomen but peritonitis had not developed. Microscopic examination revealed no evidence of local infection. The unruptured area showed almost complete absence of muscle and great distention of blood vessels. These appeared larger and more numerous than usual, but the main abnormality seems to have been a congenital defect of muscle coats.

APPENDICITIS

This condition, although rare in early infancy, was observed at the Chicago Lying-in Hospital in two infants of a few days old. Both had pronounced abdominal distention, and it was interesting that both had congenital heart disease. The infants died at 6 and 23 days of age, respectively, presumably of the heart lesions, although blood cultures were not made and the abdominal pathology was not suspected antemortem. The appendixes were swollen, reddened and surrounded by an exudate that extended over the loops of intestine in the lower abdominal cavity. In one case the appendix was coiled and bound to the cecum (Fig. 18–22). No obstruction of the lumen could be found in either appendix. The muscularis and serosa of both were infiltrated by leukocytes.

Of 30 cases in children aged under 36 months gathered by Fields and Cole over a 10-year period only one was under 1 year of age; these investigators cited another report of five fatal cases, all in infants under 1 year of age.

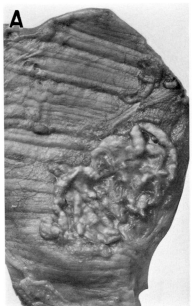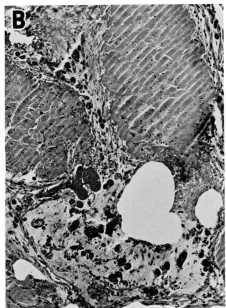

Fig. 18–20.—Calcified area on the diaphragm. **A,** circinoid calcified area on peritoneal surface of the diaphragm. Similar smaller areas were present on the surface of the liver, adrenal glands and kidneys. **B,** photomicrograph showing calcified areas surrounded by smooth muscle fibers. Intervening tissue contains innumerable small vascular channels. The entire structure bears considerable resemblance to a hemangioma that has undergone thrombosis and calcification.

ERYTHROBLASTOSIS

At the Chicago Lying-in Hospital lesions were observed in the intestinal tract of several infants with erythroblastosis. They consisted of slightly elevated cherry-red areas in the walls of the stomach and intestine. Visible from both the mucosal and serosal surfaces, they were round or oval, measured 2–10 mm in greatest diameter and were composed of masses of immature red blood cells (Fig. 18–23, A). No lymphoid structures could be found in the intestinal wall, and these red areas seemed to be Peyer's patches and solitary lymph follicles that had been completely replaced by erythropoietic cells (Fig. 18–23, B).

Orme and Eades reported six infants with perforation of the bowel due to necrotizing enterocolitis, chiefly of the colon, who had undergone exchange transfusion for erythroblastosis. They found extensive areas of mucosal and submucosal necrosis, ulcerations and inflammation. In one case vascular thrombi were present. A similar case was observed at the Boston Lying-in Hospital. It has been suggested that the lesions are caused by a severe fall in blood pressure.

STENOSIS AND ATRESIA

Malformations of the intestine are common, and most of those found in young infants cause obstruction. Persistent vomiting or absence of stools is highly suggestive of intestinal stenosis or atresia. Complete atresia always causes symptoms in the first few days of life. Mild degrees of stenosis may not be evident until solid food is introduced into the diet.

Obstruction may be caused by a variety of lesions. A thin membrane may extend across part or all of the lumen, especially in the duodenum or lower part of the rectum. A local narrowing of the lumen with hypoplasia of the mucosa and musculature may cause partial or intermittent obstruction. Complete atresia may be associated with complete discontinuity of the two ends (Fig. 18–24), or the ends may be connected by a fibrous cord (Fig. 18–25).

Atresia of the esophagus or duodenum is ordinarily recognized promptly because of the rapidity with which emesis follows the intake of food. With obstruction lower in the intestine vomiting comes later; rarely, there is no vomiting for several days,

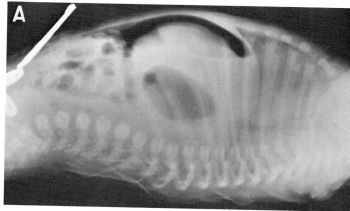

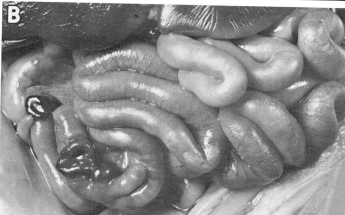

Fig. 18—21.—Rupture of the intestine on the 2d day of life. **A,** pneumoperitoneum giving evidence of a ruptured viscus. **B,** intestine showing areas of spontaneous rupture, one in the ileum at the cecal junction, another adjacent to a Meckel's diverticulum. A third area, distended but unruptured, is present in close proximity. There was no infection and the only abnormality in the unruptured distended area was an extreme thinning of the muscle and dilatation of the blood vessels.

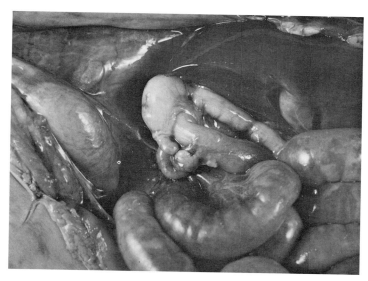

Fig. 18—22.—Acute appendicitis in infant aged 6 days associated with extreme abdominal distention clinically thought to have been caused by an intestinal malformation.

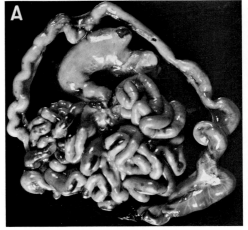

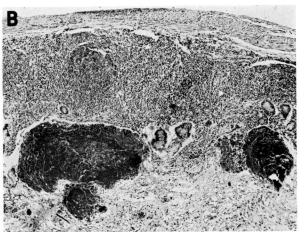

Fig. 18—23.—Erythroblastosis. **A,** stomach and intestine showing conversion of Peyer's patches and solitary lymph follicles into cherry-red areas of erythropoiesis.

B, photomicrograph showing such an area of erythropoiesis. The lower black masses are meconium.

and abdominal distention and absence of stools are the first symptoms. With all malformations the symptoms rapidly become more severe, and with low intestinal obstruction the vomiting may be fecal in character. The presence of bile in the vomitus indicates a point of obstruction below the papilla of Vater. Distention of the abdomen, especially with low intestinal occlusion, is often excessive.

Among 211 infants and children reported by

Gross who were treated surgically because of intestinal obstruction one third had an area of atresia in the ileum. This site was over twice as common as the duodenum, where similar lesions were found with the next greatest frequency. For stenosis the reverse was true, and the duodenum was the site of greatest predilection, with the ileum second. The distribution as given by Gross is found in Table 18—1.

Fig. 18—24 (left).—Agenesis of part of the ileum with discontinuity of the two segments. Operation was refused by the parents but the infant survived for 18 days. Note hypoplasia of the distal bowel and overdistention of the proximal portion.

Fig. 18—25 (right).—Atresia of the ileum with two segments connected by a fibrous cord.

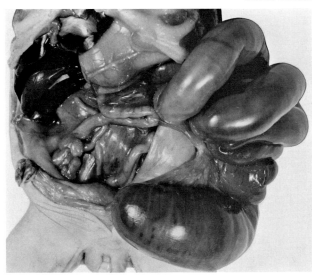

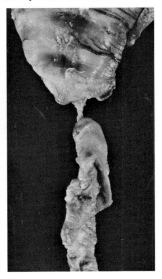

TABLE 18–1.—LOCATION OF
INTESTINAL ATRESIA AND STENOSIS
AS DETERMINED AT OPERATION (GROSS)

LOCATION	ATRESIA	STENOSIS
Duodenum	32	39
Jejunum	19	5
Ileum	72	19
Ileocecal valve	2	6
Colon	6	1
Multiple	9	1

Lynn and Espinas found a thirteenfold predominance of small intestinal over colonic atresias among 930 cases obtained by combining three reported series.

Atresia or stenosis of any portion of the intestine results in distention of the proximal part and narrowing of the distal part. This is especially noticeable in involvement of the terminal portion of the duodenum, where the size of the duodenum often approximates or exceeds that of the stomach (Fig. 18–26). This sacculated structure may be mistaken for the lower half of the stomach, and the pylorus may be interpreted as a constriction ring. Roentgen examination after administration of radiopaque

material reveals a characteristic dumbbell-shaped shadow (Fig. 18–27). A roentgenogram taken without contrast medium shows the stomach and duodenum greatly distended by air and complete absence of air in the rest of the abdomen (Fig. 18–28, A). Polyhydramnios is often present with esophageal, pyloric or duodenal atresia, which supports the belief that the fluid intake and output of the fetus play a role in determining the volume of amniotic fluid. A prenatal amniogram would be diagnostic although such a procedure is not recommended because radiopaque material injected into amniotic fluid enters the lungs as well as the stomach.

Obstruction of any portion of the jejunum is also associated with great dilatation of the more proximal part (Fig. 18–29). Air can be demonstrated in this part of the intestine on x-ray examination, which differentiates it from duodenal atresia (Fig. 18–28, B).

Obstruction of the ileum is more often due to complete atresia than to stenosis and the two segments are often separated. X-ray examination reveals air in much of the small intestine and none in the large intestine (Fig. 18–28, C).

Bremer's widely accepted theory of the formation of intestinal atresias has been disturbed by the

Fig. 18–26.—Duodenal stenosis and atresia. **A,** stenosis of the duodenum producing a sacculation between pylorus and area of stenosis. Colon terminates at the splenic flexure. Sirenomelus monster. **B,** atresia at the duodenal-jejunal junction with separation of the two segments. The greatly dilated duodenum can be seen anterior to the stomach. Laparotomy was performed but anastomosis was not attempted. Infant survived 21 days.

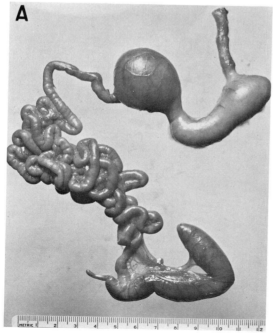
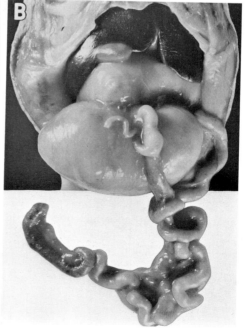

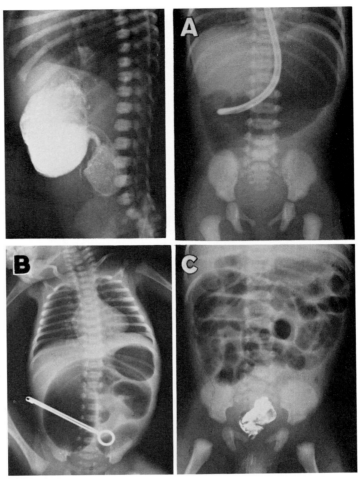

Fig. 18–27 (top left).—Characteristic roentgenogram of infant with duodenal stenosis. Barium fills stomach and pylorus, and intermixture of a small amount with contents of the duodenal pouch permits visualization of that structure.

Fig. 18–28 (top right and bottom).—Roentgenograms without contrast medium showing air above region of atresia. **A,** atresia of terminal portion of the duodenum. Stomach and duodenum are greatly distended and no air is present in remaining portion of the intestine. **B,** atresia of jejunum with distention of the stomach and bowel proximal to the point of atresia. Death followed attempted anastomosis. **C,** atresia of ileum with air above point of obstruction and small amount of barium in lower sigmoid colon. Infant survived following surgical anastomosis.

reports of Lynn and Espinas, and Santulli. Bremer believed that the embryonic intestine normally develops an epithelial plug with recanalization and secondary formation of a new lumen and that incomplete formation of the secondary lumen leads to atresia. Lynn and Espinas disputed this observation, and Santulli and Blanc found that in 27 of 43 cases of atresia evidence existed of previous injury caused by prenatal volvulus, umbilical hernia, persistent omphalomesenteric duct, perforation or meconium ileus secondary to cystic fibrosis of the pancreas. The meconium contained numerous squa-

mous cells distal to the atresia in all 43 cases which seemed to indicate a previous continuity of the intestine.

IMPERFORATE ANUS

Failure of the terminal portion of the large bowel to establish a communication with the exterior of the body is somewhat more common than loss of continuity in other parts of the intestine. It may be an isolated abnormality or it may be found with malformations of other parts of the body. The skin

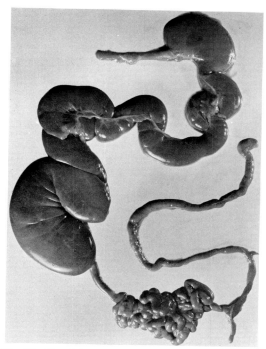

Fig. 18–29.—Jejunal atresia with pronounced dilatation of proximal segment.

tures to which it gives rise. Normally the vesicorectal septum reaches the cloacal membrane and effects a separation of the urogenital sinus from the rectum during the 7th week of gestation. After this the urogenital opening appears, followed slightly later by the perforation of the anal orifice. If the urogenital orifice fails to rupture, the genital ridges ordinarily do not develop and the clitoris or penis does not appear. The anal portion may rupture normally or it too may remain closed (Fig. 18–32, A). In one infant observed at the Chicago Lying-in Hospital no structures that normally come from the cloaca could be identified. Ovaries, kidneys and ureters were present but the bladder, urethra, clitoris, vagina, uterus, fallopian tubes and major part of the large intestine were missing. The intestine ended blindly about 4 cm distal to the ileocecal valve. The ureters emptied into the intestine a short distance from its termination (Fig. 18–32, B).

Abnormalities in the downgrowth of the urorectal septum are responsible for fistulous communications between the rectum and the bladder, urethra or vagina.

Santulli divided anal abnormalities into four groups and gave their frequency as follows: Type I (7%), anal closure incomplete; type II (0.025%),

over the anal region may be smooth and give little indication of the expected site of the anus, or it may be invaginated, the degree varying from a shallow dimple to a depth of 1 cm or more (Fig. 18–30). Stimulation of the area often reveals the presence of sphincteric muscle even though a depression is not visible.

The terminal portion of the intestine may end blindly or open into the urethra, bladder or vagina. If it ends blindly, the lumen may be separated from the exterior by only a thin membrane or it may terminate at varying distances from the surface. Valuable information concerning the distance between the end of the intestine and the body surface can be obtained by taping a lead shot to the approximate location of the anus and taking a roentgenogram of the infant in an inverted position. Air swallowed by the infant reaches the lower part of the bowel within a short time of birth, and when the child is held with the head down, the air rises to fill the terminal part of the rectum. By measuring the distance between the air and the point marking the external surface of the body the extent of the abnormality can be estimated (Fig. 18–31).

Disturbances in the evolution of the cloaca may be responsible for profound alterations in the struc-

Fig. 18–30.—Imperforate anus.

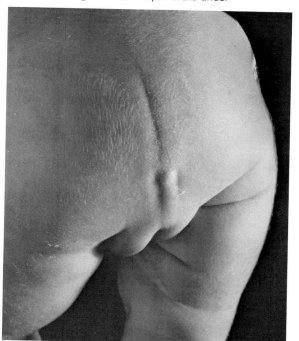

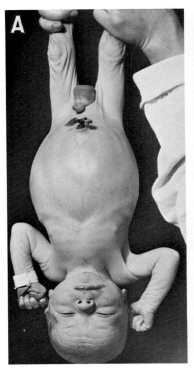

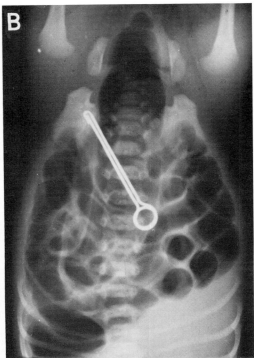

Fig. 18–31.—Imperforate anus. **A,** infant with marked abdominal distention inverted in preparation for x-ray demonstration of air in terminal portion of intestine. **B,** air in dilated rectum; roentgenogram made with infant suspended by feet.

Fig. 18–32.—Absence of anus and penis. **A,** external view. **B,** interior of abdomen showing communication of ureters with cecum and termination of colon at the hepatic flexure. Kidneys are polycystic.

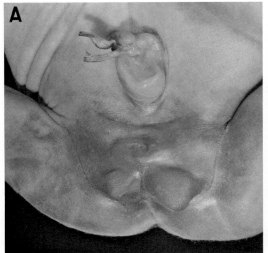

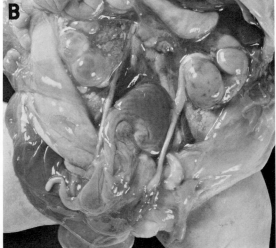

imperforate anus closed by a thin membrane; type III (91%), combined anal and rectal agenesis with 80% complicated by persistent cloacal communications; type IV (the remainder), anal atresia alone. A fistula, if present, opens onto the perineum except when the atresia also involves the rectum, in which case it usually opens into the urethra in the male or the vagina in the female.

Associated anomalies were reported in 97–100% of cases by both Santulli, and Moore and Eades. A fifth to a quarter of these were important and life threatening. Urinary anomalies including hydronephrosis, aplasia of the kidneys, hypospadias and extrophy of the bladder were first in order of frequency, with those of the nervous system including spina bifida and hydrocephalus next. Third in frequency were alimentary tract anomalies in areas other than the anus and rectum, including tracheoesophageal fistula, abnormalities of the gallbladder and malrotation of the intestine. Vertebral malformations were fourth, and cardiovascular malformations, chiefly congenital heart disease, fifth.

ABNORMAL ROTATION

Incomplete rotation of the intestine is common in association with other malformations, especially those involving the genitourinary system. It may, however, be an isolated anomaly in infants who die of unrelated causes or it may produce symptoms of obstruction and be diagnosed at operation.

In the early period of embryonic development the intestine elongates more rapidly than the abdominal cavity enlarges and the intestine protrudes into the base of the umbilical cord, where it proceeds to develop (see Fig. 3–50, B). The part to which the yolk sac is attached leads in the outward movement of the intestine in the 5th week and is the last part to return to the abdominal cavity in the 10th week. As the intestine is withdrawn into the abdominal cavity it normally moves in a counterclockwise direction around the superior mesenteric artery, which acts as an axis. On first reentering the abdomen, the terminal ileum and all of the colon, which are the parts distal to the yolk sac attachment, lie in the left side of the abdomen while the jejunum and the rest of the small bowel lie to the right. The cecum at this stage is high in the middle of the abdomen just below the stomach. Rotation normally continues and the cecum moves to the right and downward, finally taking up its permanent position in the right lower quadrant. After rotation is completed the cecum and ascending colon become fixed

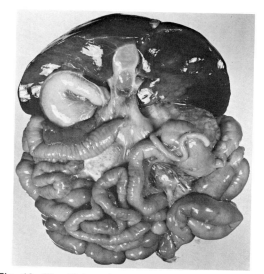

Fig. 18–33.—Malrotation of the intestine associated with dextroposition of stomach. Entire colon lies in left side of the abdomen, and ileum enters the cecum from right to left. Thoracic organs in normal position.

in position by the fusion of the mesentery with the posterior abdominal wall, while the small bowel below the duodenum is free to move because of its wide mesentery.

The movement of the intestine after it returns to the abdominal cavity may be brought to an end at any stage. If it returns to the abdomen as a single mass, no rotation occurs and the jejunum and ileum lie on the right, the large intestine lies on the left and the ileum enters the cecum from right to left

Fig. 18–34.—Incomplete rotation with small intestine lying to right of midline and large intestine attached by a wide mesentery.

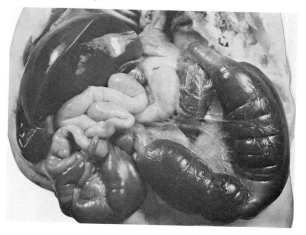

(Fig. 18–33). More commonly, partial rotation, so-called malrotaton, occurs, in which case the loops of small bowel occupy the right side of the abdomen, the large bowel occupies the left and the cecum lies in the epigastrium. The large intestine retains a wide mesentery and is freely movable.

The cecum may be found in any position between the middle portion of the upper abdomen and the right lower quadrant, depending on the degree of nonrotation. Even though it attains a normal position, fixation may not occur and the wide mesentery to which it is attached may be fixed only in the midabdominal region. This condition is commonly called *cecum mobile* (Fig. 18–34). Occasionally, all of the large intestine is attached to a wide mesentery (Fig. 18–35). Haller and Morgenstern gathered several reports of malrotation in which the primitive gut rotated in a clockwise direction, the splenic flexure passing behind the superior mesenteric artery and duodenum.

In complete situs inversus the appendix is in the left lower quadrant, and the entire intestine, like the rest of the viscera, is in a position resembling a mirror image of the normal. Situs inversus, particularly if incomplete, is associated with an increased incidence of intestinal stenosis, atresias and malrotations (Fonkalsrud *et al.*).

VOLVULUS

If development is arrested in any stage, the attachment of the mesentery of the small intestine to the posterior abdominal wall is incomplete and does not extend much below the origin of the inferior mesenteric artery. Such a state allows the entire intestinal mass to swing on this pedicle and the mesentery may become twisted several times. By this mechanism the intestine becomes closed off in the distal portion of duodenum and the middle part of the descending colon. This condition is known as volvulus (Fig. 18–36). Blood flow through the superior mesenteric artery is partially or completely cut off and unless the volvulus is promptly relieved, infarction of the involved intestine soon follows. Early symptoms are those of acute intestinal obstruction.

Incomplete rotation may be responsible for duodenal obstruction even in the absence of volvulus. When the cecum lies in the right side of the upper abdomen, bands of peritoneum may extend from it to the right posterior part of the abdominal wall and, in extending over the duodenum, may interfere with passage of material through that organ. With still less rotation the cecum is present in the middle portion of the upper abdomen,

Fig. 18–35 (left).—Entire intestine possessing wide mesenteric attachment.

Fig. 18–36 (right).—Intestinal obstruction caused by volvulus resulting from torsion in region of duodenum and hepatic flexure of the colon. Infant aged 44 hours.

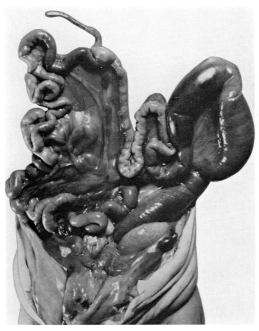
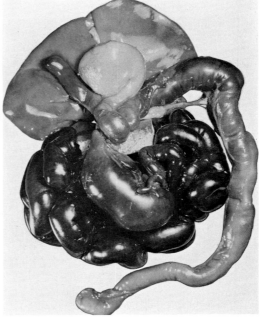

and the duodenum may be compressed by direct pressure.

MESENTERIC HERNIATION WITH OBSTRUCTION

Defects may occur in any part of the mesentery through which the intestine may be herniated. Loops of intestine may also pass through the foramen of Winslow or any of the preformed openings in the broad ligament or omentum. One of the more common sites through which intestine may herniate is an opening a short distance below the ligament of Treitz. This is a defect left in the attachment of the mesentery to the posterior abdominal wall a little below the junction of duodenum and jejunum. A pocket may exist behind the mesentery to either the right or the left into which intestinal loops may extend. Pressure from the contents of the bowel often increases the size of the pouch and it may contain several loops of intestine before there is evidence of obstruction. Small bands extending from two points of peritoneum or between peritoneum and mesentery may also cause obstruction. We have seen one infant with a peritoneal band producing partial obstruction in the proximal portion of the cecum associated with local distention and infection.

INTUSSUSCEPTION

This condition is rare in the newborn. Although it may be found toward the end of the 1st month, it is most frequent in infants of 4–10 months, with a peak at 7 months. The cause is usually unknown, but since the age at which it occurs most commonly is the time when solid food is being introduced into the diet, a possible relationship must be considered.

Intussusception consists of the invagination of one part of the intestine (intussusceptum) into an adjacent portion (intussuscipiens) (Fig. 18–37). Any part of the large or small bowel may be involved but, according to Ravitch, about 95% occur in the region of the ileocecal valve with invagination of the cecum into the colon. It is most often found in previously healthy, well-nourished infants, with males more frequently affected than females.

The first symptom is generally severe abdominal pain recurring at frequent intervals. In the early stages the infant may seem well between attacks, but if the obstruction continues, symptoms of severe illness develop and the infant may go into shock and die within a few days. One or two normal stools may be passed after the onset of symptoms,

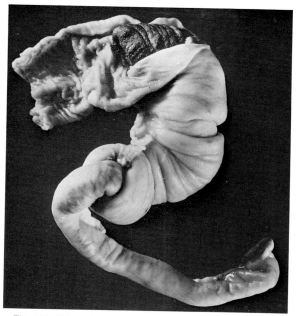

Fig. 18–37.—Intussusception of cecum into the colon. Infant aged 3 months.

but subsequently the stools are blood-tinged or frankly bloody. Palpation of the abdomen usually reveals a sausage-shaped, firm, painless mass in the upper abdomen. If the ileocecal valve is the leading point of the intussusceptum, the right lower quadrant will feel empty because of the upward movement of the cecum into the colon.

The amount of invagination varies, but it is often progressive until it is diagnosed and surgically corrected. Insertion of a finger into the rectum may reveal a doughnut-shaped mass, or at times the intussusceptum protrudes through the anus. It may resemble a prolapsed rectum, but careful examination easily differentiates the conditions.

The blood supply to the invaginated portion is seriously impaired, and if the condition is not promptly corrected the wall becomes necrotic and ruptures (Fig. 18–38). Pathologic examination reveals edema, engorgement of blood vessels, extravasation of blood cells and necrosis of mucosa and muscularis. In about 8% of cases, according to Ravitch, an anatomic abnormality such as Meckel's diverticulum can be demonstrated as a leading point of the intussusception. Although lymph nodes in the intussuscepted bowel mesentery may become enlarged, this is usually secondary to the changes in the bowel wall and its blood supply and are not to be regarded as the cause of the intussusception.

Intussusception may occur as a terminal condition unrelated to the primary cause of death. In such cases little or no histologic alteration is visible and the invaginated portion is easily withdrawn, leaving no evidence of antemortem change.

RECTAL PROLAPSE

Prolapse of the rectum is uncommon except when the nerve supply to the lower part of the body is defective. It is seen most often with severe spina bifida. The prolapsed bowel is congested and edematous (Fig. 18–39). Necrosis and ulceration take place soon after the prolapse occurs.

PATENT OMPHALOMESENTERIC DUCT

The omphalomesenteric duct is the last point to close during the separation of the intestine from the yolk sac during embryonic development. The communication is gradually reduced during the early weeks, and while the intestine is outside the abdominal cavity from the 5th to the 10th weeks, closure is completed. Temporarily, a fine fibrous cord remains to connect the two structures but even this soon disappears. The point of final closure is 8–10 cm above the ileocecal valve in the infant at birth. Development may be halted at any time during the final closure and the communication between the intestine and yolk sac may not be obliterated. Occasionally the omphalomesenteric (vitelline) duct

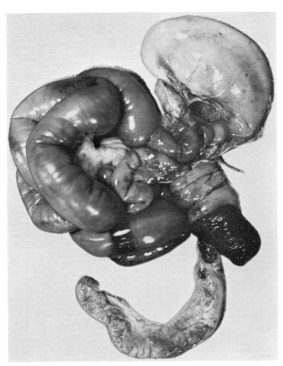

Fig. 18–38.—Rupture of the bowel with protrusion of intussusceptum. Appendix was the leading point in the intussusception. Infant aged 4 months.

Fig. 18–39 (left).—Rectal prolapse in infant with hydrocephalus and spina bifida.
Fig. 18–40 (right).—Patent omphalomesenteric duct

(A) connecting intestine with umbilicus. Infant aged 30 hours with multiple malformations.

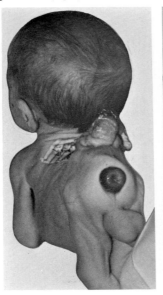
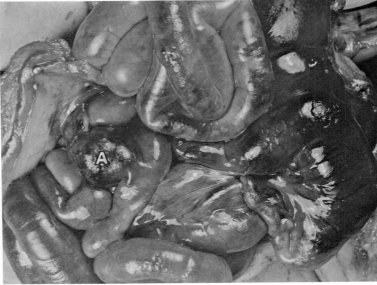

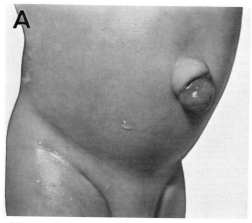
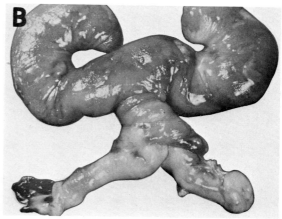

Fig. 18–41.—Patent omphalomesenteric duct. **A,** early prolapse of tissue of the duct. **B,** late prolapse. Surgically removed specimen showing two-horned mass *(above)* that was evaginated through the umbilicus *(center)* and segments of the adjacent intestine *(below).* (Courtesy Drs. C. F. Kittle, H. P. Jenkins and L. R. Dragstedt.)

remains patent and forms an open tubelike connection with the umbilicus. It may be of approximately the same caliber as the intestine (Fig. 18–40) and may be either completely lined by mucosa resembling that in the ileum or partially lined by tissue similar to gastric or duodenal mucosa. If the diameter is as great as that of the intestine, it is usually not more than 2–3 cm long. If the duct remains open at the umbilicus and communicates with the exterior, it produces an umbilical fistula and permits escape of fecal material from the umbilicus. A not uncommon complication of such a fistula is intestinal obstruction due to prolapse and evagination of both the proximal and the distal loop of bowel through the opening at the umbilicus (Fig. 18–41). This can be relieved only by resection of the involved portions of bowel. Fatal infarction of a patent omphalomesenteric duct that formed a

Fig. 18–42.—Meckel's diverticulum. **A,** wide, cone-shaped diverticulum. **B,** narrow, elongated diverticulum. Position in relation to cecum and appendix the same.

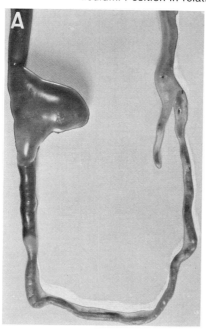
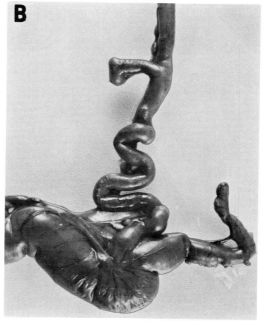

large, necrotic, partially calcified mass lying between and attached to the umbilicus and terminal ileum was observed at the Boston Lying-in Hospital.

MECKEL'S DIVERTICULUM

Only rarely does the omphalomesenteric duct remain widely patent and in communication with the exterior of the body. More often only the portion immediately adjacent to the bowel remains open and forms a pouchlike diverticulum 1–2 cm in length on the antimesenteric side of the intestine (Fig. 18–42). At times, however, it has a much smaller lumen and may be several centimeters long, even in the newborn. Rarely, it remains attached by a fine cord to the umbilicus, in which case loops of bowel may be strangulated by being caught underneath it. The mucosal lining may be similar to that of the rest of the ileum, it may contain areas resembling the mucosa of stomach, duodenum or colon or it may have small masses of pancreatic tissue.

Meckel's diverticulum is usually symptomless in young infants and is often discovered only on postmortem examination. According to Jackson and Bird, it is found in 2–3% of otherwise normal individuals but may occur in conjunction with abnormal development of any part of the body. The symptoms most often produced in older infants and children are hemorrhage, pain and intestinal obstruction. Such a diverticulum may be a leading point in intussusception. Zones of gastric mucosa may develop ulcers similar to those occurring in the stomach.

DUPLICATION OF THE GASTROINTESTINAL TRACT

Duplications are cystic structures composed of intestinal mucosa and sometimes muscle that are closely adherent to some part of the gastrointestinal tract. The cyst may lie between mucosa and muscle of the intestine, the muscle of the cyst may be fused with that of the normal bowel or occasionally the muscle of the intestine splits and the cyst is found between the layers. The mucosa is often similar to that in the portion of bowel to which it is attached, but part or all may resemble the mucosa of distant parts of the gastrointestinal tract. The duplications vary in length from a few to several centimeters. The lumen is generally greater than that of the bowel to which it is attached and is

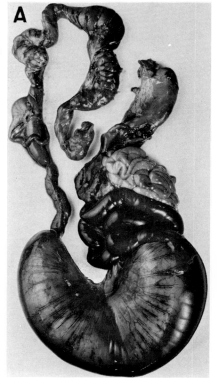
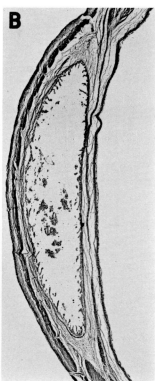

Fig. 18–43.—Duplication of part of the distal ileum. **A,** the duplicated area forms a large elongated cyst with the intestine flattened over the surface. **B,** cross-section of the intestine and part of the cyst wall. Note continuation of intestinal musculature around the cyst wall and minimal amount of muscle between mucosa of intestine and cyst. Stillborn fetus.

filled with clear mucus secreted by the cells of the mucosal lining. Occasionally the contents are discolored as a result of hemorrhage. The cyst wall is usually complete and only rarely is there a communication between it and the intestine, although at least one case has been reported in which there was a duplication of most of the intestine with both parts seeming to be functionable.

Such duplications may be symptomless or they may cause obstruction of the adjacent intestine or bleeding and necrosis from pressure by the cyst on mesenteric blood vessels. Pain may result from distention of the cyst by excessive mucosal secretion.

These lesions are rare and only two were found in the series of autopsies at the Chicago Lying-in Hospital. One was a cyst 6 cm in diameter and 8 cm in length, the lower end of which was 10 cm above the ileocecal valve. The intestine was flattened over its surface and the two could not be separated. The muscle layers surrounding the cyst were split in the region of the bowel, with a small part of the muscle extending between the cyst and the intestine and the major part surrounding the outer surface of the two structures (Fig. 18–43). The lining mucosa was similar to that of the ileum. The other duplication was a small cyst in the pyloric end of the stomach (see Fig 18–17).

Gross *et al.* reported 67 patients from the Boston Children's Hospital with duplications distributed as follows: stomach and duodenum 6, jejunum 4, ileum 20, ileocecum 8 and colon 13. As in the case illustrated in Figure 18–43, the duplication was almost always on the mesenteric border of the intestine. They found other malformations in 27 of the 67 patients.

MEGACOLON (HIRSCHSPRUNG'S DISEASE)

This is a congenital disorder in which a total absence of ganglion cells in a portion of the large intestine interferes with function and prevents normal movement of fecal content so that the abdomen becomes severely distended (Fig. 18–44). In the classic form, which makes up about 90% of cases, absence is limited to a small segment of the terminal colon and is designated "short segment" disease. In a less common form making up only 10% of cases the deficiency of ganglion cells may extend throughout the descending colon or even the entire large bowel with rare extension into the ileum. The more proximal portions of the bowel may be hypertrophied and dilated but, except for occasional ulceration produced by scybalous feces, they are normal. In the involved portions of the colon

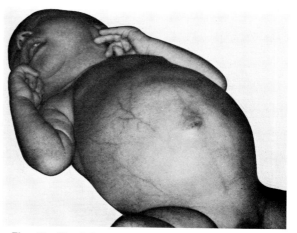

Fig. 18–44.—Infant aged 4 weeks with abdominal distention resulting from congenital megacolon.

the myenteric neural plexus lying between the circular and longitudinal muscle coats is strikingly hypertrophied although devoid of ganglion cells, as is the submucous plexus (Fig. 18–45). The line of division between normal and abnormal bowel is usually sharp and at a right angle to the longitudinal axis although at times it is irregular or runs across the bowel at a slant.

The diagnosis is best established by roentgen examination, followed by biopsy in which enough of the mucosa, submucosa and muscularis must be removed to include the myenteric plexus. It must be remembered that in infants the lowest 2 cm of the rectum is normally devoid of ganglion cells.

Removal of the affected portion restores bowel

Fig. 18–45.—Hypertrophy and hyperplasia of the myenteric plexus; ganglion cells are absent in this segment. The surrounding smooth muscle is hypertrophied.

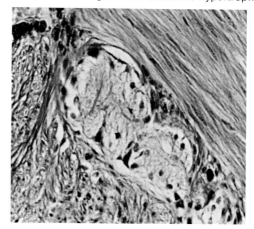

function to normal. If the small bowel is involved, the mortality is very high.

Megacolon is thought to be a familial disease although the exact method of transmission has not been established. In the short segment form of the disease there is a frequency among male sibs of 1 in 10, in female sibs of 1 in 100. In the long segment form there is a preponderance of females, but the difference is not as striking as in the short segment form (Edelman *et al.*). It is a relatively common disorder and in England occurs once in 2,000 births (Bodian and Carter).

REFERENCES

Aitken, J.: Case of colon and ileum duplication, Br. J. Surg. 37:349, 1950.

Aldridge, A. T., and Campbell, P. E.: Ganglion cell distribution in normal rectum and anal canal, J. Pediatr. Surg. 3:475, 1968.

Ardran, G. M., and Kemp, F. H.: Aglossia congenita, Arch. Dis. Child. 31:400, 1956.

Belding, H. H., and Kernohan, J. W.: A morphologic study of the myenteric plexus of the pylorus with special reference to hypertrophic pyloric stenosis, Surg. Gynecol. Obstet. 97:322, 1953.

Bell, R. S., Graham, C. B., and Stevenson, J. K.: Roentgenologic and clinical manifestations of neonatal necrotizing enterocolitis, Am. J. Roentgenol. 112:123, 1971.

Berdon, W. E., *et al.*: Necrotizing enterocolitis in premature infant, Radiology 83:879, 1964.

Bernstein, J., *et al.*: The occurrence of intestinal atresia in newborns with meconium ileus, Am. J. Dis. Child. 99:804, 1960.

Bodian, M., and Carter, C. O.: A family study of Hirschsprung's disease, Ann. Hum. Genet. 26:261, 1963.

Bremer, J. L.: *Congenital Anomalies of the Viscera* (Cambridge, Mass.: Harvard University Press, 1957).

Brown, M. J.: Intussusception in infancy and childhood, Arch. Surg. 84:459, 1962.

Burmeister, R. E., and Hamilton, H. B.: Infantile hypertrophic pyloric stenosis in four siblings, Am. J. Dis. Child. 108:617, 1964.

Charif, P.: Perforated appendicitis in premature infants. A case report and review of the literature, Johns Hopkins Med. J. 125:92, 1969.

Clifford, S. H.: Diarrhea of the newborn: Causes and prevention, N. Engl. J. Med. 237:969, 1947.

Corcoran, W. J.: Prenatal rupture of the appendix, Am. J. Dis. Child. 39:277, 1930.

Edelman, S., *et al.*: Universal aganglionosis of the colon, Surgery 47:667, 1960.

Ehrenpreis, T.: Hirschsprung's disease in the neonatal period, Arch. Dis. Child. 30:8, 1955.

Evans, W. A., Jr.: Obstructions of the alimentary tract in infancy, Radiology 51:23, 1948.

Farber, S.: Congenital atresia of alimentary tract: Diagnosis by microscopic examination of meconium, J.A.M.A. 100:1733, 1933.

Farber, S.: Relation of pancreatic achylia to meconium ileus, J. Pediatr. 24:387, 1944.

Fields, I. A., and Cole, N. M.: Acute appendicitis in infants 36 months of age or younger, Am. J. Surg. 113:269, 1967.

Fields, I. A., Naiditch, M. J., and Rothman, D. E.: Acute appendicitis in infants, Am. J. Dis. Child. 93:287, 1957.

Filler, R. M., Randolf, J., and Gross, R. E.: Esophageal hiatus hernia in infants and children, J. Thorac. Cardiovasc. Surg. 47:551, 1964.

Fonkalsrud, E. W., Tompkins, R., and Clatworthy, H. W., Jr.: Abnormal manifestation of situs inversus in infants and children, Arch. Surg. 92:79, 1966.

Friesen, S. R., and Pearse, A. G. E.: Pathogenesis of congenital pyloric stenosis—histochemical analysis of ganglion cells, Surgery 53:604, 1963.

Graivier, L., and Siefer, W. K.: Hirschsprung's disease and mongolism, Surgery 60:458, 1966.

Gray, A. W.: Triplication of the large intestine, Arch. Pathol. 30:1215, 1940.

Gross, R.: *The Surgery of Infancy and Childhood* (Philadelphia: W. B. Saunders Co., 1953).

Gross, R. E., Holcombe, G. W., Jr., and Farber, S.: Duplication of the intestinal tract, Pediatrics 9:949, 1954.

Gross, R. E., and Ware, P. F.: Intussusception in childhood, N. Engl. J. Med. 239:645, 1948.

Gruenwald, P., and Marsh, M. R.: Acute esophagitis in infants, Arch. Pathol. 9:1, 1950.

Guthrie, K. J.: Peptic ulcer in infancy and childhood, with review of the literature, Arch. Dis. Child. 17:82, 1942.

Haight, C.: Tracheoesophageal Fistula, in Mustard, W. T., *et al.* (eds.): *Pediatric Surgery* (Chicago: Year Book Medical Publishers, Inc., 1969), p. 357.

Haller, J. P., and Morgenstern, L.: Anomalous rotation and fixation of the left colon, Am. J. Surg. 108:331, 1964.

Halpert, B., and Patzer, R.: Maxillary tumor of the retinal anlage, Surgery 22:837, 1947.

Hardy, J. D., Savage, T. R., and Shirodia, C.: Intestinal perforation following exchange transfusion, Am. J. Dis. Child. 124:136, 1972.

Haymond, H. E., and Dragstedt, L. R.: Anomalies of intestinal rotation, Surg. Gynecol. Obstet. 53:316, 1931.

Holder, T., *et al.*: Esophageal atresia and tracheoesophageal fistula, Pediatrics 35:542, 1964.

Holinger, P. H., Johnston, K. C., and Potts, W. J.: Congenital anomalies of the esophagus, Acta Otolaryngol. (supp.) 100:100, 1952.

Howell, L. M.: Meckel's diverticulum, Am. J. Dis. Child. 71:365, 1946.

Inouye, W. Y., and Evans, G.: Neonatal gastric perforation, Arch. Surg. 88:791, 1964.

Jackson, R. H., and Bird, A. R.: Meckel's diverticulum in childhood, Br. Med. J. 2:1399, 1961.

Jones, T. W.: Congenital pyloric stenosis: Experience in diagnosis and therapy, Q. Rev. Surg. 13:209, 1956.

Judge, D. J., Cassidy, J. E., and Rice, E. C.: Intestinal emphysema in infants, Arch. Pathol. 48:206, 1949.

Kiesewetter, W. B., and Nixon, H. H.: Imperforate anus and its surgical anatomy, J. Pediatr. Surg. 1:60, 1967.

Kittle, C. F., Jenkins, H. P., and Dragstedt, L. R.: Patent omphalomesenteric duct and its relation to diverticulum of Meckel, Arch. Surg. 54:10, 1947.

Klinefelter, E. W.: Congenital absence of colon, Am. J. Dis. Child. 50:454, 1935.

Lafer, D. J., and Kottmeier, P. K.: Congenital gastric obstruction, Am. J. Dis. Child. 107:202, 1964.

Lee, M. J.: Congenital anomalies of the lower part of the

rectum, Am. J. Dis. Child. 68:182, 1944.

Leix, J., and Greaney, E. M., Jr.: Surgical experience with peptic ulcer in infancy and childhood, Am. J. Surg. 106: 173, 1963.

Lynn, H. B., and Espinas, E. E.: Intestinal atresia, Arch. Surg. 79:357, 1959.

Lyon, G. M., and Folsom, T. G.: Epidemic diarrhea of the newborn, Am. J. Dis. Child. 61:427, 1941.

Marton, L. W., and Perrin, E. V.: Neonatal perforation of appendix associated with Hirschsprung's disease, Ann. Surg. 166:799, 1967.

McCormack, W. F.: Rupture of the stomach in children, Arch. Pathol. 67:416, 1959.

McIntosh, R., and Donovan, R. J.: Disturbances in rotation of intestinal tract: Clinical picture based on observation of 20 cases, Am. J. Dis. Child. 57:116, 1939.

Merriam, J. C., and Benirschke, K.: Esophageal erosions in the newborn, Lab. Invest. 8:39, 1959.

Mizrahi, A., *et al.*: Necrotizing enterocolitis in premature infants, J. Pediatr. 66:697, 1965.

Moore, T. C., and Eades, S. M.: Congenital malformations of the rectum and anus: Associated anomalies in 120 cases, Surg. Gynecol. Obstet. 95:781, 1952.

Oberhelman, H. A., and Condon, J. B.: Acute intussusception in infants and children, S. Clin. North Am. 27:3, 1947.

Orme, R. L., and Eades, S. M.: Perforation of bowel in newborn as a complication of exchange transfusion, Br. Med. J. 4:349, 1968.

Passarge, E.: Gastrointestinal hemorrhage in Turner's syndrome due to telangiectasia in intestinal walls, Dtsch. Med. Wochenschr. 93:204, 1968.

Ravitch, M. M.: Intussusception, in Mustard, W. T., *et al.* (eds.): *Pediatric Surgery* (Chicago: Year Book Medical Publishers, Inc., 1969), p. 914.

Rector, L. E., and Connerly, M. L.: Aberrant mucosa in the esophagus in infants and children, Arch. Pathol. 31: 285, 1941.

Santulli, T. V.: Malformations of Rectum and Anus, in Mustard, W. T., *et al.* (eds.): *Pediatric Surgery* (Chicago: Year Book Medical Publishers, Inc., 1969), p. 983.

Santulli, T. V., and Blanc, W. A.: Congenital atresia of the intestine: Pathogenesis and treatment, Ann. Surg. 154:939, 1961.

Shaw, A., *et al.*: Spontaneous rupture of the stomach in newborn; a clinical and experimental study, Surgery 58: 561, 1965.

Shwachman, H., Pryles, C. V., and Gross, R. E.: Meconium ileus, Am. J. Dis. Child. 91:223, 1956.

Smith, B., and Clatworthy, H. W., Jr.: Meconium peritonitis: Prognostic significance, Pediatrics 27:967, 1961.

Spock, A., Schneider, S., and Boylin, G.: Mediastinal gastric cysts, Am. Rev. Chest Dis. 94:97, 1966.

Stowens, D.: A pigmented tumor of infancy. The melanotic progonoma, J. Pathol. Bacteriol. 73:43, 1957.

Strong, R.: Intussusception in infancy and childhood, Br. J. Surg. 46:484, 1959.

Sturim, H. S., and Ternberg, J. L.: Congenital atresia of the colon, Surgery 485, 1965.

Walker, A. W., Kempson, R. L., and Ternberg, J. L.: Aganglionosis of the small intestine, Surgery 60:449, 1966.

Wallgren, A.: Incidence of hypertrophic pyloric stenosis, Am. J. Dis. Child. 62:751, 1941.

Willis, R. A.: *Pathology of Tumors* (4th ed.; New York: Appleton-Century-Crofts, 1967), pp. 316, 700.

Wiseman, H. J., Celano, E. R., and Hester, F. C., III: Spontaneous rupture of the esophagus in a newborn, J. Pediatr. 55:207, 1959.

Witzleben, C. L.: Aplasia of trachea, Pediatrics 32:31, 1963.

Wolman, I. J.: Congenital stenosis of the trachea, Am. J. Dis. Child. 61:1263, 1941.

Zuelzer, W. W., and Wilson, J. L.: Functional intestinal obstruction on congenital neurogenic basis in infancy, Am. J. Dis. Child. 75:40, 1948.

19

Diaphragmatic and Abdominal Hernias

Defects of the Diaphragm

THE DIAPHRAGM arises from four sources which appear at different times during embryonic life. The first part to appear is a single anterior portion, the septum transversum, which extends dorsally from the central part of the anterior body wall and temporarily forms a shelflike arrangement separating the heart from the liver. Much of the superior surface of this portion becomes the floor of the pericardial cavity. For a considerable time the open areas posterior to the septum transversum form a communication between thoracic and abdominal cavities. These openings are the pleuroperitoneal

Fig. 19–1.—Left diaphragmatic hernia. **A,** chest plate removed to show intestine and part of left lobe of the liver lying within left thoracic cavity. Stomach is distended with air because of pressure on duodenum associated with malposition of intestine. **B,** viscera drawn out of chest permitting visualization of defect in posterior portion of left diaphragm. Death at 8 days.

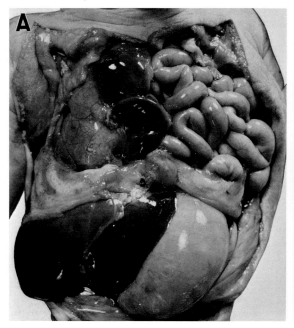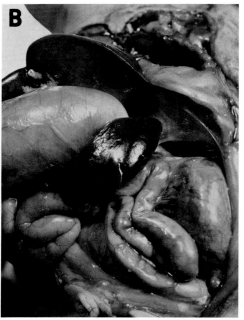

canals known as the foramina of Bochdalek. Gradually they are obliterated by the outgrowth of the pleuroperitoneal folds from the posterolateral portions of the body wall. From the beginning these folds are continuous with the dorsal margin of the septum transversum, and when their posterior borders meet and fuse with each other and with a small persisting part of the primary mesentery at about 8 weeks, the diaphragm is complete. Considerably later a secondary ingrowth of muscle from the body wall forms a narrow ridge around the posterolateral margins of the diaphragm.

One of the most common malformations found in newborn infants is a failure of the pleuroperitoneal folds to effect a complete separation of the abdominal and thoracic cavities. The disturbance is usually unilateral and involves the left side more often than the right. The pleuroperitoneal fold of the affected side may be completely absent, or only the posterior portion may be missing. Occasionally it is entirely formed but fails to unite dorsomedially with the mesentery and with its mate on the opposite side. If part or all of the fold fails to develop, the peritoneum and parietal pleura are usually also absent from the defective area, and the thorax and abdomen remain in open communication. The pleura and peritoneum covering the posterior body wall are continuous, with no line of demarcation between them.

As a result of the diaphragmatic defect the intestine, on its return into the abdomen from its temporary period of development in the umbilical cord, rises into the chest. If the defect is large and on the left side, the stomach, spleen and part of the left lobe of the liver (Fig. 19–1) may also lie in the chest. The only intraperitoneal viscera remaining in the abdomen may be the descending colon and part of the liver. If the opening is only a narrow posterior slit, nothing but part of the intestine may be displaced into the chest. If the defect is on the right, the intestine and part of the right lobe of the liver are usually present in the thorax (Fig. 19–2). A defect on the right is usually smaller than one on the left, and, in addition, the liver forms a partial obstruction to the ascent of the intestine into the chest so that often the only structure protruding through the opening is a portion of the liver.

Rarely, a defect is present in both leaves of the diaphragm, and the intestine may ascend into the left side, and part of the liver into the right (Fig. 19–3). The kidneys and adrenal glands often lie higher than is normal and extend up into the area that belongs to the thorax.

Since the major defects of the diaphragm present

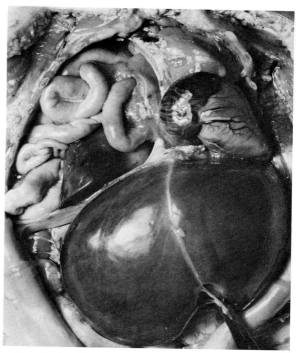

Fig. 19–2.—Right diaphragmatic hernia showing intestine and part of right lobe of the liver in right thoracic cavity.

at birth are almost invariably posterior, the greatest pressure from the abdominal viscera is exerted against the posterior mediastinum. The heart is pushed anteriorly and a hernial sac is produced in the area between the descending aorta and the esophagus (Fig. 19–4). The thoracic contents are greatly compressed and the heart, both lungs and some of the intestine occupy the side of the chest with an intact diaphragm.

Large defects are more common than small ones. With a large defect the infant's respiration at birth is already compromised because of pulmonary hypoplasia, even before swallowed air has distended the intestine and caused further distortion of the mediastinum and compression of the opposite lung. Extrauterine respiration may never be established. The usual clinical picture is of a mature well-developed infant who appears normal at birth except for a scaphoid abdomen and makes a few gasping attempts at breathing but dies in a short time despite all attempts at resuscitation. If the infant does breathe, air can be heard entering only one side of the chest. Soon after birth swallowed air passes into the intestine and can be visualized in the chest on x-ray examination. Even before it is present in the intestine it may be seen in the

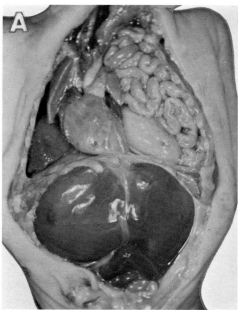
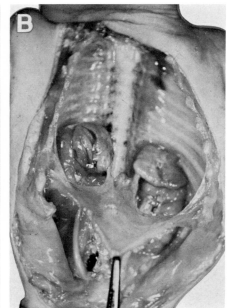

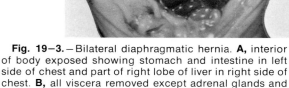

Fig. 19–3.—Bilateral diaphragmatic hernia. **A,** interior of body exposed showing stomach and intestine in left side of chest and part of right lobe of liver in right side of chest. **B,** all viscera removed except adrenal glands and kidneys and diaphragm drawn forward to show defects on both sides. Adrenal glands and upper poles of kidneys lie in the thoracic cavity because of the absence of the posterior portions of the diaphragm.

Fig. 19–4.—Left diaphragmatic hernia with herniation of posterior mediastinum. **A,** viscera withdrawn from chest showing absence of left diaphragm. The cystlike structure is the sacculated posterior mediastinum that was ballooned into the left chest by a right pneumothorax. **B,** interior of the chest showing extremely hypoplastic left lung and posterior mediastinal hernia between the descending aorta and esophagus. This was the area that was ballooned out by the pneumothorax. Hernia was caused by pressure of viscera against the left posterior mediastinum. Infant aged 45 minutes.

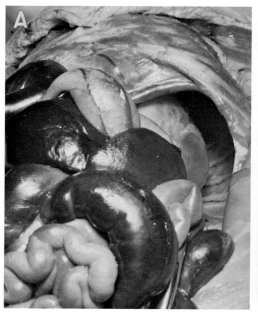
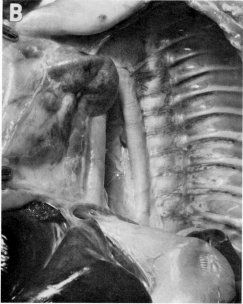

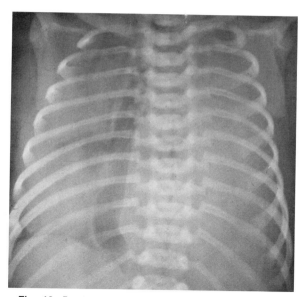

Fig. 19–5.—Roentgenogram showing air-filled esophagus displaced into the right chest by pressure of viscera.

esophagus (Fig. 19–5), and if the esophagus is displaced, the diagnosis should always be suspected.

According to Gross, when the lungs are sufficiently developed to permit immediate postnatal survival, and surgical attack is possible, recovery

Fig. 19–6 (left).—Small diaphragmatic defect covered by pleura and peritoneum through which bulges a small elevated mass of liver.

Fig. 19–7 (right).—Large defect of left diaphragm, the margins of which are attached to a sac composed of pleura and peritoneum. The membrane is transparent

can be expected in 89% of cases. Even a markedly hypoplastic lung develops postnatally to such an extent that no physiologic defect can be detected.

The survival of infants with diaphragmatic hernias is largely related to the degree of pulmonary hypoplasia. Johnson et al., who studied 34 cases of diaphragmatic hernia, found that of 11 infants with hypoplastic lungs only two survived, but all of 14 with no hypoplasia survived. When the defect is small and the passage of abdominal viscera through the opening is limited, the onset of symptoms may be delayed for weeks or years. Among 60 cases of diaphragmatic hernia reported by Butler and Claireaux 21 were stillborn and 37 died in the 1st week of life. There was a preponderance of females (60%) in the latter group, and 92% of the hernias were on the left side. Forty-seven percent had additional lethal malformations (95% among the 21 who were stillborn). The most frequently associated anomaly was anencephaly; other malformations included hydrocephalus, iniencephaly, congenital heart disease and esophageal atresia.

Herniation through the foramen of Bochdalek is the most frequent diaphragmatic defect encountered in infants and children. According to Baffes, this accounts for 59% of cases and is the only form ordinarily diagnosed at birth. He found the next most frequent defect to be eventration of the dia-

and the apparent opacity is caused by cotton used to distend it. The left diaphragm, sac and left half of the chest plate are included in the photograph. (Specimen obtained in Rio de Janeiro, courtesy Dr. Martagão Gesteira.)

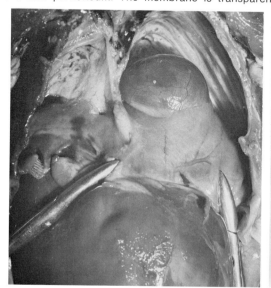

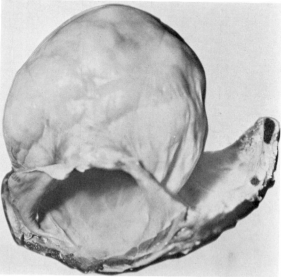

phragm (14%). Here the area from which muscle and fascia are absent is covered by pleural and peritoneal membranes. When the defect is small a portion of the liver or intestine fills a saclike protrusion above the normal level of the diaphragm (Fig. 19–6). When a large opening is covered by a membrane, the effect of the muscular defect is not altered. The sac cannot withstand the pressure of the abdominal viscera and becomes so distended that it lies in contact with the inner surface of the chest wall (Fig. 19–7). It is inconspicuous and easily overlooked unless the inner surface of the thorax is carefully investigated.

Hernias through the small anterior retrosternal foramina of Morgagni accounted for only 2.6% of Baffes' series of congenital diaphragmatic hernias. Baran *et al.* described eight cases, three in infants aged under 1 year. The liver was the herniated organ in all. Dextrocardia, tetralogy of Fallot and ventricular septal defects were present in some.

Hiatus hernia, i.e., the herniation, usually of the stomach upward through the opening in the diaphragm, through which normally only the esophagus passes, is usually small. Alone or associated with a congenitally short esophagus, such herniation of the stomach fundus accounted for 23% of Baffes' series.

Defects of the Abdominal Wall

The anterior abdominal wall arises principally from four folds of the somatic mesoderm. The cephalic fold forms the thoracic-epigastric wall and septum transversum, the two lateral somatic mesodermal folds form the midlateral portions of the abdominal wall and the somatic-caudal fold forms the ventral abdominal wall. Any part may fail to develop and result in eventration of subjacent parts, giving rise to such conditions as ectopia cordis, omphalocele and extrophy of the bladder.

The simplest and most common form of disturbance in the anterior abdominal wall is an umbilical hernia caused by an enlargement without actual defect of the umbilical ring. The ring, which may be 1–2 cm in diameter, is covered with normal skin and bulges with increased abdominal pressure. It has a natural tendency to contract and usually the hernia disappears in the first 2 years of life. According to Sibley *et al.*, there is a slight genetic predisposition; they found that 9% of infants with umbilical hernias have siblings, a parent or offspring with similar defects.

There is a somewhat more serious abnormality similar to the above but with herniation of the intestine into the umbilical cord. Here the umbilical

Fig. 19–8 (left).—Herniation of intestine and part of the liver into sac composed of amniotic membrane. **A,** newborn infant. **B,** same child at 3 years of age showing successful surgical repair.

Fig. 19–9 (right).—Herniation of intestine. The sac covering the intestine ruptured during delivery and the intestine has become greatly distended by air and fluid. Discoloration is due to interference with blood supply.

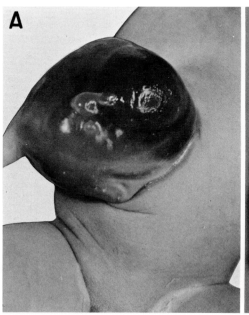
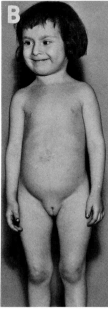
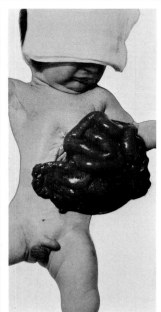

ring is variably dilated and the base of the cord is enlarged and contains one or more loops of intestine. It is not covered by skin and there is no sac except the dilated cord itself. This is easily repaired at birth.

The most frequent severe malformation of the anterior abdominal wall is omphalocele (exomphalos). Here part of the abdominal wall is missing and the umbilical cord runs over the surface or arises from the apex of a membranous sac composed of amnion and peritoneum and filled with intestine.

Other anomalies were present in 67% of 58 cases of omphalocele reported by Hutchin. At least half of these were gastrointestinal malformations, with malrotation and volvulus being the most frequent. This is not surprising since the intestine is outside the abdominal cavity at the usual time of rotation and fixation to the posterior abdominal wall. Other less commonly associated anomalies included duplication of the intestine, atresia, stenosis, agenesis of the terminal bowel and tracheoesophageal fistula. Omphalocele is one of the abnormalities found in Beckwith's syndrome.

The sac is very thin and may rupture during delivery or soon afterward (Figs. 19–8 and 19–9). The abdomen is usually small, and replacement of the herniated bowel soon after birth may be impossible or may cause sufficient elevation of the diaphragm to interfere seriously with respiration. Conservative therapy with intestinal decompression, intravenous feeding and prevention of infection for several weeks greatly improves the chance of survival by allowing the abdominal cavity to grow sufficiently to accommodate the intestines. The probability of survival is inversely proportional to the size of the defect.

Gastroschisis and eventration are terms applied to extensive absence of the abdominal wall where no sac is present and the umbilical cord is attached to one side of the defect, usually the left. This lesion is much more severe but less common than omphalocele. The serosal surfaces of the herniated intestines are often opaque and thickened because of their exposure to amniotic fluid. The intestine is usually shortened and malrotation is almost always present, but volvulus is less common than in omphalocele. If there is failure of fusion of the lateral somatopleure combined with a similar failure of union of the cephalic and caudal folds, very extensive and usually lethal malformations involving the esophagus, sternum, pericardium and/or urachus and bladder are produced. In both omphalo-

cele and gastroschisis about one half of all affected infants are delivered prematurely.

The most serious type of abdominal wall defect — absence of the body stalk (sometimes also designated gastroschisis) — results from a profound alteration in development in early embryonic life in which the body stalk fails to form. Normally a cleft appearing in the mesoderm between the amniotic sac and the wall of the blastocyst during the 3d week enlarges until the embryo is attached to the blastocyst only by a small mass of mesoderm that gradually elongates to form the umbilical cord. When the area of cleavage is incomplete, the umbilical cord is rudimentary or absent and a portion of the embryo remains in contact with the wall of the blastocyst. This is in the area of the yolk sac, and as a result the region of the anterior abdominal wall is not covered by skin but remains open and adjacent to the placenta, the latter being derived from the portion of the blastocyst wall to which the body stalk is attached. The abdominal viscera lie outside the abdominal cavity in a sac made up of placenta on one side and amnion on the other. There is no true umbilical cord, and the umbilical vein and arteries usually course over the amniotic

Fig. 19–10. — Intestine and liver outside the abdominal cavity as a result of abnormal formation of body stalk and umbilical cord. Viscera are covered on one surface by amnion and on the other by chorion.

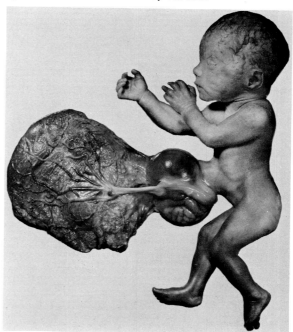

portion of the sac. They are seldom more than 8–10 cm long and are usually grouped together in a mass simulating the cord.

Rarely, the intestine lies in a sac between the placenta and abdomen of the fetus, and the fetus is otherwise normal (Fig. 19–10). Much more often the abdominal portion of the fetus is attached directly to the placenta and, consequently, to the uterine wall; the spine is then severely kyphotic and scoliotic owing to forward protrusion and fixation of the abdomen (Fig. 19–11). The limbs are abnormal as a result of their cramped position (Fig. 19–12) and one or more may be entirely missing. Partial amputations of extremities associated with amniotic bands have been observed (see Fig. 27–39). Defects in the chest wall, diaphragm and pericardium may also be present, as well as abnormalities in the structure of the heart, lungs and liver. Anencephalus is not uncommon. Occasionally, part of the fetus develops outside the amniotic sac (Fig. 19–13).

This type of gastroschisis is always fatal. Since the fetus cannot be delivered until the placenta is detached, symptoms suggesting abruptio placentae may occur and the fetus may die of anoxia before birth. The malformation is so great that even fetuses born alive die within a few hours.

In an extremely rare malformation the umbilical ring and adjacent intestine appear normal, with intestine forming a mass in the cord several centimeters from the abdominal wall. In one case 10 cm of normal-appearing umbilical cord extended from the umbilicus to a mass about 5 × 7 cm with an opaque red wall. From external inspection this was diagnosed as a hematoma from a ruptured varix, but further investigation showed that it contained a large Meckel's diverticulum, appendix, cecum, ascending colon and 40 cm of ileum. All structures appeared hypoplastic and gave no evidence of having contained meconium. Microscopic examination, however, revealed normally developed mucosa and muscularis but with necrosis and mild infection of the Meckel's diverticulum and neighboring intestine. The origin of this anomaly appears to be different from that of the usual omphalocele in which extrusion of the intestine is secondary to a defect in the anterior abdominal wall; here an abnormality of the omphalomesenteric duct produced a Meckel's diverticulum and prevented part of the intestine from returning to the abdomen normally as it

Fig. 19–11.—Scoliosis of the spine and other skeletal and visceral abnormalities usually accompany eventration (gastroschisis) caused by abnormal formation of the body stalk. **A,** external view. Placenta is attached 4 cm from the edge of the liver. **B,** roentgenograms showing abnormalities of spine, ribs and pelvis.

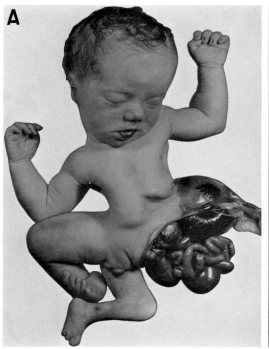
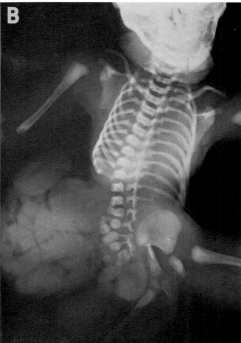

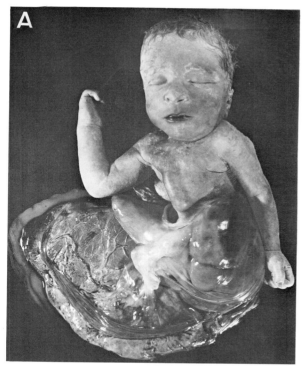

Fig. 19–12.—Extreme malformation associated with abnormal formation of body stalk. **A,** anterior view showing abdominal viscera between amnion and chorionic surface of the placenta. **B,** posterior view showing malformation of left leg which overlies the right shoulder. Right leg is absent.

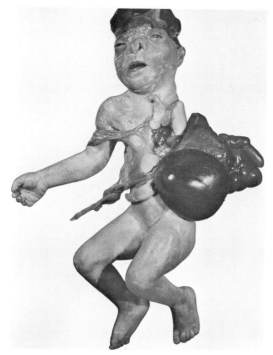

Fig. 19–13.—Severe malformation associated with abnormal formation of body stalk. Lower half of fetus developed outside the amniotic sac. Left arm absent except for one finger. Anencephalus.

should during early embryonic life. In this case the portion of intestine in the cord was removed when the cord was cut following delivery, but subsequent anastomosis of the ends of the remaining bowel was followed by normal function and the child was well when last seen at 3 years of age (Potter).

Congenital lumbar hernias occur in the newborn. Large soft compressible masses appear in the flank. Butler and Shafer reported that an unusual thinning of the transversalis abdominis and internal oblique muscle is responsible.

Internal hernias through mesenteric defects of the small bowel may be seen in the newborn. Of 11 cases reported by Murphy for a period of 2 years at the Boston Children's Hospital Medical Center seven were associated with nearby atresia or stenosis of the bowel.

REFERENCES

Baffes, T. G.: Diaphragmatic Hernia, in Mustard, W. T., *et al.* (eds.): *Pediatric Surgery* (Chicago: Year Book Medical Publishers, Inc., 1969), p. 342.

Baran, E. M., *et al.*: Foramen of Morgagni hernias in children, Surgery 62:1076, 1967.

Bill, A. H.: Hernias of the Abdominal Wall Other Than Inguinal, in Mustard, W. T., *et al.* (eds.): *Pediatric Surgery* (Chicago: Year Book Medical Publishers, Inc., 1969), p. 677.

Bremer, J. L.: The diaphragm and diaphragmatic hernias, Arch. Pathol. 36:439, 1943.

Butler, B. W., and Shafer, A. D.: Bilateral congenital lumbar hernia, Ohio Med. J. 62:577, 1966.

Butler, N., and Claireaux, A. E.: Congenital diaphragmatic hernia as a cause of perinatal mortality, Lancet 1: 659, 1962.

Gross, R.: *The Surgery of Infancy and Childhood* (Philadelphia: W. B. Saunders Co., 1953), p. 444.

Hutchin, P.: Somatic anomalies of the umbilicus and anterior abdominal wall, Surg. Obstet. Gynecol. 120:1075, 1965.

Izant, R. J., Brown, F., and Rothman, B. F.: Current embryology and treatment of gastroschisis and omphalocoele, Arch. Surg. 93:49, 1966.

Johnson, D. G., Deaver, R. M., and Koop, C. E.: Diaphragmatic hernia in infancy. Factors affecting mortality rate, Surgery 62:1082, 1967.

Liebow, A. A., and Miller, H. C.: Congenital defects in the diaphragm, Am. J. Pathol. 26:707, 1940.

Murphy, D. A.: Internal hernias in infancy and childhood, Surgery 55:311, 1964.

Nunn, I. N., and Stephens, F. D.: The triad syndrome—a composite anomaly of the abdominal wall, urinary system and testes, J. Urol. 86:782, 1961.

Sibley, W. J., III, Lynn, H. B., and Innis, L. E.: A twenty-five year study of umbilical hernia, Surgery 55:463, 1964.

Wells, L. J.: Development of the human diaphragm and pleural sacs, Carnegie Contrib. Embryol. 35:109, 1954.

20

Liver and Gallbladder

THE LIVER is first visible during the 4th week of development in the 2.5 mm embryo as an outgrowth from the anterior wall of the entodermal tube cephalad to the yolk sac in the region of the future duodenum. It divides almost immediately into a caudal branch, which differentiates into the extrahepatic ducts and gallbladder, and a cephalic branch, which becomes part of the liver. The latter branch penetrates the septum transversum and begins differentiating into masses and plates of cells. Within the mesenchyme of the septum transversum capillary plexuses of isolated endothelial vesicles arise that subsequently unite with small branches of the omphalomesenteric vein; the entodermal masses invest the branches of this plexus and become single-layer plates of hepatic parenchymal cells, while the vascular channels become hepatic sinusoids. Further growth is by simultaneous formation of new sinusoids and plates.

According to Elias, not all of the hepatic cells come from the entoderm. He believed that mesodermal cells enter the spaces between the capillary plexuses and are transformed into parenchymal cells that intermingle indistinguishably with those of entodermal origin. According to this idea, the anterior part of the liver is entodermal, the posterior portion mesodermal and the intermediate portion an intermixture of the two. The mesenchyma of the septum transversum forms the serosal capsule and portal connective tissue and, according to Elias, the stimulus of contact with portal connective tissue causes hepatic cells to differentiate into canaliculi, ductules and intrahepatic bile ducts that subsequently unite with one another and with the extrahepatic ducts. The hepatic cells are each encircled by a canaliculus. Bile from the liver flows through the meshwork of canaliculi, empties into ductules (canals of Hering) and then into portal bile ducts.

A secretory lobule of the liver consists of hepatic cells arranged radially around a branch of the bile duct into which ductules and canaliculi drain. Each portal triad consists of connective tissue embedding one or more branches of the hepatic bile duct, hepatic artery and portal vein.

The vascular lobules are arranged around branches of the hepatic (central) vein and are composed of portions of several secretory lobules. The central veins lie in the interstices between secretory units, and in each lobule blood from the branch of the portal vein flows peripherally to reach different hepatic veins at the edges of the lobule.

By custom the vascular pattern is used as the basis for designating portions of the lobule, with the area around the central vein considered the center and that adjacent to the portal triads the periphery.

The branches of the hepatic artery are not ordinarily distinguishable beyond the portal triads but they extend into the lobules for varying distances and empty into sinusoids. The arteries do not anastomose but are end branches, a fact that must be taken into account in any surgical procedure.

During intrauterine life the fetus is supplied with oxygenated blood through the umbilical vein. After the umbilical vein enters the liver it gives off numerous branches to the left lobe before it joins the portal vein. The portal vein and umbilical vein meet and become the short ductus venosus, which is joined by the hepatic veins from the right lobe of the liver just before it enters the inferior vena cava. After birth the umbilical vein atrophies in its more proximal portions and becomes the ligamentum teres; some of the branches to the left lobe of the liver may persist and supply that lobe postnatally, the blood flow being the reverse of that in intrauterine life. The ductus venosus also closes after birth, thus obliterating the communication between the portal system and the inferior vena cava.

The junction of the portion that will remain open (the portal area) and the portion that will become obliterated (the ductus venosus) is marked by a constriction that often impedes the passage of a catheter during exchange transfusion. The structure of the vascular wall on the two sides of the constricting point is different, as is true for all permanent and temporary vessels. The ductus venosus contains proportionately less muscle and elastic tissue than the portal vein.

It has been said that in one third of all livers some portion of the umbilical vein remains patent without producing symptoms. If any portion of the portal vein becomes thrombosed, portal hypertension with splenomegaly and esophageal and hemorrhoidal varices results. Such a process is usually preceded by infection of the umbilicus although the liver remains normal. Occasionally, branches of the portal vein become thrombosed while proximal portions of the umbilical vein remain open or recanalize. Then dilatation of the superficial abdominal veins may occur, forming a *caput medusae* about the umbilicus. In cases of primary cirrhotic liver disease with portal hypertension, recanalization of the umbilical vein may also take place with the same production of a caput as in primary vascular disease.

Among 98 cases of portal hypertension in children reported by Voorhees *et al.* 58 were ascribed to portal system thromboses and 40 were secondary to cirrhosis of the liver. In 27, symptoms began in the 1st year of life. In most instances the etiology of the thromboses was obscure, and 49 of the 58 had no known etiology although in 28 there was a vague history of abdominal pain. Five were secondary to omphalitis, two to neonatal sepsis and two to trauma. In the series of patients with portal hypertension of Hsia and Gellis only four of 21 had symptoms beginning before the end of the 1st year of life. Omphalitis, diarrhea, peritonitis, osteomyelitis or pneumonia in the first weeks of life were believed to be precipitating episodes. Only one patient died in the 1st year. Five of six autopsied cases had obstruction caused by thrombi or atresia somewhere in the portal system.

Another consequence of the developmental relationship of the umbilical and portal veins in the liver can be observed immediately after birth in stillborn and liveborn infants as well as in older infants. Because before birth the left lobe of the liver is supplied directly with highly oxygenated blood from the umbilical vein, liver cells in the left lobe are better nourished and show fewer changes as a result of anoxia than those in the right lobe, which are supplied by the portal vein (Fig. 20–1). In the newborn the right lobe may have more erythropoiesis, fat, nonlipid vacuoles and iron than the left lobe but less congestion and shrinkage of parenchymal cell cytoplasm. Frequently a sharp line of demarcation between the two portions can be recognized on gross examination. Gruenwald found differences in lobar cytology in 15% of autopsies on stillborn fetuses and infants up to 2 months of age. He also found multiple foci of necrosis limited to the right lobe of the liver and suggestive of a vascular origin. Similar changes have been observed at the Boston Hospital for Women.

Fig. 20–1.—Liver from newborn infant with erythroblastosis. **A,** left lobe shows fat and few immature red blood cells. **B,** right lobe shows less fat and more immature red blood cells. Difference presumed to result from differences in antenatal blood supply to right and left lobes.

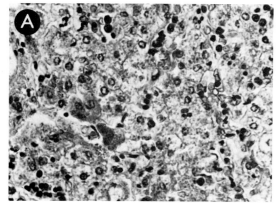 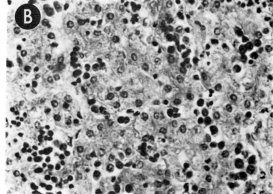

Since at birth the right and left lobes of the liver are nearly equal in size, the left lobe must grow more slowly than the right, presumably because of the relatively poorer blood supply (Emery). Hence, later in infancy the left lobe may show the same lesions that are found in the immediate postnatal period in the right lobe.

Normal Liver

The normal liver at birth varies in weight in relation to total body weight but averages 170 gm in a 3,500 gm infant. It is firm, the margins are sharp and smooth and the color is dark red-purple. In comparison with the adult it is larger in relation to total body size and the left lobe is proportionately larger than the right. The edge of the right lobe is generally about 3 cm below the costal margin in the right midclavicular line, although the level of the liver is determined to some extent by the level of the diaphragm. With pneumothorax, pleural effusion or any condition causing a depression of the diaphragm the resultant depression of the liver may be mistaken for hepatomegaly. The reduction of intrathoracic volume often found in achondroplasia, anencephalus and other malformations produces the same result.

The liver comes from a part of the entodermal tube closely adjacent to the yolk sac and, like the yolk sac, is an important source of red blood cells. In the fetus erythrocytes arise in the liver from endothelial cells lining the sinusoids and from mesodermal cells closely associated with them. Red cells in all stages of maturation are found in the liver throughout intrauterine life (Fig. 20–2), although in the last few weeks, as erythropoiesis in the bone marrow is accelerated, that in the liver is decreased. At term, only widely separated small groups of cells normally remain.

In the young fetus connective tissue containing numerous immature leukocytes surrounds the portal triads (Fig. 20–3). Eosinophilic myelocytes are

Fig. 20–2 (left).—Liver of infant weighing 700 gm who survived 1½ hours, showing normal erythropoiesis. Immature red blood cells in all stages of differentiation are diffusely distributed throughout the sinusoids. They are formed only from reticuloendothelial cells.

Fig. 20–3 (right).—Normal liver of an infant weighing 710 gm who survived 1 hour. Wide bands of connective tissue containing immature leukocytes are present in the periportal spaces.

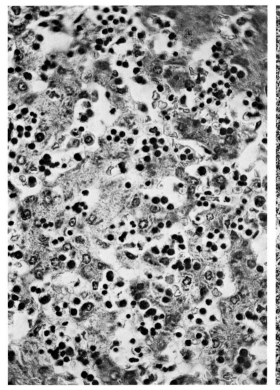
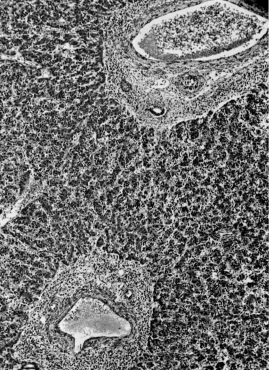

often especially prominent. This source of leukocytes gradually diminishes and at birth only a few immature cells can be found.

In unusually large infants weighing 4,500 gm or more at birth erythropoiesis is occasionally somewhat more pronounced than in those weighing considerably less. This has been described as a change characteristic of infants of mothers with diabetes mellitus, but it seems to be related to this condition because infants of such mothers are often unusually heavy in relation to length of gestation and are more immature than their weight would indicate. Moreover, the large size and relative immaturity of the placentas of infants of diabetic mothers result in an increase in the perfusion distance between the maternal sinusoids and the fetal villous capillaries. Some investigators believe that this leads to anoxia with a resultant increase in erythropoiesis in the fetus. Red blood cells formed in the liver appear to be able to escape into the circulation in a more immature form than do those produced in the bone marrow, and infants weighing over 4,500 gm at birth often have slightly more cells in the circulation that are immature than infants weighing 3,000–3,500 gm.

The histologic appearance of the liver of the fetus and young infant differs from that of the older child or adult. This is exaggerated during much of intrauterine life by the presence of erythropoiesis, but even in the mature fetus in whom erythropoiesis has largely disappeared the liver is easily distinguishable from that of an older individual. The lobules are poorly delineated and the margins often indistinguishable. Hepatic cells rapidly degenerate, and even when tissues are placed in fixing fluid soon after death, the cytoplasm is more granular and stains less uniformly than does that of older infants and adults.

Nuclear size in the infant as well as in the adult is normally fairly uniform but may vary considerably in any pathologic condition. Irregular enlargement is sometimes found following irradiation for a Wilms' or other malignant tumor.

Nucleolar size has been related especially to nutrition and functional activity of the cell. Although some investigators have found a decrease in nucleo-

Fig. 20–4 (left).—Normal liver of 2,660 gm newborn infant. With hematoxylin-eosin stain hepatic cells appear to contain only a little finely granular cytoplasm because of the presence of large amounts of glycogen. Erythropoiesis almost entirely absent.

Fig. 20–5 (right).—Best's carmine stain for glycogen on same liver as shown in Fig. 20–4.

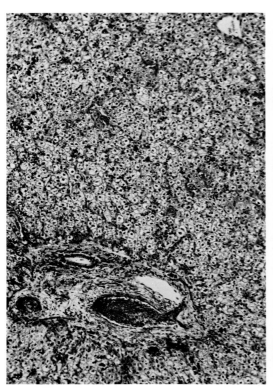
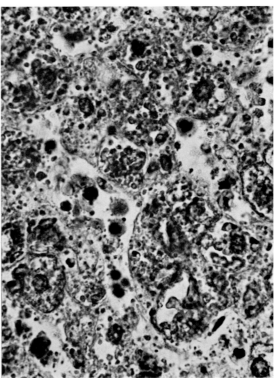

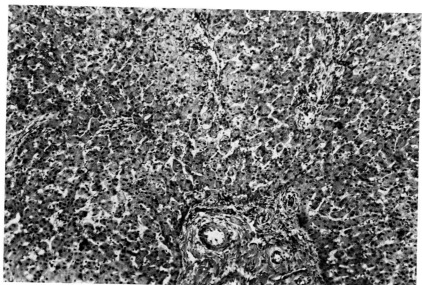

Fig. 20—6.—Normal liver in which glycogen has disappeared except for small amounts around the central veins. Infant weighed 2,890 gm and died on 5th day from rupture of the stomach. Compare staining reaction of liver containing little glycogen to that containing much glycogen (Fig. 20—4).

lar size following protein depletion, others have reported an increase to as much as three times the normal size and have described the "hunger nucleolus" as one in which much of the basophilic material of the nucleus is concentrated into a prominent central mass.

The presence of glycogen is often responsible for a seeming emptiness of hepatic cells when the liver tissue of a mature newborn infant is stained with hematoxylin-eosin. Glycogen is not present in the liver of young fetuses, but it appears at about the 30th week and gradually increases in amount. In a mature fetus who dies suddenly during labor or soon after birth the hepatic cords are usually composed of uniform large pale cells that, when stained with hematoxylin-eosin, show only a few fine granules in the cytoplasm (Fig. 20—4). Best's carmine stain reveals large amounts of glycogen in all cells (Fig. 20—5). Infants who survive for even a short time after birth show some depletion of glycogen at the periphery of the lobules, or almost all glycogen may disappear and leave the hepatic cells with a uniform deeply staining cytoplasm (Fig. 20—6) closely resembling that of the adult. Glycogen in premature infants may be limited to the areas immediately surrounding the central veins. It seems to be formed first and to disappear last in the central portions of the lobules.

Glycogen has been thought to disappear from tissues fairly soon after death and to be fixed satisfactorily only by alcohol, but Morrione and Mamelok found that any of the common fixatives are satisfactory and that following a delay in fixation of as much as 10 hours the amount of glycogen stainable by Best's carmine and periodic acid-Schiff (PAS) technics is not appreciably decreased. However, for best preservation an alcohol, picric acid and formalin mixture such as Rossman's fluid should be used.

The variation in staining reaction between the center and the periphery of the lobules has been attributed by some authors to degeneration of the central areas as a result of anoxia. We have been unable to find such a correlation and believe that since anoxia frequently is rapidly lethal and death occurs suddenly before glycogen stores are depleted, the appearance associated with the presence of glycogen may be mistaken for degeneration (Fig. 20—7). Chronic anoxia, however, will lead to depletion of glycogen due to anaerobic glycolysis.

Congestion of the liver causing extreme distention of the sinusoids is not uncommon in fetuses who die before birth. So much blood may be present that the hepatic cords are compressed into narrow strands between greatly distended vascular channels. This occurs because blood from the placenta often continues to enter the liver through the umbilical vein and accumulates in the hepatic sinusoids when the heart is unable to distribute it to the peripheral parts of the body (see Fig. 7—3).

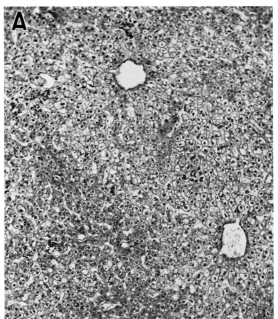

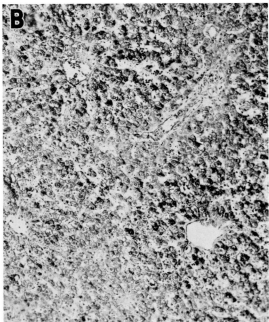

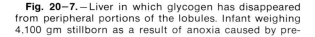

Fig. 20–7.—Liver in which glycogen has disappeared from peripheral portions of the lobules. Infant weighing 4,100 gm stillborn as a result of anoxia caused by premature separation of the placenta. **A,** hematoxylin-eosin stain after Zenker fixation. **B,** Best's carmine stain for glycogen after alcohol fixation.

Local distention may accompany focal areas of necrosis.

Fatty Metamorphosis

Fine fat droplets are often found in the hepatic cells of stillborn fetuses, although they are more common in infants who survive for a time after birth. Fat has been described as physiologic during the latter weeks of intrauterine life, but it is seldom demonstrable in infants who die during or immediately after birth of trauma or acute anoxia. Some fat, however, is present in the majority who live more than a few hours (Dorkin and Weinberg). It is always present in association with infection or malnutrition. One probable reason for its frequent occurrence in the first few days after birth is that food is often withheld from infants who are not doing well and some degree of malnutrition exists.

In tissues stained with hematoxylin–eosin, fat is usually visible as sharply circumscribed vacuoles of varying size. It is always most pronounced in the periportal areas at the periphery of the lobules (Fig. 20–8, A), the region from which glycogen first disappears. Sometimes there are many small vacuoles; at other times a single vacuole fills the cell and compresses the nucleus against one side of the cytoplasmic membrane (Fig. 20–8, B). Vacuoles in the liver cells secondary to anoxia do not always contain fat. As discussed in Chapter 7, the so-called anoxic vacuoles are largely empty; some have a small, centrally placed, round, sudanophilic droplet surrounded by an empty space, not stainable by any known method.

FATTY LIVER ASSOCIATED WITH SUDDEN DEATH.—A serious, often fatal, clinical condition in infants and young children, which develops after partial recovery from viral infections, has been recognized with increasing frequency in the past 10 years. This is *Reye's syndrome;* it consists of vomiting followed by coma or convulsions. At autopsy there is marked fatty metamorphosis of the liver and the tubules of the kidney (Becroft). The brain shows only anoxic changes. Abnormal liver function tests (serum glutamic oxaloacetic transaminase [SGOT]), and elevated ammonia levels have been demonstrated during the height of the illness (Huttenlocher *et al.*). The exact nature of the disturbance is not understood.

KWASHIORKOR.—This condition is uncommon in infants under 1 year of age, since weaning in the societies in which kwashiorkor is prevalent usually takes place late in the 2d or early in the 3d year of life. It is found in all parts of the world, especially

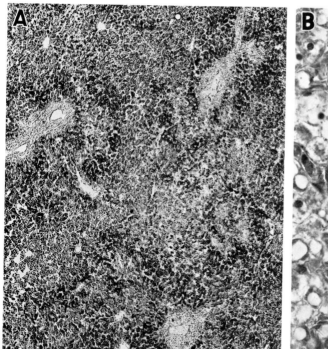

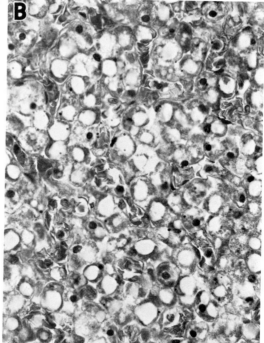

Fig. 20—8.—Fatty metamorphosis of the liver in infant aged 6 days with death due to tracheoesophageal fistula. Fat is common in hepatic cells of periportal areas in infants who die of infections. These are the areas from which glycogen disappears first. **A,** Sudan III stain for fat. **B,** high power view showing many hepatic cells with large amounts of fat causing lateral displacement and compression of nuclei.

the tropics and subtropics, where protein foods are scarce and their importance in the diet not recognized. It has been called by many names but is the same in Uganda and India and Central America.

It develops only when protein intake is very low in relation to carbohydrate. With reduction in total calories it does not occur, so affected children are not emaciated and, because of the frequently associated edema, often seem quite plump. However, they may be undersized, are hyperirritable and photophobic and often have patches of hyperpigmented desquamating skin in the groins and other flexures. The hair is dry, brittle and easily pulled out; among Negroes partial depigmentation may give it a reddish color. In Guatemala, bands of complete depigmentation have been observed to mark periods of exacerbation. Diarrhea is frequently associated with an increase in symptoms and is considered by some to be the precipitating factor and by others to be one of the symptoms of the disease.

In some countries in which kwashiorkor is not recognized the intestinal tracts of many infants who die of diarrhea show no evidence of infection at autopsy. It is probable that this also has a nutritional component.

The cause of kwashiorkor is lack of protein, generally with associated vitamin deficiency, but the latter is probably of secondary importance. Whole milk will generally effect a cure, although sudden overfeeding, especially if carbohydrates are added, may cause death.

Liver obtained by biopsy or at autopsy shows no

Fig. 20—9.—Kwashiorkor. Liver with hepatic cells distended by single fat droplets.

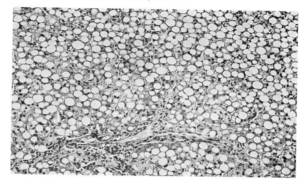

change except severe fatty metamorphosis. The majority of the cells are distended by a single fat globule with the nucleus flattened against the cell membrane (Fig. 20–9). Glycogen is said to persist in the thin rim of cytoplasm. Thymus, pancreas and intestinal mucosa are usually atrophic.

The question of whether the fat in the liver causes cirrhosis is not definitely settled. Workers in Africa have claimed that it does. Equally well-trained observers in India and other parts of the world have insisted that with recovery fat disappears and the liver resumes and retains a normal appearance.

Congenital Metabolic Disorders with Hepatic Involvement

Many of the disorders considered at greater length under inborn errors of metabolism (Chapter 10) are responsible for marked enlargement of the liver as a result of the deposit of abnormal metabolites in parenchymal or Kupffer cells.

Glycogen storage disease types I, II, III and IV are accompanied by an increase in liver size. In type I the liver cells and in types II and IV the liver and Kupffer cells are abnormal. The hepatic cells are large and pale with the nucleus eccentrically placed or seemingly hung in the center of an empty cell. Occasional cells are distended with fat. Glycogen can usually be demonstrated in abnormal amounts after simple formalin fixation if specifically fixed tissue is not available.

Gaucher's disease is characterized by a proportionately larger spleen than liver, but the latter is also enlarged by aggregates of large closely packed polyhedral phagocytes that distort and compress the parenchyma (see Fig. 10–13). They are 40–80 μ in diameter, with a small eccentric nucleus, and tend to accumulate around central veins and in portal areas. The cytoplasm is opaque, slightly basophilic, often reticulated and positive with Sudan and PAS stains. Hemosiderin is common in interstitial tissues.

In older patients with chronic disease cirrhosis may follow the earlier development of fibrous strands around clusters of Gaucher cells. The characteristic picture is that of a nodular liver in which clusters of Gaucher cells are embedded in fibrous scars associated with atrophic nonregenerated nodules of residual parenchyma and deposits of hemosiderin without proliferation of bile ducts or inflammatory exudate in portal areas.

In *Niemann-Pick disease* the liver is proportionately larger, yellower and more fatty-appearing than in Gaucher's disease. Characteristic are the large number of "foam" cells filled with numerous small refractive droplets of sphingomyelin that, although lipoid in character, resist ordinary fat solvents. They are positive with Sudan black, PAS, leukofuchsin and Hale stains in tissue embedded in paraffin as well as in frozen tissues. Although the lipoid material is more common in phagocytes, it may also be found in parenchymal cells and the two may be difficult to distinguish (see Fig. 10–15) from each other. Cirrhosis may develop as an advanced manifestation. Fibrous trabeculae are regularly distributed and clusters of lipoid-containing histiocytes persist. Liver cells may show giant cell transformation, and jaundice, even in newborn infants, has been ascribed to Niemann-Pick's disease (Landing).

Gargoylism is generally associated with mild hepatomegaly, and the liver contains abnormal cells similar to those found in other parts of the body. Both endothelial and parenchymal cells are pale and swollen and often cannot be distinguished from each other. They have been described as resembling decidual cells or the cells of a granular cell myoblastoma. Stains for fat and carbohydrate are usually negative or very weakly positive following formalin fixation, but the PAS stain is usually positive following Lindsay's dioxane–picric acid fixation. Cirrhosis is said to be an occasional complication in older patients.

Letterer-Siwe disease (histiocytosis X) is usually accompanied by considerable enlargement of the liver. The principal abnormality is proliferation and increase in size of reticulum cells. These may be in groups, especially around the portal areas, or diffusely distributed throughout the parenchyma. They are often accompanied by an infiltration of mononuclear leukocytes. Abnormal liver function tests and icterus may be found in rapidly advancing cases.

Cystinosis is occasionally accompanied by enlargement of the liver, and the histologic changes are variable. Usually there is no abnormality except for scattered small groups of histiocytes filled with granular material which under ordinary light is brown but under polarized light is brilliant red, purple or white, depending on the degree of polarization (see Fig. 10–9). At other times the liver also contains varying amounts of fat, and cirrhosis has been reported.

Hemosiderosis in infants is most often associated with excessive destruction of red blood cells such as occurs in erythroblastosis (see Fig. 20–24, B) and cytomegalic inclusion disease with multiple transfusions for anemia. It is more marked in the liver than in other organs, is present as granular masses in the center of parenchymal cells and may fill enlarged Kupffer cells. Whether it ever represents an early stage of endogenous hemochromatosis is questionable although iron deposits associated with changes in parenchymal cells including giant cell formation have been described under this title.

Thalassemia may produce large masses of hemosiderin in hepatic cells in infants over 1 month of age. Kupffer cells also may be abnormal and may contain PAS-positive material, which Landing believed is related to breakdown of erythrocytes.

Galactosemia produces a more profound disturbance in the liver parenchyma and at an earlier period than any of the other congenital metabolic disorders. If completely intolerant to galactose, the infant may deteriorate rapidly before any anatomic changes are visible (Smetana *et al.*). In a large proportion of infants jaundice appears early and there are also early alterations in the indicators of liver function such as alkaline phosphatase, cephalin flocculation and SGOT.

A fairly large amount of fat is found throughout the parenchyma, often in small droplets at the periphery of the cells, pushing the nucleus toward the center; this is in contrast to the usual distribution, which is central, pushing the nucleus peripherally. There also appear to be cases in which extreme fatty metamorphosis masks all other changes. Such metamorphosis has been observed in siblings of children who have had a typical liver pattern and proved galactosemia. For the most part this seems to occur in younger infants, especially those who die a few days after birth, and there seems little doubt that it is a severe, acute form of the disease.

Bile canalicular stasis and severe fatty metamorphosis, which comprise the "pseudoacinar change" that is characteristic of the disease, are seldom found in infants except in this disorder (see Fig. 10-6). Tranquilizers and certain stimulant drugs will produce a similar change although they need not usually be considered in young infants. Focal liver atrophy, fibrosis and early regenerative nodules, together with the "pseudoacinar change," are characteristic of galactosemia. In more chronic cases the periphery of the lobules is generally greatly altered and wide bands of connective tissue containing many young bile ducts divide the liver into nodules.

The white blood cells and tissues of both homozygotes and heterozygotes have decreased amounts of diphosphate galactose transferase (Hsia).

Cystic fibrosis of the pancreas causes obstruction and proliferation of the intrahepatic bile ducts and, later in childhood, is occasionally responsible for focal biliary cirrhosis with gross distortion of the liver. Jaundice occasionally occurs in the 1st year of life and may even be a presenting symptom (Farber and Craig). In such cases inspissation of bile, proliferation of bile ducts and some periportal inflammation can be recognized (Craig *et al.*; Di Sant'Agnese and Blanc). Fatty infiltration of the liver parenchymal cells may be present toward the end of the 1st year.

In *inherited forms of abnormal bilirubin metabolism* such as the Crigler-Najjar, Rotor and Dubin-Johnson syndromes jaundice may be one of the main symptoms. It may begin in the 1st year of life although the disorders are rarely if ever fatal at this time.

Crigler-Najjar syndrome, or congenital nonhemolytic jaundice with kernicterus, is due to a failure of conversion of indirect bilirubin to the glucuronide, or direct-acting bilirubin. The liver alterations, which are minimal, consist of inconstant canalicular or intrahepatic duct stasis and slight periportal fibrosis. A high level of indirect bilirubin is responsible for staining of the basal ganglia of the brain (Crigler and Najjar).

In *Rotor's syndrome* (chronic nonhemolytic jaundice with conjugated bilirubin) there is both conjugated and unconjugated bilirubin in the serum. The liver histology is normal and a normal life is possible (Vest *et al.*).

Dubin-Johnson syndrome is characterized by bilirubin in the serum that is also partly conjugated; here, however, lipofuchsin pigment is present in the liver cells. Jaundice may begin as early as at 3 months (Farber and Craig), and Dubin reported six cases with onset in the 1st year of life. All patients had abdominal pain, fatigue, dark urine and slight hepatomegaly, with symptoms aggravated by intercurrent infection. The liver is dark green. The pigment in the liver cells is Sudan black and Schmorl positive and is bleached by 30% hydrogen peroxide.

Byler's disease (fatal familial intrahepatic cholestasis), named after the couple from whom a large kindred of affected Amish have descended, is characterized by conjugated hyperbilirubinemia with onset before 4 months of age, hepatosplenomegaly in the 1st year, foul-smelling stools, failure to thrive and death secondary to liver failure (Clayton *et al.*). The liver cords appear tubular because of bile thrombi in the canaliculi; there is periportal inflammation and fibrosis, bile duct proliferation and small foci of parenchymal necrosis. The chemical defect appears to be a reduction in trihydroxybilirubin salt conjugate. It occurs only in homozygotes.

Another form of familial nonhemolytic hyperbilirubinemia was reported in Norway by Aaegenaes *et al.* In this condition jaundice begins in the 1st week of life and both direct and indirect bilirubin serum levels are elevated. Cholestasis is prominent in the liver, with bile in liver cells, Kupffer cells and multinucleated giant cells, which are frequently present. A high proportion of cases are familial but the exact pattern of inheritance and details of the metabolic defect are not known.

A recently recognized hereditary metabolic disorder that causes liver dysfunction in early life with a histologic picture of "neonatal hepatitis" and cirrhosis in late infancy is *serum alpha-1 antitrypsin deficiency*. Patients may present with jaundice, and the histologic appearance of the liver may resemble neonatal hepatitis (see page 413) (Lynch *et al.*; Favera *et al.*). Electron microscopic photographs at 10 weeks of age may show bile stasis and the presence of membrane-bound amorphous masses of material, which later, by 5–13 months, are visible with the light microscope as intracellular hyaline cytoplasmic bodies. The Kupffer cells may also be swollen and contain hyaline material. Postnecrotic cirrhosis has been recognized as early as at 5–13 months. Some cases may be complicated by lung infections.

Necrosis

Acute necrosis unaccompanied by evidence of infection is occasionally found at autopsy in young infants, especially newborns. It varies from minute areas involving only small portions of lobules to large areas involving many lobules. With small zones of necrosis the entire liver may be equally affected, but with more extensive changes some parts may be severely disturbed while others remain normal. Necrosis is rarely limited to areas around central veins as it is in adults with passive congestion or pneumonia. Instead, it tends to run irregularly from one lobule to the next (Fig. 20–10), although it often includes the parenchyma around the central veins. In some such cases fibrin thrombi can be recognized in the sinusoids of affected areas. The zones of necrosis may be either ischemic or hemorrhagic. In the former there is loss of cellular cytoplasm and nuclei with collapse of reticulum; in the latter the sinusoids are distended with blood, and hepatic cells are so compressed between them that they may not be identifiable.

Severe necrosis has been observed in infections caused by herpes simplex, Coxsackie B, Echo and variola viruses and by Listeria, Pyocyaneus and other bacteria. Severe hemorrhagic necrosis may be associated with the Waterhouse-Friderichsen syndrome. It has also been described occasionally in

Fig. 20–10.—Midzonal necrosis and hemorrhage in infant weighing 1,750 gm who died on the 3d day of life without other pathologic lesions.

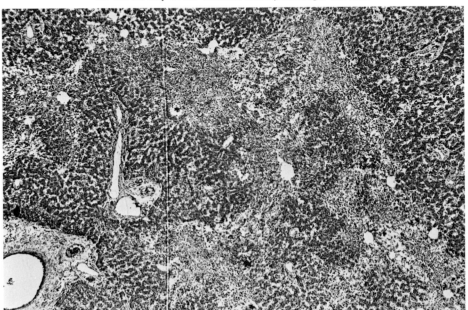

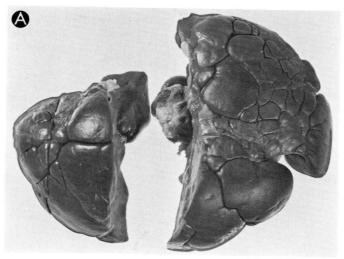

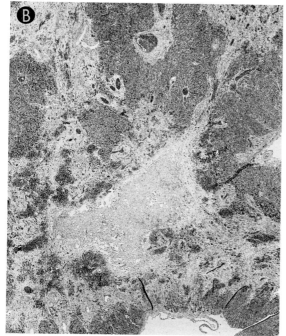

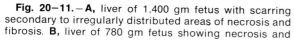

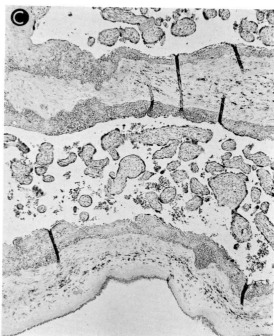

Fig. 20–11.—**A,** liver of 1,400 gm fetus with scarring secondary to irregularly distributed areas of necrosis and fibrosis. **B,** liver of 780 gm fetus showing necrosis and umbiliform depression; gross appearance similar to that shown in A. **C,** placenta with leukocytes on surfaces of chorion and villi from fetus shown in B.

the infants of women with eclampsia but we have not observed it in this connection. Intrauterine anoxia does not appear to be a cause of hepatic necrosis, but, rarely, fairly extensive multilobular necrosis, usually limited to the right lobe of the liver, has been seen in cases of severe erythroblastosis.

Weinberg and Bolande, Coen and MacAdams, and Shiraki all found an increased frequency of acute liver necrosis in infants with a hypoplastic left heart syndrome. Weinberg and Bolande found that 37% of infants with such heart lesions had liver pathology. In infants dying in the first 2 days of life at the Boston Hospital for Women fewer than

20% of those with left heart syndrome had significant necrosis; when present, it involves areas immediately beneath the capsule and is associated with intense congestion of the parenchyma. Shiraki found that the classic lesion is rarely present in the first 2 days of life, which probably accounts for the low incidence at a lying-in hospital.

NECROSIS AND PSEUDOLOBULATION. — Necrosis with secondary scarring was observed at the Chicago Lying-in Hospital in two very young fetuses (780 and 800 gm) and two mature infants, one of whom was a twin with a normal mate. Irregular linear and umbiliform depressions caused by connective tissue replacement of necrotic parenchyma were present on all surfaces of each liver, producing pseudolobulation (Fig. 20–11, A). The necrosis extended in irregularly branching areas throughout the liver and seemed to have no relation to lobular pattern. The zones of necrosis were irregularly infiltrated by moderate numbers of mononuclear leukocytes and immature red blood cells. Small islands of normal liver cells were still present within some of the areas of necrosis (Fig. 20–11, B). Proliferation of the bile ducts and bile stasis had not

occurred. In one instance in which the spleen was similarly involved the fetal zone of the adrenal glands had been replaced by edematous fibrinoid material and the placenta had encircling masses of leukocytes on the surfaces of some villi (Fig. 20–11, C). One of the small fetuses was one of twins, the other twin having a normal liver; the pregnancy was accompanied by extreme polyhydramnios. One mature infant (2,500 gm) had severe ascites and the process seemed of longer duration; fibrosis was more marked and the distortion of the lobular pattern could be considered true cirrhosis (Fig. 20–12). The fourth infant, also one of twins, showed a similar gross appearance of the liver, but in addition to the zones of necrosis there were many areas in which liver cells existed only as syncytial masses similar to the giant cells found in so-called neonatal hepatitis. The other twin was normal and survived.

The cause of this irregular necrosis is not known and one can only note that it operated early in pregnancy and that in two cases scarring had already occurred by approximately 26 weeks. No inclusion bodies could be found but the general ap-

Fig. 20–12. — Cirrhosis of the liver in mature stillborn infant with massive peritoneal effusion. **A,** view of opened abdomen after removal of fluid. Liver and spleen are both enlarged. Liver contains several depressed fibrotic areas, the largest of which is on the anterior surface of the right lobe. **B,** diffuse necrosis and increase in connective tissue and proliferation of bile ducts throughout the liver.

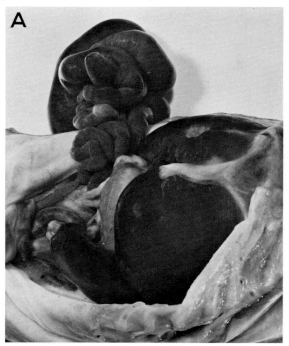

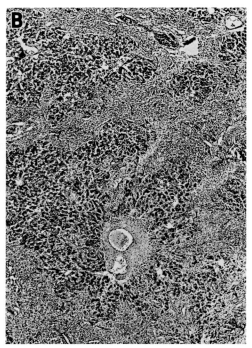

pearance seemed compatible with a viral etiology. Reubner and Mujai reported five similar cases with negative viral cultures and no known etiology.

Infection

General aspects of diseases caused by infectious agents are discussed at more length in Chapter 9. Only the pathologic lesions observed in the liver are included here.

BACTERIAL INFECTION. — Before the introduction of modern technics into delivery rooms and nurseries omphalitis and accompanying infections of the liver were common causes of infant death. In some parts of the world this is still true but fortunately in the United States such infections are now almost never observed in well-run hospital units. In omphalitis polymorphonuclear leukocytes are diffusely distributed throughout the hepatic sinusoids and are often associated with small foci of necrosis. More rarely, larger abscesses may develop (Fig. 20–13). On rare occasions leukocytes are present without a demonstrable source of infection, although in the newborn infant microscopic evidence of infection can usually be found in the region of the umbilicus even when it is not visible grossly. In older infants mild infection of the liver is commonly secondary to appendicitis.

Listeriosis. — The liver, which is usually not enlarged, is characterized by small well-delineated zones of necrosis present in any part of the lobule and scattered diffusely throughout the parenchyma. Sinusoids may be distended by deposits of homogeneous granular material, and moderately

Fig. 20–13. — Abscess of the liver in a very young infant with omphalitis and ascending infection.

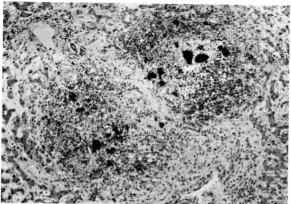

degenerated hepatic cells may be compressed between them, or hepatic cells may be completely absent and only the granular-appearing material may remain (see Fig. 9–18). Early lesions can usually be distinguished from necrosis caused by other agents by the complete absence of cellular reaction and the lack of a transitional zone between normal and necrotic tissue. The organisms are long slender rods that may be visible in ordinary stains but are more easily demonstrated with a Levaditi stain. They are limited to the necrotic areas, where they exist in large numbers. They can be identified positively in tissue sections by use of the fluorescent antibody technic. Culture of the Listeria organisms is not difficult, although identification may fail because of unfamiliarity with characteristics of the organisms.

Syphilis. — The principal change in the liver caused by intrauterine syphilitic infection is an increase of connective tissue with consequent enlargement of the liver. When localized zones of fibrosis are visible on gross examination, they may be present anywhere in the liver but are most common in the right lobe immediately adjacent to the ductus venosus (Fig. 20–14). In such areas hepatic cells are almost completely replaced by connective tissue (Fig. 20–15). In the early stages diffuse increase of connective tissue is often limited to portal areas, but when more advanced, it extends throughout the lobules and produces a diffuse intralobular cirrhosis rarely found in any other condition. At times the connective tissue is so increased that the hepatic cords are disrupted and the hepatic cells resemble multinucleated giant cells embedded in a connective tissue matrix (Fig. 20–16). Localized areas of mononuclear cell infiltration, either with or without necrosis, are frequently present and are often incorrectly designated miliary gummas.

TUBERCULOSIS. — When tuberculosis is of intrauterine origin, the liver is the organ most constantly affected inasmuch as organisms are brought here before they reach other parts of the body. The liver is ordinarily not enlarged and the lesions are generally visible on the external and cut surfaces as circumscribed yellow nodules 3–5 mm in diameter. They may be typical tubercles with epithelioid and giant cells, but more often they resemble soft tubercles that consist of sharply demarcated zones of necrosis without cellular reaction. Acid-fast organisms can be demonstrated in the necrotic areas and their identity proved by animal inoculation.

TOXOPLASMOSIS. — Although the brain is the or-

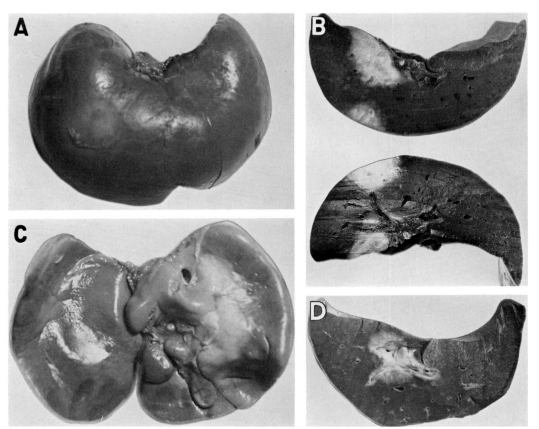

Fig. 20–14.—Syphilitic cirrhosis of liver. **A,** external surface of liver showing an area of fibrosis on anterior surface of right lobe. **B,** cross-section of same liver, showing two areas of complete fibrosis in right lobe. **C,** inferior surface of the liver with zone of fibrosis extending to the surface from area shown in D. **D,** cross-section showing distribution around proximal portion of the ductus venosus and its branches. A and B from stillborn infant. C and D from infant who survived 2 days. (Specimens obtained in Rio de Janeiro, courtesy Dr. Martagão Gesteira.)

gan most severely affected by Toxoplasma, the liver may also be involved. Lelong and co-workers reported an infant icteric from birth on whom a diagnosis was made at 10 days and who died a month later. A biopsy 10 days before death revealed pigment in hepatic cells, distention of bile canaliculi and new connective tissue isolating islands of hepatic cells. A few cells were multinucleated and others were atrophic. At autopsy all changes, including fibrosis and intralobular bile retention, were more pronounced. Cellular infiltration was limited to a few lymphocytes.

HISTOPLASMOSIS.—While this disease is rare in infants, hepatosplenomegaly diagnosed by biopsy as being due to histoplasmosis was reported by Stowens. There was little necrosis, but massive numbers of organisms were present in reticuloendothelial cells.

VIRAL INFECTIONS.—The significance of certain disturbances in the liver has not yet been definitely determined. A few viral infections produce inclusion bodies and characteristic patterns of necrosis, but others have no inclusions and no way has been found of proving a viral origin. This is especially true of a generalized abnormality in the liver characterized by large syncytial giant cells and of the lesion described earlier in four fetuses that was associated with massive necrosis in early intrauterine life.

Herpes simplex.—In most of the cases described the surface of the liver has exhibited numerous irregular grayish-yellow to pale brown nonelevated areas measuring 1–6 mm in diameter. Microscopically, as much as 70–95% of the total parenchyma has appeared to be necrotic although individual lesions are usually small (see Fig. 9–11).

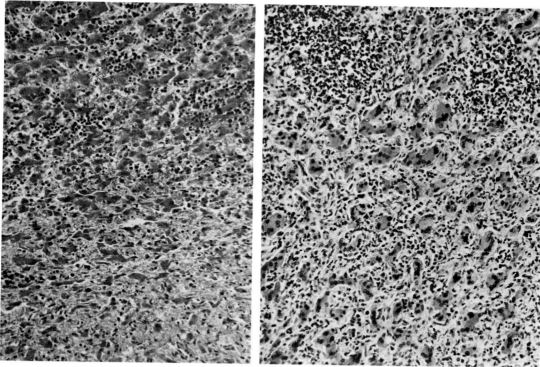

Fig. 20–15 (left). — Syphilitic cirrhosis showing junction of a liver area in which hepatic cells are still present and a fibrotic area in which the liver cords have been largely replaced by connective tissue. Infant aged 2 days.

Fig. 20–16 (right). — Syphilitic cirrhosis showing typical intralobular distribution of connective tissue. Remaining liver cords resemble multinucleated giant cells. Focal areas of leukocytes are present.

The necrosis is generally fairly complete, with endothelium and parenchyma losing affinity for stains. Nuclear inclusions are present at the margins of necrotic areas where structure is still fairly well preserved. Most characteristically the cells contain a prominent, sharply circumscribed, strongly acidophilic amorphous mass surrounded by a clear zone that separates it from marginated chromatin. Leukocytic infiltration is minimal and proliferation of bile ducts or connective tissue has not been observed. The adrenal glands frequently also show isolated zones of necrosis without inflammatory reaction, and lungs and bone marrow may rarely also be the site of massive necrosis. It is curious how seldom lesions are seen in the brain.

Coxsackie B virus infection.—Infection with Coxsackie B virus may be responsible for a devastating necrosis of the liver, ordinarily associated with very little cellular response (see Fig. 9–13, A). Parenchymal cells and sinusoids can usually be distinguished but nuclei and cytoplasm may retain their affinity for stains only in the cells immediately adjacent to the portal areas. Intranuclear in-

clusions are rare but have been found in parenchymal cells surrounding the zones of necrosis. Portal areas are usually normal and bile ducts are not increased. Myocarditis is rare in infants but if found in conjunction with hepatic necrosis is almost pathognomonic of a Coxsackie B virus infection.

Cytomegalic inclusion disease.—As a cause of death this infection ordinarily appears to be limited to the newborn period. The most outstanding feature in the liver is marked generalized erythropoiesis similar to that found in infants with severe erythroblastosis. The distention of bile canaliculi, the presence of bile pigment and iron in hepatic cells and the absence of necrosis are also similar to erythroblastosis. The main histologic difference between the two conditions is the presence of giant intranuclear inclusions in cytomegalic inclusion disease. They are of variable frequency, sometimes being numerous and prominent, at other times requiring considerable search, and are usually limited to bile ducts, especially those at the periphery of the portal areas (Fig. 20–17). These ducts are often somewhat enlarged and their appearance

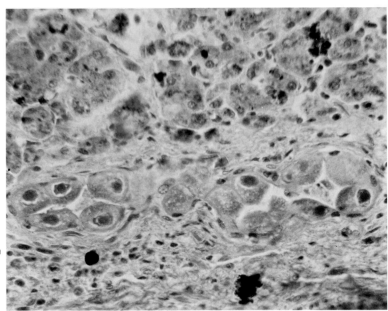

Fig. 20–17.—Cytomegalic inclusion disease. Characteristic inclusions are present in cells of bile ducts.

suggests that they are young and possibly newly formed as a result of the infection. Generally, from one to four cells in cross-section of any involved duct are enlarged and the equally enlarged nuclei contain prominent, sharply outlined inclusions separated from the nuclear membrane by a clear zone. These inclusions are more characteristic than those of any other viral infection and their size and staining characteristics ordinarily make them easy to identify.

Multinucleated giant cells have been reported in this condition but are usually not present in appreciable numbers in early fatal cases. Later, when erythropoiesis decreases and inclusions become less frequent, multinucleated giant cells become more prominent and the liver may take on the appearance of neonatal hepatitis. Inclusions are almost always more prominent in the kidney, and failure to find them in the liver has occasionally led to the erroneous diagnosis of erythroblastosis complicated by the virus of cytomegalic inclusion disease, the diagnosis of erythroblastosis being based on the extensive hepatic erythropoiesis.

Echo virus.—This was isolated by Benirschke from one case of massive liver necrosis in which only the portal areas still persisted.

Homologous serum hepatitis.—Designated type B hepatitis, this has a long incubation period and is associated with the Australian antigen. It has long been suspected as a cause of "neonatal" hepatitis

(see next section) but proof of transmission from mother to infant had been lacking until recently (Schweitzer *et al.*). It has been postulated that the infant becomes infected either by way of the placenta or directly during passage through the birth canal. Although the presence of the antigen (hepatitis B) has been demonstrated in mothers and in some of their infants who have also had abnormal levels of transaminase in the liver, the search for the antigen in infants presenting with overt clinical hepatitis and the histologic picture of "neonatal hepatitis" has been disappointing. The ultimate prognosis for such infants is still unclear.

Infectious hepatitis.—Designated hepatitis type A, this has a short incubation period and gives little evidence of being transmitted to the fetus or young infant from an affected mother. Although it is ordinarily a relatively mild process in the very young, it has produced a histologic pattern in infants identical to that in adults. Some investigators believe that the giant cell involvement of the liver described in the next section is caused by the intra-uterine transmission of such a virus, but this has not been satisfactorily proved, and almost none of the offspring of women with infectious hepatitis during pregnancy have had evidence of the disease.

The characteristic picture of nonfatal infectious hepatitis is one of irregular degeneration and regeneration of individual liver cells associated with varying degrees of cellular infiltration. No part of the lobule is exempt. Destroyed cells disappear and reticulum collapses; injured cells may swell and become "balloon cells" or may shrink, become hyalinized and form the "acidophilic bodies" that are considered especially characteristic of this condition. The general contour of the lobules and the structures in the portal areas appear to be normal. Deposition of fat is rare and bile stasis is not common even though jaundice may be present. Occasionally there are areas of complete necrosis that may lead to postnecrotic cirrhosis but, except for this, recovery is complete.

The typical picture in fatal cases is devastating necrosis affecting all of the lobule except possibly a few cells immediately adjacent to portal areas. This is the picture that has been described as acute yellow atrophy and only fairly recently recognized as one aspect of viral hepatitis. The pattern of the liver is preserved; central veins and portal areas remain, the latter infiltrated by a variety of cells.

Rubella syndrome liver changes are not common but include cellular swelling and vacuolization and giant cell formation.

Hyperbilirubinemia

Approximately half of all infants who are carefully examined have some degree of jaundice during the 1st week of life although all have bilirubin levels that would produce jaundice in adults. This appears to be true regardless of when the cord is cut or whether the child is mature or premature. The bilirubin is normally almost entirely unconjugated, indicating an increased red cell breakdown and/or a failure of conjugation of the pigment by the liver. This failure prevents excretion of bile pigment and often infants with high total serum bilirubin levels have only a small amount of bile in the intestine.

The average serum bilirubin level at birth is ordinarily under 2 mg per 100 ml and in mature infants reaches a maximum at about the 3d day; although starting at about the same level at birth, bilirubin in premature infants continues rising a little longer and generally reaches a somewhat higher level at about the 4th or 5th day. In all infants the higher the bilirubin level in cord blood, the higher the subsequent rise. There is no critical level of bilirubin above which jaundice will invariably be visible, nor is there a definite level above which the bilirubin value can be considered pathologic. The possibility that variation in level may depend on difference in laboratory technics must always be considered in comparisons of results.

Allen and Diamond considered a cord blood bilirubin level above 7 mg per 100 ml a specific indication for exchange transfusion in an infant with a positive Coombs test, and Brown and Zuelzer considered that blood levels above 12 mg per 100 ml in mature infants or above 15 mg per 100 ml in premature infants at any age indicate bilirubinemia significantly above a physiologic level. Since the premature infant generally has a greater proportion of bilirubin in the unconjugated form and is susceptible to kernicterus at lower levels of serum bilirubin than the full-term infant, exchange transfusion should be considered for premature infants at levels of serum bilirubin that might be ignored in mature infants.

Conversion of indirect- to direct-reacting bilirubin has been shown to take place in the liver through the action of glucuronyl transferase, which converts free bilirubin into the direct-reacting bilirubin glucuronide by conjugation with glucuronic acid. Free bilirubin is fat soluble and has a higher affinity for binding to protein, particularly albumin. Because of its fat solubility and protein-binding properties unconjugated bilirubin can pass the blood brain barrier and enter the brain cells; this occurs when serum levels of indirect bilirubin reach about 15 mg per 100 ml. The level of the enzyme glucuronyl transferase increases rapidly in the first days after birth and soon reaches adult levels. In premature infants the initial level is lower and the postnatal increase in activity is at a slower rate than in mature infants.

Although bilirubin levels may not be directly related to visible jaundice, there is little evidence that bilirubin will reach a harmful level under natural conditions without producing jaundice. The use of ultraviolet light in the treatment of postnatal icterus may reduce the visible jaundice of the treated skin to a level not commensurate with the plasma level. Rarely, unexpected kernicterus is found at autopsy in premature infants with sepsis when no visible jaundice was observed before death and when bilirubin levels were 12 mg per 100 ml or lower. It is impossible to set a definite level above which serum bilirubin can be expected to exert a damaging effect on the brain, which is the only organ that appears to be permanently injured by the high concentration. The sooner bilirubin becomes elevated after birth, the more potentially dangerous it is considered to be, largely because the more rapid the rise, the higher the level it can be expected to reach. Indirect-reacting bilirubin of 30 mg per 100 ml frequently appears to be damaging, and it is recommended that an attempt be made to prevent the level from rising above 17 mg per 100 ml in order to allow a little margin of safety.

Jaundice considered physiologic, or nonpathologic, is caused by elevations of both conjugated and nonconjugated moieties. Such jaundice does not ordinarily appear until the 2d or 3d day and generally disappears by the end of the 1st week.

Pathologic jaundice in the newborn is most often caused by indirect-reacting bilirubin and is usually a result of blood destruction by Rh, AB or related antibodies. Jaundice appearing in the first 24 hours of life should be considered evidence of erythroblastosis until proved otherwise. Very infrequently it is due to blood destruction by cytomegalic or other virus, and rarely no cause can be found.

Later in infancy an increase in indirect-reacting bilirubin usually results from some other variety of hemolytic anemia, such as bacterial sepsis, or an inborn error of metabolism of red cells, such as glucose-6-phosphate dehydrogenase deficiency. Liver injury, either toxic or infectious, may be responsible for elevation of indirect as well as direct bilirubin if there is sufficient damage to interfere with conjugation of bilirubin and inhibit excretion.

Direct-reacting bilirubin usually does not become sufficiently elevated to cause jaundice until several days after birth. Then, as well as later in childhood, jaundice is most often due to an obstruction to passage of bile through intra- or extrahepatic bile ducts and is usually accompanied by acholic stools. Atresia of extrahepatic bile ducts is the most common cause and any infant with prolonged jaundice due to direct-reacting bilirubin without other demonstrable etiology probably warrants an exploratory laparotomy, although those with any portion of hepatic duct that can be anastomosed to the intestine are few. Gross reported that of 146 infants with bile duct atresia, in only 27 could the hepatic duct be anastomosed.

On autopsy of 750 infants Nakai and Landing found that 42 had evidence of intrahepatic bile stasis with bile in cells, canaliculi or bile ducts, although nearly twice that number had had visible jaundice before death. The infants were immature or suffered from infection, liver cell damage, hemolysis (either intravascular or secondary to internal bleeding), dehydration or, in rare instances, upper gastrointestinal obstruction with extrinsic pressure on the bile ducts. The discrepancy between the degree of intrahepatic bile stasis and the degree of jaundice was greatest in those with external pressure on the ducts. A group of infants with congenital heart disease, particularly those with the hypoplastic left heart syndrome, had icterus and parenchymal bile stasis, the latter presumably resulting from anoxic changes in the liver. The most common cause of intrahepatic bile stasis was prematurity. These workers also found that intrahepatic bile stasis could not be correlated with elevated levels of conjugated bilirubin in the peripheral blood, although at the Boston Hospital for Women extraction studies on liver sections and chromatographic analysis of homogenates of livers with bile stasis have suggested that much of the bile present in the liver is direct acting. At the Chicago Lying-in Hospital distention of bile canaliculi was often found in infants who died of erythroblastosis at 2–3 days of age before modern methods of treatment were instituted. Since then it has rarely been encountered.

The differential diagnosis of obstructive jaundice in the neonatal period, however, is still difficult. Hays and Snyder reported that of 137 cases followed for 36 months an accurate distinction could be made between neonatal hepatitis and atresia of the bile ducts in only 60%, even with the use of the needle or open biopsy. With an operative cholangiogram the distinction between the two conditions rose to 79%. Brough and Bernstein reported 62% accuracy for liver biopsy in cases of biliary atresia and 79% in hepatitis.

All cases of prolonged jaundice (196) occurring at the Boston Children's Hospital Medical Center between 1940 and 1951 were analyzed by Hsia and co-workers, who found 60% due to biliary atresia, 15% to inspissated bile caused by erythroblastosis, 19% to inspissated bile syndrome of unknown origin and 6% to other causes (hepatitis, hemangioendothelioma, node compression, portal vein thrombosis, Niemann-Pick disease and unknown cause, one each). On the other hand, Hays *et al.* found biliary atresia responsible for only 28% of their cases of obstructive jaundice; Danks and Bodian found 41% caused by neonatal hepatitis.

NEONATAL HEPATITIS. — Among young infants presenting with symptoms of obstructive jaundice there are, as noted above, a fairly large number whose livers have characteristic identifiable changes generally designated neonatal hepatitis for which a specific etiology has never been found. There is much overlap in the microscopic appearance of biliary atresia and neonatal hepatitis, although at the ends of the spectrum the changes are clearly distinguishable. The description given by Craig and Landing in 1952 still appears valid in most of its features. The picture is one of moderate to severe disorganization of liver cell columns, diffuse lobular infiltration, chiefly of mononuclear cells, focal necrosis of liver cells and evidence of

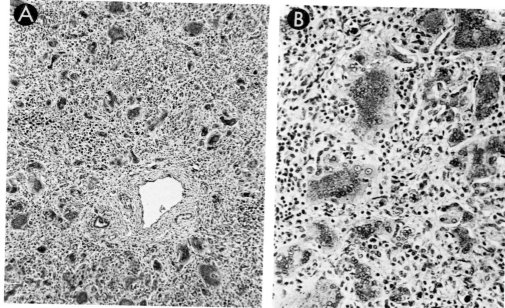

Fig. 20–18.—Liver with giant cell transformation. Innumerable irregular syncytial masses containing large numbers of nuclei with increased connective tissue and cellular infiltration. No normal parenchyma. **A,** low magnification showing normal bile ducts in portal area and general distribution of liver giant cells. **B,** high power view of giant cells.

bile stasis in liver cells, Kupffer cells and bile canaliculi, but rarely in intrahepatic ducts. There is often inflammation in portal triads, and frequently small foci of erythropoiesis remain after the usual time of disappearance. Multinucleated parenchymal giant cells are ordinarily present, sometimes in large numbers, but are not specific or necessary for the diagnosis (Fig. 20–18). Their nonspecificity suggests that giant cells represent a form of degen-

eration; at least they are a far more frequent manifestation of abnormal liver cell physiology in the young infant than in any other age group. Bile duct proliferation is not a usual feature of the disorder, although in rare cases much of the parenchyma seems to be converted into abnormal bile ducts as a result of secondary liver destruction or repair (Fig. 20–19).

It seems almost certain that necrosis and giant

Fig. 20–19.—Liver with no normal parenchyma or bile ducts. Entire liver converted into abnormal structures resembling abortive attempt at formation of bile ducts.

A, low magnification showing portal area to left and central vein to right. **B,** high magnification of abnormal liver parenchyma.

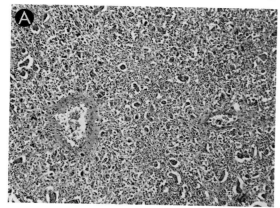

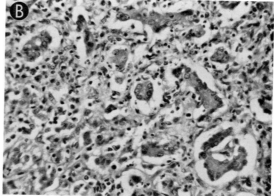

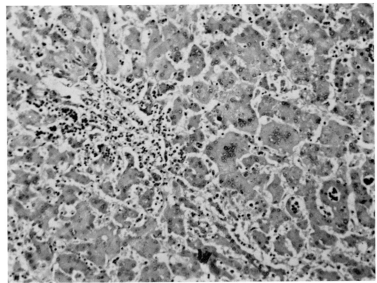

Fig. 20–20.—Liver with giant cells similar to those thought by Smetana *et al.* to be caused by failure of development of intralobular bile ducts. Bile ducts are also lacking in portal areas. Age 10 weeks.

cell formation do not represent a change due to a single etiology. Some cases of herpes simplex, cytomegalic inclusion disease (Weller and Hanshaw), the congenital rubella syndrome (Strauss and Bernstein) or alpha-1 antitrypsin deficiency may have the same picture. The histologic similarity to epidemic and serum hepatitis is suggestive although proof of such infection in the newborn is generally lacking.

In several series (Danks and Bodian; Cassady *et*

Fig. 20–21.—Diagram showing variations in abnormalities of extrahepatic bile ducts.

COMMON VARIETIES OF ATRESIA OF THE BILE DUCTS AND GALL BLADDER

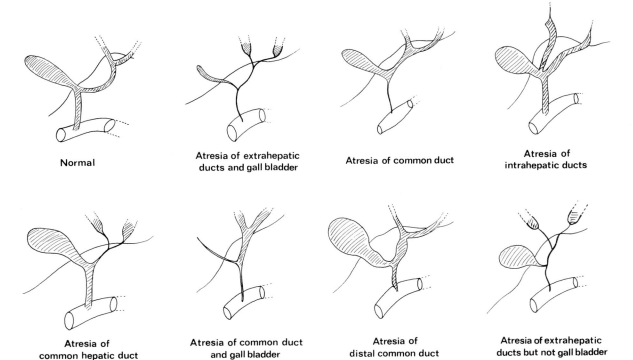

Normal

Atresia of extrahepatic ducts and gall bladder

Atresia of common duct

Atresia of intrahepatic ducts

Atresia of common hepatic duct

Atresia of common duct and gall bladder

Atresia of distal common duct

Atresia of extrahepatic ducts but not gall bladder

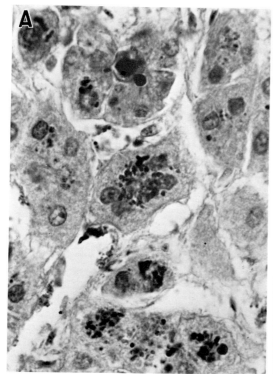

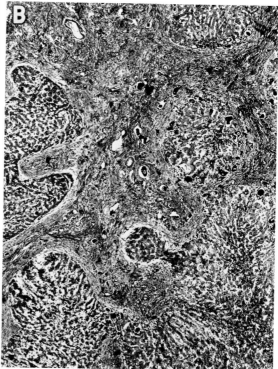

Fig. 20–22.—Congenital atresia of extrahepatic bile ducts. **A,** bile thrombi in bile capillaries and pigment granules in hepatic cells. Infant aged 1 month. **B,** marked proliferation of connective tissue causing isolation of islands of hepatic cells. Infant aged 3 months.

al.; Hsia *et al.*) the frequent occurrence of familial cases and of consanguinity in the parents raises the question of a congenital metabolic disorder such as alpha-1 antitrypsin deficiency.

The variation in outcome of patients with this histologic picture also suggests a variable etiology. In the series of Hays *et al.*, of 37 patients 15 died, 13 recovered and five had either early or well-established cirrhosis with known complications. However, in these cases jaundice was sufficiently severe and persistent to warrant exploration and biopsy.

Smetana *et al.* and others believed that a form of liver disease exists that is probably congenital in which the liver cell cords are transformed into masses of syncytial giant cells associated with failure of canalicular formation (Fig. 20–20). It has been suggested that in cases with a favorable outcome abnormal areas are eventually replaced with normal elements. These must comprise a special group of cases because in our experience at the Boston Hospital for Women adenosine triphosphatase reactions on livers with neonatal hepatitis containing many giant cells revealed canaliculi within the giant cells.

ATRESIA OF THE EXTRAHEPATIC BILE DUCTS. — Prolonged jaundice in the newborn period is usually a result of atresia of the extrahepatic bile ducts. Duct pattern may be a variable, as depicted in Figure 20–21, and the etiology is uncertain. Alpert *et al.* reported a few cases associated with trisomy E but some of these infants had hepatitis, and some investigators believe that many atresias of the bile ducts are secondary to postnatal infection inasmuch as the diagnosis is not made even at autopsy on stillborn and rarely on newborn infants.

The histologic changes of classic extrahepatic atresia may be minimal in the first few weeks of life. Somewhat later, bile stasis in intrahepatic bile ducts, ducts of Hering and canaliculi is a prominent feature (Fig. 20–22, A). In the parenchyma, bile lakes may be prominent and portal triads may be widened by duct proliferation. Inflammation, if present, is often limited to the ducts and surrounding connective tissue. Since bile duct proliferation in biliary atresia appears stimulated by and largely dependent on bacterially induced cholangitis, the absence of proliferation in the early weeks of life is not surprising. Necrobiosis of parenchymal cells and necrosis are often limited to the periportal areas. Multinucleated giant cells can be identified in very young infants in about one third of the cases. They are not seen in later stages.

Bile duct proliferation may become less marked in children living for more than a year, and at times many portal areas must be searched for the presence of ducts. They may be absent or increased in different parts of the same liver. Severe cirrhosis occurs before death (see below).

Operation can seldom relieve the obstruction caused by atresia of the bile ducts. Danks and Bodian reported successful repair in only four of 32 infants, Hays *et al.* in two of 71 and Gross in 27 of 146. Hays *et al.* gave 19 months as the average duration of life for infants with extrahepatic atresia.

ATRESIA OF INTRAHEPATIC BILE DUCTS. — The diagnosis of primary intrahepatic biliary atresia can be made with certainty only at autopsy, when many sections of the liver taken from various areas can be examined. Some pathologists conversant with pediatric material do not believe such an entity as congenital intrahepatic atresia exists (Brent). In putative cases absence of observable duct structures has often been the only abnormality, and periportal fibrosis and inflammation have been minimal or absent. Infants with a diagnosis of intrahepatic atresia may survive considerably longer than those with extrahepatic atresia and may have associated hypercholesterolemia (Ahrens *et al.*). Congenital extrahepatic obstruction may be accompanied by intrahepatic atresia.

Cirrhosis

Cirrhosis is often erroneously used as a synonym for fibrosis of the liver. It is applied correctly only to a condition in which (1) there is necrosis of liver cells, (2) the necrosis is followed by nodular parenchymal regeneration with fibrous tissue joining central veins and portal tracts, thus producing a disorganization of hepatic architecture, and (3) all parts of the liver are involved.

Since the possible response of the liver to injury is limited, the ultimate histologic appearance is much the same regardless of cause and consists principally of collapse of hepatic lobules, formation of fibrous septa and nodular regeneration of hepatic parenchyma. The impediment to portal blood flow resulting from distortion of the vascular tree by fibrous strands and nodules of regeneration is responsible for portal hypertension, one of the prominent symptoms of cirrhosis.

In adults, three principal types are recognized: (1) portal, most commonly associated with alcoholism and characterized by thick, regular bands of connective tissue, by regenerating small nodules of fairly uniform size and by involvement of every lobule; (2) postnecrotic, often secondary to viral hepatitis and characterized by bands of connective tissue of varying thickness, by nodules within the larger nodules and by bizarre, often multinucleated liver cells; and (3) biliary, resulting from prolonged obstructive jaundice, characterized by marked proliferation of bile ducts within bands of connective tissue encircling intact liver lobules with maintenance of a normal relationship between central vein and portal areas. In late stages the changes are identical to those found in portal cirrhosis.

According to Sherlock, the most commonly accepted etiologic factors are viral hepatitis, alcoholism, obstruction of the extrahepatic biliary tract, cardiac failure, hemachromatosis, hepatolenticular degeneration and congenital syphilis; rare or questionable causes include malnutrition, chemical poisons, infections and granulomatous lesions. In over 50% of her patients no cause could be found.

In infants and small children most cirrhosis is either postnecrotic or biliary, although it may be a sequel to metabolic disease or of unknown cause. Craig *et al.* reviewed the literature on cirrhosis in infants and children and summarized 30 years' experience at the Children's Medical Center in Boston. They found no examples of classic Laennec's (portal) cirrhosis, and, although this may be due to the absence of alcoholism and severe nutritional deficiencies, they thought it should more probably be interpreted as a difference in the way the liver responds to injury during infancy and childhood. They found congenital malformations of the biliary tree and hepatitis to be the primary causes in their cases; 61 were secondary to biliary obstruction, 30 were thought to be associated with hepatitis (although in 13 no previous illness had been recognized) and seven were due to miscellaneous causes. Sixty-seven of the patients in this series had symptoms within days or weeks of birth and almost all of these died during the 1st year. By far the most common cause was atresia of the extrahepatic bile ducts; one child was treated successfully, 39 died within the 1st year, five died at 12–60 months and in four the outcome was unknown. Nine cases followed neonatal hepatitis, in all but two of whom symptoms appeared within the 1st month of life; two of these patients also had erythroblastosis and died at 1 month. Two cases followed viral hepatitis at ages 5 and 5½ months. The miscellaneous causes with symptoms in the 1st year included glycogen storage disease (two), galactosemia (two), cardiac cirrhosis (one), cholangitis (one) and hemosiderosis (one).

The cirrhosis following neonatal hepatitis was relatively mild in most instances, probably because the condition was fulminating and death occurred early; periportal fibrosis was variable but there was marked distortion of liver cords in spite of lack of regenerative nodules. Inflammation and degeneration were present but bile ducts were not proliferated, although bile stasis was present in over half of the cases. Craig *et al.* believed that cirrhosis frequently follows neonatal hepatitis, having found it in 11 (27%) of 41 infants in whom neonatal hepatitis had been diagnosed previously. They suggested that the high incidence might be due to immaturity of the liver, infection by homologous serum hepatitis virus and the added insult of anesthesia and trauma to the liver during the surgical exploration undertaken in most of these infants.

Cirrhosis following viral hepatitis did not present symptoms until 7 months to 4 years after the initial infection, and only two patients had their infection and presented the first symptoms of cirrhosis during the 1st year. The livers of these children had many intact lobules though some regenerative nodules were found, and in some cases evidence of active hepatitis was still present, as demonstrated by infiltration of chronic inflammatory cells in periportal areas. Bile ducts were seldom increased although they seemed to be so at times because of collapse of parenchymal lobules. Portal areas were irregularly broadened by fibrous bands. The spleen was usually enlarged. In most cases it was impossible to determine whether a first attack of jaundice was due to viral hepatitis or was the first sign of hepatic failure in cirrhosis, so this cause of cirrhosis cannot be considered proved. It is interesting too that of 200 children with viral hepatitis observed by Craig *et al.* none developed evidence of cirrhosis within 3 years of the infection.

Among the children with cirrhosis without a history of probable hepatitis only one child was less than a year old. The histologic appearance was similar to that observed when cirrhosis followed viral hepatitis.

Of the congenital metabolic diseases only galactosemia and type IV glycogen storage disease would be likely to cause symptomatic cirrhosis in the 1st year of life (Gall and Landing). Although cirrhosis is occasionally found following erythroblastosis fetalis, the assumption that this is due to the erythroblastosis needs further proof (Craig; Lightwood and Bodian). In cystic fibrosis of the pancreas periportal fibrosis, duct proliferation,

jaundice and intrahepatic duct obstruction may be found in the 1st year although true cirrhosis has not been identified during that time. Jaundice, rather than the usual respiratory symptoms, may be the first evidence of the disease (Farber and Craig).

A curious form of cirrhosis that is seen only in India and is a common ailment among higher caste Hindus is called *infantile cirrhosis* (Smetana *et al.*). Some cases begin with jaundice in the 1st year of life and have established cirrhosis by the age of 1–3 years. This form is marked histologically by the presence of focal to massive acute necrosis, regenerative nodules and Mallory bodies. It has many features of the nutritional cirrhosis of the alcoholic but lacks the fatty metamorphosis. Its cause is unknown.

Cirrhosis secondary to atresia of extrahepatic bile ducts exhibits the usual changes of cirrhosis. The liver is uniformly enlarged, is green or yellow on the cut surface and has a smooth outer surface until the patient is about 5 months of age. After this, nodularity increases simultaneously with an increase in the fibrotic perilobular tissue (Fig. 20–22, B). By 3–4 months of age liver cell cords are generally distorted as a result of irregularity in size, the presence of occasional multinucleated giant cells and swelling of the Kupffer cells. The extent of portal infiltration, width of periportal connective tissue and increase in bile ducts seem to have little correlation with length of life although, with increasing age, ducts in the center of the triads tend to disappear and new ducts form at the periphery. In some lobules bile ducts may be difficult to identify, giving an appearance suggestive of absence of intrahepatic bile ducts, while at other times lobules seem to consist of nothing but proliferated ducts. Bile stasis is prominent in all cases, especially in ducts and portal triads. Bile plugs in the canaliculi are often placed nearer the center of the lobule than the periphery. Stasis in the cytoplasm of liver cells is present in only about half of the cases and in Kupffer cells only when bile is present in liver cells. Ascites, esophageal varices and splenic enlargement are often present, indicating some degree of portal obstruction.

The importance of obstruction and infection in the production of biliary cirrhosis in both infants and adults has been debated. It has been suggested that the atresia of extrahepatic ducts found in young infants may be a result of fetal cholangitis, but the evidence appears to be overwhelmingly in favor of a congenital malformation unassociated with infection. It has also been thought that the principal cause of biliary cirrhosis is an increase in intraductal pressure and that the extensive production of new bile ducts is an attempt to compensate for the obstruction and consequent obliteration of the intrahepatic bile ducts and to restore the continuity between the main biliary passages in the portal spaces and the bile capillaries in the parenchyma.

Sherlock, in describing the histologic differences in occlusion of intra- and extrahepatic ducts, stressed the fact that in intrahepatic obstruction the bile passages are inconspicuous and empty, while in extrahepatic obstruction they are long and tortuous with wide lumens filled with bile and lined by cuboidal cells.

Veno-occlusive disease has been described from Jamaica, Egypt, Israel and South Africa as a condition affecting young infants in which nonportal cirrhosis follows occlusion of the radicles of the hepatic veins. In the acute stage the small hepatic veins are involved, with the medium-sized and larger vessels normal. The block is said to be caused by subendothelial edema with subsequent collagenization. Massive congestion of central zones leads to loss of liver cells, with fibrosis, thickening and narrowing of the lumen of hepatic veins. Nonportal cirrhosis develops as the disease becomes chronic. The cause is generally ascribed to "bush teas" or related substances taken for medicinal purposes (Jelliffe *et al.*; Brooks *et al.*).

Blood Dyscrasias

LEUKEMIA.—Erythroblastosis and leukemia are the only two blood disturbances in the fetus and newborn that produce characteristic changes in the liver. Leukemia is rare at this age, but several

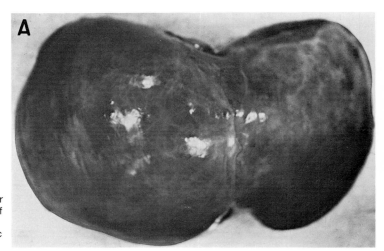

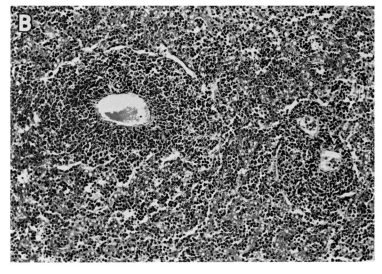

Fig. 20–23.—Leukemia. **A,** anterior surface of liver showing a network of interlacing fine white bands caused by periportal distribution of leukemic cells. **B,** photomicrograph showing immature myeloid cells filling all sinuses and present in masses around portal areas. Infant aged 2 days. External surface of body is shown in Fig. 28–9.

cases have been reported. Two were observed at the Chicago Lying-in Hospital, one infant dying at the age of 3 days of myelogenous leukemia and one at 6 weeks of the lymphatic form of the disease (see Chapter 28). In the former the liver was enlarged and the external surface had a white, irregularly branching fernlike pattern (Fig. 20–23, A). This was caused by the wide bands of immature myeloid cells that surrounded the portal triads and separated the lobules. The parenchyma was also diffusely infiltrated by immature myeloid cells (Fig. 20–23, B). There was no necrosis, evidence of bile stasis or proliferation of bile ducts.

ERYTHROBLASTOSIS.—Until the last trimester of pregnancy the liver of the fetus is seldom enlarged, and the diagnosis on anatomic grounds of serologically proved erythroblastosis may be impossible. In mild cases, even in older fetuses, the size of the liver is usually within normal limits. In severe cases it may be increased 50–75%; only rarely does it exceed this. When death occurs before delivery or in the first few hours after birth, erythropoiesis in the liver may be profoundly increased, but when death does not occur until later, formation of blood cells may have ceased and at times the liver ap-

pears normal. Even though cell destruction continues at an abnormally rapid rate, ectopic areas of erythropoiesis ordinarily disappear soon after birth.

When cells have been produced in the liver at an increased rate, a differential diagnosis of erythropoiesis resulting from erythroblastosis, prematurity and other conditions in which erythropoiesis is unusually active may be impossible. The principal differential point is the variation in the stage of development attained by the cells in any localized area. In normal premature infants, cells varying from early erythroblasts to late normoblasts are diffusely distributed throughout the parenchyma. In erythroblastosis the foci of erythropoiesis are usually more sharply circumscribed and all cells in any one area are frequently in approximately the same stage of maturation (Fig. 20–24, A). The earliest forms of erythroblasts are proportionately more numerous than in the normal erythropoiesis of prematurity. Erythropoiesis in the liver, whatever its cause, disappears soon after birth.

The liver of an infant stillborn because of erythroblastosis often indicates that erythrocyte destruction has exceeded the ability of the liver to

Fig. 20–24.—Erythroblastosis. **A,** erythropoiesis in the liver of mature hydropic infant surviving 1 hour. Foci of cells are larger and more circumscribed than those in the normal liver of a premature infant, and the cells in each focus are at a more uniform stage of development (compare with Fig. 20–2). **B,** hemosiderin in the liver of a mature infant with erythroblastosis who survived 1½ hours. Hemosiderin is most concentrated in periportal areas.

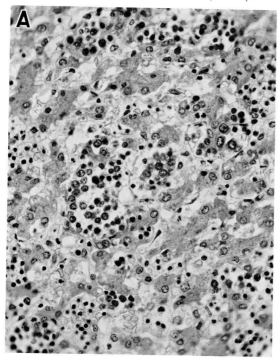
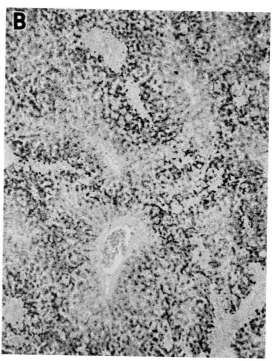

handle the circulating iron-containing substances that result from hemoglobin breakdown. Large amounts of hemosiderin are visible with ordinary stains as brown pigment in hepatic and endothelial cells. Erythropoiesis in such instances is usually overwhelming. When the infant is born alive, changes are rarely as severe except among hydropic infants who ordinarily die very soon after birth (Fig. 20–24, B).

In the days before exchange transfusions were made, many infants died a few days after birth, most often with kernicterus and pulmonary hemorrhage, and in most of these the liver showed stagnation of bile and deposits of hemosiderin. This was due not only to excessive blood destruction but to inability of the liver to excrete bile. Direct- as well as indirect-reacting serum bilirubin was high and the stools were often acholic. This was known as the inspissated bile syndrome because of the belief that the bile becomes so thick that it cannot pass normally through bile ducts.

Such a picture is almost never seen today in adequately treated infants, and even earlier some infants with this clinical appearance survived. Whether or not they have persisting liver damage has been the subject of disagreement. Harris and her co-workers reported that in some infants with erythroblastosis multinucleated giant cells were present that were indistinguishable from those in giant cell "hepatitis." Craig reported cirrhosis in two of 141 infants with erythroblastosis. One infant was observed who died at 14 months of age with advanced cirrhosis (Fig. 20–25) and had had many transfusions (not exchanges) for erythroblastosis (Potter). Whether this was a sequel of the erythroblastosis or a result of serum hepatitis contracted

Fig. 20–25.—Liver from infant with erythroblastosis who was jaundiced throughout life. Death at age 14 months. **A,** external surface showing severe atrophy. **B,** photomicrograph showing extreme fibrosis. (Courtesy Dr. Anadil Cavalcanti.)

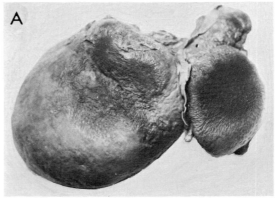

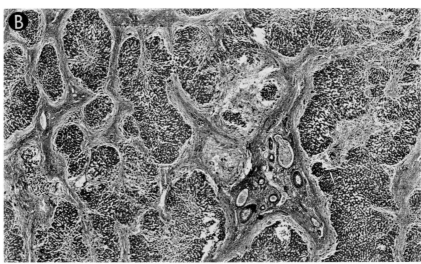

from one of the many transfusions it is impossible to say.

Trauma

The liver is the principal abdominal organ subject to injury. If the upper abdomen is grasped too firmly during delivery, the surface of the liver may be traumatized. The capsule usually remains intact and blood escaping from the injured sinusoids collects beneath it, at times raising it 1 cm or more above the surface. The usual history is of breech delivery with difficulty in extraction of the head. The infant often appears normal at birth and remains so for 2 or 3 days. Then, while it is being bathed or otherwise handled, it suddenly goes into shock and may die within a few minutes. The sudden onset of symptoms is associated with rupture of the delicate capsule enclosing the hematoma. Release of pressure permits fresh hemorrhage and the infant becomes exsanguinated by loss of blood into the abdominal cavity. One infant observed at the Chicago Lying-in Hospital lived several hours after the capsule ruptured. Soon after the rupture the hemoglobin value fell abruptly from loss of blood into the abdomen, and if a correct diagnosis had been made, operation might have saved the child's life.

By far the most frequent site of the hematoma is the anterior surface of the right lobe. It reaches to the liver margin inferiorly, and the upper extent is determined by the volume of extravasated blood. Hemorrhage rarely extends into the liver substance (see Fig. 8–16).

Subcapsular hematomas of the liver are less common since methods of resuscitating apneic infants have become more rational. Vigorous handling of infants, especially such procedures as jack-knifing in an attempt to inflate and deflate the lungs, has probably cost the lives of far more infants than it has saved.

Malformations

Absence of the liver is incompatible with survival and has rarely been observed except in acardiac twins. Abnormalities of position are ordinarily secondary to malformations of other structures except in situs inversus, in which the shape and position of the liver are reversed right to left. Fluid or air in the right pleural cavity or reduction of thoracic volume such as often occurs in chondrodystrophy or anencephalus may displace the liver downward, giving a false impression of hepatomegaly. Absence

of the anterior abdominal wall permits extrusion outside the body cavity.

Abnormal lobulation is variable and ordinarily has no functional significance. With large diaphragmatic defects in which much of the abdominal mass lies within the thoracic cavity, part of the liver is ordinarily also carried upward, and a deep depression is usually produced by pressure against the edge of the diaphragm. Such partially detached portions of liver often have an increase in connective tissue that simulates cirrhosis and is presumably caused by interference with circulation.

CYSTIC DISEASE OF THE LIVER. – The coexistence of multiple cysts in kidneys and liver is well recognized in infants as well as adults, as is also the occurrence of one without the other. All infants with type I cystic kidneys and one third of those with type III have abnormalities of the liver, but the liver seldom contains cysts in the absence of cystic changes in the kidneys.

Several kinds of polycystic kidneys can be distinguished but in only one are liver changes invariably present. This is the variety designated type I (see Chapter 22), in which fundamental structure is normal but increase in length and diameter of all collecting tubules produces giant, symmetrically enlarged kidneys. The livers of these infants are not grossly altered but all have striking microscopic changes. Bile ducts lined by well-differentiated cuboidal cells make up a proportionately much greater part of the liver than normal. Connective tissue is not appreciably increased but the blood vessels and lymphatics in portal areas are unusually prominent. The bile ducts are greatly increased in length and tortuosity, are often dilated and frequently have blunt papillary projections extending into the lumens. Although most concentrated in portal areas and at the periphery of lobules, they generally extend at random throughout the liver in direct contact with parenchymal cells (Fig. 20–26). At times small clusters of ducts suggest an independent origin rather than an outgrowth from existing ducts.

The livers of infants with other varieties of cystic kidneys are variable. The majority are normal, although a few that seem normal when stained with hematoxylin-eosin show a slight increase in connective tissue radiating outward from portal areas on differential staining for collagen. Type II seldom has distinguishable changes of any kind, but in about two thirds of type III cases there is marked periportal proliferation of connective tissue, and in about half of these the number of bile ducts is increased. Bile ducts generally consist of multiple

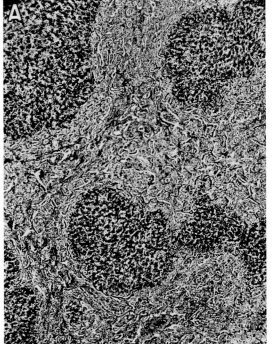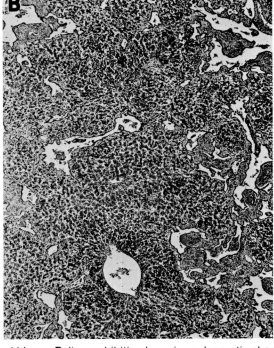

Fig. 20–26.—Cystic disease of the liver. **A,** liver exhibiting wide bands of connective tissue in which there are innumerable tubular structures resembling bile ducts. Newborn infant with atresia of larynx and type III cystic kidneys. **B,** liver exhibiting large irregular cystic channels and only slight increase in connective tissue. This appearance is found only in association with type I cystic kidneys. Same case as in Fig. 22–21.

short tubules with small undilated lumens. The increase in connective tissue often far outshadows the proliferation of bile ducts (Fig. 20–26).

In the absence of other abnormality of the liver

Fig. 20–27.—Liver with increase in size and number of bile ducts at periphery of portal areas and between lobules. Portal connective tissue also increased. Newborn infant with normal kidneys.

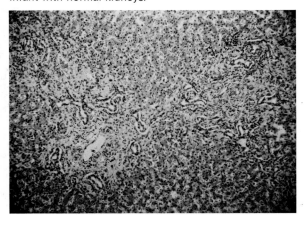

or kidneys proliferation of bile ducts with or without increase in connective tissue is extremely rare in infants. It has been observed at the Chicago Lying-in Hospital on only two occasions and then the proliferation of ducts and connective tissue was mild and ducts were undilated (Fig. 20–27).

CONGENITAL HEPATIC FIBROSIS.—In this rare condition portal areas and the periphery of lobules are altered by what appears to be loss of parenchymal cells and replacement by loose connective tissue mildly infiltrated by histiocytes and other mononuclear cells but without increase in bile ducts.

Neoplasms

Tumors of the liver are more common in the first 2 years of life than at any other time in childhood. The first symptom is usually an abdominal mass, and the diffuse enlargement that may occur in liver disease often cannot be distinguished by palpation from that found with neoplasia; nor can a tumor of the liver be differentiated by palpation from a Wilms' tumor or a neuroblastoma.

The most common tumors in the newborn are hemangioendotheliomas, cavernous hemangiomas and solitary cysts; after 2 years of age they are carcinomas, mesenchymomas and solitary cysts. Solitary cysts and hemangioendotheliomas are said to be more common in girls and carcinomas in boys. Between the newborn period and age 2 years a tumor that is large enough to cause abdominal distention and be visible on x-ray is most likely to be a solitary cyst, mesenchymal hamartoma, mixed tumor or teratoma. Tumors that may contain calcium visible in roentgenograms include liver cell carcinomas, cavernous hemangiomas, adrenal rest tumors, mixed tumors and occasionally solitary cysts.

Pedicles are usually limited to benign tumors such as focal nodular hyperplasia, solitary cysts and mesenchymal hamartomas. Focal nodular hyperplasia, which is benign, is firm, cirrhotic and nodular, in contrast to the soft friable character of carcinomas and the fleshy appearance of sarcomas. Any cystic tumor is usually benign.

The following review has been modified from the excellent survey by Edmondson.

Benign Tumors

Tumorlike epithelial lesions. — The lesion of nodular hyperplasia (hamartoma, isolated solitary nodular hyperplasia) is generally gray to gray-brown, solitary and sharply demarcated. It may be deep in the liver, superficial or pedunculated. The center is often occupied by a stellate mass of connective tissue that becomes less conspicuous toward the periphery and contains many small bile ducts and lymphocytes that give it the appearance of cirrhosis. Near the periphery circumscribed groups of hyperplastic cells surround central areas of connective tissue, bile ducts and blood vessels, producing a microscopic appearance helpful in distinguishing this lesion even on biopsy.

Resection should be considered only for those that are superficial or pedunculated. They must be distinguished from multiple areas of nodular hyperplasia secondary to acute necrosis of the liver and from accessory lobes.

Epithelial tumors. — Adenomas are rare in infancy and should be diagnosed only after examination of several microscopic sections. They are encapsulated, are usually in the right lobe and consist of tissue resembling normal liver cells but lacking bile ducts and portal tracts. They can easily be confused with low-grade liver cell carcinomas.

Adrenal rest tumors usually located on the lower surface of the liver beneath the capsule have been described but are also rare.

Cysts and tumorlike mesenchymal lesions. — Mesenchymal hamartomas (cavernous lymphangiomatoid lesion, hamartoma, lymphangioma, solitary bile cell fibroadenoma) are not true neoplasms. They consist chiefly of extremely edematous, relatively acellular collagenous connective tissue and fluid-filled spaces lacking lining cells. A few liver cells, either as solid cords or as larger masses with bile ducts but without Kupffer cells, are generally present, and occasionally angiomatous and hematopoietic foci are associated with masses of primitive mesenchyme. They are poorly demarcated from the surrounding normal liver since the connective tissue of the hamartoma merges with that of the portal triads (Fig. 20–28). These tumors usually present as symptomless masses in the upper abdomen, usually located near the lower margin of the liver. They often increase rapidly in size because of accumulation of fluid.

Tumors of supporting structures. — These include fibromas, hemangiomas, hemangioendotheliomas and lymphangiomas. The fibromas and hemangiomas are usually microscopic and incidental. The *nodular hemangioendotheliomas* are often multiple and are responsible for hepatomegaly (Dehner

Fig. 20–28. — Mesenchymal hamartoma of liver showing poorly circumscribed areas of mesenchymal tissue that replaced much of the liver parenchyma in a large portion of the right lobe.

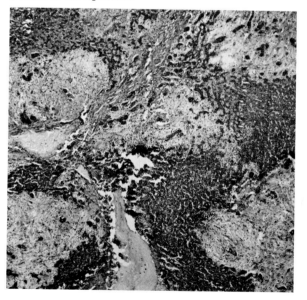

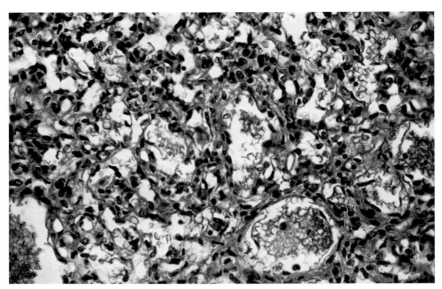

Fig. 20—29.—Hemangioendothelioma of the liver composed of numerous spaces filled with blood separated by intervening solid masses of endothelial cells.

and Ishak). They may present with jaundice or cardiac failure and may cause pulsation in the liver. Grossly, they form irregular nodules on the liver surface and in the parenchyma; they have the same structure as hemangioendotheliomas elsewhere (Fig. 20—29). Aicardi and Nezelof reported that most will regress spontaneously by 6 months of age if the symptoms of cardiac failure can be controlled. In the series of Dehner and Ishak one third of the cases occurred in premature infants and the lesion may have been the cause of premature birth.

The fluid-filled cystic spaces seen in hamartomatous connective tissue tumors of the liver are often regarded as lymph spaces and the tumors designated lymphangiomas. Edmondson, however, found no cells lining these spaces and did not believe that they should be considered lymphatics. Clatworthy *et al.* described two lymphangiomas in the 1st year of life.

TERATOMAS.—These are extremely rare in the liver but, like teratomas in other locations, are composed of elements derived from all three germ layers and contain epithelium, nerve cells and other tissues foreign to the liver.

MALIGNANT TUMORS

HEPATOBLASTOMAS (MIXED TUMORS).—These make up the majority of malignant tumors found in early infancy. Ishak and Glienz, in a report of 35 malig-

nant tumors of the liver in infants and children, found 25 to be hepatoblastomas, and 21 of these were in infants in the 1st year of life. One was in a premature infant born at 34 weeks' gestation. The tumor appears in males 2.5 times as frequently as in females. It presents with an abdominal mass, fever, failure to thrive and pallor and is firm, smooth and usually nontender. Ishak and Glienz divided the hepatoblastomas into epithelial and mixed types. The epithelial form, which they found in 16 cases, is believed to be derived from entoderm

Fig. 20—30.—Hepatoblastoma of the mixed type, with primitive liver cells, fibroblastic tissue and an area of osteoid.

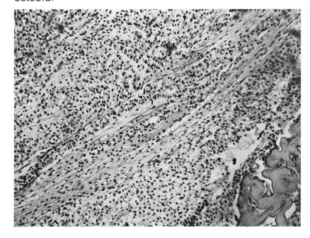

and consists of small cells, some of which are arranged in columns having many aspects of liver cells while others resemble immature bile ducts. Six of these 16 tumors had smaller, more embryonal cells that had few of the tinctorial properties of liver cells (granular cytoplasm, glycogen). The mixed type (19 cases) had the same epithelial components plus primitive mesenchymal derivatives such as connective tissue, osteoid and blood vessels (Fig. 20–30). In four of the cases of this type squamous cells were also present. All hepatoblastomas tend to have vascular metastases (Fig. 20–31). Some produce gonadotropin responsible for virilization.

MESENCHYMOMAS.—These tumors are generally composed of a variety of mesodermal derivatives including an intermixture of fibrous, angiomatous and undifferentiated mesenchymal cells. They are fleshy masses beneath the capsule of either lobe of the liver and may attain a considerable size. In Andersen's series from Babies Hospital at the Columbia Medical Center all were malignant but some have been reported with no recurrence following resection.

SARCOMAS.—These are usually of an undifferentiated spindle cell—mesenchymal variety that is

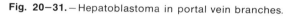

Fig. 20–31.—Hepatoblastoma in portal vein branches.

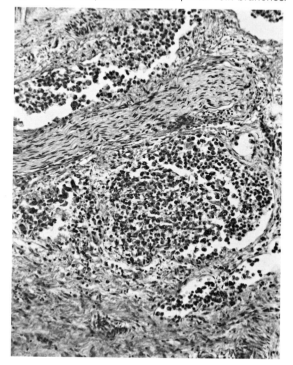

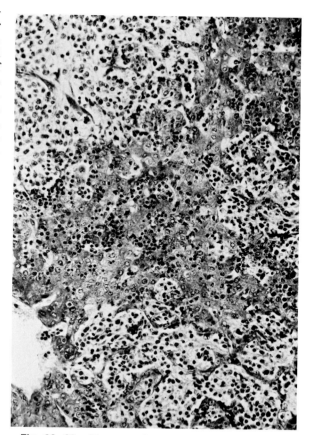

Fig. 20–32.—Masses of sympathicoblasts diffusely disseminated throughout the liver. The small dark cells are erythropoietic foci. The pale-staining cells with round central nuclei make up the tumor masses. Gross appearance shown in Fig. 12–46.

difficult to subdivide. In Andersen's material they were more frequent than carcinomas.

METASTATIC TUMORS.—Metastatic tumors of the liver in infants and children have about the same frequency as primary tumors and, like them, are most common before the age of 2 years. The majority are secondary to neuroblastomas (Fig. 20–32) or Wilms' tumors. The fact that they are more diffusely distributed through the liver and rarely cause local enlargement may be of help in differential diagnosis.

Gallbladder

The gallbladder is rarely abnormal at birth except in association with atresia of the extrahepatic bile ducts. It may vary slightly in position, at times being deeply embedded in the liver substance with the lower end several millimeters from the liver margin; at other times it may protrude beyond the lower edge of the liver. Its size is mildly variable and, although ordinarily containing only a small amount of bile, it is occasionally considerably distended. The color of bile varies from that of honey to dark amber.

If the cystic duct or the common bile duct is atretic, the gallbladder is ordinarily underdeveloped or is a small slender structure containing only a small amount of mucus and no bile. Rarely, stenosis or atresia of the common duct produces a choledochal cyst. Fonkalsrud and Boles reported four choledochal cysts in infants under 12 weeks of age. These infants were jaundiced, with acholic stools but without palpable abdominal masses. Such cysts have a lining of biliary epithelium and have smooth muscle in the wall. A palpable mass was present in 76% of cases in older children described by Horne. Complete absence of the gallbladder has been reported in association with absence of the bile ducts and also in some instances in which the remainder of the biliary system was normal.

Rhabdomyosarcoma of the bile ducts has been observed in older children but not in the very young (Hays and Snyder). One was seen at the Boston Hospital for Women with dilatation of the common duct and numerous small excrescences of tumor protruding into the lumen. These tumors have the usual mixture of primitive muscle and connective tissue.

REFERENCES

Aagenaes, Ø., Van den Hagen, C. B., and Refsum, S.: Hereditary recurrent intrahepatic cholestasis from birth, Arch. Dis. Child. 43:646, 1968.

Ahrens, E. H., Jr., Harris, R. C., and MacMahon, H. E.: Atresia of the intrahepatic bile ducts, Pediatrics 8:628, 1951.

Aicardi, J., and Nezelof, C.: Multinodular hemangiomatosis of the liver in infants: Anatomico-clinical comments with respect to four cases, Arch. Fr. Pediatr. 20:933, 1963.

Allen, F. H., Jr., and Diamond, L. K.: *Erythroblastosis Fetalis* (Boston: Little, Brown and Co., 1957).

Alpert, L. I., Strauss, L., and Hirschhorn, K.: Neonatal hepatitis and biliary atresia associated with trisomy, N. Engl. J. Med. 280:16, 1969.

Andersen, D. H.: Tumors of infancy and childhood, Cancer 4:890, 1951.

Becroft, D. M. O.: Syndrome of encephalopathy and fatty degeneration of viscera in New Zealand children, Br. Med. J. 2:135, 1966.

Benirschke, K.: Personal Communication.

Brent, R. L.: Persistent jaundice in infancy, J. Pediatr. 61:111, 1962.

Brock, J. F., and Autrel, M.: *Kwashiorkor in Africa* (Geneva: World Health Organization, 1952), p. 22.

Brooks, S. E. H., Miller, C. G., McKenzie, K., Audretsch, J. J., and Bras, G.: Acute veno-occlusive disease of the liver, Arch. Pathol. 89:507, 1970.

Brough, A. J., and Bernstein, J.: Liver biopsy in diagnosis of infantile obstructive jaundice, Pediatrics 43:519, 1969.

Brown, A. K., and Zuelzer, W. W.: Studies in hyperbilirubinemia. I. Hyperbilirubinemia of newborn unrelated to isoimmunization, Am. J. Dis. Child. 93:263, 1957.

Cassady, G., Morrison, A. B., and Chen, M. M.: Familial "giant cell hepatitis" in infancy, Am. J. Dis. Child. 107:456, 1964.

Clatworthy, H. W., Jr., Bales, E. T., Jr., and Newton, W. A.: Primary tumors of the liver in infants and children, Arch. Dis. Child. 35:22, 1960.

Clayton, R. J., *et al.*: Byler disease: Fatal familial intrahepatic cholestasis in an Amish kindred, Am. J. Dis. Child. 117:112, 1969.

Coen, R., and MacAdams, A. J.: Visceral manifestations of shock in congenital heart disease, Am. J. Dis. Child. 19:383, 1970.

Craig, J. M.: Sequences in the development of cirrhosis of the liver in cases of erythroblastosis fetalis, Arch. Pathol. 49:665, 1950.

Craig, J. M., Gellis, S. S., and Hsia, D. Y.: Cirrhosis of liver in infants and children, Am. J. Dis. Child. 90:299, 1955.

Craig, J. M., Haddad, H., and Schwachman, H.: The pathology of the liver in cystic fibrosis of the pancreas, Am. J. Dis. Child. 93:357, 1957.

Craig, J. M., and Landing, B. H.: Form of hepatitis in the neonatal period simulating biliary atresia, Arch. Pathol. 54:321, 1952.

Crigler, J. F., and Najjar, V. A.: Congenital familial nonhemolytic jaundice with kernicterus, Pediatrics 10:169, 1952.

Danks, D., and Bodian, M.: A genetic study of neonatal obstructive jaundice, Arch. Dis. Child. 38:378, 1963.

Danks, D. M., and Campbell, P. E.: Extrahepatic atresia: Comments on frequency of patently operable cases, J. Pediatr. 61:21, 1966.

Dehner, L. P., and Ishak, K. G.: Vascular tumors in infants and children, Arch. Pathol. 92:101, 1971.

Di Sant'Agnese, P. A., and Blanc, W. A.: Distinctive type of biliary cirrhosis of the liver associated with cystic fibrosis of the pancreas. Recognition through signs of portal hypertension, Pediatrics 18:387, 1956.

Dorkin, J. R., and Weinberg, T.: Normal occurrence of histologically demonstrable fat in liver of newborn infant, Arch. Pathol. 48:578, 1949.

Dubin, I. N.: Chronic idiopathic jaundice, Am. J. Med. 24:268, 1958.

Edmondson, H. A.: Differential diagnosis of tumors and tumorlike lesions of the liver in infancy and childhood, Am. J. Dis. Child. 91:168, 1956.

Elias, R. L.: Re-examination of structure of main mammalian liver, Am. J. Anat. 84:311, 1949.

Emery, J. L.: Asymmetrical liver disease in infancy, J. Pathol. Bacteriol. 69:219, 1955.

Emery, J. L.: The functional symmetry of the liver, Ann. N. Y. Acad. Sci. 111:37, 1963.

Enders, J. F. (ed.): Seminar on viral hepatitis, Am. J. Dis. Child. 123:275, 1972.

Farber, S., and Craig, J. M.: Clinical pathological conference: Chronic idiopathic jaundice, J. Pediatr. 49:91, 1956.

Favera, B. E., Franciosi, R. A., and Silverman, A.: Serum alpha-1 antitrypsin deficiency and infantile liver disease, Pediatr. Res. 6:378, 1972.

Fonkalsrud, E. W., and Boles, E. T., Jr.: Choledochal cysts in infancy and childhood, Surg. Obstet. Gynecol. 121:733, 1965.

Gall, E. A., and Landing, B. H.: Hepatic cirrhosis and hereditary disorders of metabolism, Am. J. Clin. Pathol. 26:1398, 1956.

Gellis, S. S., Craig, J. M., and Hsia, D. Y.: Prolonged obstructive jaundice in infancy, Am. J. Dis. Child. 88:285, 1954.

Gross, R. E.: *Surgery of Infancy and Childhood* (Philadelphia: W. B. Saunders Co., 1963).

Gruenwald, P.: Degenerative changes in the right half of the liver resulting from intrauterine anoxia, Am. J. Clin. Pathol. 19:801, 1949.

Harris, R. C., Andersen, D. H., and Day, R. L.: Obstructive jaundice in infants with normal biliary tree, Pediatrics 13:293, 1954.

Hays, D. M., *et al.*: Diagnosis of biliary atresia. Relative accuracy of percutaneous liver biopsy, open liver biopsy and operative cholangiography, J. Pediatr. 77:598, 1967.

Hays, D. M., and Snyder, W. H., Jr.: Botryoid sarcoma (rhabdomyosarcoma) of bile ducts, Am. J. Dis. Child. 110:595, 1965.

Hays, D. M., and Snyder, W. H., Jr.: Life span in untreated biliary atresia, Surgery 54:373, 1963.

Horne, L. M.: Congenital choledochal cysts: Report of three cases and discussion of etiology, J. Pediatr. 50:30, 1957.

Hsia, D. Y.: *Human Developmental Genetics* (Chicago: Year Book Medical Publishers, 1968).

Hsia, D. Y., *et al.*: Prolonged obstructive jaundice in infancy, Pediatrics 10:243, 1952.

Hsia, D. Y., and Gellis, S. S.: Portal hypertension in infants and children, Am. J. Dis. Child. 90:290, 1955.

Huttenlocher, P. R., Schwartz, A. D., and Klatskin, G.: Reye's syndrome—ammonia intoxication as a possible factor in encephalopathy, Pediatrics 43:443, 1969.

Ishak, K. G., and Glienz, P. R.: Hepatoblastoma and hepatocarcinoma in infancy and childhood, Cancer 20:396, 1967.

Jelliffe, D. B., Bras, G., and Mukerjee, K. L.: Veno-occlusive disease of liver and Indian childhood cirrhosis, Arch. Dis. Child. 32:369, 1957.

Kasai, M., and Watanabe, I.: Histologic classification of liver cell carcinoma in infancy and childhood and its clinical evaluation. A study of 70 cases collected in Japan, Cancer 25:551, 1970.

Landing, B. H.: Lesions of the liver in hereditary metabolic disease, Ann. N. Y. Acad. Sci. 111:399, 1963.

Lelong, M., Lepage, F., Alison, F., and Tan-Vinh, L.: Toxoplasme du nouveau-né avec ictère et cirrhose du foie, Arch. Fr. Pediatr. 10:173, 1953.

Levick, C. B., and Rubie, J.: Hemangioendothelioma of the liver simulating congenital heart disease in an infant, Arch. Dis. Child. 28:49, 1958.

Lightwood, R., and Bodian, M.: Biliary obstruction associated with icterus gravis neonatorum, Arch. Dis. Child. 21:209, 1946.

Lin, T. Y., Chen, C. C., and Liu, W. P.: Primary carcinoma of the liver in infancy and childhood, Surgery 60:1275, 1966.

Lynch, M. J., Glasgow, J. F., Hercz, A., Levinson, H., and Sass-Kortsak, A.: The pathology of alpha-1 antitrypsin deficiency in children: A study of 10 cases. Occurrence of both liver and lung disease in 2 siblings, Am. J. Pathol. 66:20a, 1972.

McClean, R. M., *et al.*: Multinodular hemangiomatosis of liver in infancy, Pediatrics 49:563, 1972.

Morrione, T. G., and Mamelok, H. L.: Observations on persistence of hepatic glycogen after death, Am. J. Pathol. 28:497, 1952.

Nakai, H., and Landing, B. H.: Factors in the genesis of bile stasis in infancy, Pediatrics 27:300, 1961.

Porter, C. A., Mowat, A. P., Cook, P. J. L., and Haynes, D. W. G.: Alpha-1 antitrypsin deficiency and neonatal hepatitis, Br. Med. J. 2:435, 1972.

Powell, L. W., *et al.*: Idiopathic unconjugated hyperbilirubinemia (Gilbert's syndrome), N. Engl. J. Med. 277:1108, 1967.

Reubner, B. H., *et al.*: Neonatal hepatic necrosis, Pediatrics 43:963, 1969.

Reubner, B. H., and Mujai, K.: The pathology of neonatal hepatitis and biliary atresia with particular respect to hemapoiesis and hemosiderin deposition, Ann. N. Y. Acad. Sci. 111:375, 1963.

Reye, R. D. K., and Morgan, G., and Boral, J.: Encephalopathy and fatty degeneration of the viscera, Lancet 2:749, 1963.

Schaffner, F., and Popper, H.: Morphologic studies in neonatal cholestasis with emphasis on giant cells, Ann. N. Y. Acad. Sci. 111:358, 1963.

Schweitzer, I. L., Wing, A., McPeak, C., and Spears, R. L.: Hepatitis and hepatitis-associated antigen in 56 mother-infant pairs, J.A.M.A. 220:1092, 1972.

Sherlock, S.: *Diseases of the Liver and Biliary System* (London: Blackwell Scientific Publications, 1968).

Shiraki, K.: Hepatic cell necrosis in the newborn, Am. J. Dis. Child. 119:395, 1960.

Silverberg, M., and Gellis, S. S.: Problems in diagnosis of biliary atresia, Am. J. Dis. Child. 99:574, 1960.

Smetana, H., Edlow, J. B., and Glienz, P. R.: Neonatal jaundice, Arch. Pathol. 80:553, 1960.

Smetana, H. F., Hadley, G., and Sirsat, S. M.: Infantile cirrhosis. An analytic review of the literature and report of 50 cases, Pediatrics 28:107, 1961.

Stowens, D.: *Pediatric Pathology* (Baltimore: Williams & Wilkins Co., 1959).

Stowens, D.: Congenital biliary atresia, Am. J. Gastroenterol. 32:577, 1959.

Strauss, L., and Bernstein, J.: Neonatal hepatitis in the congenital rubella syndrome, Arch. Pathol. 86:317, 1968.

Thaler, M. M.: Fatal neonatal cirrhosis, entity or end result? Comparative study of 24 cases, Pediatrics 33:721, 1964.

Vest, M. F., Kaufmann, H. J., and Fritz, E.: Chronic nonhemolytic jaundice with conjugated bilirubin in the serum and normal liver histology: A case study, Arch. Dis. Child. 35:600, 1960.

Voorhees, A. B., Jr., *et al.*: Portal hypertension in children, Surgery 58:540, 1964.

Weinberg, A. G., and Bolande, R. G.: The liver in congenital heart disease, Am. J. Dis. Child. 119:390, 1970.

Weller, T. W., and Hanshaw, J. B.: Virologic and clinical observations on cytomegalic inclusion disease, N. Engl. J. Med. 266:1233, 1962.

Wolfrom, I.: Rupture of the liver in the newborn, Arch. Dis. Child. 34:302, 1959.

Zuelzer, W. W., and Brown, A. K.: Neonatal jaundice, Am. J. Dis. Child. 101:87, 1961.

21

Spleen

THE SPLEEN appears first in the 10 mm embryo as a condensation of mesenchymal cells in the dorsal mesogastrium near the dorsal pancreatic bud. It grows slowly and until miduterine life seems disproportionately small in relation to other abdominal organs. During the early months it is closely associated with the stomach wall, lying on the lateral surface of the cardiac portion. As growth proceeds, the posterior part of the dorsal mesogastrium attaches the spleen to the left kidney as the lienorenal ligament, and the anterior portion attaches it to the stomach as the gastrosplenic ligament. The dorsal pancreas grows to come in contact with the spleen, and the splenic branch of the celiac artery extends through the pancreas to supply the spleen with blood. During the first 2 trimesters of intrauterine life the spleen is made up chiefly of connective tissue and reticulum cells. There are few lymphocytes, and the later perivascular concentrations of lymphoid cells are not present. It seems probable that some time after the 20th week there is an inward migration of lymphocytes from the thymus and intestinal centers, the former having to do with cellular and the latter with humoral antibody formation. The spleen lags far behind the liver in the inception of erythropoiesis. As late as 24 weeks of gestation, even in the presence of severe erythroblastosis fetalis, erythroid cells are not increased in number. By the time of birth the appearance of the spleen is fairly similar to that of the adult spleen except that less connective tissue is present. The details of structure are not completely known, and whether the arteries and veins communicate through a system of sinusoids or whether there is discontinuity, with blood flowing through open intermediate spaces not lined by endothelium, has not been settled.

The white pulp of the spleen consists of lymphoid cells arranged in a sheathlike manner around all but the major divisions of the splenic artery. In localized areas, especially near the points at which the vessels branch, the cells are in larger masses known as malpighian corpuscles. Germinal centers are not present in the corpuscles of the fetus or newborn. The small lymphocytes in the newborn spleen undergo destruction as a result of the release of excessive adrenal cortical hormone, just as do the small lymphocytes in the lymph nodes and thymus. However, acute reaction centers in the primary follicles, consisting of areas of cellular necrosis with a marked karyolytic reaction but without polymorphonuclear reaction, are rarely seen. Such reactions, followed by a proliferation of lymphocytes and plasma cells, are common in later life and may occur before the end of the 1st year. Granulomatous centers in the follicles that are indicative of the stage of antigen-antibody equivalence in which serum levels of circulating antigen and antibody neutralize each other may be found for the first time late in the 1st year. The absence of both of these features may be related to the inability of the newborn to make gamma globulin at a normal rate.

The red pulp makes up the major portion of the spleen and is composed of endothelium-lined sinusoids that are often much more prominent at birth than in later life. Between the sinusoids is a fine meshwork of reticulum cells containing many erythrocytes.

The average weight of the spleen at birth is 11 gm. Most clinicians find it impossible to palpate the spleen in the majority of normal infants, but Akerren reported being able to make out the lower pole in 32% of 1,062 infants at birth and in 45% on the

3d day. He thought that there was often a physiologic increase in size in the first few days of life that made it possible to palpate the rounded lower pole under the costal margin.

Abnormalities of the spleen, in comparison with other organs, are rare in intrauterine life as well as in the first few months after birth. Syphilis and erythroblastosis both cause outstanding changes, but other diseases seldom affect the spleen at this time.

Malformations

Agenesis is rare as an isolated malformation in an otherwise normal individual, more often being part of a diffuse involvement of thoracic or abdominal viscera. According to Ivemark, it is especially associated with septation defects in the heart and great vessels and with situs inversus of the heart and lungs. An interventricular septal defect is found in virtually all such cases and, in the majority, is associated with an intra-atrial defect. About one sixth of the cases have a persistent ductus arteriosus and those not so affected almost always have transposition of the great vessels. Over one third of the cases of asplenia have cardiac situs inversus, usually associated with anomalies of lung lobation and of pulmonary and systemic venous return to the heart. Over one half of those with transposition of the great vessels also have pulmonary stenosis or atresia and a patent ductus arteriosus. Since venous return to the heart is frequently abnormal, the transposition is often "corrected," in that venous blood from the "aorta" goes to the lungs and oxygenated blood from the "pulmonary artery" goes to the peripheral vessels. Gilbert et al. believed that such anomalies are a result of changes occurring in embryonic life when the heart, omentum and major mesenteries are being formed. They also found that absence of the spleen was often associated with partial situs inversus of the thoracic viscera and abnormal septation of the heart. In some similar cases, instead of being absent, the spleen is composed of several small nodules (Ivemark).

The problem of sepsis in young patients with a congenitally absent spleen or following splenectomy has been disturbing. One of the largest series in which cases were followed carefully is that of Eraklis et al. who followed 417 infants and children in whom splenectomy was performed for periods of 3–10 years. Twenty-five deaths occurred, a frequency of 5.4%. The incidence of infection varied with the indications for the splenectomy; no deaths followed removal for trauma or thrombocytopenic purpura.

Thalassemia, cirrhosis and dysgammaglobulinemia were the indications for removal in nearly two thirds of the patients who died, and the storage diseases for the remaining one third. Overwhelming sepsis with or without meningitis accounted for 60% of the deaths and severe pneumonia for the remainder. Most of the deaths took place in the first 2 years of life. Since all other immunologic functions are normal, the lack of protection against overwhelming sepsis appears to lie in the absence of fixed macrophages of the spleen with their phagocytic blood-clearing ability. Because the phagocytic function of the spleen includes removal of degenerated hemoglobin and nuclear fragments, individuals without a spleen have remnants of altered hemoglobin (Heinz bodies) and nuclear debris (Howell-Jolly bodies) in their red blood cells (Polhemus and Schafer).

A rapid rise in the number of organisms in the bloodstream of asplenic individuals almost invariably causes death. Murphy and Mitchell described one case in which congenital absence of the spleen was the only malformation. Death occurred from the Waterhouse-Friderichsen syndrome at 15 months as a result of severe pneumococcal infection.

The position of the spleen is altered in any condition that disturbs the relationships of the viscera in the abdomen. With a diaphragmatic hernia or omphalocele the spleen is often in the thoracic cavity or outside the body, and in situs inversus it is found on the right side of the abdomen.

The shape may be altered by pressure or by intrinsic changes. The most common variation consists of numerous indentations giving a scalloped anterior margin. Accessory nodules of splenic tissue are often found around the hilus of the spleen or lower in the abdomen. Rarely, the spleen is composed of several small round masses of approximately equal size. Portions of the splenic tissue are occasionally incorporated into the tail of the pancreas.

Infarction

Infarcts of the spleen are rare and, when present in newborn infants, a cause can rarely be discovered. They are conical white areas with a base at the capsular surface and are similar in structure to those found in older individuals. Evidence of infection is rarely demonstrable and the areas of vascular obstruction responsible for cutting off the blood supply can seldom be identified. The normal spleen lies well protected by the lower part of the thoracic cage and is seldom traumatized. Gruenwald, reporting an infant with a laceration of both liver and spleen, suggested that compression of the chest during breech delivery might have caused abnormal descensus of these organs, permitting the spleen to be traumatized. He also thought that it might have been injured by too vigorous attempts at resuscitation.

Injury is somewhat less rare if the spleen is so enlarged as to extend well below the costal margin and is therefore more fragile and susceptible to injury. Rupture has been reported most often in infants with erythroblastosis. Three cases of avulsion of an enlarged spleen associated with erythroblastosis have been observed at the Boston Lying-in and Children's Hospital Medical Center. These were thought to have been the result of birth trauma, and death was due to massive abdominal hemorrhage.

When the spleen is lacerated, hemorrhage is usually profuse, and, as with lacerations of the liver, death occurs from massive intraperitoneal hemorrhage. Operative repair is difficult because of the fragility of the capsule and the friability of the parenchyma, and splenectomy is usually the preferred procedure.

With internal tears of the spleen, organization of the resulting hematoma may give rise to zones of highly vascular fibrous tissue; some cases of fibroangioma such as those reported by Grove may be examples of this; similar lesions have also been called splenomas.

In a few recorded cases rupture of the spleen in early life has led to multiple implantations of the splenic pulp on the peritoneal surfaces, forming small tumorlike masses.

Infection

NONSPECIFIC INFECTION. — Enlargement of the spleen may occur with any infectious process in the newborn but is especially common with septicemia. Often there is no direct microscopic evidence of local infection and the enlargement is caused by an increase in volume of blood. Multiple abscesses are sometimes present with known septicemia, and rarely they are found when no other evidence of infection can be demonstrated. They may be discovered only on microscopic examination, or they may be visible through the capsule or on the cut surface as multiple small white areas. In a newborn spleen grossly similar to that in Fig. 21–1 we have found massive infiltration of polymorphonuclear cells in the cords of Billroth (Craig); these were not true abscesses for complete necrosis was lacking. Both *Staphylococcus aureus* and *Escherichia coli* have been cultured from such spleens.

In a severe infection such as pneumonia, particularly with bacteremia, the spleen of the newborn, like that of the adult, usually has a marked increase in polymorphonuclear leukocytes in the red pulp. Occasionally the capsule and trabeculae are invaded by the same cells.

SYPHILIS. — The spleen of an infant in whom syphilis has caused prenatal pathologic changes is always enlarged (Fig. 21–2). If clinical evidence of the disease is lacking, even though the infant is subsequently proved to be affected, the spleen is

Fig. 21–1 (left). — Multiple abscesses in spleen of infant aged 5 days. Infant was thought clinically to have erythroblastosis because of splenomegaly and increase in circulating nucleated red blood cells in spite of having an Rh-positive mother. Moderate erythropoiesis was seen in many organs at autopsy, although no evidence of infection could be found except in the spleen. The mother subsequently had two normal infants.

Fig. 21–2 (right). — Syphilic enlargement of the liver and spleen. Gross appearance of these organs is identical to that found in erythroblastosis. Fetus stillborn at term.

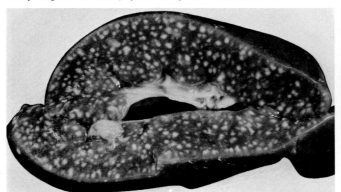
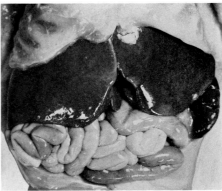

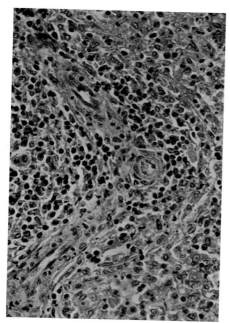

Fig. 21–3.—Syphilis. Spleen in which malpighian follicles are depleted of lymphocytes and partially replaced by polymorphonuclear and mononuclear cells.

usually of normal size. The white pulp is ordinarily not affected although occasionally malpighian corpuscles are partially depleted of lymphocytes (Fig. 21–3). The principal change consists of an increase in the amount of circulating blood and in the width of intersinusoidal spaces from proliferation of connective tissue and presence of numerous macrophages.

HISTOPLASMOSIS.—In young infants with fatal systemic infection with the yeast organism *Histoplasma capsulatum* the reticuloendothelial cells in the spleen as well as those in other parts of the body (lungs, lymph nodes, liver and bone marrow) are filled with unicellular organisms (see Fig. 9–24).

Erythroblastosis

The spleen is always enlarged in infants with erythroblastosis. The degree varies with the severity of the disease and the age of the infant. When symptoms are mild at birth the spleen may not be palpable, but when they are severe it often extends several centimeters below the costal margin and may reach the iliac crest (Fig. 21–4). When other symptoms of the disease abate, the size of the spleen decreases. The average weight in severe

erythroblastosis is 35–50 gm, but it may weigh up to 80 gm.

The characteristic microscopic changes consist of reduction in the volume of the white pulp and distention of the splenic sinusoids. In severe forms of the disease the white pulp is greatly reduced and only a few lymphocytes can be found around the arteries, or so few are present that the arteries lie naked in the red pulp (Fig. 21–5). This is part of the general lymphoid hypoplasia that is characteristic of erythroblastosis.

The distention of the sinusoids coupled with the fact that they are usually empty gives a lacy, spongelike appearance to the pulp (Fig. 21–6). Sinusoids are lined by large endothelial cells, the nuclei of which bulge prominently into the lumens. Groups of immature red blood cells may be present both in sinuses (Fig. 21–6, B) and pulp in variable numbers depending on the severity of the disease and the ability of the fetus to respond with an increased rate of hematopoiesis. The immature red cells are usually much more numerous than at any

Fig. 21–4.—Massive enlargement of the spleen in stillborn fetus with erythroblastosis. The cardiac hypertrophy, ascites and edema of the anterior abdominal wall are also commonly seen in the hydropic form of erythroblastosis.

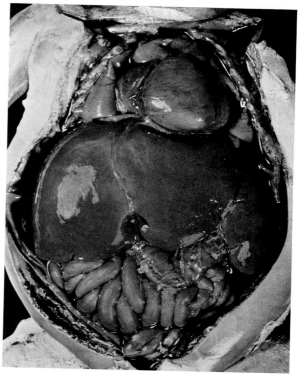

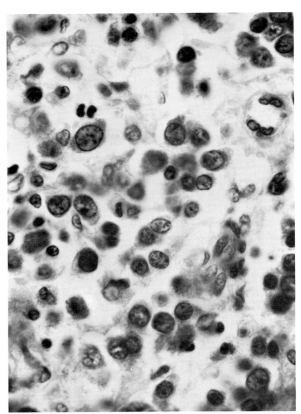

Fig. 21–5.—Spleen in erythroblastosis showing absence of lymphocytes around a vessel (upper right) that normally should be sheathed with these cells. Most of the cells in the surrounding tissue are erythroblasts. Fetus stillborn at term.

period of normal development. After birth erythropoiesis quickly disappears from the spleen.

In normal individuals hemosiderin deposition in the spleen before birth is not marked but rapidly increases postnatally. In infants with erythroblastosis there may be considerable hemosiderin in the spleen even at birth (Fig. 21–7) because of excessive destruction of red cells by the fetus.

Occasionally erythrophagocytosis can be demonstrated in severe erythroblastosis (Potter) but we have never seen pigments other than hemosiderin in the splenic reticulum cells.

Leukemia

The spleen is usually considerably enlarged in congenital leukemia. The architecture is obscured by great numbers of immature myeloid or lymphoid cells, usually the former since lymphoid leukemia is even more rare then myeloid leukemia in the

newborn. Malpighian corpuscles are inconspicuous or absent and the entire substance has a remarkably uniform appearance (Fig. 21–8). Sinusoids are filled with immature cells and do not stand out prominently as in erythroblastosis.

Hypersplenism

In hypersplenism there is an excess of the phagocytic and destructive activity that is normally directed toward circulating blood cells. This may occur with enlargement of the spleen due to congestion, infection or an auto-immune reaction. In auto-immune reactions such as congenital hemolytic anemia and idiopathic thrombocytopenic purpura, an identifying lesion of the malpighian follicles can be seen in older infants. This consists of a ring of immature lymphocytes in the secondary center surrounded by a rim of adult lymphocytes, and this in turn by another circular collection of immature lymphocytes, giving rise to the term "inside-out follicles." When hypersplenism is secondary to portal obstruction and hypertension, the follicles are normal but the capsule and the trabeculae as well as the reticulum of the sinusoids are greatly thickened. Frequently, large blood-filled spaces, "peripenicillar lakes," are present. In older children these become thrombosed and form an analogue of the gamma gandy body seen in malaria; this is a fibrous mass encrusted with iron phosphates formed from degenerating hemoglobin.

Reticuloendothelioses

Although the reticuloendothelioses of the young infant, child and adult have many features in common, individual variations are frequent in both clinical behavior and pathologic change; because of this and the absence of an established etiology for any of the group, it is believed that they may represent different diseases that have a common clinical and pathologic mode of expression. The reticuloendothelioses fall into three general groups. The first, *Letterer-Siwe's* disease, begins before birth or within the 1st year of life and frequently has a rapid downhill course (Cohen *et al.*; Ahnquist and Holyoke). The second, *Hand-Schüller-Christian syndrome,* often has an onset in the 1st year of life and a more benign, prolonged course with healing of many of the multiple lesions. The third, *eosinophilic granuloma,* more often is restricted in distribution and may be an isolated lesion, although it also may involve more than one organ system. Letterer-Siwe's disease is usually fatal, Hand-Schüller-Christian syndrome only if a vital organ is in-

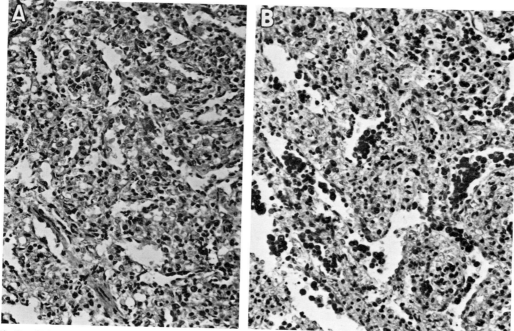

Fig. 21–6.—Spleen in erythroblastosis. **A,** distended empty sinusoids with prominent endothelial nuclei. Malpighian corpuscles could not be distinguished. This is the most common appearance in severe erythroblastosis. **B,** sinusoids distended by erythroblasts.

Fig. 21–7.—Spleen of newborn erythroblastotic infant. A stain for iron shows a large amount of hemosiderin peripheral to the depleted malpighian follicle.

Fig. 21–8.—Spleen from newborn infant with leukemia. The distinction between pulp and sinusoids is obscured by the dense infiltration of immature myeloid cells. Malpighian corpuscles could not be identified. Same infant as in Fig. 28–9.

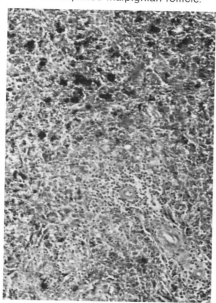

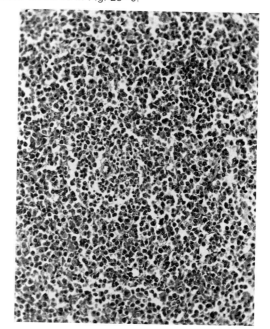

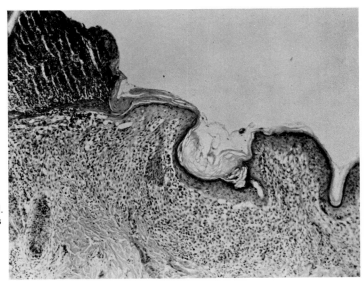

Fig. 21–9.—Letterer-Siwe's disease. Epithelium thin and crusted. Histiocytes present in large numbers in a localized area immediately beneath the epidermis.

volved, and the lesions of eosinophilic granuloma often heal with radiation therapy.

In the 1st year of life Letterer-Siwe's disease is the most important although not the most frequent. It is characterized by seborrheic dermatitis particularly involving the scalp, a maculopapular rash, hepatosplenomegaly, pulmonary infiltrations, lymphadenopathy, fever, cough and failure to thrive. Roentgenograms may show punched-out areas in the skull and long bones.

Pathologically, the lesions are characterized by a massive infiltration of mononuclear cells, histiocytes and occasional eosinophils. In the skin they have a particular location in the dermis immediately below the dermal-epidermal junction (Fig. 21–9). Infiltration of the alveolar spaces in the lungs may cause airway obstruction, and then cystically dilated emphysematous spaces may develop in the interstitium. In the lymph nodes the infiltrate destroys and obscures the normal architecture; in the spleen the red pulp may be heavily infiltrated but the white pulp and the trabeculae are spared (Fig. 21–10). The bone marrow may be extensively replaced, and infiltration of the solid organs such as the pancreas, ovaries, liver and salivary glands is common. Occasionally the brain and meninges are similarly involved.

Familial reticuloendotheliosis, a disorder that has some histologic similarity to Letterer-Siwe's disease, has been described in several sibships (Farquhar and Claireaux; Miller; Schoeck *et al.*). The onset may occur later in childhood although cases have been seen in early infancy. The cellular

infiltration is more aggressively invasive especially in the meninges, and the bone lesions may be less prominent. Active erythrophagocytosis by the proliferated reticuloendothelial cells has been a prominent feature of these cases. None of the classic cases of Letterer-Siwe's disease has been familial. The exact relationship of the two processes is still unclear.

Onset of the Hand-Schüller-Christian syndrome may occur in the 1st year but is proportionately

Fig. 21–10.—Spleen in Letterer-Siwe's disease. Normal cells of the spleen are largely absent and are replaced by histiocytes having the marked variation in form and size characteristic of this disease. (Courtesy Dr. G. Vawter.)

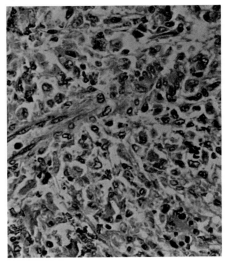

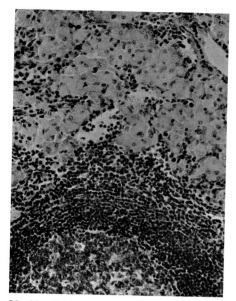

Fig. 21—11.—Spleen in Gaucher's disease. The malpighian corpuscle is normally reactive with a central primary follicle surrounded by the secondary follicle. The red pulp is nearly replaced by swollen histiocytes of the Gaucher type. (Courtesy Dr. G. Vawter.)

less common (six of 29 cases in the series of Avery *et al.*), and a fatal outcome is less frequent (two of six with onset in the 1st year) than in Letterer-Siwe's disease. The lesions are more often limited to bones and are less aggressive with less cellularity and less monotony of cell type than in Letterer-Siwe's disease but with more fibrosis and evidence of healing.

The least aggressive of the three forms, eosinophilic granuloma, is usually limited to a single bone but may be found in adults in the skin and lungs as well (see also under bone).

In *Gaucher's disease* the abnormal accumulation of cerebrosides in reticuloendothelial cells is responsible for great enlargement of the spleen (Fig. 21–11). The condition is discussed in Chapter 10.

REFERENCES

Ahnquist, G., and Holyoke, J. B.: Congenital Letterer-Siwe's disease (reticulo-endotheliosis) in a term stillborn infant, J. Pediatr. 57:897, 1960.

Akerren, Y.: Occurrence of palpable spleens in healthy newborn and older infants, Acta. Paediatr. 34:184, 1947.

Avery, M. E., McAfee, J. G., and Guild, H. G.: The course and prognosis of reticuloendotheliosis (eosinophilic granuloma, Schüller-Christian disease, Letterer-Siwe's disease), Am. J. Med. 22:636, 1957.

Cohen, D. N., Mitchell, C. B., and Alirondes, J. W.: Letterer-Siwe's disease in a newborn, Arch. Pathol. 86:347, 1966.

Conant, N. F.: *Manual of Clinical Mycology* (Philadelphia: W. B. Saunders Co., 1954), p. 119.

Eraklis, A. J., Kevy, S. V., Diamond, L. K., and Gross, R. E.: Hazard of overwhelming infection after splenectomy in childhood, N. Engl. J. Med. 276:1225, 1967.

Farquhar, J. W., and Claireaux, E. E.: Familial haemophagocytic reticulosis, Arch. Dis. Child. 27:519, 1952.

Gilbert, E. F., Nishimura, K., and Wedum, B. G.: Congenital malformation of heart associated with splenic agenesis—report of five cases, Circulation 17:72, 1958.

Grove, L. W.: Fibroangioma of spleen, Ann. Surg. 105:969, 1937.

Gruenwald, P.: Rupture of liver and spleen in newborn infant, J. Pediatr. 33:195, 1948.

Ivemark, B.: Implications of agenesis of the spleen on the pathogenesis of cono-truncus anomalies in childhood, Acta Paediatr. (supp.) 44:104, 1955.

Lichenstein, L.: Histiocytosis X, Arch. Pathol. 56:84, 1953.

Miller, D. R.: Familial reticuloendotheliosis: Concurrence of disease in five siblings, Pediatrics 38:986, 1966.

Murphy, J. W., and Mitchell, W. A.: Congenital absence of spleen, Pediatrics 20:253, 1957.

Polhemus, D. W., and Schafer, W. B.: Absent spleen syndrome—hematologic findings as aid to diagnosis, Pediatrics 24:254, 1959.

Potter, E. L.: *Rh: Its Relation to Erythroblastosis and Fatal Intragroup Transfusion Reactions* (Chicago: Year Book Medical Publishers, Inc., 1947).

Schoeck, V. W., Peterson, R. D. A., and Good, R. A.: Familial occurrence of Letterer-Siwe's disease, Pediatrics 32:1055, 1963.

22

Kidneys, Ureters,
Urinary Bladder and Urethra

Kidneys

DEVELOPMENT

TWO SETS of primitive kidneys develop in the human embryo before the third set appears that persists throughout life. The pronephros, or first kidney, is first visible in the early part of the 4th week in embryos of 9–10 somites as a group of cell masses lying between the coelom and the ventrolateral border of the somites on both sides of the embryo. Each mass of cells becomes subdivided into medial vesicular and lateral tubular portions, and before the end of the 4th week about seven pairs of tubules and vesicles are present between the level of the fourth and the fourteenth somites. The ends of the tubules turn downward and grow caudally, each uniting with and opening into the one immediately

Fig. 22–1.— Section through a 2 cm embryo of about 7 weeks showing, on the right, a group of mesonephric glomeruli and tubules with three portions of the mesonephric duct lateral to them. The left side is cut at a slightly different level and shows only a few mesonephric glomeruli. Visible above these glomeruli is the primitive metanephros composed of branches of the metanephric bud surrounded by metanephric blastema. The gonads are slightly medial to the lower ends of each mesonephros.

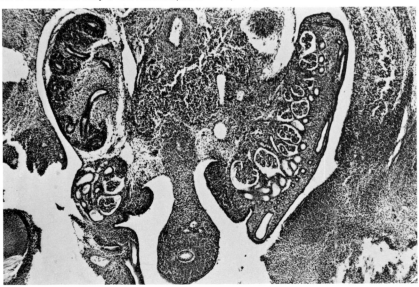

adjacent to it. The longitudinal channels thus formed are the pronephric ducts.

In some primitive forms of life these structures persist as the permanent kidneys, but in man the earliest pronephric tubules begin to degenerate before the last appear. Vesicles (glomeruli) and lateral tubules continue to be formed in the region caudal to the pronephros and to be attached to the mesonephric (wolffian) ducts, which are elongations of the pronephric ducts. The mesonephric ducts reach the cloaca late in the 4th week at about the 4 mm stage of embryonic development. Somewhat over 40 pairs of tubules appear, but since those in the more cephalic region degenerate as the more caudal ones develop, not more than 30–32 pairs are present at any one time. The group of glomeruli, tubules and connecting ducts present on each side of the body is known as a wolffian body or mesonephros (Fig. 22–1).

The fate of the mesonephric ducts and tubules differs in the two sexes. In the female the ducts degenerate, but a few of the tubules persist to form the small cystic structures called epioöphoron and paroöphoron found almost constantly in the mesosalpinx between the fallopian tube and medulla of the ovary. In the male, part of the tubules persist to form the rete and epididymis of the testes. The mesonephric ducts become the ductus deferentia.

During the 5th week a small outgrowth known as the metanephric bud appears near the lower end of each mesonephric duct. The final kidney, or metanephros, develops by the simultaneous differentiation of this bud and the metanephrogenic tissue into which it grows. The terminal end of the bud, known as the ampulla, expands almost immediately after it first appears and quickly begins to divide dichotomously. Early division progresses more rapidly at the poles than in the intermediate zone and is the cause of the elongated shape of the kidney. The first three to five generations of branches eventually expand to produce the renal pelvis, the next three to five form the calices and papillae and the succeeding seven to eight produce the collecting tubules. The rate of ampullary division decreases when the fetus is 13–14 weeks old, and little division takes place after 20 weeks.

In addition to being responsible for dichotomous division, the ampullae induce the formation of nephrons from the metanephric blastema. Nephrons appear first as solid round or oval masses at the sides of the ampullae. They develop slitlike cavities and by variable cell proliferation each quickly assumes the shape of a letter S. One end fuses with the ampulla by which it was induced, and a contin-uous lumen is established between nephron and collecting tubule (Fig. 22–2). The portion of the nephron in communication with the collecting tubule is the connecting piece; the distal convoluted tubule, loop of Henle, proximal convoluted tubule and malpighian corpuscle come from the remainder. Eight to 12 generations of nephrons are formed.

As long as new tubules are being produced each ampulla divides into two parts, one of which retains the attachment of the nephron formed at the time of the preceding division while the other induces the formation of a new nephron, which, when it reaches the S-stage, attaches to and communicates with that ampulla. Both of these ampullae repeat this process and this continues until six to eight generations of nephrons are formed, one nephron always remaining attached to one of the two ampullae produced at each division while the other ampulla induces formation of a new nephron. Consequently, when ampullary division ceases, each ampulla has a single attached nephron. These are of different ages depending on when in the course of ampullary division they were produced.

Fig. 22–2.—The ampullae of a collecting tubule with adjacent nephrons of different ages. On the right the ampulla has an attached S-stage nephron; on the left the nephron is still in the vesicle stage.

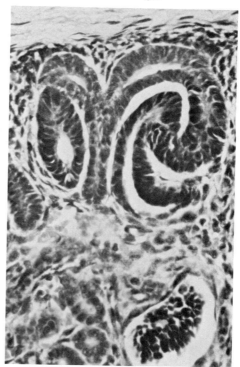

At about midpregnancy the ampullae stop dividing but each one continues to induce the formation of nephrons. Each nephron attaches to the ampulla by which it was induced but when the next nephron to be formed also attaches, the connecting piece of the first nephron shifts slightly so that it is attached to the connecting piece of the new nephron instead of directly to the ampulla. This produces a succession of nephrons attached to one another by their connecting pieces, with only the youngest attached directly to an ampulla. Known as arcades, these consist of four to six nephrons (Peter; Osathanondh and Potter).

While arcades are being formed the peripheral growth of ampullae is arrested, but when the arcades are completed, forward growth is resumed and then, as nephrons are induced, each attaches directly to its ampulla so that an additional four to six nephrons become distributed at regular intervals along the terminal portion of each collecting tubule (Fig. 22–3).

As long as new nephrons are being induced, S-forms and metanephric blastema are visible microscopically as the nephrogenic zone adjacent to the capsule of the kidney (Fig. 22–4, A and B). Nephron induction normally ends at 32–36 weeks and the nephrogenic zone disappears (Fig. 22–4, C). Because of this the kidney makes an excellent histologic index of fetal maturity.

When birth takes place before the full complement of glomeruli has developed, they continue to form until an approximately normal number exists (Fig. 22–4, D). This is probably responsible for the great variability in statements concerning the time at which glomerular formation normally ceases.

Once nephron production is brought to a halt, it is never resumed. Increase in kidney size is a result of interstitial growth of tubules and an increase in blood vessels and connective tissue. At birth all portions of the nephrogenic tubules are much shorter, both actually and in relation to length of collecting tubules, than they are in later life. The difference in the ratio of the number of glomeruli to the surface area of tubal epithelium in the adult and the newborn can be expected to result in marked differences in kidney function.

Urine is produced in the early months of fetal life as soon as the first glomeruli assume a definitive form. In fetuses measuring only a few centimeters the bladder is globular and filled with a clear fluid. The urine is voided into the amniotic sac and is a source of amniotic fluid. What part of the total is composed of fetal urine has not been determined. Amniotic fluid is present before the metanephros

originates, and the amount of fluid surrounding the fetus in the first few months of pregnancy, when proportionately few nephrons have yet developed, is greater in relation to total body size than in the later months. The great reduction or absence of fluid found in association with urethral obstruction or complete renal agenesis suggests that urine may be a more important constituent of amniotic fluid in the latter part of pregnancy.

For the first few days after birth the urine often contains epithelial cells, red blood cells, leukocytes, a little albumin and large amounts of uric acid. In living infants uric acid crystals precipitated from voided urine may be found on the diaper as a fine deposit resembling brick dust. In infants dying at 5–10 days of age precipitates of uric acid may be

Fig. 22–3.—Microdissection of the terminal portion of a collecting tubule (arrow) and its attached nephrons from the kidney of a normal mature newborn infant. There is a single nephron attached at A, followed by an arcade at B consisting of four nephrons, and this is followed by 6 nephrons attached individually at C to H. This is the typical form of nephron attachment except for nephron A. Most often no nephrons are attached proximal to arcade.

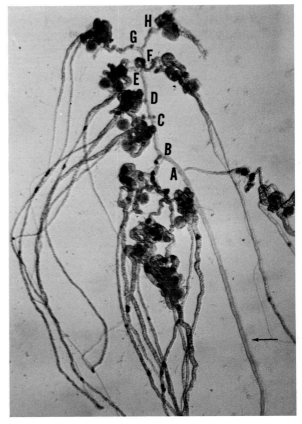

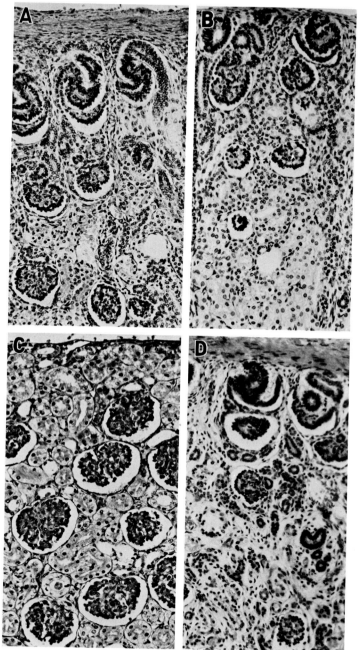

Fig. 22–4.—Nephrogenic zone of the kidney. **A,** fetus weighing 1,000 gm. Adjacent to the capsule is a layer of immature tubules and glomeruli arising from the metanephric blastema. Two layers of definitive glomeruli are also visible. **B,** fetus weighing 2,000 gm. The nephrogenic zone is still present but is less immature than in A. **C,** mature newborn infant weighing 3,550 gm. The nephrogenic zone has disappeared and tubular development is considerably more advanced. **D,** infant aged 34 days weighing only 1,010 gm at death. The nephrogenic zone is still present and glomeruli are still being formed. When an infant is born prematurely, glomerular formation continues until the normal complement of glomeruli is produced.

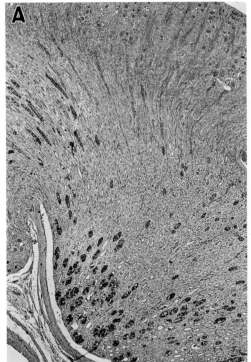

Fig. 22–5.—Uric acid deposits in the collecting tubules of the kidney of an infant aged 6 days. They were grossly visible as bright orange streaks. **A,** view showing general distribution in the kidney. **B,** higher magnification showing crystalline nature of the deposits.

grossly visible in the collecting tubules. They are distinguishable as fine yellow-orange lines radiating from the kidney pelvis. Microscopic examination reveals sheetlike masses of crystals distending the collecting tubules (Fig. 22–5).

Tubular degeneration is usually a result of postmortem decomposition and can rarely be considered evidence of disturbed kidney function. Hyaline degeneration, although rarely encountered, was present in one infant at the Chicago Lying-in Hospital who died of leukemia at 2 days of age.

Hyaline or cellular casts are rare. Even in erythroblastotic infants who are destroying large numbers of red blood cells, casts or evidence of hemoglobin precipitate in the tubules is unknown.

Sclerotic glomeruli have been reported in varying numbers in the absence of other renal lesions in infants a few months of age and occasionally in newborns (Fig. 22–6). Most frequently observed in the periphery of the kidney, they are occasionally found in small groups immediately beneath the capsule, sometimes in sufficient numbers to cause small pits. Groups of sclerotic glomeruli often ap-

Fig. 22–6.—Kidney of a newborn infant showing two of several sclerotic glomeruli in an otherwise normal cortex.

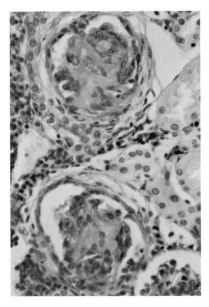

pear to be supplied by a single arcuate artery. Such involvement of a large number of glomeruli may be a rare cause of the nephrotic syndrome.

Vascular Disturbances

Renal vein thrombosis is a lesion most often seen in infants of diabetic mothers, in whom the incidence among those autopsied may be as high as 5.8%, compared to 0.8% in infants of nondiabetic mothers (Oppenheimer and Esterly). The renal vein thrombosis may extend to nearby vessels in the adrenal gland. The thrombi may be fresh or old but do not often lead to renal infarction (Fig. 22–7). Renal vein thrombosis has also been described in infants with the congenital nephrotic syndrome (Norio). Predisposing maternal states include difficult labor, dehydration, shock, maternal hydramnios and toxemia.

Renal cortical and medullary necrosis may occur rarely in infants with the same background of shock, sepsis, dehydration and asphyxia. Hematuria and renal insufficiency are the chief clinical manifestations. In some cases fibrosis and calcification are present, suggesting that the lesions occurred in utero, possibly even before glomerular production was completed. Disseminated intravascular coagulation has been postulated as a cause of some cases of cortical necrosis in the newborn (Moore *et al.*).

Infection

Infections of the urinary system are uncommon in newborn infants. Kidney infections are most often pyelitis or pyelonephritis beginning as cystitis and ascending from the bladder. Rarely, the kidneys are the principal site of involvement in septicemia, or infection may exist without known cause. Malformations that interfere with urinary outflow may be predisposing factors. Abscesses are occa-

Fig. 22–7.—Infarction of the renal cortex secondary to renal vein thrombosis.

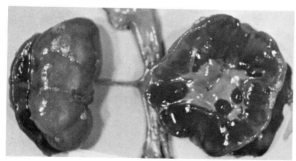

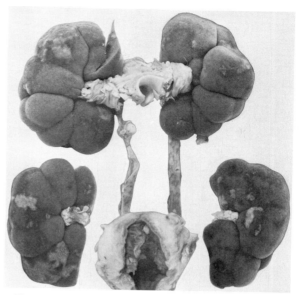

Fig. 22–8.—Multiple kidney abscesses associated with cystitis and pyelonephritis in an infant aged 12 days. Source of infection unknown.

sionally encountered (Fig. 22–8) and are thought to be more common in hematogenous than in ascending infections. Pyelitis or pyelonephritis must be considered in the differential diagnosis of any unexplained fever in young infants.

Pyelonephritis originating before birth or in the first few weeks of life was described at length by Pasternack and other investigators. In some kidneys Pasternack found dysplastic structures similar to those occurring in some cases of type II polycystic kidneys, but the majority of investigators have considered the presence of leukocytes alone sufficient to warrant a diagnosis. A so-called thyroid-like appearance caused by the presence of a protein-rich fluid in mildly dilated tubules is present in some cases (Fig. 22–9) and has been described as characteristic of this condition. However, Bell ascribed it to tubular atrophy and thought it nonspecific.

Glomerulonephritis is rare in infancy, but lesions thought to be indicative of both acute and chronic stages of the disease have been described. Fison reported acute nephritis in two siblings both dying at about 7 months. Albuminuria, hematuria and anemia were prominent symptoms. Pathologic changes included enlarged glomeruli with adhesions to Bowman's capsule, acute and chronic epithelial crescents and occasional blocking of capillary loops by hyaline.

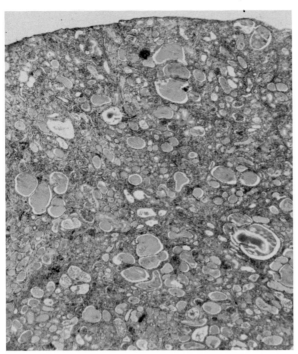

Fig. 22–9.—Kidney with dilated tubules filled with protein-rich material simulating colloid and having the appearance sometimes described as thyroidlike. Many glomeruli are small and dysplastic and there is a diffuse lymphocytic infiltration. Infant aged 90 hours.

In *syphilis* a mild increase in connective tissue is the only characteristic change in the kidney. This increase is most pronounced in the subcapsular area and may extend in fingerlike processes into the peripheral portions of the cortex between the tubules. Occasionally leukocytes or immature erythrocytes are present in the connective tissue. Hyalinization of glomeruli and degeneration of tubules have also been described.

In *cytomegalic inclusion disease* the changes are usually greater in the kidney than in any other organ. The glomeruli are ordinarily normal, but some of the cells lining the tubules are increased to several times their normal size (see Fig. 9–9). The nuclei of the affected cells contain large basophilic inclusions that are responsible for a characteristic "bird's eye" appearance. On microdissection Fetterman *et al.* found them limited to peripheral collecting tubules, distal convoluted tubules, loops of Henle and Bowman's capsules. The involvement of other organs is variable, and at times similar inclusion bodies are widely scattered throughout the body (see p. 130).

Nephrosis

Nephrosis in infants has been divided into several varieties. One, designated the *congenital nephrotic syndrome,* which is observed at birth or within a few weeks, is characterized by premature birth, large placenta, edema, proteinuria, high susceptibility to infections and a fatal outcome. Microscopically, descriptions of kidneys have varied but characteristics have included tubular dilatation, interstitial and periglomerular fibrosis, infiltration by mononuclear leukocytes and crescent formation. Paatela, who dissected kidneys of 30 infants with this condition, found that all had fat deposition and cellular hyperplasia in zones of cystic dilatation in proximal convoluted tubules. These alternated with narrow atrophic segments. Two thirds of the cases also had shortening and narrowing of the neck of the tubules. A cause has not been definitely established, but the two most widely considered possibilities have been inheritance as an autosomal recessive trait (Norio) and renal damage caused by transplacental passage of immune antibodies produced by the mother against the fetus (Kouvelainen). Oliver gave the name microcystic disease to this condition, but because such a wide variety of disturbances have been given this designation, continued use of the term seems undesirable.

Lipoid nephrosis differs from the congenital nephrotic syndrome in that it seldom has an onset before 2 years of age, and death, usually from infection, does not occur for several years. The symptoms are generalized edema, albuminuria, hyperglycemia and hypoproteinuria. On microdissection of six cases Paatela found multiple kinks in proximal convoluted tubules associated with marked deposit of fat and, on microscopic examination, intermittent zones of flattened epithelium and fatty casts in distal convoluted tubules. The cystic dilatation of proximal convoluted tubules characteristic of the congenital nephrotic syndrome was lacking.

Hemolytic Uremia Syndrome

This is a subacute disorder of infants and young children with onset often before the end of the 12th month (Gianantonio *et al.*; Lieberman *et al.*) The prodromal symptoms include abdominal pain, fever, diarrhea, vomiting and upper respiratory infections and are soon followed by petechial hemorrhages, melena, hypertension, oliguria and coma. Thrombocytopenia is common; helmet cells appear

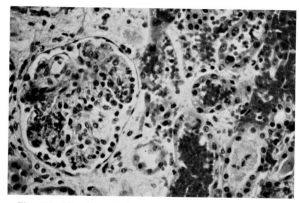

Fig. 22—10.—Hemolytic uremia syndrome. The glomerulus at left has focal areas of necrosis and the tubules on the right are filled with red blood cells.

among the erythrocytes and hemolytic crises may occur.

Pathologically, fatal cases may show bilateral cortical necrosis, but in less severe cases changes are often limited to thrombosis of glomerular capillary loops and focal glomerular necrosis. Occasionally present are tubular hyaline, red cell and heme casts and tubular necrosis (Fig. 22–10). In the most severely affected kidneys arcuate and interlobular arteries may be thrombosed. The subacute stage is remarkable for the absence of interstitial inflammation. Despite the occasional presence of severe cerebral signs, no pathologic changes other than subdural hematomas have been described.

Mortality has varied from 7 to 27% in different reports. Most survivors have normal renal function although renal biopsies of seemingly recovered patients may show not only glomerular fibrosis and tubular atrophy, but also fresh crescents, thickening and hypercellularity of nonfibrosed glomeruli.

ERYTHROBLASTOSIS

In this condition foci of erythropoiesis are commonly found in the intertubular connective tissue of the kidney, especially in the areas surrounding the blood vessels at the apexes of the pyramids (Fig. 22–11). The degree of involvement may vary from a few scattered cells to infiltration so severe that portions of kidney parenchyma are destroyed. Erythroblasts are often more numerous in capillaries and small blood vessels than in the general circulation. Occasionally they are visible in glomerular capillaries. Bile pigment is often found in tubular epithelium of infants who were intensely

jaundiced at the time of death. In severe erythroblastosis, hemosiderin and even bile can be demonstrated in large amounts in the proximal convoluted tubules.

MALFORMATIONS

BILATERAL AGENESIS. — This malformation is more common than generally believed, the incidence at the Chicago Lying-in Hospital being approximately 1:4,500 births. Fifty cases were included in the Chicago Lying-in Hospital autopsy series, 27 of which were fetuses and infants born in other hospitals. Nineteen were stillborn, 27 lived less than 4 hours and among the remaining four the longest survival was 48 hours. Death of all liveborn infants was preceded by dyspnea, cyanosis and evidence of respiratory embarrassment resulting from pulmonary hypoplasia. In none was there evidence of uremia although in a few cases with survival up to 2 weeks, described by other investigators, this may have been a cause. Thirty-six were male. In all eight sirenomelic monsters observed in this laboratory the kidneys and ureters were absent; all but one of these were male.

Fig. 22—11.—Kidney of a mature newborn infant with erythroblastosis. Immature erythrocytes are present between the tubules and in large masses in the perivascular connective tissue at the apexes of the pyramids. Age 3 hours.

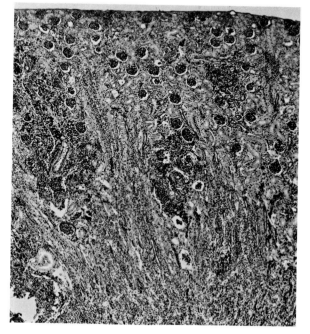

Sixty percent had gestation periods of less than 38 weeks, and of those of 38 weeks or more only three weighed over 2,500 gm. Almost all were small for the calculated length of gestation, a condition true of most infants with severe malformations.

The weight of the placenta in relation to infant weight was generally low although never less than 1:10, which is often considered the lower limit of normal. The histologic structure of the placenta was not demonstrably abnormal although the amnion usually had multiple small nodules composed of masses of squamous epithelial cells on the fetal surface (see Fig. 3–52, A). This condition was first described by Landing in renal agenesis but may be present in association with oligohydramnios from any cause.

The external appearance of all infants with renal agenesis is remarkably similar. The majority appear to have an excessive amount of skin, looking as if they were greatly dehydrated. They have an unusual bowing of the legs and inward rotation of the feet because of fixation in the uterus as a result of oligohydramnios (Fig. 22–12). The hands often seem unusually large with excessive amounts of skin and subcutaneous tissue.

The facial expression alone, generally that of extreme age, is characteristic enough to warrant a diagnosis of renal agenesis (Fig. 22–13, A). This appearance seems to be related to lack of kidney function rather than to the specific malformation because a similar facial appearance is found in infants with severe renal dysplasia (type II cystic kidneys).

The most constant facial characteristic is a prominent V-shaped epicanthic fold that arises above the eyelid, swings down to cover the medial palpebral commissure and ends on the cheek. It is different from the fold present in Down's syndrome, which ordinarily ends at the level of the commissure. The nose is flattened, the depression below the lower lip is unusually prominent and the ears are almost always abnormal although the distortion is not uniform. They generally are set somewhat low on the head and the region of the lobe is

Fig. 22–12.—Infant with bilateral renal agenesis. **A,** anterior view showing appearance of extreme age, general dehydration, bowing of legs and characteristic face. **B,** intrauterine position explaining cause of bowing of legs.

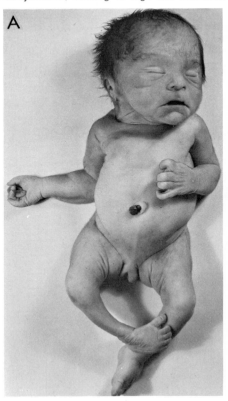
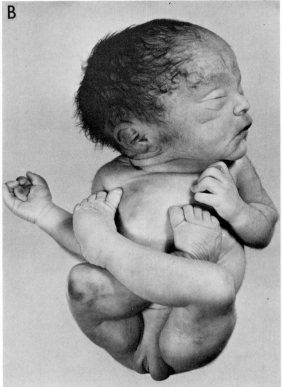

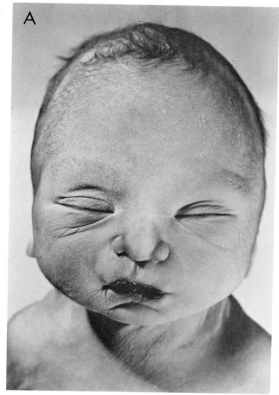
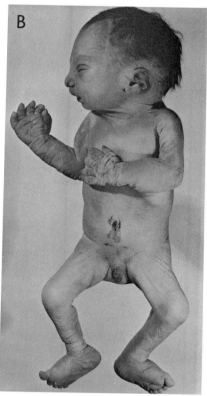

Fig. 22–13.—Infant with renal agenesis. **A,** face characteristic of renal agenesis. The inner canthus is covered by a V-shaped fold, the nose is flattened and a prominent depression is present below the lower lip. **B,** total body showing cutis laxa, especially marked on the hands.

Facial profile is characteristic. The ear is less upright than normal, the tragus is absent, the lobe and antitragus are abnormally broad and crura of the antitragus are malformed.

drawn forward, giving a less upright position than is normal. They are flaccid and often pressed against the side of the head, so that the crura antihelices and antitragus are unduly prominent. The lobe and antitragus are abnormally broad and the tragus is sometimes absent. The total ear seems excessively large but this results largely from the flaccidity and flattening (Fig. 22–13, B).

Some attempt has been made to correlate isolateral malformation of the external ear with absence or abnormality of one kidney. The ear malformations described have been variable and usually minor, and none have resembled those that accompany bilateral absence. An unsuccessful attempt was made by the Department of Urology of the University of Chicago to demonstrate such a relationship.

Almost all infants have accompanying pulmonary hypoplasia and in almost all, the lungs weigh less than one half of the normal for body weight

(Potter). The changes in the lungs may be of two types. In one described by Peale and Esterly the abnormality is much the same as that often found in infants with severe craniospinorachischisis and consists of a reduction in the number of distal airways in the lung so that there are fewer alveoli in relation to bronchi than is normal. In another variety, which was present in some of the cases in the Chicago Lying-in Hospital series, the defect consists of failure of maturation of primitive pulmonary tissue. Primitive alveolar ducts, normally present by midpregnancy, become vascularized, and alveoli develop from them during the latter half of pregnancy. The abnormality in renal agenesis consists not only of a reduction in the number of alveoli but also of a more fundamental disturbance in which there is an irregular failure of vascularization leading to failure of formation of normal alveolar ducts as well as alveoli (see Fig. 15–29). Whether compression of the chest by the uterine

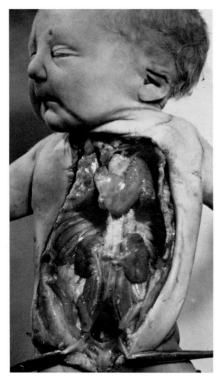

Fig. 22–14.—Bilateral renal agenesis. The adrenal glands are flat oval disks on the posterior wall of the abdominal cavity. The ovaries are the two elongated structures the upper poles of which lie at the level of the bifurcation of the aorta. The fallopian tubes are adjacent to them (indistinguishable in the photograph). The uterus and vagina are absent. Forceps are attached to the umbilical arteries. The bladder is the elongated hypoplastic structure lying between them.

wall, because of the absence of amniotic fluid, limits space for growth and is responsible for the pulmonary immaturity, or whether it is a result of inhibition of respiratory activity because of lack of amniotic fluid, is undecided.

The genital system was normal in only one of 14 females in the series reported by Potter. In two the uterus was double, and in one of these the vagina was closed, with the lower part missing. In 11 the uterus and vagina were absent or rudimentary. In all, however, fallopian tubes and ovaries were present and of normal size.

External genitalia were absent or abnormal in all of eight sirenomelic monsters and in 10 other infants. Of the latter, two females had penile urethras and in a third extreme clitoral hypertrophy gave an appearance simulating hypospadias. Among the affected males the penis was absent in two, rudimentary in one, hypospadic in one and unusually

long in two, and the scrotum was absent in one.

Adrenal glands are oval, discoid structures positioned flat against the posterior abdominal wall since there are no kidneys to exert upward pressure and give them their normal shape (Fig. 22–14). Cellular constituents, however, are normal. The lower intestine, probably because of its location in the immediate vicinity of the developing kidney, is also often abnormal. In the eight sirenomelic fetuses plus four other males and four females in Potter's series the sigmoid colon and rectum were absent and the anus was imperforate. Additional intestinal malformations were: imperforate anus with rectum present, 5; nonrotation of bowel, 3; tracheoesophageal fistula, 2; and duodenal atresia, 1.

Hydrocephalus, generally associated with spina bifida, was found in eight infants, and there were malformations in other parts of the skeleton in 11, exclusive of the sirenomeluses.

The only other malformations that occurred frequently were cardiac (11). Principally resulting from abnormal division of the truncus arteriosus, they were aortic or pulmonary stenosis, transposition of great vessels or persistent truncus arteriosus.

Absence or great reduction in amount of amniotic fluid seems an almost invariable accompaniment of renal agenesis. There is no record of amniotic fluid having been present in an amount greater than 1–2 oz in any of the cases in the Chicago Lying-in Hospital series or in many additional cases discussed by correspondence (Potter). The only cases described by other authors in which amniotic fluid was present had accompanying anencephaly. This seems to negate some of the current ideas on the origin of amniotic fluid (see p. 59) and is an experiment provided by nature that must be taken into account in any theory proposed to explain the source of amniotic fluid. The almost constant pulmonary hypoplasia is also of interest in the controversy about the relation of aspiration of amniotic fluid to alveolar development.

The cause of renal agenesis is unknown, although it seems probable from the great variation in associated malformations that all result from the action of an exogenous agent exerted at a critical time during embryonic development. Supporting this idea is the fact that it has been observed in only one of monozygotic twins. On the other hand, at least four instances of sibling involvement have been reported (Rizza and Downing). Buchts and Opitz have observed additional cases, as yet unreported, and believe that the condition could be caused by a polygenic-multifactorial trait with an extremely low empiric recurrence risk.

UNILATERAL AGENESIS.—Absence of both kidneys is more common in the Chicago Lying-in Hospital series of autopsies than is absence of a single kidney, and it seems probable that unilateral and bilateral agenesis are unrelated anomalies. Unilateral absence shows no predilection for either sex. In all of the females with complete renal agenesis in the Chicago Lying-in Hospital series both fallopian tubes were present; in none of the females lacking only one kidney was the fallopian tube present on the affected side (Fig. 22–15). However, the fallopian tube may be missing when a normal kidney is present. When one kidney is absent the entire müllerian duct ordinarily fails to develop in the affected side, and the unicornuate uterine corpus, cervix and vagina arise from a single müllerian duct.

When only one kidney is present, it is usually in a normal position and arises from a single ureter and nephrogenic mass. Rarely, it lies at or near the midline and arises from nephrogenic tissue of both right and left sides even though there is no demonstrable separation and a single ureter is present. In such cases the adrenal glands are also often fused (Fig. 22–16).

ECTOPIA.—Normally the kidneys lie retroperitoneally on each side of the lower abdomen, and at birth the lower pole is at the level of or slightly below the brim of the pelvis. Each kidney is supplied by a ureter that opens into the bladder on the same side as the kidney. In rare instances a ureter crosses the midline and opens into the bladder on the opposite side, a condition known as crossed ectopia. One or both kidneys may lie abnormally close to the midline or below the brim of the pelvis.

Changes in position are always associated with secondary changes in shape. A kidney in an abnormal position is usually more spherical than normal and the pelvis is often directed anteriorly or inferiorly instead of medially (Fig. 22–17, A).

Fusion of the kidneys is a fairly common anomaly. If the axes of the kidneys are altered by a medial shift of the lower poles they become united in the midline. The condition produced is known as horseshoe kidney, and often only the most superficial portions of the cortex are fused. The ureters cross the anterior surfaces of the kidneys to reach the bladder (Fig. 22–17, B). Fusion of the upper poles is rare.

Occasionally both kidneys develop close to the midline of the body, both pelves are rotated anteriorly and the approximated surfaces of the kidneys fuse. This may be a superficial union of the cortex (Fig. 22–18, A), or the kidneys may become so

Fig. 22–15 (left).—Unilateral renal agenesis associated with isolateral absence of the fallopian tube. Adrenal glands and ovaries are normal.

Fig. 22–16 (right).—Fused kidney with a single pelvis and ureter. Adrenal glands are also fused.

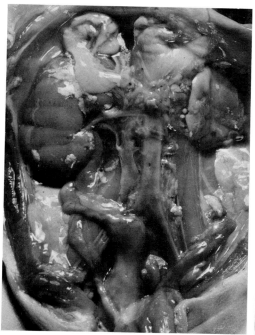

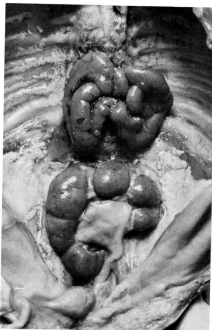

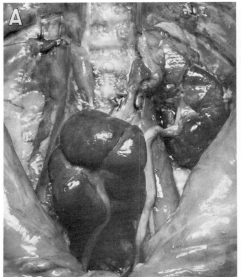
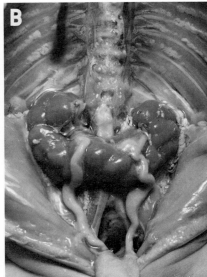

Fig. 22–17.—A, displacement of right kidney with anterior rotation of the pelvis. **B,** horseshoe kidney in situ showing typical fusion of the lower poles with ureters crossing the anterior surfaces to reach the bladder.

completely merged that the portions arising from the right and left masses of nephrogenic tissue cannot be differentiated (Fig. 22–18, B). In the latter case the fused kidneys may lie on one side of the abdominal cavity or in the midline at the brim of the pelvis. The ureters may enter united pelves (Fig. 22–19, A) or separate pelves (Fig. 22–19, B).

HYPOPLASIA.—A kidney never develops in the absence of a ureter. The stimulus afforded by the presence of the metanephric bud is essential for the

Fig. 22–18.—Fused kidneys. **A,** anterior rotation of kidney pelves with fusion of medial surfaces. Adrenal glands also fused. Aorta, which has been cut off below the adrenals, originally crossed anterior to them. Right uterine horn and fallopian tube are absent although both ovaries are present. **B,** fused kidneys with downward displacement and hydronephrosis of the left pelvis. Uterine corpus, cervix and vagina are completely duplicated.

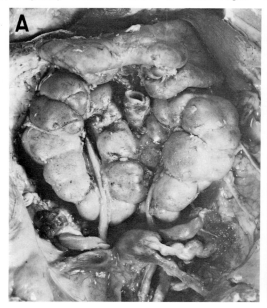
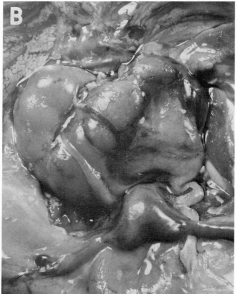

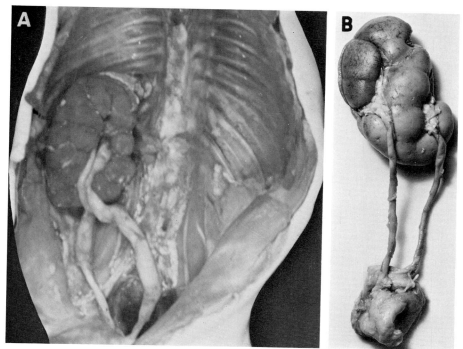

Fig. 22–19.—Fused kidneys. A, kidneys lying on right side of the abdomen with both ureters opening into a single pelvis. Crossed ectopia. B, kidneys with similar location in which ureters open into separate pelves.

elaboration of the nephrogenic tissue into glomeruli and secretory tubules, and no case has ever been observed in which normal collecting tubules or nephrons existed without a ureter.

In the large amount of material at the Armed Forces Institute of Pathology, Ashley and Mostofi found 11 cases in which a "knot" of tissue or a small group of cysts without an attached ureter was present in place of one kidney, but no normal renal parenchyma was ever observed without a ureter attached to it.

When a ureter is present there is almost invariably some semblance of kidney tissue. It may be only a rudimentary mass weighing a few milligrams and composed only of connective tissue with a few tubules, or it may also contain a few glomeruli. Glomeruli never develop in the absence of a ureter, but they do not always appear even though a ureter is present. Even a larger mass having the gross appearance of a kidney may show nothing but tubules surrounded by connective tissue, and occasionally even tubules are lacking and the mass is composed almost exclusively of connective tissue. In our experience such abnormalities are less common than complete agenesis.

Although the term hypoplasia is sometimes used for any abnormally small kidney, it is generally considered more properly limited to a kidney in which nephrons and collecting tubules are normal except for a reduction in number. The number of calices and papillae is diminished; each papilla may be composed of a normal number of normally formed collecting tubules and nephrons, or these also may be reduced in number. This condition is rare and almost all small kidneys show evidence of dysplasia.

CYSTIC DISEASE

Early writers on cystic kidneys usually considered this condition a single entity of uniform pathogenesis. With improved methods of investigation, especially microdissection, it has become evident that cysts may be found in several conditions of diverse origin. Microdissections made in the laboratories of Oliver, Fetterman, Darmady, Paatela, Baxter, Potter and others have all contributed important information. The studies of Osathanondh and Potter showed that the two widely held concepts concerning pathogenesis—(1) failure of nephrons to unite with collecting tubules and (2) persistence of cysts believed to form and later disappear as part of the normal development process—are incorrect. Instead, cysts in kidneys may result either from a primary disturbance in the function of ampullae of collecting tubules or from a secondary enlargement of portions of collecting tubules or nephrons, the original architecture of which was normal. Most of the kidneys commonly designated as polycystic, multicystic, dysgenetic or dysplastic fall in the former category; most of those in which cysts are localized to specific portions of collecting tubules or nephrons fall in the latter. From a study of 303 cases of kidneys containing cysts, many of which were examined by microdissection, Osathanondh and Potter concluded that pathogenetically the most commonly observed kidneys containing cysts can be divided into four groups—types I, II, III and IV.

TYPE I (POLYCYSTIC KIDNEY OF THE NEWBORN, SPONGE KIDNEY, HAMARTOMA).—This variety results from a secondary diffuse enlargement of collecting tubules in kidneys the fundamental architecture of which is normal. The kidneys are always bilater-

Fig. 22–20.—Type I cystic kidneys are always bilaterally enlarged and fetal lobulation is retained; they are covered with punctate dark areas that are the ends of dilated terminal branches of collecting tubules. Same kidney as shown in Fig. 22–21, B.

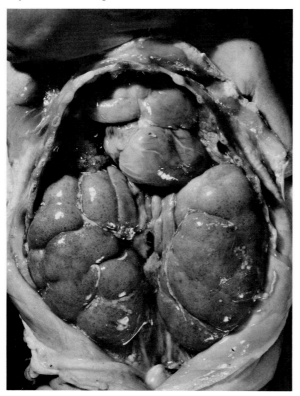

ally enlarged and equally affected (Fig. 22–20). Renal pelves, calices and papillae have a fairly normal shape although they are considerably enlarged, and the openings of papillary ducts are often grossly visible. The entire parenchyma has a strikingly uniform spongy appearance. Fetal lobation is retained and the surface is smooth although studded with very small cysts that are the ends of enlarged collecting tubules. The microscopic appearance, like the gross, is uniformly spongy (Fig. 22–21). The cortex is composed of the greatly enlarged terminal branches of collecting tubules with interspersed, normal-appearing nephrons. The medulla is composed of collecting tubules of somewhat more variable size and many are not enlarged except for local sacculations and diverticuli. Microdissection reveals that collecting tubules are normally branched and nephrons normally formed and normally attached to collecting tubules. The terminal branches of collecting tubules are diffusely enlarged; the more proximal branches are the site of local sacculations and cystic diverticulae (Fig. 22–22). Nephrons are generally of normal structure except for occasional small cysts at the angles of the loops of Henle. Connective tissue is not increased.

Intrahepatic bile ducts are increased in size and number (see Fig. 20–26, B), but malformations seldom occur in other parts of the body. Affected infants usually die soon after birth and only rarely survive into childhood. Siblings may be affected. This kidney type is believed to be caused by the homozygous state of a recessive autosomal gene.

The Chicago Lying-in Hospital series included 22 cases in 17 families with a maximum of three in one family.

TYPE II (MULTICYSTIC KIDNEY, MULTILOCULAR CYSTS, APLASIA, DYSPLASIA, DYSGENESIS).—This variety results from inhibition of the action of the ampulla of the ureteral bud or one or more of the first few generations of branches. Since the function of the ampullae is to initiate tubular division and to induce formation of nephrons, collecting tubules and nephrons in this abnormality are all reduced in number and abnormal in form. The diameter of the collecting tubules is increased and the terminations are usually cystic, the size of the cysts determining the size of the kidneys. The kidneys may be mildly or greatly enlarged (type IIA, Fig. 22–23), or if cysts are small or absent the size may be reduced (type IIB, Fig. 22–24). Some investigators have designated such kidneys when enlarged as multicystic and when small as dysgenetic,

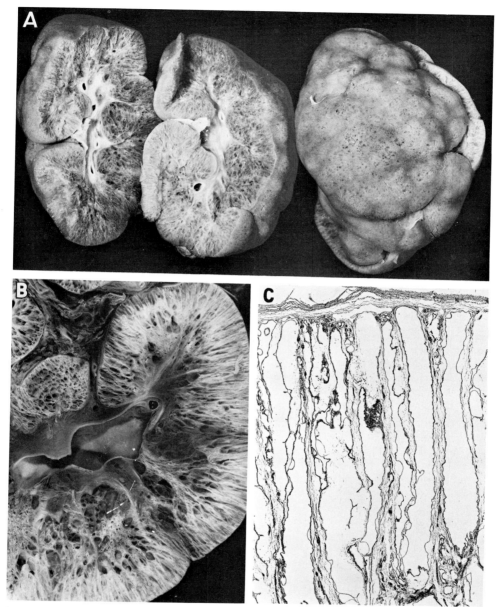

Fig. 22–21.—Identical type I cystic kidneys from siblings born 6 years apart. In both, the collecting tubules are uniformly dilated, there is no increase in connective tissue and glomeruli appear normal. Cystic hyperplasia of intrahepatic bile ducts was present in each infant. **A,** first sibling. **B,** infant born 6 years later with no intervening pregnancies. **C,** photomicrograph of portion of cortex of kidney shown in A. Terminal branches of collecting tubules are diffusely enlarged. Normal glomeruli are present throughout the cortex. Appearance identical to that observed in second sibling.

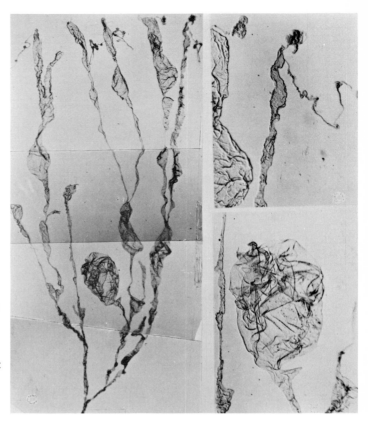

Fig. 22–22.—Cystic kidney type I. Microdissection of several generations of collecting tubules showing diverticular cysts and sacculations in early generations and diffuse enlargement of last generation. Nephrons are attached normally to last generation.

dysplastic or aplastic. They are a result of the same process, however, and there is no sharp distinction between them. At times there is great disparity in size and one may be large and the other small (Fig. 22–25); sometimes only one is abnormal (Fig. 22–26, A) and rarely only one member of a horseshoe kidney may be affected (Fig. 22–26, B). Occasionally only one or a few adjacent collecting tubules are involved so that only a segment of the kidney is abnormal. Such areas may not become cystic and may be present as one or more localized areas of dysgenesis in an otherwise normal kidney, or, more often, the involved area becomes cystic and is known as a multilocular cyst (Fig. 22–27).

The external surfaces of the enlarged kidneys are irregularly elevated by the cysts, and the cut surfaces are honeycombed by cysts of variable size (Fig. 22–28). Small kidneys are composed largely of connective tissue and show few, if any, visible cysts (Fig. 22–29). Microscopically both varieties have a great proliferation of connective tissue, and type IIA contains many thick-walled cysts (Fig.

22–30). Circumscribed groups of small tubules and incompletely formed glomeruli are sometimes present (Fig. 22–31). Islands of cartilage (Fig. 22–32) are found in about half of the cases and abnormally large nerve trunks are common. Characterizing this type of kidney is the complete absence of normal collecting tubules or nephrons.

Microdissection reveals a similar structure in all kidneys except that in type IIB the cysts are small or absent. Collecting tubules are short and thick, have few branches and terminate in variably sized cysts (Fig. 22–33). Calices are absent and the pelvis is tubular in form (Fig. 22–34), as would be expected when there is no urine to cause the early generations of tubules to expand to produce the renal pelvis as they do normally.

The condition of the ureters is variable. The part adjacent to the bladder is usually normal but that near the kidney is often narrow although seldom actually atretic. When the urethra is atretic the kidneys are often of typical type II, but when only partially occluded they are usually of type IV (see

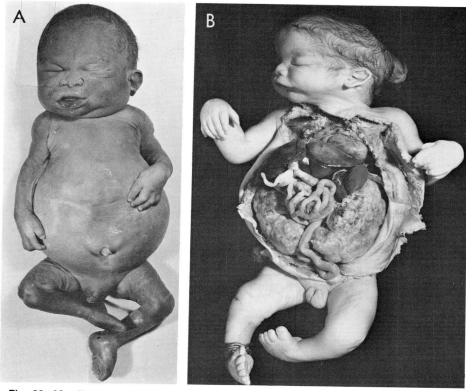

Fig. 22–23.—Two infants with greatly enlarged type IIA (multicystic) kidneys. Both have facies characteristically associated with absent or nonfunctioning kidneys.

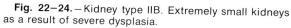

Fig. 22–24.—Kidney type IIB. Extremely small kidneys as a result of severe dysplasia.

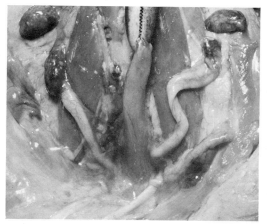

below). With urethral atresia the ureters are usually enlarged and sacculated and the bladder wall thickened.

The liver is seldom abnormal in infants with type II kidneys although malformations in other parts of the body are common and were present in half (60) of the cases in the Chicago Lying-in Hospital series. They involved all organs but especially the brain (anencephaly, cebocephaly, etc.) and the gastrointestinal tract. The liver was normal in all but one case. When both kidneys are affected, the face is usually identical to that associated with renal agenesis.

The condition, if bilateral, is always fatal soon after birth but if one kidney is normal, survival is not affected. In 92 of the 120 cases in the above series neither kidney was normal. Among those in which one was normal the other kidney had a multilocular cyst in eight cases, multiple localized zones of noncystic dysplasia in one and generalized dysplasia in 19. The distribution of the bilateral cases was 43 in type IIA, 24 in type IIB and 17 with

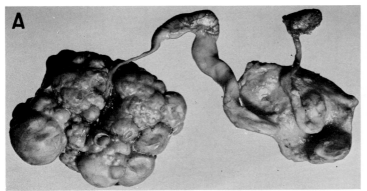
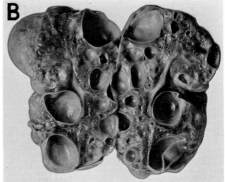

Fig. 22–25. — Type II cystic kidneys in which one is large and cystic (type IIA) and the other small with only a few minute cysts (type IIB). **A,** external surface of both kidneys, ureters and bladder **B,** cut surface of the larger kidney showing multiple irregularly sized cysts associated with diffuse increase in connective tissue.

one of each. In eight type IIB cases one kidney was absent.

This condition has been described clinically as being always unilateral, but this is only because infants with bilateral involvement do not reach the clinician. Actually, bilateral involvement is far more common than unilateral.

In the majority of cases there is no evidence of inheritance although, rarely, a familial distribution has been reported. In one family unilateral agenesis occurred in some members and unilateral type IIB kidneys in others. Juberg *et al.* reported one infant with trisomy C who had large bilateral type II kidneys.

TYPE III (POLYCYSTIC KIDNEYS, POLYCYSTIC KIDNEYS OF THE ADULT AS SEEN IN INFANTS). — This type results from a variable interference with ampullary function acting in a slightly later stage of development and with less severity than in type II. In type II the ampullae are affected so early and so severely that all tubular division is greatly inhibited and nephrons are not induced. In type III the

Fig. 22–26. — Type II cystic kidneys. **A,** right kidney has many large cysts; left kidney had a few small cysts at termination of collecting tubules on microscopic exami- nation. **B,** unilateral involvement in fused kidney; adrenal glands also fused.

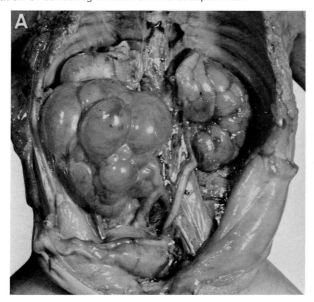
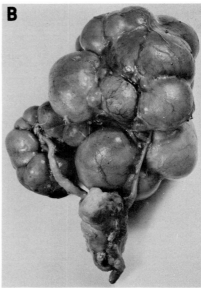

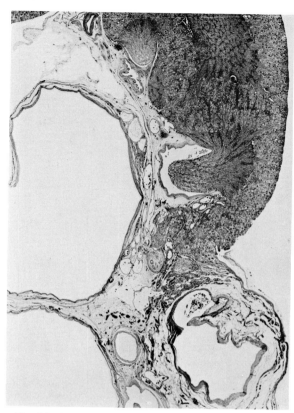

Fig. 22–27.—Type II cystic kidney with segmental involvement. Kidney normal except for multilocular cyst of the lower pole. Newborn infant.

those generally designated *polycystic kidneys.* They are ordinarily not recognized clinically until after the 3d or 4th decade and occasionally produce no symptoms during life even though anatomically similar to those responsible for death (33 cases in the Chicago Lying-in Hospital series). However, kidneys that are anatomically similar may also cause death in infants and small children; some investigators have designated these the "adult variety occurring in infants" (35 cases in the Chicago Lying-in Hospital series). Whether the abnormality is the same disease in infants and adults is not definitely known. A search of the literature fails to reveal any case in which affected parents had children who died of the disease in infancy or childhood or of children dying in infancy who had a parent or other relative with the disease. The Chicago Lying-in Hospital series, however, does include two pairs of siblings all of whom had kidney and liver involvement characteristic of this variety and all of whom died within a few months of birth. The disease, as it occurs in adults, appears to be inherited as an autosomal dominant gene of low penetrance.

Fig. 22–28.—Type IIA enlarged cystic kidney (multicystic). Cut surface shows many cysts of variable size with thick connective tissue walls.

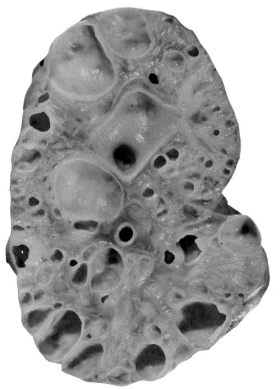

interference occurs slightly later and affects the ampullae of only part of the branches. Those affected are responsible for abnormal division and nephron induction, while those unaffected produce normally branched collecting tubules and nephrons. The number of affected ampullae is variable so that at times the majority are architecturally normal, and at other times, especially when symptoms occur in infancy, the majority are abnormal. Even structures that are architecturally normal are subject to subsequent enlargement, and cysts may develop in Bowman's capsules or any part of collecting tubules or nephrons. There is no evidence that cysts result from obstruction, and attached tubules are ordinarily of normal caliber. This is the only variety of cystic disease in which normal and abnormal collecting tubules and nephrons are intimately intermixed. Both kidneys are generally equally enlarged and only rarely is one normal or involved so slightly that it remains of normal size.

The cases of major importance in type III are

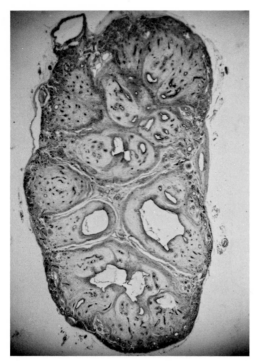

Fig. 22–29.—Type IIB extremely small cystic kidney (dysplastic). Weight 1 gm. No renal pelvis but early generations of tubules are moderately enlarged. No glomeruli and few cysts.

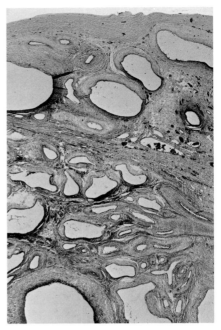

Fig. 22–30.—Photomicrograph of type IIA cystic kidney showing absence of nephrons and multiple thick-walled cysts derived from collecting tubules.

Fig. 22–31.—Photomicrograph of type IIA cystic kidney showing circumscribed zones of connective tissue containing dysplastic tubules. No normal collecting tubules or nephrons.

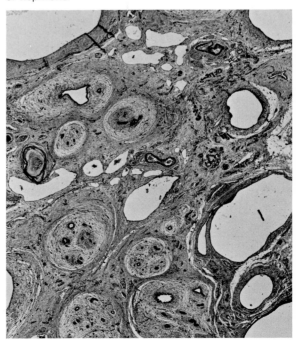

Malformations in parts of the body other than the liver are rare in patients in whom kidney disease is responsible for death.

The anatomic structure of the kidneys in the 68 cases diagnosed as clinically significant type III in the Chicago Lying-in Hospital series was much the same in infants and adults except for the size of the cysts. Cysts were visible grossly in both cortex and medulla (Fig. 22–35, A) and cysts in nephrons and collecting tubules were intermixed with normal structures (Figs. 22–35, B and 22–36). All of those subjected to microdissection, adults as well as infants, had collecting tubules that were abnormally branched (Fig. 22–37), a condition that can be produced only during early development, thus proving a prenatal origin for all cases. The time at which cysts could have been first identified in those cases not recognized until adult life is not definitely known, but here also the changes were the same in adults and infants, and both had cysts in all portions of collecting tubules and nephrons (Fig. 22–38). Cystic kidneys that produce clinical symptoms are rare during the 1st or 2d decades except for the 1st year. It appears that when cyst formation in

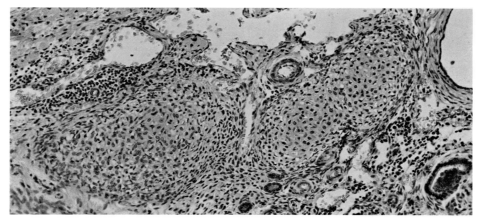

Fig. 22–32.—Islands of cartilage in type IIA cystic kidney. These are present in about 50% of both types IIA and IIB.

Fig. 22–33.—Microdissection of a portion of a type II cystic kidney showing short, poorly branched collecting tubules terminating in cysts of varying size. From same kidney as in Fig. 22–30.

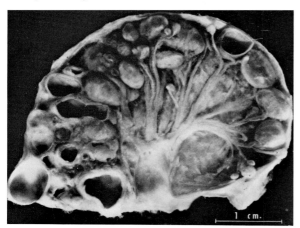

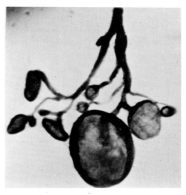

this condition does not begin during prenatal life, only the potentiality for such abnormality exists and its manifestation is held in abeyance for many years.

Because of the variability in the degree of renal change it is not surprising that one kidney may sometimes exhibit more extreme changes than the other, and when—in type III—changes are already well advanced at birth, one kidney may be so severely affected as to resemble type II. Five such cases were present in the material from the Chicago Lying-in Hospital.

The question has arisen as to whether the type III cystic kidney is ever unilateral. In the Chicago Lying-in Hospital material there were several cases in which the condition was severe in one kidney while the other was so mildly affected as to seem normal on gross inspection. Only one case was included, however, that seemed definitely unilateral. Here kidney function was normal at 8 years of age following removal of an enlarged type III kidney at the age of 4 months. In some parts of this kidney there were large areas of normal parenchyma and only localized zones of proliferated connective tissue and scattered cysts (Fig. 22–39, A), while other areas were composed largely of cysts derived from both collecting tubules and nephrons with many in Bowman's capsules, as evidenced by the presence of glomeruli (Fig. 22–39, B).

In both infants and adults the portal connective tissue of the liver is increased in about two thirds of the cases, and in about half of these the number and size of bile ducts are also increased. In young

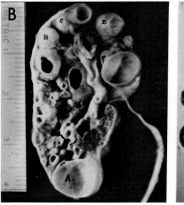
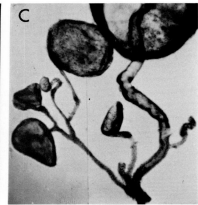

Fig. 22−34.−Type II cystic kidney with stenosis of adjacent portion of ureter. **A,** gross appearance. **B,** partial dissection showing that renal pelvis maintains tubular pattern normal for fetal kidney prior to formation of functioning glomeruli. **C,** microdissection showing characteristic tubules and terminal cysts.

infants the bile ducts are usually slender, undilated channels (see Fig. 20−26, A) but in later life are most often cystic.

The number of cysts that may be present in kidneys of this type is extremely variable. At times only a few late ampullae are affected and the cysts are few in number and of no clinical significance (28 in the Chicago Lying-in Hospital series). In several syndromes such as tuberous sclerosis, trisomy D and cerebrohepatorenal syndrome the disturbance may be somewhat more severe, but here also there are seldom symptoms attributable to the kidneys (11 in the Chicago Lying-in Hospital series).

TYPE III CYSTIC KIDNEYS WITH OTHER SYNDROMES. − In tuberous sclerosis multiple small renal cysts are usually found as an accompaniment of brain and heart lesions (see Figs. 12−38, 24−23 and 24−24). Three such cases are included in the Chicago Lying-in Hospital series of cystic kidneys. In one the cysts were of variable size (Fig. 22−40) and were demonstrated by microdissection to be located in various portions of collecting tubules and

nephrons. In another case only a few small cysts were present. They were lined by large cuboidal cells arranged in a slightly papillary pattern and showed evidence of active mucoid secretion (Fig. 22−41). Other abnormal tissues described in the kidneys of older individuals with tuberous sclerosis, but not in infants, have included Wilms' tumors or focal collections of blood vessels, fibrous tissue, fat and muscle, often designated hamartomas or angiolipomas.

Renal changes characteristic of mild type III cystic disease usually accompany the other abnormalities found as a result of trisomy D (see p. 178). Small cysts are visible beneath the capsule (Fig. 22−42). Microdissection locates them in all portions of collecting tubules and nephrons. Two such cases were included in the Chicago Lying-in Hospital material. Similar renal changes have also been described, although less often, in association with trisomy C and E (Juberg *et al.*).

A *cerebrohepatorenal syndrome* has been described in a few infants, three of whom are included

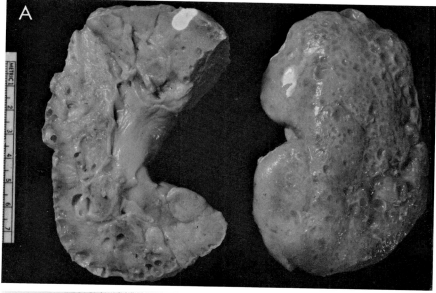

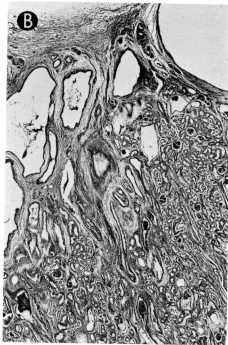

Fig. 22–35.—Type III cystic kidneys, each weighing 175 gm, from infant dying at 4 months with renal insufficiency. **A,** cysts are visible throughout cortex and medulla. **B,** cysts in superficial portion of cortex are terminations of collecting tubules. Many normal nephrons are present.

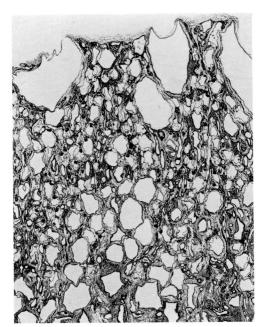

Fig. 22–36. – Type III cystic kidney with cysts in nephrons and collecting tubules. Numerous small cysts contain glomeruli. Infant aged 3 hours; each kidney weighed 220 gm.

in the Chicago Lying-in Hospital material. The infants were hypotonic and developmentally retarded, had minor skeletal malformations and died in the early weeks of life. The kidneys were mildly enlarged and had small cysts in collecting tubules and nephrons; the liver in all had large deposits of pigment in portal areas and sinusoids, producing a characteristic appearance not seen in other conditions (Potter). The brains had leukoencephalomyelopathy. The condition involved two pairs of siblings, and Opitz *et al.* thought its inheritance to be autosomal recessive.

TYPE IV (SECONDARY TO PARTIAL OR INTERMITTENT URETHRAL OBSTRUCTION). – This variety differs from that caused by complete obstruction to urinary outflow as a result of atresia or agenesis of the urethra in which the renal changes occur early and are characteristic of type II cystic kidneys (Fig. 22–43). In type IV, in which some urine escapes through the urethra, formation of collecting tubules is normal, and changes occur only after several generations of nephrons are formed and enough urine is being produced to cause sufficient increase in pressure within the bladder to damage developing nephrons by retrograde pressure exerted through the relatively short collecting tubules. At times this is accompanied by bladder distention and hydronephrosis (Fig. 22–43), especially when the ob-

Fig. 22–37. – Type III cystic kidneys showing moderate enlargement; from newborn infant. **A,** cut surface reveals a tubular pelvis with moderate demarcation into cortex and medulla, a few large and many small cysts. **B,** microdissection of a tubule arising from an abnormal tubular

calix. It gives rise to a few abnormally long branches, each of which has an abnormal cluster of branches. Other tubules had localized and diffuse enlargement, and nephrons had cysts especially in loops of Henle and Bowman's capsules.

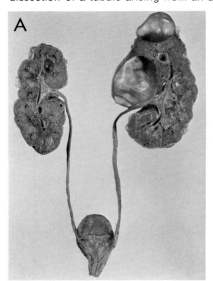

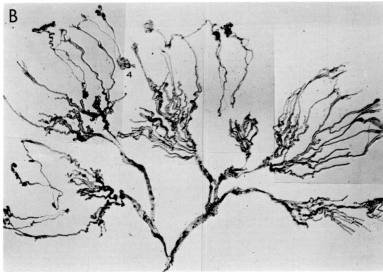

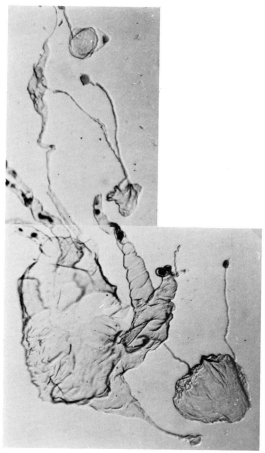

Fig. 22–38.—Type III cystic kidney. Microdissection of collecting tubule detached at renal pelvis. Several branches are dilated into a common cyst, and three nephrons with cysts in loop of Henle are attached. Note normal size of tubules proximal and distal to cysts in loop of Henle and the absence of convoluted tubules. Newborn infant; kidney weight 140 gm.

struction is caused by urethral valves (Fig. 22–44), or at times ureters are normal and the bladder wall is greatly thickened and sometimes trabeculated but not distended (Fig. 22–45). Minute cysts are visible under the capsule both grossly and microscopically (Fig. 22–46, A). They result from damage to developing nephrons while the latter are still in the S-stage of development soon after their attachment to collecting tubules (Fig. 22–46, B). Because the ampullae of the collecting tubules are frequently injured by the increased pressure, no more nephrons are induced and the nephrogenic zone disappears. Ordinarily, enough nephrons are produced before cysts begin to develop to permit the kidneys to

function normally if the obstruction is alleviated soon after birth. There is no evidence of inheritance, and malformations in other organs are rare. There were 16 such cases in the Chicago Lying-in Hospital series.

OTHER CYSTS.—Cysts other than those falling into groups I–IV are rare in infancy. All recognized at the present time appear to result from enlargement of localized portions of collecting tubules or nephrons, the original architectural development of which was normal.

Medullary sponge kidney.—This is found almost exclusively in adults although two cases in newborn infants are included in the Chicago Lying-in Hospital material. Medullary portions of collecting tubules were uniformly enlarged in some segments of all kidneys, and in one the enlargement extended into the cortex in a few places (Fig. 22–47). One infant had Turner's syndrome and fibroelastosis of the heart, the other only a cardiac malformation. Such enlargement of the tubules ordinarily produces no symptoms although in adults the condition is commonly associated with renal lithiasis.

Medullary cystic disease.—This condition was first described by Smith and Graham in an 8-year-old boy who died of renal insufficiency complicated by hyperparathyroidism. It is thought by many to be the same condition described, especially in the European literature, as nephronophthisis. In both, the cysts are limited to the renal medulla. Neither has been observed in infants.

Cysts of Bowman's capsule.—Occasional Bowman's capsules may be dilated in otherwise normal kidneys or in association with cysts in tubules. A disturbance limited to a uniform enlargement of the majority of Bowman's spaces is a rare cause of renal enlargement, but such a case was described by Roos in an 8-month-old infant (Fig. 22–48). Normal-appearing glomeruli were attached to the walls of the cysts, and all tubules appeared normal. Reconstructions were said to show no communication between Bowman's space and tubules and the case was cited as proof that the cause of polycystic kidneys is failure of nephrons to unite with collecting tubules. This is now recognized as untenable inasmuch as all collecting and nephronic tubules appeared normal and the only disturbance was enlargement of Bowman's spaces, a condition that current knowledge of renal development shows could not be caused by failure of union of nephrons and collecting tubules. The cause of interference with outflow of urine from Bowman's spaces in this case is not apparent.

Cysts in nephronic tubules.—Localized cysts in

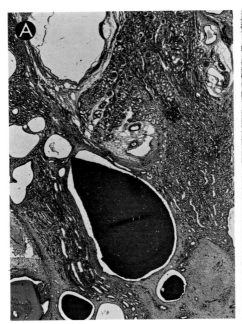
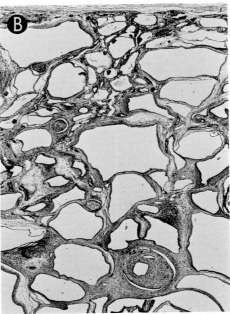

Fig. 22–39. — Unilateral type III cystic kidney removed at age 4 months from child with normal renal function at 8 years. **A,** section showing portions of large zones of normal tubules and nephrons with localized increase in connective tissue and scattered cysts. **B,** portion of peripheral cortex containing multiple cysts in collecting tubules and in nephrons, including Bowman's capsules, as evidenced by presence of glomeruli.

Fig. 22–40. — Mild type III cystic kidney from infant with tuberous sclerosis. Cysts scattered throughout cortex and medulla were present in both collecting tubules and nephrons.

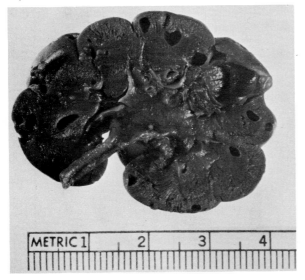

any portions of nephrons are rare except in the type III kidney. When nephrons are the only abnormal structures in the kidney, the enlargements are usually saccular and involve major portions of convoluted tubules, especially proximal convoluted tubules. Diffuse enlargement is characteristically found in galactosemia, and Fetterman *et al.* found mean volume of proximal tubules increased from 50% to 400%. Microcystic disease has been described as having enlarged proximal convoluted tubules, and this designation was used by Oliver to indicate the changes found in the congenital nephrotic syndrome. Since this same term was used by Darmady *et al.* for some type I kidneys, confusion exists as to its exact meaning. A few cases have also been described under this designation in which enlargement was limited to distal convoluted tubules. Such kidneys ordinarily produce no symptoms (Fig. 22–49).

INBORN ERRORS OF METABOLISM

Many inborn errors of metabolism are associated with excretion of abnormal substances in the urine, some because of abnormality of renal function and others only because the abnormal substances are

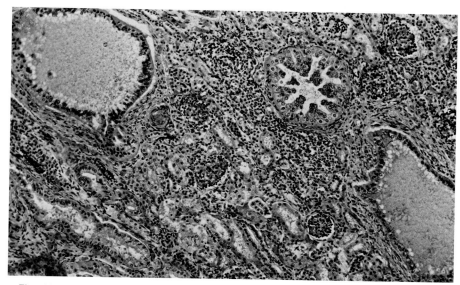

Fig. 22–41.—Kidney in tuberous sclerosis showing characteristic cysts with slight papillary proliferation. Infant aged 22 days. (Brain Lesions, Figs. 24–26 and 24–27; rhabdomyoma of the heart, Fig. 12–38.)

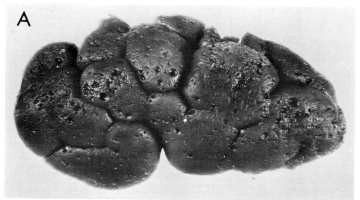

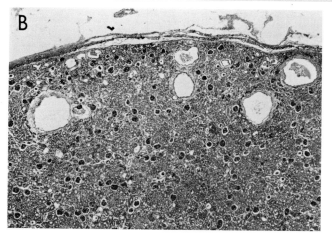

Fig. 22–42.—Kidney from infant with trisomy D with changes characteristic of mild type III cystic kidneys. Multiple small cysts were present in collecting tubules and nephrons in cortex of both kidneys. **A,** gross appearance. **B,** microscopic appearance showing a few small cysts in collecting tubules and nephrons in otherwise normal parenchyma.

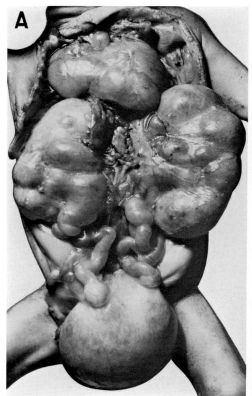
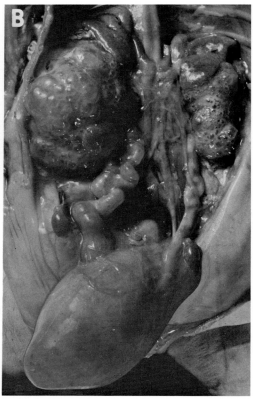
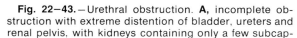

Fig. 22–43.—Urethral obstruction. **A,** incomplete obstruction with extreme distention of bladder, ureters and renal pelvis, with kidneys containing only a few subcapsular cysts. **B,** complete obstruction with distention of bladder, marked tortuosity of ureters and renal pelvis and multiple cysts in kidney similar to those of type II.

present in the blood in excessive amounts. A few, usually observed only in older children, are associated with abnormalities of renal structure. In galactosemia proximal convoluted tubules are dilated, and in the de Toni-Fanconi syndrome with cystinosis a "swan neck" accompanied by narrowing and shortening of the proximal convoluted tubule has been described. In von Gierke's disease excessive glycogen and fat are present in proximal convoluted tubules, hemosiderin is found in thalassemia and sometimes in spherocytosis, and copper has been observed in Wilson's disease.

Oculocerebrorenal Syndrome

This hereditary syndrome is marked by renal dysfunction, mental retardation, hypotonia, growth retardation, bilateral cataracts and glaucoma (Abbassi *et al.*). Most of the changes are present at birth, and by 3 months renal dysfunction is present which includes metabolic tubular acidosis, proteinuria, hyperaminoaciduria and hypophosphatemic renal rickets with osteoporosis and pathologic fractures. It is limited to males, who are short and blond and display choreoathetosis, head wagging, nystagmus and screaming. In the kidney, tubules are dilated and filled with proteinaceous material. The glomeruli are sclerotic and basement membranes thickened. In older patients there may be evidence of tubular atrophy (Richards *et al.*). In the brain there is subpial parenchymal vacuolization, diffuse endothelial proliferation and diffuse astrocytosis of the white matter. Renal insufficiency often causes death in early childhood. The affected males are heterozygotes but with full expression of the gene. Other male sibs may be unaffected.

Abnormal Numbers of Nephrons

Beckwith's syndrome.—Beckwith first described a syndrome, subsequently observed by others, in which macroglossia, omphalocele, adrenal cytomeg-

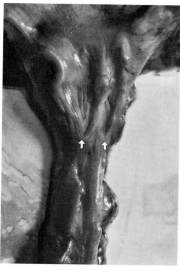
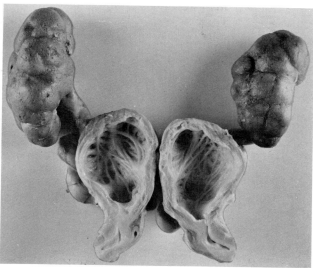

Fig. 22–44 (left).—Partial obstruction of urethra by two cusplike folds of tissue below the verumontanum. New-born infant shown in Fig. 22–43, A.

Fig. 22–45 (right).—Excessive hypertrophy of the bladder with mild hydroureter and microscopic subcapsular cysts in the kidneys secondary to urethral stenosis. Infant aged 3 weeks.

Fig. 22–46.—Type IV cystic kidney from fetus weighing 1,254 gm. **A,** photomicrograph showing subcapsular cysts located in terminal portions of immature nephrons. Previously formed parenchyma normal. Note absence of nephrogenic zone. **B,** microdissection of the last few generations of collecting tubules showing absence of normal arcades and abnormal cortical branching. Terminal cysts result from distention of S-stage nephrons.

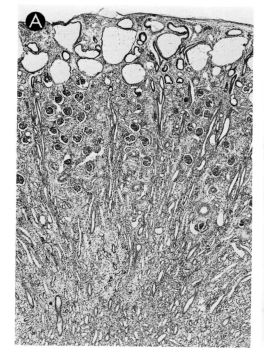
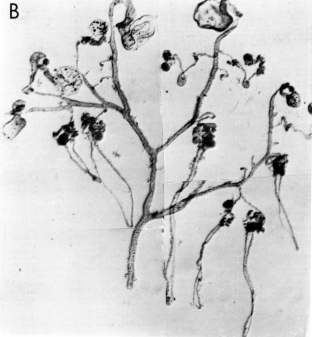

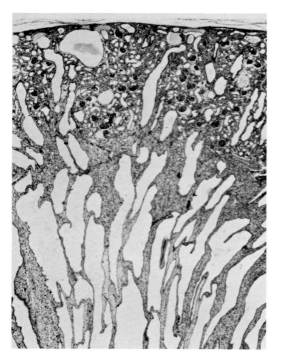

Fig. 22–47.—Medullary sponge kidney showing diffuse enlargement of medullary portions of collecting tubules. In this area cortical portions of a few tubules are also distended. Collecting tubules in some papillae were normal and cortical collecting tubules were seldom involved. Infant aged 3 days with no symptoms of kidney disease.

aly and hyperplasia of the islands and acini of the pancreas exist in conjunction with enlargement of the kidneys (see Fig. 11–4). In surviving children hypoglycemia is usually present and hemihypertrophy may develop. The kidneys have an increased number of lobes, calices and papillae, some papillae lying deep in the kidney and connected to the pelvis by tubules similar to those often found on microdissection of type III polycystic kidneys (Potter). Nephrons are normal and are normally attached to terminal branches of collecting tubules. One child with such kidneys but without the accompanying malformations was observed at the Chicago Lying-in Hospital. Large bilateral abdominal masses were present at birth, and death followed exploratory laparotomy at 2 days of age. Each kidney weighed 120 gm and was composed of normal collecting tubules and nephrons. The only abnormality was an increase and a disarrangement of papillae and calices and the structures arising from them.

OLIGOMÉGANÉPHRONIE.—Several cases were described under this name by Royer *et al.* in which kidneys were reduced in size because of a reduction both in the number of papillae and in the number of nephrons within papillae. In all, however, there was a marked increase in size of individual nephrons. Fetterman and Habib microdissected such a kidney and found the size of proximal convoluted tubules and glomeruli greatly increased. Mean length of proximal tubules was four times and volume 17 times normal; the diameter of glomeruli was twice normal, with surface area five times and volume 12 times normal. Evidence of renal insufficiency usually appears in early infancy and death occurs at 2–3 years of age. The condition has its origin in early fetal life, as evidenced by the reduced number of lobes, with the disturbance continuing into later fetal life, as indicated by the reduction in number of nephrons attached to each collecting tubule. No cases have been described in newborn infants, but since it is probable that the tubular and glomerular hyperplasia are compensatory and only occur subsequent to birth, cases in newborns may have been considered simple hypoplasia.

WILMS' TUMOR (METANEPHROBLASTOMA)

This tumor results from interference with normal maturation of metanephric blastema. Primitive nephrogenic tissue normally differentiates into nephrogenous which produces nephrons, and stromatogenous, which produces connective tissue. Abnormal proliferation of either variety may produce tumors, the former producing the highly malignant tumors of early childhood, the latter the relatively benign tumors found almost exclusively in very young infants.

Tumors arising from this primitive tissue assume several forms that appear to depend on whether tumor formation is initiated in entirely undifferentiated cells or in those already exhibiting some directional proclivity. The majority are highly malignant and are composed of cells lacking definable boundaries and having large hyperchromatic nuclei intermixed with immature tubules and primitive connective tissue. At times one cellular variety predominates, a fact that in the past has given rise to various designations for these tumors—e.g., sarcoma (Fig. 22–50, A) if the cells are completely undifferentiated or are becoming identifiable as capable of producing connective tissue; carcinomas if they are composed principally of immature tubules (Fig. 22–50, B); or carcinosarcoma if tubules and structures derived from connective tissue are both present. In the normally developing kidney stromatogenous cells produce only connective tis-

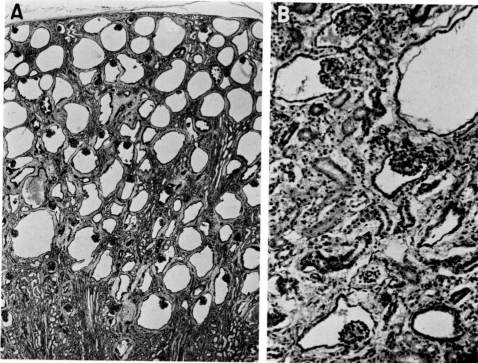

Fig. 22—48.—**A,** kidney showing pronounced dilatation of Bowman's capsules associated with enlargement of the kidneys; infant aged 5 months. (Courtesy Dr. Allan Roos and Children's Memorial Hospital, Chicago.) **B,** kidney showing mild irregular dilatation of Bowman's capsules. A few such glomeruli are not rare in newborn infants and are related to mild obstruction of outflow from Bowman's space but are not caused by failure of union of the two portions of the nephron.

sue, but in these tumors some cells often differentiate into smooth or striated muscle, cartilage or fat cells (Fig. 22–51). The organization of a normal glomerulus is a complex process that is never accomplished in these tumors, but small groups of capillaries or epithelioid cells may produce structures bearing some resemblance to glomeruli.

With few exceptions Wilms' tumors are limited to early childhood, three years being the maximum age. They are usually well-demarcated single nodules although they may be multiple, may involve much of the subcapsular cortex or may be bilateral. When more than one tumor is present, especially when located in both kidneys, they are often considered primary tumors with metastases but it is often impossible to identify any one mass as the primary, and the tumors are more probably of multicentric origin. The cellular pattern of tumors that histologically are definitely malignant cannot be correlated with degree of malignancy, and although the general outlook for survival is poor, cure by simple surgical removal has been reported even

when tumor cells have been present in the renal vein. Distant metastases are most frequent in the lungs, liver and regional lymph nodes. In general the younger the child, the better the prognosis.

Lattimer *et al.*, in compiling one of the largest published groups of nephroblastomas, found 11 in infants under 1 year of age with only one infant dying from the tumor. The diagnosis in the two youngest, aged 3 days and 6 weeks, respectively, was sarcoma; in the others it was carcinosarcoma (5) and carcinoma (4).

A few cases have been reported in newborn infants in whom the tumor was composed of an excessive number of disoriented structures bearing a strong resemblance to normal nephrons and connective tissue. Although there may not be a sharp distinction between such tumors and those containing evidence of cellular immaturity, these are for the most part benign and perhaps should be considered malformations rather than neoplasms (Nicholson).

More common in the newborn than other tumors

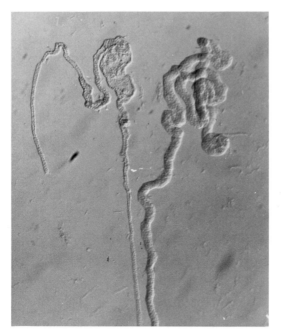

Fig. 22—49.—Saccular enlargement of a portion of a distal convoluted tubule with slight diffuse dilatation of proximal convoluted tubule and descending limb of loop of Henle which has been described as characteristic of microcystic disease. Death at 3 weeks following laparotomy for intussusception.

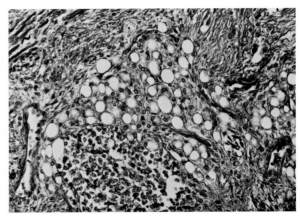

Fig. 22—51.—Wilms' tumor showing differentiation into fat cells and muscle.

of the kidney are those composed exclusively of connective tissue. Although they sometimes contain areas in which cells seem somewhat immature, they are benign tumors. They are encapsulated and ordinarily single (Fig. 22–52, A). However, there is a diffuse involvement of stromatogenous tissue within the affected areas so that normal nephrons are distributed among proliferated connective tissue fasciculi (Fig. 22–52, B).

Polycystic kidneys may rarely have interspersed solid masses of tissue resembling either stromatog-

Fig. 22—50.—Wilms' tumor from infant aged 1 year. **A,** portions of tumor composed largely of undifferentiated blastema. **B,** portion of tumor composed largely of tubules.

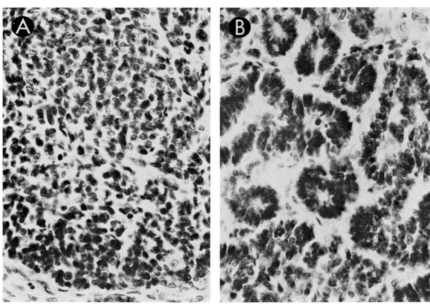

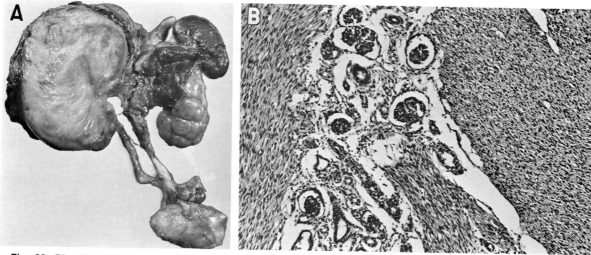

Fig. 22–52.—Solid kidney tumor resembling a fibroma. Newborn infant. **A,** gross appearance of cut surface. **B,** photomicrograph showing connective tissue with an island of normal kidney. (Courtesy Dr. Harvey D. Lynn.)

enous or nephrogenous tumors (Figs. 22–53 and 22–54).

Very small areas in which nephrogenous blastema proliferates abnormally may be found as in situ tumors in fetuses and young infants (Fig. 22–55). The in situ tumors may be single or multiple or, rarely, may involve most of the nephrogenous blastema (Fig. 22–56). They are usually composed of circumscribed masses of cells with large, hyperchromatic nuclei. A few tubules are sometimes also present but other nephroblastic derivatives such as are found in larger tumors in older children are seldom observed.

Wilms' tumors have been found in association with aniridia (Fraumeni and Glass) and with hemihypertrophy (Fraumeni *et al.*) in greater than anticipated frequency although in no case have both been present.

The Chicago Lying-in Hospital series included 11 stromatogenous tumors, 15 in situ nephrogenous tumors, 18 characteristic Wilms' tumors and two associated with polycystic kidneys.

Ureters

DUPLICATION OF URETERS.—Differentiation of kidney parenchyma from the metanephrogenic blastema depends on the stimulation afforded by the presence of the metanephric bud. If one bud fails to arise from the mesonephric duct, the ureter and kidney on that side fail to develop. If both ducts fail to appear, neither ureter nor kidney is formed.

Fig. 22–53.—In situ tumor in a polycystic kidney, the pattern suggestive of an origin in a glomerular anlage.

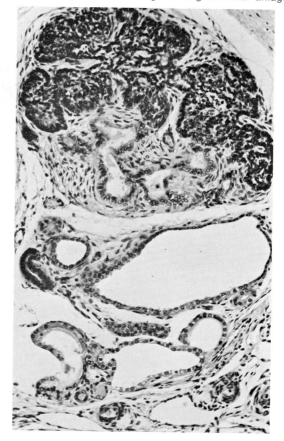

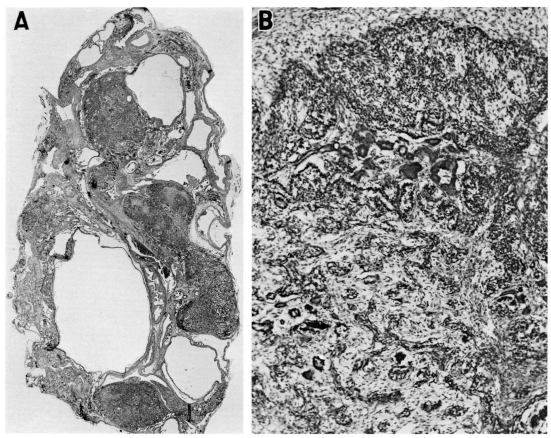

Fig. 22–54.—Small polycystic kidney from a stillborn fetus with islands of tissue resembling a Wilms' tumor. **A,** low power view. **B,** solid and tubular masses with areas of calcification and cartilage (not shown).

One or both mesonephric ducts may give rise to two metanephric buds or, after appearing in a normal manner, one or both buds may divide prematurely, giving rise to partial or complete duplication of the ureters. The two ureters on the involved side may empty separately into the bladder but more often open through a single ureterovesical orifice (Fig. 22–57, A). A single kidney pelvis may receive both ureters, but more frequently a double pelvis is present and each receives a ureter (Fig. 22–57, B). Although a kidney with a double pelvis is elongated and appears enlarged, according to Patten the number of nephrons is not increased. Very rarely, an additional rudimentary kidney is formed and is supplied by one of the accessory ureters.

Occasionally, when a ureter is completely duplicated, only one opens into the bladder. The other, in females, usually opens into the vestibule, less often into the vagina or urethra, while in males the opening may be into the prostate, urethra, seminal vesicles, vas deferens or ejaculatory duct.

The ureter supplying the upper portion of a double pelvis is most commonly the one with the lowermost origin from the bladder if the two ureters arise independently. If one ureter has an ectopic orifice it also is the one usually connected with the upper kidney pelvis. When two ureters supply a single kidney, one or both, as well as the associated kidney pelves, are usually dilated.

HYDROURETER AND HYDRONEPHROSIS.—The lumens of the ureters of the newborn are proportionately somewhat larger than those of the adult. Abnormal dilatation is common with many renal anomalies and may also be an isolated disturbance. Obstruction at the ureterovesical junction is usually partial and is generally caused by local muscular hypertrophy. It is often unilateral but, when bilateral, is usually more severe on one side than

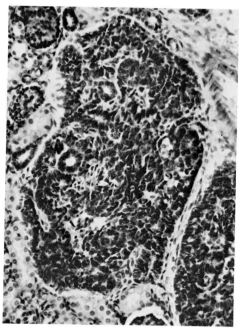

Fig. 22–55.—In situ Wilms' tumor with early tubule formation.

the other. The ureters become progressively more dilated as they ascend from the bladder, and the kidney pelvis is the site of major enlargement (Fig. 22–58, A). Such ureters are often very tortuous. They are easily demonstrated in living infants by roentgen examination.

An obstruction in the form of muscle hypertrophy, partial or complete membrane or actual atresia may exist at the junction of ureter and kidney

Fig. 22–56.—Widespread in situ tumor involving much of the subcapsular region of the kidney in a newborn infant. A similar distribution has been observed in well-developed tumors in older children.

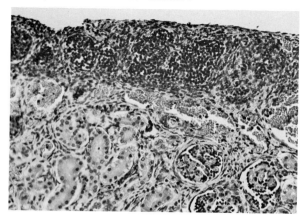

pelvis. In such cases the pelvis alone is dilated and a large saccular structure is produced (Fig. 22–58, B). Urethral obstruction produces varying degrees of ureteral dilatation. The greatest distention observed at the Chicago Lying-in Hospital was in two cases with associated urachal cysts.

MEGAURETER, MEGACYSTIS AND HYDRONEPHROSIS. — The above conditions in association with partial or complete absence of abdominal muscles and cryptorchidism comprise a well-recognized syndrome. Urethral obstruction and/or urachal cysts and renal dysplasia may also be present (see Fig. 22–61), and at other times there is partial absence of bladder musculature. (For further discussion see Absence of Abdominal Muscles, Chapter 26.)

Urinary Bladder and Urethra

DEVELOPMENT

The urinary bladder is formed in part from the allantois, which is an evagination of the hindgut appearing early in embryonic life, and in part from the terminal portion of the hindgut proper, which dilates to form the cloaca caudal to the origin of the allantois. The urorectal fold grows down from the region where the allantois and gut meet and separates the dorsal rectal portion from the anterior urogenital sinus. The upper part of the definitive bladder comes from the allantois, the lower part and the urethra from the cloaca. The upper part of the allantois normally loses its lumen during the latter half of intrauterine life and first becomes a fibrous cord extending from the apex of the bladder to the umbilicus and later disappears altogether. Many types of malformations are possible as a result of the close proximity and original communication of the bladder and rectum and, in the female, the vagina.

The bladder at birth is normally somewhat spindle-shaped, especially when it contains only a little urine. The wall is composed of well-developed muscle and is lined by transitional epithelium. It is constantly being emptied during intrauterine life. The urethral sphincter in this regard differs from the anal sphincter, which normally does not relax before birth and holds the meconium in the intestine. Despite the normal expulsion of urine, the bladder is often somewhat distended at the time of birth and urine is frequently expelled immediately after delivery. If the child dies without urinating, the bladder may be distended at the time of autopsy.

URETHRAL OBSTRUCTION. — The effect on the blad-

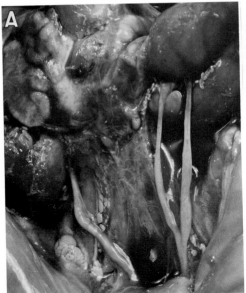

Fig. 22–57.—Double ureter. **A,** unilateral branching of one ureter a short distance from the bladder. The kidney is more spherical than normal and the pelvis is rotated anteriorly. **B,** unilateral double ureter with orifice of the double ureter opening into separate kidney pelves. The ureter emptying into the upper pelvis is moderately dilated.

Fig. 22–58.—**A,** bilateral hydroureter and hydronephrosis associated with moderate stenosis at the ureterovesical orifices. Stillborn fetus. **B,** massive dilatation of the pelvis of one kidney associated with local stenosis of the ureter. Infant aged 2 days.

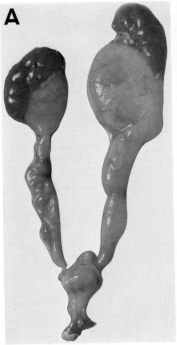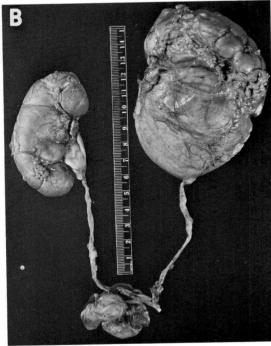

der, ureters and kidneys depends on the degree of obstruction. When partial, all structures are variably distended, the ureters ordinarily becoming progressively more dilated as they reach the kidney and terminate in a distended renal pelvis. When intermittent, as in cusplike valves in the region of the verumontanum, the ureters may not be dilated, but the bladder wall is hypertrophied and sometimes trabeculated (see Fig. 22–45) but not grossly distended. Type IV cysts are usually present in the kidneys. When obstruction is complete, as in atresia or agenesis, the bladder is distended, ureters are sacculated and the kidneys are cystic of a typical type II.

Massive Ascites of the Newborn due to Urethral Obstruction

From 300 cases of fetal ascites in the literature Dockray isolated seven in whom ascites was identified as due to leakage of urine from hydronephrosis caused by obstruction in or below the bladder. In another series collected by the same author 11 surviving infants of 17 with ascites had such obstruction. These cases can be identified by excretory urography because of the formation of a halo around the kidney with extension down the urethral sheath. The pelvis of the kidney must be drained to prevent perirenal infection.

Malformations

Agenesis of the bladder. — Absence of the bladder is rare except in association with anomalies involving other parts of the urogenital system. In sirenomelic monsters the bladder as well as kidneys, ureters, rectum and anus are invariably miss-ing. In one otherwise normal infant in our series the allantois, cloaca and genital tubercle had not developed. There was complete absence of external genitalia, urethra, bladder and urachus. The small intestine was normal, but only the cecum and a few centimeters of large intestine were present. The ureters emptied into the cecum. Both kidneys were moderately hypoplastic and one, which apparently had some obstruction to outflow through the ureter, contained many small cysts (see Fig. 18–32, B).

Abnormal configuration. — Septa in the bladder and diverticulae arising from the bladder and urethra have been reported. True duplication does not seem to exist except in conjoined twins. Abnormal communications between the bladder or urethra and the vagina or rectum may be of many varieties. In the female, communication between the rectum and bladder or urethra is less frequent than in the male; a more common anomaly in the female is a partially undivided urogenital sinus that leads to a communication between the vagina and the urethra or bladder.

Prolapse of the bladder through the vagina has been reported rarely in newborn female infants and only in association with defects of the spinal cord. Even then it is more rare than prolapse of the uterus or rectum or eversion of the urethral mucosa.

Exstrophy (ectropion) of the bladder. — This is a condition in which the interior is open to the surface of the body and the entire mucosal lining is visible above the pubis. The trigone and ureteral orifices can be made out in the lower portion of the suprapubic mass, and in the living child urine can be seen coming from the ureteral openings. The genital organs are abnormal and the pubic bones are widely separated, the latter being responsible for an unstable waddling gait when the child be-

Fig. 22—59. — Ectropion of the bladder. **A,** female with separation of the two halves of the clitoris. **B,** specimen from another newborn infant showing complete lack of fusion of müllerian ducts with a cervix visible on each side of the bladder mucosa.

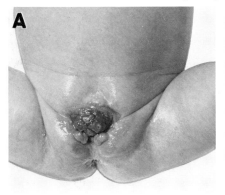
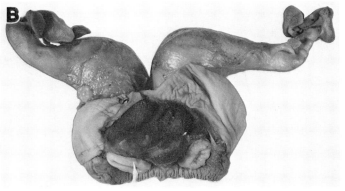

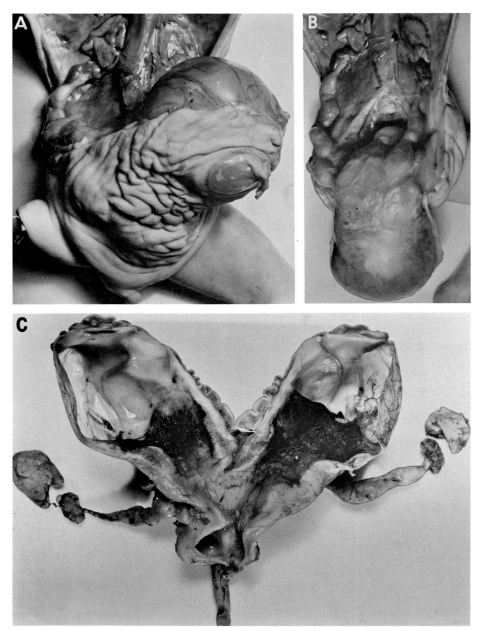

Fig. 22–60. — Urachal cyst and hypoplasia of the kidneys. **A,** cyst in situ showing dilatation of umbilical ring. Right adrenal gland, hypoplastic kidney and dilated ureter are visible. Major part of the right leg was missing; bones extending beyond the stump had penetrated abdominal cavity. Rugose appearance of the skin is due to escape of fluid originally distending the abdomen **B,** anterior abdominal wall removed showing urachal cyst continuous with the bladder; ureters are distended and kidneys are hypoplastic. **C,** opened specimen. Note thinness of the cyst wall and extreme hypertrophy of the bladder wall. Prostatic portion of the urethra is also dilated. There was no anatomic obstruction in the urethra.

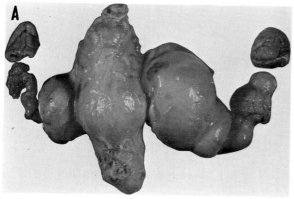
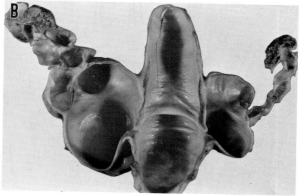

Fig. 22–61.—Urachal cyst, excessive distention of ureters and hypoplastic polycystic kidneys. **A,** exterior view. **B,** interior view. There is no demarcation between the wall of the urachus and the bladder. The urethral orifice was absent.

gins to walk. In the male there is complete epispadias or duplication of the penis and in the female the clitoris is split and develops into two parts lying either superior or inferior to the bladder mucosa (Fig. 22–59). The uterine corpus and cervix are usually double, the vagina often short with mucosa exposed to the exterior. Rarely, the lower portions of the müllerian ducts may be formed and the vagina may be in a normal position.

Ectropion of the bladder is a result of failure of the lower anterior abdominal wall to develop. The unsupported allantois ruptures and the interior is exposed to the surface of the body. This occurs so early that the genital tubercle is as yet undeveloped and the tissue from which it will originate is separated into two portions. This accounts for the apparent duplication of penis or clitoris.

TUMORS

There are almost no reports of tumors of the bladder in the newborn, although one neurinoma of the bladder in an infant who also had a widespread neuroblastoma and ganglioneuroma (see Fig. 12–46) was described by Potter and Parrish.

Urachus

The principal abnormalities of the urachus consist of retention of a lumen in all or part of its length, with or without the formation of cysts and with or without an opening at the umbilicus. The entire urachus may retain a fine lumen, and urine may drain from the umbilicus through this narrow channel. The greater part of the urachus may be obliterated with only local areas remaining patent. Secretory activity of the urachal lining leads to cystic dilatation of any portions that remain patent.

Two cases were observed at the Chicago Lying-in Hospital in which the entire urachus failed to close and was about the same size as the bladder. In both instances the bladder and urachus were greatly distended, and in one case the umbilical ring was dilated to a diameter of 2 cm by pressure of the underlying cyst. In this case one leg had an intrauterine amputation with two small bones protruding from the end. These had perforated the wall of the abdomen, which was thought to have permitted escape of ascitic fluid and to be responsible for the rugose appearance of the abdominal wall (Fig. 22–60). It is typical, however, of the abdominal muscle deficiency syndrome (prune belly syndrome) that occurs without ascites. In this case the muscle of the bladder wall was greatly hypertrophied and the lining was extremely vascular so that the bladder was easily differentiated from the thin, white, avascular wall of the urachus (Fig. 22–60). In the other case the two structures were less well demarcated and the wall of the bladder merged gradually with the urachus (Fig. 22–61). In both cases the proximal portions of the ureters were remarkably distended and the kidneys had the severe dysplasia characteristic of type II kidneys. In the first case the prostatic portion of the urethra was also dilated although no anatomic obstruction could be found in the urethra; in the second the urethra was absent, and although the urinary tract resembled that of the first case, abdominal musculature was normal.

REFERENCES

Abbassi, V., Lowe, C. U., and Calcagno, P. L.: The oculo-cerebro-renal syndrome; a review, Am. J. Dis. Child. 115:145, 1968.

Ashley, D. J. B., and Mostofi, F. K.: Renal agenesis and dysgenesis, J. Urol. 83:211, 1960.

Beckwith, J. B.: Macroglossia, omphalocele, adrenal cytomegaly, gigantism and hyperplastic visceromegaly, Birth Defects Original Article Series, No. 5 (New York: The National Foundation-March of Dimes, 1969), p. 188.

Begg, R. C.: Urachus: Its anatomy, histology and development, J. Anat. 64:170, 1929–1930.

Bell, E. T.: *Diseases of the Kidney* (2d ed.; Philadelphia: Lea & Febiger, 1951).

Burke, E. C., Shin, M. H., and Kelalis, P. P.: Prune-belly syndrome, Am. J. Dis. Child. 117:668, 1969.

Darmady, E. M., Offer, J., and Woodhouse, M. A.: Toxic metabolic defect in polycystic disease of the kidney, Lancet 1:547, 1970.

Davidson, W. M., and Ross, G. I. M.: Bilateral absence of kidneys and related congenital anomalies, J. Pathol. Bacteriol. 68:450, 1954.

Dockray, K. T.: The perirenal P sign, Am. J. Dis. Child. 119:170, 1970.

Ericsson, N. O., and Ivemark, B. I.: Renal dysplasia and pyelonephritis in infants and children, Arch. Pathol. 66:255, 1958.

Fetterman, G. H., and Fabrizio, N. S.: The application of renal microdissection to the study of kidney disease in infancy and childhood, Clin. Pediatr. 5:626, 1966.

Fetterman, G. H., Fabrizio, N. S., and Studnicki, F. M.: Generalized cytomegalic inclusion disease in the newborn. Localization of inclusions in the kidney, Arch. Pathol. 86:86, 1968.

Fetterman, G. H., Fabrizio, N. S., and Studnicki, F. M.: The Study by Microdissection of Structural Defects in Certain Examples of the Hereditary Nephropathies, in *Proceedings of the 3rd International Congress of Nephrology* (Basel and New York: S. Karger A. G., 1967), Vol. 2.

Fetterman, G. H., and Habib, R.: Congenital oligophrenic renal hypoplasia with hypertrophy of nephrons (oligomèganèphroni), Am. J. Clin. Pathol. 52:199, 1969.

Fison, T. N.: Acute glomerulonephritis in infancy, Arch. Dis. Child. 31:101, 1956.

Fraumeni, J. F., Jr., Geiser, C. F., and Manning, M. D.: Wilms' tumor and congenital hemihypertrophy: Report of five new cases and review of literature, Pediatrics 40:886, 1967.

Fraumeni, J. F., Jr., and Glass, A. G.: Wilms' tumor and congenital aniridia, J.A.M.A. 206:825, 1968.

Friedman, H. H., Grayzel, D. M., and Lederer, M.: Kidney lesions in stillborn and newborn infants: Congenital glomerulosclerosis, Am. J. Pathol. 18:699, 1942.

Geisinger, J. F.: Supernumerary kidney, J. Urol. 38:331, 1937.

Gervais, M., Richardson, J. B., Chin, J., and Drummond, K. W.: Immunofluorescent and histologic findings in hemolytic uremic disease, Pediatrics 47:352, 1971.

Gianantonio, C. A., Vitacco, M., Mendelaharzen, F., and Gallo, G.: The hemolytic uremic syndrome, J. Pediatr. 72:757, 1968.

Giles, H. M., Pugh, R. C. B., Darmady, E. M., Stranack, F., and Woolf, L. I.: Nephrotic syndrome in early infan-cy: Report of three cases, Arch. Dis. Child. 32:167, 1957.

Hildebrand: Weiterer Beitrag zur pathologischen Anatomie der Nierengeschwulste, Arch. Klin. Chir. 48:343, 1894.

Juberg, R. C., Gilbert, E. F., and Salisbury, R. S.: Trisomy C in an infant with polycystic kidneys and other malformations, J. Pediatr. 76:598, 1970.

Kampmeier, O. F.: Hitherto unrecognized mode of origin of congenital renal cysts, Surg. Gynecol. Obstet. 26:208, 1923.

Kouvelainen, K.: Immunological features in the congenital nephrotic syndrome: A clinical and experimental study, Ann. Paediatr. Fenn. (supp. 22) 9:1, 1963.

Landing, B. H.: Amnion nodosum: A lesion of the placenta apparently associated with deficient secretion of fetal urine, Am. J. Obstet. Gynecol. 60:1339, 1960.

Lathrop, D. B.: Cystic disease of the liver and kidney, Pediatrics 24:215, 1959.

Lattimer, J. K., Melicow, M. M., and Uson, A. C.: Wilms' tumor: Improved results with modern therapy; review of seventy-one cases, N.Y. State J. Med. 59:415, 1959.

Lieberman, E., Heuser, E., Donnell, G., Landing, B. H., and Hammond, G.: Hemolytic uremic syndrome, N. Engl. J. Med. 275:227, 1966.

Moore, C. M., McAdams, A. J., and Sutherland, J.: Intra-uterine disseminated intravascular coagulation: A syndrome of multiple pregnancy with a dead twin fetus, J. Pediatr. 74:523, 1969.

Nicholson, G. W.: Studies on tumour formation: V. The importance of congenital malformations in tumour formation, Guy's Hosp. Rep. 73:37, 1923.

Norio, R.: Heredity in the congenital nephrotic syndrome, Ann. Paediatr. Fenn. (supp. 27), 12:1, 1966.

Oliver, J.: Microcystic renal disease and its relation to "infantile nephrosis," Am. J. Dis. Child. 100:132, 1960.

Opitz, J. M., et al.: *The Zellweger Syndrome (Cerebro-Hepato-Renal Syndrome)*, Birth Defects Original Article Series, No. 5 (New York: The National Foundation-March of Dimes, 1969), p. 144.

Oppenheimer, E. H., and Esterly, J. R.: Thrombosis in a newborn: Comparison between infants of diabetic and nondiabetic mothers, J. Pediatr. 67:549, 1965.

Osathanondh, V., and Potter, E. L.: Development of the human kidney as shown by microdissection. I. Preparation of tissue with reasons for possible misinterpretation of observations. II. Renal pelvis, calyces and pelvis. III. Formation and interrelationship of collecting tubules and nephrons, Arch. Pathol. 76:271, 277 and 290, 1963.

Osathanondh, V., and Potter, E. L.: Development of the human kidney as shown by microdissection. IV. Development of tubular portions of nephrons. V. Development of vascular pattern of the glomerulus, Arch. Pathol. 82:391 and 403, 1966.

Osathanondh, V., and Potter, E. L.: Pathogenesis of polycystic kidneys: Type I due to hyperplasia of interstitial portions of collecting tubules. Type II due to inhibition of ampullary activity. Type III due to multiple abnormalities of development. Type IV due to urethral occlusion, Arch. Pathol. 77:466, 459, 485, and 502, 1964.

Paatela, M.: Renal microdissection in infants with special reference to the congenital nephrotic syndrome, Ann. Paediatr. Fenn. (supp. 21), 9:1, 1963.

Parker, R. A., and Piel, C. F.: Nephrotic syndrome in the first year of life, Pediatrics 25:967, 1960.

Parkkulainen, K. V., Hjelt, L., and Sirola, K.: Congenital

multicystic dysplasia of kidney: Report of 19 cases with discussion on etiology, nomenclature and classification of cystic dysplasias of kidney, Acta Chir. Scand. (supp.) 244:1, 1959.

Pasternack, A.: Microscopic structural changes in macroscopically normal and pyelonephritic kidneys of children. Ann. Paediatr. Fenn. (supp. 14), 6:1, 1960.

Patten, B. M.: *Human Embryology* (3d ed.; Philadelphia: Blakiston Co., 1968).

Peter, K.: *Untersuchungen uber Bau and Entwicklung der Niere* (Jena: Gustave Fischer, 1909, 1927).

Porter, K. A., and Giles, H. M.: Pathological study of five cases of pyelonephritis in newborn, Arch. Dis. Child. 31:303, 1956.

Potter, E. L.: Bilateral absence of ureters and kidneys: A report of 50 cases, Obstet. Gynecol. 25:3, 1965.

Potter, E. L.: Bilateral renal agenesis, J. Pediatr. 29:68, 1946.

Potter, E. L.: Development of the human glomerulus, Arch. Pathol. 80:241, 1965.

Potter, E. L.: Facial characteristics of infants with bilateral renal agenesis, Am. J. Obstet. Gynecol. 51:855, 1946.

Potter, E. L., and Osathanondh, V.: Medullary sponge kidney, J. Pediatr. 62:901, 1963.

Potter, E. L., and Parrish, J. M.: Neuroblastoma, ganglioneuroma and fibroneuroma in a stillborn fetus, Am. J. Pathol. 18:141, 1942.

Potter, E. L., and Thierstein, S.: Glomerular development in kidney as index of fetal maturity, J. Pediatr. 22:695, 1943.

Reale, P. R., and Esterly, J. R.: Pulmonary development in infants with anencephaly and renal malformations, Am. J. Pathol. 66:19a, 1972.

Richards, W., *et al.*: The occulo-cerebro-renal syndrome of Lowe, Am. J. Dis. Child. 109:185, 1965.

Rizza, J. M., and Downing, S. E.: Bilateral renal agenesis in two female siblings, Am. J. Dis. Child. 121:60, 1971.

Roos, A.: Polycystic kidney: Report of case studied by reconstruction, Am. J. Dis. Child. 61:116, 1941.

Royer, P., Habib, R., and Leclerc, F.: L'hypoplasie Renale Bilaterale and Oligomèganèphronie, in *Proceedings of the 3rd International Congress of Nephrology* (Basel and New York: S. Karger A. G., 1967), Vol. 2, p. 251.

Smith, C. H., and Graham, J. B.: Congenital medullary cysts of the kidneys with severe refractory anemia, Am. J. Dis. Child. 69:369, 1945.

Smith, D. W., Opitz, J. M., and Inborn, S. L.: A syndrome of multiple developmental defects including polycystic kidneys and intrahepatic biliary dysgenesis in 2 siblings, J. Pediatr. 67:617, 1965.

Uson, A. C., Lattimer, J. K., and Melicow, M. M.: Types of exstrophy of urinary bladder and concomitant malformations: Report based on 82 cases, Pediatrics 23:927, 1959.

Verhagen, A. P., Hamilton, J. P., and Genel, M.: Renal vein thrombosis in infants, Arch. Dis. Child. 40:214, 1965.

Welch, K. J.: Abdominal Muscular Deficiency Syndrome, in Mustard, W. T., *et al.* (eds.): *Pediatric Surgery* (Chicago: Year Book Medical Publishers, Inc., 1969), p. 1191.

Williams, P. I., and Eckstein, H. B.: Obstructive valves in posterior urethra, J. Urol. 93:236, 1965.

Zuelzer, W. W., *et al.*: Circulatory diseases of kidney in infancy and childhood, Am. J. Dis. Child. 81:1, 1951.

23

Reproductive Organs and Breast

FOR MANY YEARS it was assumed that all individuals, if sufficiently well investigated, could be designated male or female and that when a discrepancy existed between gonadal and somatic sex, extraneous influences had been responsible for "sex reversal." The structure of the gonad has been accepted as the principal criterion on which to base a diagnosis of sex, and although in general this is still true, recent developments in the study of chromosomes indicate that it is not always possible to assign a definite sex to an individual even when the structure of the gonad is known. The existence of an intersex must be recognized. Since in our society it is not possible for a person to live comfortably without a designation of sex, it is important that the best decision possible be made at the time of birth. In most instances this is fairly easily accomplished, but at times chromosome studies must be made, the structure of the gonads and internal and external genitalia must be known and one factor weighed against another before a decision as to which sex is probably the more appropriate can be reached. In too many instances an adequate evaluation of the sexual status of the newborn is not made and only years later is an abnormality discovered.

Determination of Sex

SEX CHROMOSOMES. — The normal number of chromosomes in human cells has been established as 44 plus two sex chromosomes, XX or XY. Abnormality in number is thought to result from nondisjunction during the first or second stage of meiosis in primi-

tive ova or sperm cells, or in the first mitotic division in the zygote. This could result in the existence of one chromosome too few or too many, depending on whether it was the one that received the nondisjoined pair. Nondisjunction occurring later results in mosaicism, in which part of the cells are normal and part abnormal. Any abnormality in number is associated with some abnormality of development.

The role of the sex chromosomes has been determined by correlations of their presence or absence in normal and abnormal situations. The normal female possesses two X chromosomes, and the normal male has X and Y chromosomes. The loss of one of the two chromosomes during meiotic division gives an XO constitution with a total of 45 chromosomes and produces gonadal dysgenesis (Turner's syndrome). Development, even of the embryo, however, requires the presence of at least one X chromosome, so that a YO (45 total) constitution is lethal and has never been found.

The Y chromosome has a very strong effect on sex determination, and a single Y chromosome will override the effect of two, three or more X chromosomes. An XXY constitution gives rise to a variable phenotype and may be responsible for gonadal immaturity or ambiguity.

Most true hermaphrodites, i.e., individuals with one ovary and one testis or an ovotestis have an XX karyotype, which is normal for the female (Jones *et al.*). When multiple tissues have been typed, mosaicism has sometimes been found, with some cells having an XX constitution and others having a Y in some combination with X, such as

XXY. However, enough hermaphrodites have been karyotyped who had only two X chromosomes in multiple tissues to require some explanation other than mosaicism to account for the presence of gonads of both sexes.

SEX CHROMATIN. — In some of the cells of all females a mass of chromatin within the nucleus, next to the nuclear membrane, has a slightly different staining quality from the rest of the nuclear material. This "heterochromatic" material is called a Barr body after its discoverer (Fig. 23–1). In most tissues some cells of the male also contain these bodies, although they are less common than in the same tissue in the female. A normal female complement of X chromosomes (XX) is necessary for the presence of a normal female quota of Barr bodies. A normal male as well as an individual with Turner's syndrome (XO) has few or no Barr bodies and hence is said to be chromatin negative. In Klinefelter's syndrome (XXY), the Barr body count approaches that of the normal female (XX) because of the presence of two X chromosomes. When the karyotype contains three or more X chromosomes, the number of Barr bodies in a single cell is one less than the number of X chromosomes, so that with three X chromosomes two Barr bodies are present and with 4 X chromosomes there are three.

Buccal smears, which are most frequently used for the determination of sex chromatin, have from 15% to 25% positive cells in normal females and zero to 2% in normal males.

The Barr body is believed to be segregated heterochromatic genetic material that has been inactivated. According to the Lyon hypothesis there is a final segregation of all active genetic material into

Fig. 23–1. — Cell from buccal mucosa showing sex chromatin as a small crescentic mass adjacent to nuclear membrane.

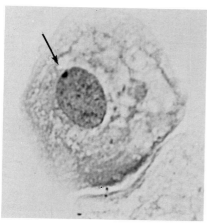

one X chromosome in normal females early in embryonic life. The active chromatic material has derivatives from both maternal and paternal sources; the inactivated chromatic material makes up the Barr body.

GONADS. — The morphology of the gonad is a far more reliable criterion to use in determining the appropriate sex of an individual than is the structure of the internal or external genitalia. This is because hormonal secretion, and consequently secondary sex characteristics, are most often directly related to the type of gonad. There are exceptions, the best recognized being found in individuals with the testicular feminization syndrome (see below).

A few rare cases have been reported in which seminiferous tubules and ova were found in the same gonad. In these cases, as well as those in which one gonad of an individual may resemble an ovary and one a testis, the gonads cannot be used as a means of identifying sex. Individuals possessing such sex glands have often been considered true hermaphrodites, although if this term is limited to individuals capable of functioning as both male and female, none has ever been observed in the human species.

ABNORMALITIES OF SEX DIFFERENTIATION

There are a number of syndromes in which there is a deviation from the normal relationships of the internal and external genitalia, the structure of the gonad and sex chromosomes.

TURNER'S SYNDROME. — Occurring in females, this syndrome is most often associated with an XO karyotype, but it has also been reported in association with mosaics of 45–46 and 45–47 chromosomes. These include:

Mosaic of 45–46 chromosomes
with XX/XO

Mosaic of 45–46 chromosomes
with XO/XY

Mosaic of 45–47 chromosomes
with XO/XYY

Mosaic of 45–47 chromosomes
with XO–XXX

Normal 46 chromosomes with XX

The characteristics of this syndrome include short stature, web neck, a broad shield chest with widely spaced nipples, cubitus valgus and cardiac malformations, particularly coarctation of the aorta (Lemli and Smith). In the newborn, peripheral edema and redundant skin folds in the posterior cervical region may be the only visible signs. The gonads are slender "streaks" of connective tissue which, in the adult, is arranged in whorls reminiscent of the ovarian cortex but without recognizable germ cells or granulosa cells (Fig. 23–2). Although the anlage for the female genital structures is present, without treatment the fallopian tubes, uterus, vagina, external genitalia and breasts remain infantile throughout life. They are capable of responding to exogenous estrogen, however.

A normal complement of two X chromosomes appears necessary to suppress the group of anomalies associated with Turner's syndrome as well as to permit the normal development of the gonads and the attainment of normal growth. Since most patients with Turner's syndrome have a mosaic pattern (Federman), or rarely even have an XX karyotype, considerable variation in phenotype is encountered. The autosomal defects seen in Turner's syndrome have been described in males with a normal karyotype (Avin; Myerson and Swinup). Such individuals have small, often undescended, testes and a small scrotum and prostate.

Only one infant in the Chicago Lying-in Hospital series of autopsies was believed to have had Turner's syndrome. This infant, who weighed 3,600 gm at birth, had an excessive amount of skin over the back and sides of the neck (see Fig. 27–25). The infant appeared to have generalized edema, which on postmortem examination was found to be largely the result of connective tissue increase. The heart was moderately hypertrophied and part of the endocardium and myocardium were hyalinized and slightly calcified (see Fig. 14–13). The striking disturbance was in the ovaries. Like those described in adults, they were cordlike structures approximately the length of the normal newborn ovary but only a fraction of the normal width. Microscopic examination failed to disclose germ cells and/or developing follicles. There seems no doubt that this was an example of Turner's syndrome (Fig. 23–2, A).

Germ cells have been described more often than not in the ovaries of infants with Turner's syndrome. Although Bove described what he thought was only the third case in which no germ cells could be found, the few cells that are ordinarily present appear to be arrested in the prophase of meiosis and incapable of undergoing the further maturation required for follicle development (Manotaya and Potter). Since most of the stroma of the ovary, even before birth, comes from regressed follicles (Potter), the ovary fails to assume a normal size and retains the "streak" appearance throughout life (Fig. 23–2, B).

An increase in X chromosomes is less common

Fig. 23–2.—Turner's syndrome. **A,** ovary from infant aged 10 days with no identifiable germ cells; same infant as in Fig. 27–25. **B,** adult "streak ovary" composed of ovarian stroma with no germ cells.

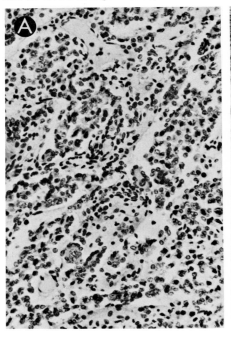
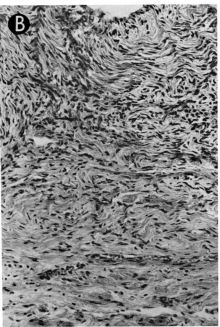

than a decrease. This does not produce a structural abnormality, but fertility is impaired and mental retardation is often associated. One, two or three X chromosomes may be present in addition to the normal two, giving a total of 47, 48 or 49 chromosomes.

KLINEFELTER'S SYNDROME. — Occurring in males, this syndrome is most often associated with the karyotype XXY, but a greater variety of chromosomal abnormalities has been described than in any other condition. These include:

48 chromosomes with XXXY

48 chromosomes with XXYY

49 chromosomes with XXXXY

Mosaic 47 – 46 chromosomes with XXY/XX

Mosaic 47 – 46 chromosomes with XXY/XY

Normal 46 chromosomes with XY

The principal symptom is infertility secondary to gonadal dysgenesis although mental retardation is commonly also present. When occurring with an extra Y chromosome beyond the usual XXY, there is often an increase in height. When additional X chromosomes are added to an XXY karyotype, as in XXXY (48 chromosomes) or XXXXY (49 chromosomes), skeletal anomalies may be present and mental and testicular deficiencies are more severe.

Affected individuals have a phallus of normal size but the testes are small and have sclerotic tubules and no spermatogonia. Leydig cells are normal. There are no somatic abnormalities other than occasional gynecomastia and increase in height.

Unless searched for by examination of buccal smears or karyotyping of large numbers of infants, it is rarely diagnosed in the newborn, although Edlow *et al.* identified such a case in a Negro infant who had a great reduction in the number of spermatogonia in the testicular tubules. Other anomalies of a minor nature were also present such as hypertelorism, long fingers and a simian crease.

TESTICULAR FEMINIZATION SYNDROME. — Occurring in genetic males with morphologically recognizable testes, this is an inherited metabolic disorder in which there is a failure of end-organ response to secreted androgens. The anlage of the prostate, seminal vesicles and phallus fail to develop early in intrauterine life, even though the organizer effect of the testis is present, so that the development of the fallopian tubes is suppressed and the ductus deferens forms normally. Also, as a result of ineffective androgen secretion a uterus, vagina and female external genitalia form. The uterus is small and the vagina short, but the external genitalia are those of a normal female. The testes of patients with testicular feminization are usually cryptorchid and as a result, after the age of 5 or 6 years, have the small tubules and decreased spermatogenesis characteristic of undescended testes.

Such individuals would not be recognized in the 1st year of life unless older siblings had been previously identified as affected.

GONADAL AGENESIS. — Here no gonads develop and the internal and external genitalia resemble those of the female. Some patients have an XY karyotype. These cases, those with testicular feminization and those with lipid adrenal hyperplasia and an XY karyotype but without androgen production all serve to illustrate the point that unless a normal amount of androgen is secreted and endorgan response is normal, internal and external genitalia have a female pattern.

FEMALE PSEUDOHERMAPHRODITISM. — Affected individuals are genetic females (XX) with congenital adrenal hyperplasia and abnormal androgen production (Bongiovanni and Root); if the onset of the excess androgen production is early and of sufficient degree, changes in the vagina and external genitalia result. In the extreme case a phallic urethra develops, the external vaginal orifice is absent because of complete labial fusion and the vagina opens into the posterior urethra. With later onset and less active secretion of androgens by the adrenal gland the phallus is enlarged but labial fusion is incomplete so that the vagina and urethra may open independently at the base of the phallus. When excess adrenal production of androgens is late in onset and only slightly above normal, no abnormalities may be recognized until investigation as to the cause of absence of menses may reveal an enlarged clitoris.

In the male the adrenogenital syndrome rarely causes genital abnormality recognizable at birth except for increased rugosity and pigmentation of the scrotum. Later in the 1st year of life an increase in the size of the penis may call attention to the metabolic defect if electrolyte disturbances have not already done so. Sexual hair develops early, and the testes, though usually in the scrotum, remain small and immature and spermatogenesis does not occur.

The oral ingestion of androgenic progestins or pure androgens (Wilkins) by the mother from the 13th gestational week may cause labial fusion and clitoral hypertrophy, or only clitoral hypertrophy if taken after this time. The three compounds indicated by Grumbach as causing genital abnormalities in 18 affected newborns included 19-nor-17 alpha ethynyltestosterone, norethynodel and 17-alpha-ethynyltestosterone. The internal organs of these infants are presumed to be normal.

LIPID ADRENAL HYPERPLASIA. — In genetic males lipid adrenal hyperplasia gives rise to male pseudohermaphroditism. This condition, found only in newborns, is due to a metabolic block in the conversion of cholesterol to active steroid precursors. Such infants fail to produce not only sex steroids but also adrenal hormone and consequently die of adrenal insufficiency. The adrenal glands are large, heavily infiltrated with lipid, particularly cholesterol, and have focal calcification in the inner cortex. While such individuals have intra-abdominal, histologically normal, small testes and seminiferous ducts, the latter due to the presence of the local organizing activity of the embryonic testis, they have female external genitalia and a short blind vagina. They lack a uterus and fallopian tubes (Prader and Sievernmann; O'Doherty). In two of the three cases described by Prader and Sievernmann a rudimentary prostate was present; in the third it was absent. Females with the same metabolic block have normal genitalia consistent with their XX genotype.

MIXED GONADAL GENESIS. — Here the development of the external genitalia may vary from that of a normal male with slight hypospadias, through partial fusion of the labioscrotal folds, to the hypoplastic external genitalia of Turner's syndrome. Affected individuals have an XO, XX mosaicism, and a significant number have the somatic malformations found in Turner's syndrome, having a pure XO constitution. Most of the individuals in this group are raised as females, but many become masculinized at puberty. A few individuals with excessive hormonal activity because of later developing gonadal tumors are feminized precociously and never become masculinized (Sohval).

TRUE HERMAPHRODITISM. — A testis and an ovary may be present on opposite sides of the body, one of each on both sides or one or the other on one side and an ovotestis on the other. The location in the peritoneal cavity or scrotum tends to follow the usual disposition for the particular gonad. Ovotestes are present with about equal frequency in the abdominal cavity and scrotum. In most cases the external genitalia more nearly resemble the male, but hypospadias occurs in nearly all. A uterus is usually present but a fallopian tube develops only when a testis is not present on that side. Inguinal hernias are common. After puberty, ovulation and menstruation may occur but spermato-genesis is rare. Ovotestes have ovarian stroma and primitive oogonia near the surface of the organ and immature tubules with some spermatogonia in deeper portions covered by a fairly well-defined capsule. Interstitial cells are present.

The relative frequency of many of the above disorders encountered in an endocrine clinic serving patients of all ages was given by Wilkins as follows: Of 324 cases Turner's syndrome accounted for 87, Klinefelter's syndrome 12, mixed gonadal dysgenesis 11, true hermaphroditism 4, male pseudohermaphroditism 66 (of whom 46 had ambiguous genitalia) and female pseudohermaphroditism 138 (of whom 100 had the adrenogenital syndrome and 38 had a nonadrenal origin).

Female Sex Organs

The fallopian tubes, uterus and most of the vagina arise from the müllerian ducts, which make their first appearance in embryos of both sexes during the middle of the 2d month. The ducts are formed by an invagination of the celomic epithelium into the mesenchyme adjacent to the cranial end of the mesonephric duct. They grow downward, lateral to the mesonephric ducts, until they approach the caudal end of the embryo. There they turn anteromedially, meet in the midline and continue to grow downward to open into the urogenital sinus. Although the ducts are initially the same, the subsequent pattern of growth is different in the two sexes. In the female the most cephalic portions remain separate to form the two fallopian tubes. The lower portions fuse and the cavities of the two ducts become confluent and differentiate into the uterine corpus, cervix and major portion of the vagina. The lowermost part of the vagina is formed by an invagination of surface ectoderm. In the male the müllerian ducts largely disappear and persist only as rudimentary vestiges without function.

At birth the anatomic structure of the uterus and vagina is far from being a miniature replica of the adult. The uterine corpus is proportionately small and makes up only one third or less of the total length of the uterus (Fig. 23–3). The muscular layer is thin and the endometrium is composed of a single layer of low columnar cells, with endometrial glands indicated by a few shallow indentations and stroma by a few specialized connective tissue cells. In a few cases some secretory activity may be seen in the endometrium, and a decidua-like change is occasionally found (Fig. 23–4). The cervix makes up about two thirds of the length of the uterus and the wall is at least twice as thick as the

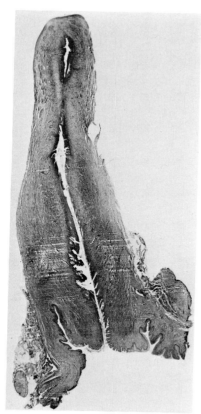

Fig. 23–3.—Uterine corpus, cervix and small portion of vagina of a mature stillborn fetus. The uterine corpus occupies approximately one third of the total length. The endocervical glands extend out onto the vaginal portion of the cervix.

Fig. 23–4.—Decidual change in the endometrium of an infant of a diabetic mother.

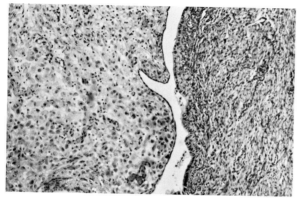

wall of the corpus. The endocervical glands are racemose structures lined by columnar cells that are actively secretory during the latter part of fetal life. The portio of the cervix is covered by a thick layer of squamous epithelium that continues uninterruptedly over the inner surface of the vagina. At birth the endocervical canal is ordinarily distended by a large plug of tenacious mucus. When the mucus plug is removed, the lower end of the cervix is widely patent and the external os may be as much as 1 cm in diameter. The os is poorly defined, and endocervical glands often extend out onto the portio a considerable distance beyond the canal. The poor delineation of the external os and the extension of glands onto the portio are responsible for so-called congenital erosions. Following birth the cervix shrinks, and as the external os becomes better delineated, the portion containing glands is ordinarily withdrawn into the canal. Glandlike structures or cysts measuring several millimeters in diameter are occasionally found in the depths of the cervical tissue. They are lined by low columnar cells and are persistent portions of the mesonephric ducts. In this location they are designated Gartner's duct cysts and may be found in older individuals as well as in newborn infants.

The cervix at birth usually extends almost a centimeter into the vagina, the posterior lip being somewhat longer than the anterior, as in the adult. The vaginal walls are approximated but they have a remarkable distensibility and are easily stretched to a circumference of 4–5 cm. In the undilated state the vaginal wall is thrown into rugae and the epithelium appears exceedingly thick, but when the vagina is distended and the folds are separated, the epithelium becomes considerably thinner. Even then it is somewhat thicker than in the older child and the cells are richer in glycogen. It is believed that passage of maternal hormones to the fetus during pregnancy is responsible for the state of the vaginal epithelium at birth as well as for the size of the uterus. The uterus shrinks gradually after birth and at 6 months is only about half the size it is at birth. This shrinkage is proportionately greater in the cervix than in the corpus, but the cervix remains larger than the corpus until the child is several years old. The length of the entire uterus at birth is about 4 cm.

At birth the hymen forms a thick cuff-shaped fold of tissue protruding out from the lower margin of the vaginal orifice instead of being a flat membrane closing the lower end of the vagina as it is in later life. It will usually admit the little finger without excessive stretching.

Abnormalities in the development of the perineal body, vagina, labia and clitoris are fairly common but usually no chromosomal or hormonal abnormality can be demonstrated. In a few instances, though, abnormalities of the clitoris or labia may be an effect of masculinizing hormones present in the fetus prenatally. Hyperactivity of the fetal adrenals as in Cushing's disease, the existence of a virilizing tumor or the administration to the mother during pregnancy of certain hormones containing testosterone-like substances may be responsible for hypertrophy of the fetal clitoris (see Fig. 16–23, A). This may be accompanied by partial fusion of the posterior portions of the labia. Hypertrophy of the clitoris accompanied by fusion of the labia, so that the vaginal orifice is obscured, constitutes the most common abnormality designated female pseudohermaphroditism.

Infection

Infections of the genitalia are uncommon in infancy but have been reported as having been caused by a variety of organisms. One infant observed at the Chicago Lying-in Hospital had a diphtheritic membrane in the vagina. The mother's disease was at its height at the time of delivery and the infant was not treated until a vaginal membrane developed a few days later. The infant died at 7 days of age.

Gonorrheal infection of the vagina may take place at the time of delivery, although this area is less commonly affected than the eyes. Most infants have a little mucoid exudation from the vagina, but if it is copious or purulent, a gonorrheal infection should be suspected. Smears or cultures will establish the diagnosis. Gonorrheal septicemia has been observed following a local infection.

The genital organs are rarely infected with *Candida albicans* despite the frequent exposure to maternal organisms in the birth canal. The mouth appears to be much more susceptible, and Candida infections occur there fairly commonly unless prophylactic steps are taken.

Abscesses of the vulva, usually from nonspecific infections, are occasionally observed.

Malformations

INTERNAL ORGANS. — The fact that the uterus and vagina normally are formed by the fusion of two tubelike structures permits many departures from

Fig. 23–5. — Abnormal uteri. **A,** absence of the right fallopian tube and uterine cornu due to failure of development of the right müllerian duct. **B,** double uterine corpus with single cervix and vagina; double left ureter.

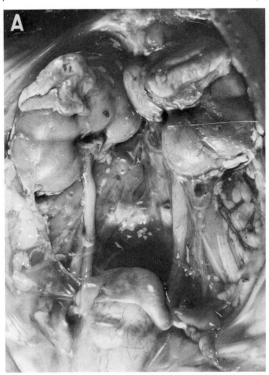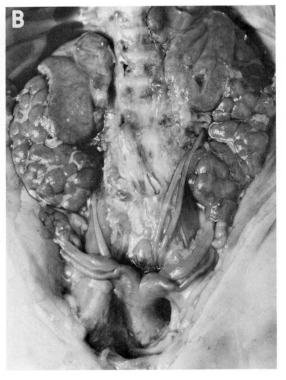

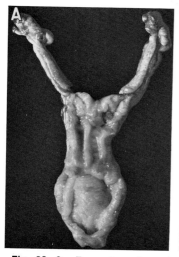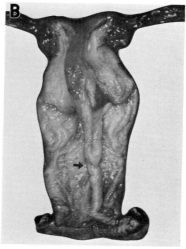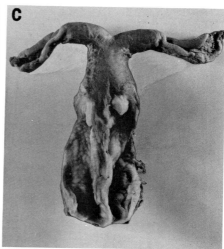

Fig. 23–6.—Examples of varying degrees of lack of fusion of müllerian ducts. **A,** double uterine corpus. A ridge extends the length of the cervix but it and the vagina both have single cavities. **B,** duplication of uterine corpus, cervix and upper half of vagina. *Arrow* indicates the lower border of the vaginal septum. **C,** complete duplication of uterine corpus, cervix and vagina; two vaginal orifices.

the usual configuration. The superior portions of the müllerian ducts, which do not fuse and which develop into the paired fallopian tubes, are less often affected than the lower portions. A uterus is rarely present without at least one fallopian tube attached to it. Both fallopian tubes, however, may be present without evidence of a uterus. In such cases the tubes usually end blindly without reaching a midline. Such an abnormality is most often an accompaniment of bilateral renal agenesis.

Complete failure of development of both müllerian ducts is rare except in sirenomelic monsters. Not infrequently, however, only one müllerian duct develops and produces a uterus that appears fairly normal except for the absence of one uterine cornu and the tube that should be connected with it (Fig. 23–5, A). The upper part of both müllerian ducts may develop but the lower part of one may be abnormal or absent. In such cases the fallopian tube on the affected side usually communicates with a rudimentary uterine cornu or ends blindly in the wall of the upper part of the corpus.

Incomplete fusion of the parts of the müllerian duct that give rise to uterus, cervix and vagina is of variable extent. The lack of fusion may be slight, resulting in an arcuate uterus with a fundus only slightly less rounded than normal. Progressive degrees of lack of fusion produce a bicornuate uterus that has a mild but definite division of the upper portion of the fundus, a uterus duplex in which the entire corpus is duplicated (Figs. 23–5, B and 23–6, A) and a uterus didelphys in which the cervix as

well as the corpus is double and in which there may be a septum extending a variable distance through the vagina (Fig. 23–6, B and C). When the corpus is double, the two parts may be fused into a single mass or they may be separate and each be surrounded by its own peritoneal covering. The cervix and vagina, if double, are almost always fused except in association with ectropion of the bladder, in which a fallopian tube, uterus, cervix and vagina are present on each side of the exposed bladder mucosa (see Fig. 22–59).

At times one müllerian duct remains underdeveloped and fuses incompletely with its normal mate. In such instances one part of a double uterus is of about normal size and the other is hypoplastic.

Duplication of the uterus and the vagina is usually such that the two parts lie side by side and the dividing partitions extend anteroposteriorly. In rare instances a septum in the vagina or cervix extends laterally, and one structure lies in front of the other. This is almost never true of the divided corpus.

A septum may partially or completely divide the vagina, cervix or both into right and left halves even though the corpus is single. This is less common than the reverse, in which the corpus is double and the cervix and vagina are single.

The vagina, in addition to being abnormal because the müllerian ducts fail to fuse, may also be affected by disturbances in differentiation of the cloaca and urogenital sinus. Even though the lower portions of the müllerian ducts are absent, an in-

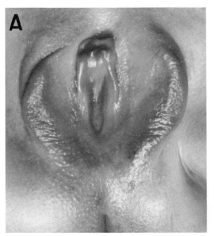

Fig. 23–7.—Abnormal vaginal orifices. **A,** agenesis of urethra and vagina associated with complete agenesis of kidneys and uterus. Indentation between labia minora represents the ectodermal component of the vagina. **B,** a fold of perineum extends anteriorly and covers the vaginal and urethral orifices This abnormality has been reported in association with hyperadrenalism or as a result of maternally administered hormones. Adrenals in this case appeared normal. The probe extends into the vagina.

dentation of varying depth is found at the usual site of the vagina if the urogenital sinus develops normally (Fig. 23–7, A). This comes from ectodermal elements normally producing the lower portion of the vagina and hymen.

Abnormalities in the development of structures that normally open to the exterior through separate channels may lead to various malformations. Rarely, a modified cloaca persists, and intestine, urinary tract and vagina may open to the exterior through a single channel. The urethra or rectum may empty into the vagina, or the lower end of the vagina may communicate with either of these structures. Rarely, the urethra opens into a vagina with a closed external orifice. Flow of urine into the vagina ordinarily causes extreme distention, not only of this structure but of the uterine corpus. If the vagina opens into the urethra or rectum or if a fold of perineum grows forward and hides the orifices of both vagina and urethra, as it does in some forms of female pseudohermaphroditism, the vagina may erroneously be thought to be absent (Fig. 23–7, B).

Abnormal separation of the vaginal canal from the vulva can take one of three forms. The first is a transverse septum, which is present immediately below the cervix and is a remnant of the urogenital sinus (Fig. 23–8). The second is atresia of the lower 2–3 cm of the vagina. McKusick et al. described this as an hereditary defect in two Amish sibships descended from a single ancestral couple. The third form is an imperforate hymen, which may have minute defects or be entirely imperforate.

In any one of these forms of vaginal obstruction marked dilatation of the vagina (hydrocolpos), or vagina, cervix and uterus (hydrometrocolpos) (Figs. 23–9 and 23–10, A), may occur. The uterus may enlarge sufficiently to cause intestinal obstruction or respiratory distress. This unusual distention of the reproductive tract occurs most commonly either in the immediate postnatal or premenarchal periods when cervical secretion is most active. Spencer and Levy gathered 62 cases of hydrometrocolpos from the literature; 40 were due to an imperforate hymen, 13 to vaginal atresia and seven to a transverse vaginal septum. After puberty similar obstruction gives rise to hematocolpos.

Fig. 23–8.—Vagina closed by a transverse septum and associated with duplication of uterine corpus, cervix and upper vagina in infant with bilateral renal agenesis.

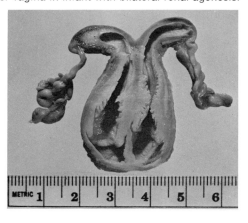

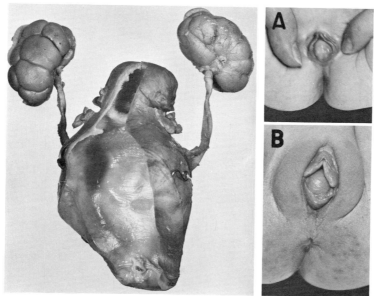

Fig. 23–9 (left).—Hydrometrocolpos. Extreme distention of the uterine corpus, cervix and vagina with occlusion of the vaginal orifice. The cavity was filled with mucoid material, presumably a result of hypersecretion of the endocervical glands. (Courtesy Dr. Jack Kirschbaum.)

Fig. 23–10 (right).—Cystlike protrusions through vaginal orifice. **A,** imperforate hymen with hydrocolpos in infant aged 7 weeks. (Courtesy Dr. Rustin MacIntosh.) **B,** cyst in wall of the vagina, presenting at the vaginal orifice. Presence of the hymenal ring, the edge of which is visible posteriorly, differentiates this condition from protrusion caused by an imperforate hymen.

For a few days after birth the vagina is normally filled with a thick yellow material consisting of mucus and masses of desquamated mature squamous cells. This desquamation accompanies the sharp fall in estrogen that occurs after birth because of withdrawal of maternal hormones. By 10 days of age smears from the newborn vagina consist only of immature intermediate and basilar squamous cells; by 4–7 months the cells have assumed the normally atrophic character of the premenarchal child (Elstein).

A cyst arising in the wall of the vagina may be confused with an imperforate hyman. The cyst may protrude through the introitus, and, unless carefully investigated, the overlying hymenal membrane may not be observed (Fig. 23–10, B). Such cysts are most often the result of abnormal development of the lower part of the mesonephric duct. Small cysts may also be found on the margin of the hymenal ring or attached to it by a small pedicle (Fig. 23–11).

Fig. 23–11.—Cyst of the hymenal ring.

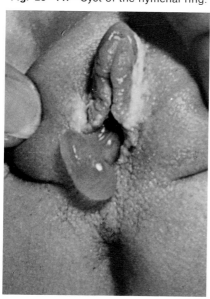

Prolapse of the vagina may occur rarely in an otherwise normal infant. The diagnosis is usually made without difficulty, although it is occasionally confused with a vaginal cyst. It was described in the newborn by Cottons, who associated it with urinary obstruction; the latter may be relieved by replacement of the fallen organs and the prolapse seldom recurs.

A groove extending from the posterior labial commissure to the anus is another anomaly seen in the newborn infant (Fig. 23–12). It remains practically unchanged throughout life.

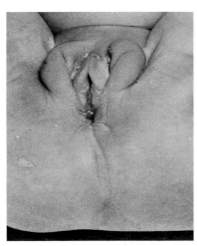

Fig. 23—12.—Perineal groove connecting vaginal orifice and anus. The anus is more anterior in location than normal. Newborn infant.

Abnormalities of the clitoris and labia may cause difficulty in establishing the sex of small infants. Hypertrophy of the clitoris, particularly if associated with absence of the vagina or with a concealed vaginal orifice, may lead to an erroneous assumption that the infant is a hypospadic male (Fig. 23–13, A). Clitoral hypertrophy may be associated with other anomalies, and on rare occasions the urethra penetrates the clitoris and produces a structure closely resembling a penis (Fig. 23–13, B). This was observed in four infants at the Chicago Lying-

in Hospital, all of whom had complete bilateral renal agenesis and absence of the uterine corpus and cervix although the ovaries and fallopian tubes were present.

Tumors

Malignant tumors of the female genitalia in the 1st year of life appear to be limited to the cervix and vagina. The most common is sarcoma botryoides of the cervix and upper vagina, which has primitive myoblasts mixed with other more undifferentiated sarcomatous elements in an edematous, papillary type of growth. The presence of malignant stroma beneath benign cervical epithelium is a characteristic feature. The tumors grow rapidly within the vagina but in early stages remain localized to the pelvis. Similar tumors arise in the prostate in the male, and together they account for about 25% of all rhabdomyosarcomas observed in children. In infants under 1 year of age such tumors are usually fatal regardless of location. All seven patients of this age reported by Grosfield *et al.* died, although in their series of children of all ages 30% with pelvic rhabdomyosarcomas survived.

The other important tumor of the genital tract at this age is a poorly differentiated papillary adenocarcinoma of the cervix and vagina (Fig. 23–14). Bayes *et al.* reported a case and cited four from the literature, all in infants under 1 year of age. This tumor had rarely been seen after puberty until recently when Herbst *et al.* described them in young

Fig. 23—13.—Pseudohermaphrodites. **A,** hypertrophied clitoris resembles hypospadic penis, Vaginal orifice is absent, and labia resemble a bilobate scrotum. Internal sex organs were those of a normal newborn female. **B,** female infant with renal agenesis. Ovaries and fallopian tubes normal. No vagina or uterine corpus except small nodule adjacent to lower end of left tube. Phallus 2 cm long with central urethra. Sex chromatin positive

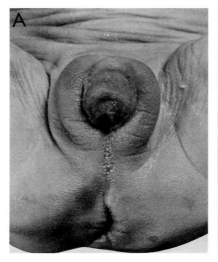
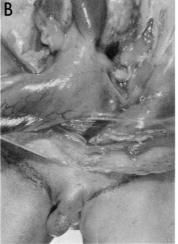

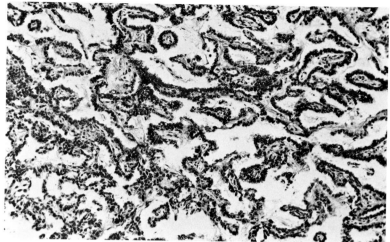

Fig. 23–14.—Papillary carcinoma of the vagina composed of papillary epithelial growths with little stroma. Death occurred from metastases a short time after removal of the tumor at 2 months of age.

postmenarchal women whose mothers had received large doses of stilbestrol early in gestation. The epithelium in the tumors of young infants as well as in adolescents is composed of cells with enlarged nuclei protruding beyond constricted bases. It resembles the epithelium in the glomerular tufts of the mesonephros and suggests a mesonephric origin. Similar tumors have been reported as arising in the vagina and vulva (Hoge and Benn; Norris *et al.*). Most have been rapidly fatal.

Male Sex Organs

As the mesonephroi degenerate and lose their function as excretory organs, the principal ducts and part of the tubules are converted into channels for the discharge of sperm cells. A few of the tubules nearest the testes form the efferent ducts that communicate with the seminiferous tubules, and these together with the portions of mesonephric ducts into which they empty become the epididymides. The remainder of each mesonephric duct becomes a ductus deferens through which sperm cells are discharged into the prostatic portion of the urethra. Early in fetal life the mesonephric ducts open into the urogenital sinus, but as growth proceeds, the relationships are altered and they communicate with the urethra a short distance below its origin from the bladder.

The seminal vesicles arise as small outpouchings from the ductus deferentes near their insertion into the urethra. Repeated branching takes place, and at birth the glands are flat, somewhat elliptic struc-

tures closely adherent to the posterior bladder wall (Fig. 23–15). If a kidney is absent, the corresponding epididymis, ductus deferens and seminal vesicle may also be missing.

The prostate arises by an evagination of glands from the urethral wall near the region where it is joined by the ductus deferentes. The glands grow into mesenchyme, which becomes converted into fibromuscular tissue (Fig. 23–16). At birth the prostate is a globular mass almost 1 cm in diameter. Anterior and posterior lobes are moderately well demarcated. The prostatic utricle is lined by and filled with squamous cells as a result of the high levels of circulating estrogens. As in the cervix, with a postnatal fall in estrogen level these squamous cells desquamate and are replaced by low cuboidal or transitional cells (Fig. 23–17).

The urethra arises from the anterior portion of the urogenital sinus. As the genital tubercle elongates, the sinus that lies on its inferior surface is gradually enclosed by the urethral folds lying at its margins. Normally it becomes completely enclosed and the urethral orifice is located at the distal end of the penis. The shaft of the penis is made up of the urethra and the corpora cavernosa, which also come from the genital tubercle.

MALFORMATIONS

HYPOSPADIAS. — The abnormal location of the urethral meatus, which is the most common malformation of the male sex organs, results from incomplete or abnormal fusion of the urethral folds on

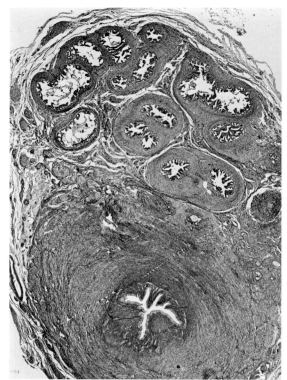

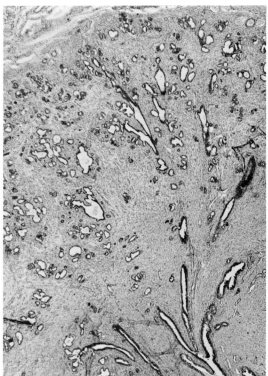

Fig. 23–15 (left).—Normal seminal vesicles adjacent to the posterior wall of the lower part of the urinary bladder from mature newborn infant.

Fig. 23–16 (right).—Portion of normal prostate from mature newborn infant.

the inferior surface of the genital tubercle. In a mild form of hypospadias the urethral orifice is located on the inferior surface of the glans near the attachment of the prepuce (Fig. 23–18, A). In a more severe form the defect extends along part or all of the inferior surface of the penis. If it extends

Fig. 23–17.—Ejaculatory ducts just before their entry into the upper urethra. They are filled with squamous cells whose desquamation shortly after birth results in canalization of the ducts.

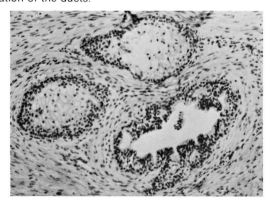

the entire length, the condition is designated complete hypospadias, and the urethral orifice is located at the junction of the penis and scrotum (Fig. 23–18, B). With such a severe defect the corpora cavernosa are frequently smaller than normal and the size of the penis is reduced, sometimes being mistaken for a hypertrophied clitoris. If the region of the median raphe of the scrotum is indented and the scrotum is bilobate, the two parts of the scrotum are often interpreted as labia associated with absence of the vagina. If the testes are in the scrotum, they can usually be palpated and the mistake avoided. If they are undescended, it may be impossible to ascertain the sex from external examination. This is the most common anomaly giving rise to confusion as to sex.

EPISPADIAS.—In this condition the urethral meatus is on the dorsum of the penis. It is much less common than an opening on the inferior surface. In its most extreme form it is associated with exstrophy of the bladder, and the urethra is open to the exterior throughout its length. Occasionally, in an otherwise normal organ a secondary meatus is present on the dorsal surface which is supplied by an

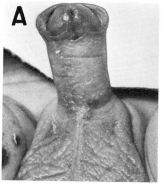
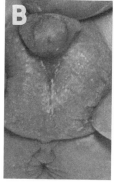
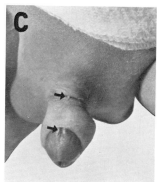

Fig. 23–18.—Abnormal location of urethral meatus. **A,** mild hypospadias with slight downward displacement of urethral meatus. **B,** complete hypospadias with urethral meatus at the base of an abnormally short penis. **C,** epi-spadias with two accessory urethral orifices on the dorsum of the penis, one at the junction of the glans and prepuce and one in the area visible as a fold of skin near the base of the penis.

accessory canal arising from the urethra near its distal end (Fig. 23 – 18, C).

PENILE AGENESIS AND HYPOPLASIA. — Absence of the penis is uncommon except in sirenomelic monsters, in whom it is associated with an imperforate anus and absence of kidneys and all genital organs except testes. When the penis is absent in infants with normally developed lower extremities, the bladder may also be absent and the ureters then open individually into the intestine or end blindly; if the bladder is normal, the urethra usually opens into the rectum (Fig. 23 – 19). Other anomalies that may accompany penile agenesis are cryptorchidism and agenesis of the prostate.

Hypoplasia of the penis is also rare except in association with other anomalies; most of the cases observed at the Chicago Lying-in Hospital were in infants with severe skeletal or renal malformations.

URETHRAL OBSTRUCTION. — Obstruction in the ure-

Fig. 23–19.—Agenesis of penis in mature newborn infant. **A,** external view. **B,** view showing communication between urethra and rectum.

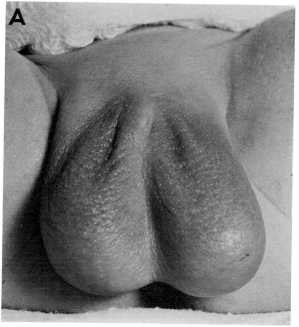
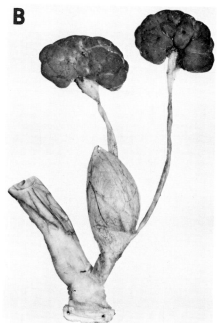

thra may be located at the meatus or in any part of
the canal. One or two cusplike folds of mucosa in
the region of the verumontanum may prevent outflow of urine (see Fig. 22–44). Urine coming down
from above fills the cusps and occludes the lumen.
The results of prenatal obstruction vary from trabeculation of the bladder and the presence of small
subcapsular cysts in the kidneys, when the obstruction is partial, to dilatation of the bladder and severe cystic dysplasia of the kidney, when it is complete.

INFECTIONS, CYSTS AND TUMORS

Abscesses of the prostate caused by Staphylococcus infections were reported in newborn infants by
Mann; they caused urinary obstruction or dribbling
and for the most part were adjacent to the urethra.

A congenital utricular cyst of the infant prostate
in conjunction with hypospadias and partial cryptorchidism was reported by Myers *et al.* The cyst

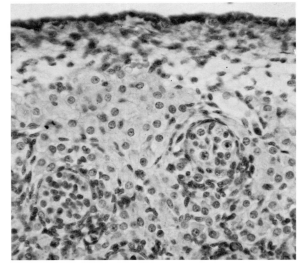

Fig. 23–20.—Normal testis from 530 gm fetus with
numerous cells of Leydig surrounding the two seminiferous tubules present in the section.

Fig. 23–21.—Testis of mature newborn infant. **A,** low
power view showing testis, epididymis and portions of
ductus deferens. **B,** high power view showing seminiferous tubules. Intervening cells of Leydig are reduced in
size and number compared to those of young fetus shown
in Fig. 23–20.

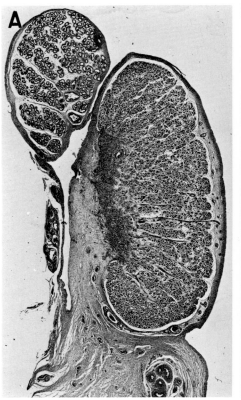

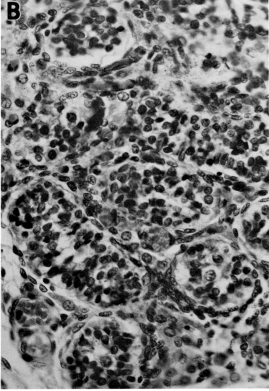

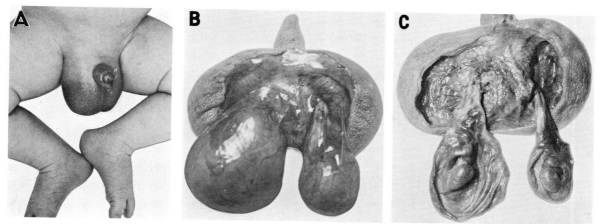

Fig. 23—22.—Bilateral hydrocele with greater involvement of right than left. **A,** external view. **B,** opened scrotum showing surface of tunicae vaginalis within which the fluid is contained. **C,** opened tunicae vaginalis showing relation to testes. Newborn infant.

opened just below the sphincter and obliterated the verumontanum.

Rhabdomyosarcomas of the prostate may occur in young infants, presumably arising from the striated muscle present on the posterior surface of the prostate or the base of the bladder. They usually involve the ureters, and urinary obstruction is often the presenting symptom. Because of this they are discovered late and cure is rare.

Gonads

The first indication of the presence of gonads is a slight enlargement of cells lining the celomic cavity in localized areas overlying the caudal ends of the mesonephroi while these are still the principal excretory organs of the embryo. Subjacent tissue proliferates and very quickly is invaded by large pale primitive germ cells that are generally believed to

Fig. 23—23.—Ovarian cortex. **A,** from 540 gm fetus, composed of primitive germ cells, few of which have been converted into primordial follicles. Separated into clusters by blood vessels but stroma not yet developed. **B,** from 350 gm fetus, showing majority of germ cells in pachytene stage of meiotic division.

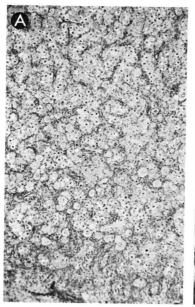

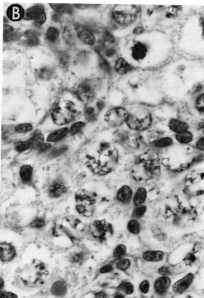

have migrated into this area by passage down the germ track from their origin in the entoderm near the junction of the yolk sac with the primitive gut. Local tissue proliferates and germ cells divide mitotically to provide the large number that are present at birth.

TESTES

The differentiation of the gonads into testes is apparent at about the 7th gestational week, when cords of cells extending at right angles to the longitudinal axis of the gonad become delineated. They are the seminiferous tubules whose peripheral ends merge into intercommunicating channels known as the rete testis; the latter open into mesonephric tubules, which in turn unite to join the wolffian duct which differentiates into the vas deferens. Germ cells comprise a large share of the cells of the primitive seminiferous tubules. During most of intrauterine life the tubules appear solid, and only near fetal maturity can any evidence of a lumen be made out. Large numbers of interstitial (Leydig) cells surround seminiferous tubules in the small fetus (Fig. 23–20); with increasing fetal age the tubules come to occupy an increasingly greater share of the total gonad, and interstitial cells become reduced in size and number and come to resemble fibroblasts (Fig. 23–21). There is little further change in the structure of the testis until puberty, when part of the cells comprising the seminiferous tubules begin to proliferate and differentiate into mature sperms. In male infants of diabetic mothers the interstitial cells retain their prominence for a longer period than in normal infants.

The fetal testis plays two important roles in the development of the sexual apparatus. The first is a local function that suppresses the formation of the fallopian tube; if one testis is absent a fallopian tube will be formed on that side. Also it fosters the development of the seminiferous tubules from the mesonephric anlage. The second role is manifested later in the 1st trimester, when the testicular androgens are required for the proper development of the prostate, seminal vesicles, phallus, penile urethra and scrotum. If no male hormone is produced at this time, development follows the female pattern with formation of a uterus and vagina. This is the pattern seen in the testicular feminization syndrome in which there is a testis and seminiferous tubule on each side but no prostate, seminal vesicle or phallus. Here the organizing effect of the testis is present but the end-organs do not respond to androgen and consequently the other male elements do

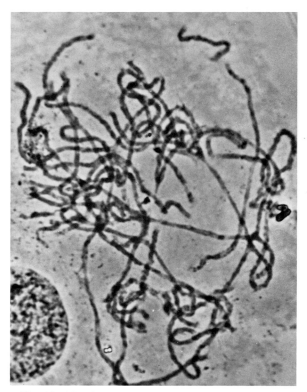

Fig. 23–24.—Chromosomes in late pachytene stage of meiosis obtained from squash preparation of ovary from fetus of 24 weeks.

not develop in spite of an XY chromosome pattern.

The gonads in the male embryo, when first formed, are located in the posterior part of the mid-abdominal cavity. In the succeeding months they move somewhat lower but do not begin their actual descent into the scrotum until about the 7th month. They are then drawn through the inguinal canals into the scrotum by the gubernaculum testes and for a time may be found intermittently in the canals or in the scrotum. As the position in the scrotum becomes established, the canals close and each testis is surrounded by the isolated portion of the peritoneum that has been carried along with it into the scrotum. The inguinal canal remains a weak spot and at any period of life may give way under excessive pressure from above and permit passage of intestine or fluid into the scrotum from the abdominal cavity. In the young infant, intestine rarely passes through the inguinal ring, but fluid under pressure in the abdomen may dilate the canal and distend the tunica vaginalis. The only inguinal hernia in a newborn infant observed at the Chicago Lying-in Hospital was in a premature chondrodystrophic dwarf. The inguinal ring was greatly dilated and the bowel was in the scrotal sac (see Fig. 25–2, D).

Hydrocele is the term given the accumulation of fluid in the tunica vaginalis surrounding the testis (Fig. 23–22). If bilateral, it is sometimes difficult to differentiate externally from edema of the scrotum. Edema is usually found only in infants delivered from a breech position and disappears promptly.

Testes that fail to descend are often abnormal in structure but this is probably not a primary abnormality. In the two series of Gross *et al.* of 43 cryptorchid infants who were subjected to operation and followed to adult life, 75–80% were known to be fertile. While testes remaining in the abdomen until puberty are known to be defective, the majority of those placed in the scrotum before the age of 5 years may be expected to function. The usual cryptorchid testes of long standing have small tubules with no spermatogonia; the interstitial cells are usually normal.

Absence of a gonad is unknown except in grossly malformed infants. However, the epididymis and ductus deferens may be absent on either side if the mesonephros fails to develop on that side or if the anterior portion undergoes complete regression.

Ovotestes are rare at any age and have not been reported in newborn infants. The Chicago Lying-in Hospital series of autopsies includes an infant whose gonads contained tubules resembling those of the rete testis as well as ova. A few similar tubules can often be found in the normal ovary, but without further evidence of male elements it seems unwise to consider such a structure an ovotestis.

Splenogonadal fusion has been described in both sexes. In males it is most often discovered when the inguinal canal is examined during hernial repair. The testis and ovary arise close to the spleen and if the two organs adhere, the subsequent descent of the gonad gives rise to the anomaly. The fusion may be continuous, with splenic tissue running from the spleen to the gonad, or discontinuous, with small isolated splenic nodules along the spermatic cord or in immediate juxtaposition to a gonad in the pelvis or inguinal canal (Putschar and Manion). In some cases the ovary does not descend and lies next to the spleen. Wolson pointed out that about 20% of patients with splenogonadal fusion

Fig. 23–25.—Ovarian cortex. **A,** mature newborn infant with the cortex composed chiefly of primordial follicles. **B,** infant aged 6 months with primordial follicles separated by slightly more stroma than in the newborn. Graafian follicles (not shown) were also present.

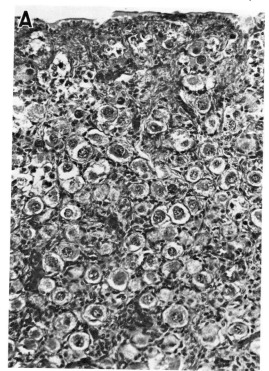
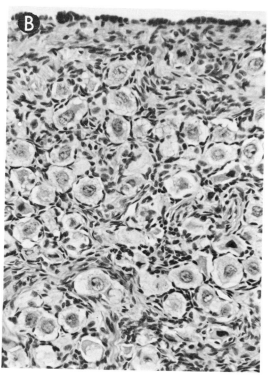

have additional somatic defects such as deformed limbs, micrognathia or inguinal hernia.

Infarction of the testis in the newborn is usually associated with torsion of the testis on the spermatic cord (Longino and Martin), although it may be caused by a strangulated hernia; at times no cause can be found (Pinto and Kiefer). Although prompt operation may be helpful, it is not necessary to remove the infarcted testis since it will not cause further trouble even if it does not recover.

The *tumors of the testis* found in the 1st year of life are thought to be derived from germinal cells; these are *embryonal carcinomas, orchioblastomas* and *teratomas.* The first consist of medullary masses or cords of epithelial cells that have polygonal, low columnar or peg-shaped outlines. The cytoplasm is pale and the nuclei, which are large and vesicular, may distend the superficial end of the cell. Considerable proteinaceous fluid is often present between the columns of epithelial cells. In such tumors occasional "embryoid bodies" may be present, so called because of their resemblance to developing blastocysts. The second tumor, orchioblastoma (called clear-celled carcinoma by Teoh *et al.*), consists of clear cells with a small amount of cytoplasm arranged in sheets, poorly formed acini and papillary masses.

Teratomas of the testis in this age group usually consist of partially differentiated epithelial and mesenchymal elements, although some areas may appear carcinomatous. Of the 35 testicular tumors of germinal origin in infants aged under 1 year collected by Hauser *et al.*, 12 were embryonal carcinomas, 15 were orchioblastomas and eight were teratomas.

The only tumor of the testis not of germ cell origin found in the 1st year of life is the Sertoli-Leydig cell tumor (Holtz and Abell). These tumors have small tubules lined by Sertoli cells but contain no spermatogonia. Leydig cells are usually poorly developed.

Burros and Mayock described a single case in a newborn of an adenomatoid tumor in the epididymis of the testis that resembled the so-called adenomatoid tumor of the fallopian tube found in adult women. It was composed of confluent spaces lined by flattened cuboidal epithelium, often suggesting a lymphangioma.

OVARIES

In the female embryo cords of cells do not appear in the early gonad as they do in the male, and germ cells make an almost solid mass merging with the surface epithelium (Fig. 23–23, A). In a study based on squash preparations and histologic sections of fetal ovaries, Manotayo and Potter found oogonia in active mitosis at 6 to 12 weeks, with early stages of meiosis first visible at about 13 weeks. According to them, meiosis begins at about the same time that mitosis becomes less frequent and occurs first in the deeper portions of the gland. By midpregnancy many germ cells are in meiosis, which can be well demonstrated both in histologic sections (Fig. 23–23, B) and squash preparations (Fig. 23–24). By fetal maturity division by mitosis has usually ended and almost all oogonia have become oocytes. The majority of cells have passed through the initial stages of meiosis (leptotene, zygotene, pachytene and diplotene) and are in the dictyotene, or resting, stage of meiosis (Fig. 23–24). They have become surrounded by a layer of small flat cells, probably derived from mesenchyme brought into the small ovary along with hilar blood vessels (Potter) and converted into primordial follicles (Fig. 23–25, A). During fetal life little stroma is present but it gradually begins to develop during infancy (Fig. 23–25, B). The follicles remain in this stage until further follicular development is stimulated and they are converted into graafian follicles weeks, months or years later. Following formation of a graafian follicle the contained oocyte usually dies and the follicle regresses. Not until after puberty is meiotic division completed and the ovum expelled from the ovary.

During the latter weeks of intrauterine life some of the primordial follicles invariably develop further. Some ova enlarge as they do in the postpubertal female, the peripheral layer of cells proliferates

Fig. 23–26.—Ovary showing normal development of follicles in deeper portions of the cortex. The perifollicular hemorrhage was a result of intrauterine anoxia. Mature stillborn fetus.

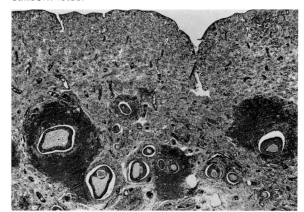

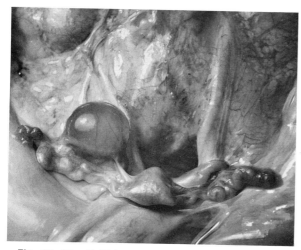

Fig. 23—27.—Follicle cyst. Estrogenic hormone was present in the fluid. Mature stillborn fetus.

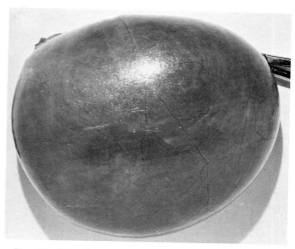

Fig. 23—28.—Ovarian cyst of follicular origin removed soon after birth. It measured 12 cm in greatest diameter. (Courtesy Dr. G. Vawter.)

Fig. 23—29.—**A,** ovary from infant aged 10 weeks showing numerous graafian follicles. Although here a few follicles are slightly larger than usual, many follicles in all stages of development are present throughout the entire prepubertal period. **B,** ovary from child aged 7 years showing normal follicular activity.

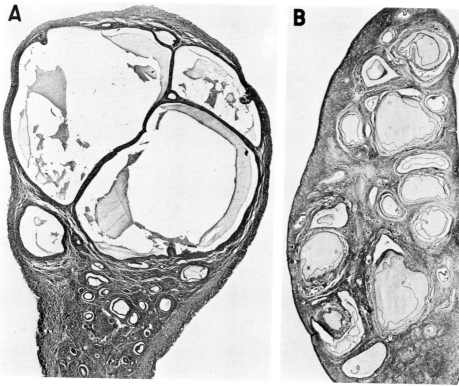

into a thick layer of granulosa cells and the follicles develop central cavities of varying sizes. At birth follicles may be visible grossly as structures several millimeters in diameter, or they may remain smaller and be visible only on microscopic examination. The layer of granulosa cells of the larger cavities is always surrounded by a richly vascularized layer of well-developed theca interna and a thinner layer of theca externa. In infants who die of anoxia the tissue immediately surrounding the more mature follicles is often infiltrated by red blood cells (Fig. 23–26). Follicles developing during fetal life undergo atresia in the same manner as those formed in infancy and later life.

Rarely, follicles are so numerous that the ovary is conspicuously enlarged. The largest number of follicles ever observed at the Chicago Lying-in Hospital were in a chondrodystrophic dwarf who died at the age of 2 days. Each ovary measured 1.5 × 1 × 0.5 cm.

Occasionally, single follicles may contain more than the usual amount of fluid and may measure several centimeters in diameter. In the fluid of a 2 cm follicle (Fig. 23–27) estrogenic hormone was demonstrated, and in another that was 12 cm in greatest diameter the lining resembled granulosa cells (Fig. 23–28).

It is generally stated that the growth of follicles beyond the primordial stage in the fetus is a direct result of stimulation by maternal hormones. This cannot be entirely true because follicles normally continue to develop during infancy and childhood and are present throughout the prepubertal period (Fig. 23–29) (Potter).

Despite the frequency with which developing and retrogressing follicles are present, further development is uncommon in the young infant. It is possible, however, for the cells of the theca interna to become luteinized. We have seen ovaries in a few infants at birth in which there were remarkable numbers of follicles composed of wide bands of luteinized theca interna (Fig. 23–30). Granulosa

Fig. 23–30.—Ovary from a 5,100 gm stillborn fetus showing excessive follicular activity with remarkable luteinization of theca interna. **A,** low power view. **B,** high power view of the wall of a follicle showing luteinized theca interna.

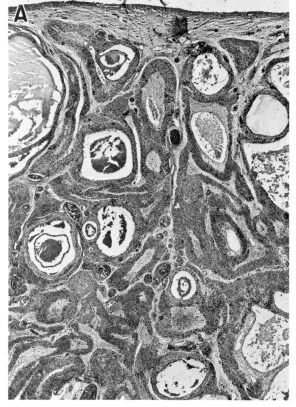
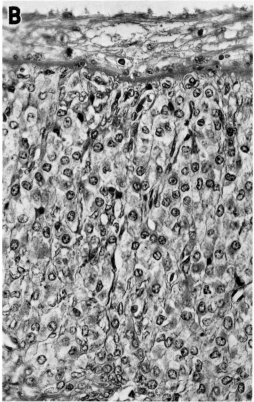

cells were not luteinized and were often absent, the inner surface of the layer of theca cells being covered or the entire cavity filled with loose connective tissue. Similarly luteinized follicles are found at other ages, and it is apparent that such luteinization may occur in the absence of ovulation. The reported cases of corpus luteum cysts in the 1st year of life bear scrutiny since ovulation must be a most rare event at this period of life (Marshall).

Hypoplasia of ovarian tissue is seldom recognized at birth except in Turner's syndrome, and complete absence of gonadal tissue is one of the rarest anomalies. Absence of müllerian or mesonephric duct derivatives does not cause absence of the gonads. Enlargements of the ovary in the newborn as well as in the 1st year of life are most often caused by cystic development or atretic follicles, or a cyst may have no specific lining. Marshall reported 45 cases of enlarged ovaries in children, with 23 having the diagnosis established in the first 37 days of life. Seven had follicular cysts, nine serous or simple cysts, two theca lutein cysts, four corpus luteum cysts and one a "granulosa cell cyst." Among 16 cysts diagnosed in the remainder of the 1st year the distribution was similar except for four cystic teratomas and one malignant mesonephroma.

Among 113 true neoplasms of ovaries of germ cell origin in children, Abell and Holtz found two embryonal carcinomas occurring in the 1st year of life. They had the same characteristics as the corresponding tumor of the testis. Of the 75 non–germ cell tumors of the ovary in childhood, Abell and Holtz found none in the 1st year. Reis and Koop reported granulosa cell tumors accompanied by evidence of pseudoprecocious puberty in the 1st year. These tumors were composed of typical sheets of granulosa cells and some contained Call-Exner bodies. Granulosa–theca cell tumors appear to be limited to older children (Pedowitz *et al.*).

Mammary Glands

The first indication of mammary glands appears during the 6th gestational week as narrow band-like thickenings of ectoderm extending over each side of the ventral surface of the embryo from a point near the origin of the anterior limb buds to a similar point near the posterior limb buds. These are known as the milk lines and are common to all mammals. In the human being only a small area near the upper portion of each line normally develops into a breast. Supernumerary breasts are not uncommon, however, and are found most often in locations compatible with an origin from the milk line. They have been described on rare occasions on the trunk, arms and legs, but in these areas are almost never visible at birth.

The major ducts of the breast originate as solid cords of cells growing down from the surface ectoderm into the underlying connective tissue. They gradually develop lumens, and in the last weeks of intrauterine life acinar buds arise from the terminal portions. At about the time of birth some of the acini become cannulated and the lumens often contain desquamated epithelial cells and a secretion similar to the colostrum that is present in the maternal breast at the termination of pregnancy (Fig. 23–31).

In a mature fetus of either sex the glands are firm button-shaped masses of tissue about 1 cm in diameter and about 7 mm thick. Each weighs about 1 gm. They are usually dark red because of great vascularity and are easily differentiated from the surrounding fat and connective tissue. After birth they may increase in size and become elevated 2 cm or more above the chest surface. A few drops of an opalescent gray fluid known colloquially as witch's

Fig. 23–31.—Breast of a newborn infant showing distention of major ducts.

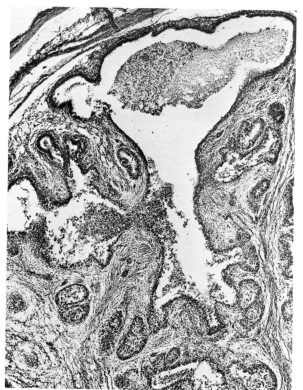

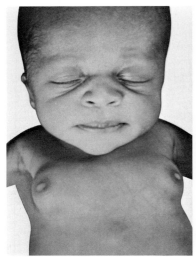

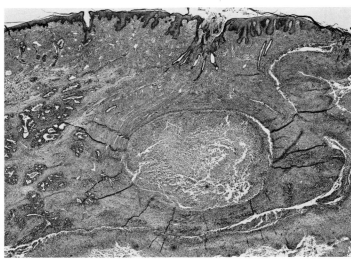

Fig. 23–32 (left).—Engorgement of the breasts. "Witch's milk" is exuding from the nipples. Infant aged 5 days. (Courtesy Drs. Lewis K. Sweet and John L. Parks.)

Fig. 23–33 (right).—Abscess of the breast located in the region of the major ducts. Infant aged 9 days.

milk may exude from the nipple (Fig. 23–32). Occasionally the breasts become severely engorged and enlarge to cover much of the anterior chest wall. Rarely, they become infected and abscesses develop (Fig. 23–33). This is the only true mastitis, although clinically the term is often applied to noninfectious engorgement.

Complete absence of breast tissue or nipples is extremely rare.

REFERENCES

Abell, M. R., and Holtz, F.: Ovarian neoplasms in childhood and adolescence. II. Tumors of the non-germ cell origin, Am. J. Obstet. Gynecol. 93:850, 1965.

Abell, M. R., and Holtz, F.: Testicular neoplasms in infants and children. I. Tumors of germ cell origin, Cancer 16:965, 1963.

Abell, M. R., Johnson, V. J., and Holtz, F.: Ovarian neoplasms in childhood and adolescence. I. Tumors of germ cell origin, Am. J. Obstet. Gynecol. 92:1059, 1965.

Avin, J.: Male Turner syndrome, Am. J. Dis. Child. 91:630, 1956.

Bayes, D. A., Hardre, M., and Agnew, A. M.: Carcinoma of the cervix in an infant, Am. J. Obstet. Gynecol. 72:1053, 1956.

Bongiovanni, A. M., and Root, A. W.: The adrenal genital syndrome, N. Engl. J. Med. 268:1283, 1342, 1391, 1963.

Bove, K. E.: Gonadal dysgenesis in a neonate with XO karyotype, Am. J. Dis. Child. 120:363, 1970.

Burros, H. M., and Mayock, P. P.: Adenomatoid tumor of the epidydimis: Report of a case in a newborn, J. Urol. 63:712, 1950.

Committee of Cytologists: A proposed standard system of nomenclature of human mitotic chromosomes (letter to the editor), Am. J. Hum. Genet. 12:384, 1960.

Cottons, D.: Procidentia in the newborn, J. Obstet. Gynaecol. Br. Commonw. 72:131, 1965.

Dennison, W. M., and Bacsich, P.: Imperforate vagina in newborn: Neonatal hydrocolpos, Arch. Dis. Child. 36:156, 1961.

Edlow, J. B., et al.: Neonatal Klinefelter's syndrome, Am. J. Dis. Child. 118:788, 1969.

Elstein, M.: Vaginal cytology of the newborn, J. Obstet. Gynaecol. Br. Commonw. 70:1050, 1963.

Federman, D. D.: Abnormal Sexual Development (Philadelphia: W. B. Saunders Co., 1967).

Ford, C. E., et al.: A sex chromosome anomaly in a case of gonadal dysgenesis (Turner's syndrome), Lancet 1:711, 1959.

Grosfield, J. L., Clatworthy, H. W., Jr., and Newton, W. A.: Combined therapy in childhood rhabdomyosarcoma, J. Pediatr. Surg. 6:637, 1969.

Gross, R. E., and Jewett, T. C., Jr.: Surgical experiences from 1,222 operations for undescended testis, J.A.M.A. 160:634, 1956.

Grumbach, M. M., Ducharme, J. R., and Moloshok, R. E.: On the fetal masculinizing action of certain oral progestins, J. Clin. Endocrinol. 19:1369, 1959.

Hauser, R., Isant, Q. J., Jr., and Persky, L.: Testicular tumors in children, Am. J. Surg. 110:876, 1965.

Herbst, A. L., and Scully, R. E.: Adenocarcinoma of the vagina in adolescence, Cancer 25:745, 1970.

Hoge, R. H., and Benn, V. A.: Carcinoma of vulva and vagina in infancy, Am. J. Obstet. Gynecol. 46:286, 1943.

Holtz, F., and Abell, M. R.: Testicular neoplasms in infants and children. II: Tumors of non–germ cell origin, Cancer 16:982, 1963.

Johnston, J. H.: The undescended testis, Arch. Dis. Child. 40:113, 1965.

Jones, H. W., Jr., et al.: Pathologic and cytogenetic findings in true hermaphroditism. Report of 46 cases and review of 23 from the literature, Obstet. Gynecol. 25:435, 1965.

Keitel, H. G., and Chu, E.: Breast nodules in premature infants, Am. J. Dis. Child. 109:121, 1965.

Kowlessar, M., and Orti, E.: Complete breast absence in siblings, Am. J. Dis. Child. 109:121, 1965.

Lemli, L., and Smith, D. W.: The XO syndrome: Study of differential phenotypes, J. Pediatr. 63:577, 1963.

Longino, L. A., and Martin, L. W.: Torsion of the spermatic cord in the newborn infant, N. Engl. J. Med. 253:695, 1955.

Mann, C.: Prostatic abscess in the newborn, Arch. Dis. Child. 35:396, 1960.

Manotaya, T., and Potter, E. L.: Oocytes in prophase of meiosis from squash preparations of humal fetal ovaries, Fertil. Steril. 14:378, 1963.

Marshall, J. R.: Ovarian enlargements in the first year of life: Review of 45 cases, Ann. Surg. 161:372, 1965.

McCrea, L. E.: Congenital absence of the penis, J. Urol. 47:818, 1942.

McKusick, V. A., *et al.*: Hydrometrocolpos as a simply inherited malformation, J.A.M.A. 189:813, 1964.

Myers, G. H., Lynn, H. B., and Kelanis, P. D.: Giant cyst of utricle, J. Urol. 101:369, 1969.

Myerson, L., and Swinup, G.: Turner's syndrome in the male, Arch. Intern. Med. 116:125, 1965.

Norris, H. J., Bagley, G. P., and Taylor, H. B.: Carcinoma of the infant vagina, Arch. Pathol. 90:473, 1970.

Ober, W. B., and Bernstein, J.: Observations on the endometrium in the newborn, Pediatrics 16:445, 1955.

O'Doherty, N. J.: Lipid adrenal hyperplasia, Guys Hosp. Rep. 113:368, 1964.

Pedowitz, P., Telmus, L. B., and Mackles, A.: Precocious puberty due to ovarian tumors, Obstet. Gynecol. Surv. 10:633, 1958.

Pinto, P., and Kiefer, J. N.: Infarction of the testicle in the newborn infant, J. Pediatr. 51:80, 1957.

Potter, E. L.: The Ovary in Infancy and Childhood, in *The Ovary*, International Academy of Pathology Monograph no. 3 (Baltimore: Williams & Wilkins Co., 1962).

Prader, A., and Sievernmann, R. E.: Lipoid hyperplasie der Nebennierren, Helv. Paediatr. Acta 12:569, 1957.

Putschar, W. G. J., and Manion, W. C.: Splenic gonadal fusion, Am. J. Pathol. 32:15, 1956.

Reis, R. L., and Koop, C. E.: Ovarian masses in infants and children, J. Pediatr. 60:96, 1962.

Richert, R. M., and Benirschke, K.: Penile agenesis, Arch. Pathol. 70:252, 1960.

Sohval, A. R.: Hermaphroditism with atypical or mixed gonadal dysgenesis, Am. J. Med. 36:381, 1964.

Sohval, A. R.: Testicular dysgenesis in relation to neoplasms of the testicle, J. Urol. 75:285, 1956.

Sohval, A. R.: The syndrome of pure gonadal dysgenesis, Am. J. Med. 38:615, 1965.

Spencer, R., and Levy, D. M.: Hydrometrocolpos: Report of three cases and review of the literature, Ann. Surg. 155:558, 1962.

Teoh, T. B., *et al.*: The distinctive adenocarcinoma of the infant's testicle: An account of 15 cases, J. Pathol. Bacteriol. 80:147, 1960.

Wilkins, L.: *Diagnosis and Treatment of Endocrine Disorders in Childhood and Adolescence* (2d ed.; Springfield, Ill.: Charles C Thomas, 1966).

Wilkins, L., *et al.*: Masculinization of the female fetus associated with administration of oral and intramuscular progestins during gestation: Non-adrenal female pseudohermaphroditism, J. Clin. Endocrinol. 18:559, 1958.

Wolson, R. J.: Splenogonadal fusion, Surgery 63:853, 1968.

24

Central Nervous System

THE NERVOUS SYSTEM makes its first appearance as a groove in the ectodermal component of the embryonic disk during the 3d week after fertilization. The groove becomes deeper and the upper edges gradually unite to produce a hollow tube. This becomes detached from the surface, and the edges of the overlying ectoderm fuse to form a continuous sheet of cells covering the tube beneath. The anterior part of the neural groove develops into the brain, the posterior part becomes the spinal cord and motor nerves appear as local outgrowths from both regions. Cells coming from the neural crest, which is derived from the neural plate lateral to the neural tube, migrate outward to form the chromaffin tissue of the adrenal medulla and much of the peripheral nervous system, especially the cells of sensory nerves and sympathetic ganglia.

Development progresses rapidly and the brain of the average mature newborn infant weighs about 430 gm, almost one third as much as the adult brain. By the time of birth the cell layers are well differentiated, the basal nuclei and conduction paths can be identified and the general pattern that will persist throughout life is established.

Cerebrospinal Fluid

The water content of the brain of the fetus is high in comparison with that of the adult but is proportionately lower at term than it is earlier. The amount of cerebrospinal fluid is inversely related, both actually and relatively, to the age of the fetus. During most of intrauterine life the brain develops in a fluid-filled space, and in early fetal life as much as 26% of the cranial cavity may be filled with fluid (Lanman *et al.*). It is evident that the growth of the brain is not responsible for the growth of the skull. As the fetus matures, the amount of fluid decreases in relation to brain size, and according to Scammon the brain of the mature fetus occupies 97% of the cranial cavity and fills the skull more completely than at any other time of life. This statement should probably be limited to infants delivered vaginally, for fluid seems to be forced out of the meninges during passage through the birth canal and larger amounts are present in the heads of infants delivered by cesarean section. Since so little fluid is found when delivery is by the vaginal route, the convolutions often appear to be flattened against the skull (see Fig. 6–2). There is no evidence that true edema of the brain ever exists in the newborn, and this normal characteristic of the brain is usually responsible for such a diagnosis.

An excessive amount of fluid is occasionally found in the heads of infants who die a short time after delivery, especially when delivery has been by cesarean section. The fluid is held in the subarachnoid space, and the meningeal vessels that normally lie directly on the brain substance are raised 2–3 mm above the surface. If the skull is opened over a pan so that the fluid and blood that escape may be saved, and if the brain and the fluid content of the pan are strained through dampened cheesecloth, the amount of fluid can be measured. From the cell volume of the fluid the amount of blood in the specimen can be calculated and subtracted from the total amount in order to determine the actual volume of cerebrospinal fluid. No fluid can be obtained by this method from the head of a normal infant delivered at term through the vagina. Ten to 15 ml can be obtained from infants weighing 1,500–2,000 gm (Potter and Rosenbaum). From the heads of some infants, either mature or premature, delivered by cesarean section this method will yield

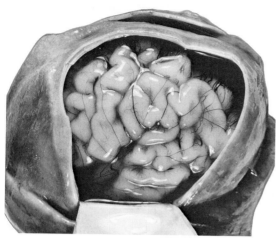

Fig. 24–1.—Increase in intracranial fluid associated with delivery by cesarean section. Fifty ml of cerebrospinal fluid was obtained from this head. Death at 18 hours from pulmonary failure caused by respiratory distress syndrome. Weight 2,790 gm.

30–60 ml or even more of cerebrospinal fluid (Fig. 24–1).

Most infants delivered by cesarean section appear normal at the time of birth and remain normal. In a few, however, respiratory distress develops in a short time and becomes rapidly progressive. In our experience almost all infants who die following cesarean section, except those who had been severely anoxic before birth or who are malformed or erythroblastotic, show both an increase in intracranial fluid and the pulmonary changes designated the respiratory distress syndrome (see p. 288). Premature infants who are delivered vaginally may have similar pulmonary changes, but among mature infants this pulmonary abnormality is largely limited to those delivered by cesarean section who also have marked meningeal edema. Whether there is a direct causal relationship between an increase in subarachnoid fluid and the respiratory distress syndrome is unknown. It is possible that the increase in fluid elevates intracranial pressure and interferes with respiratory function, but since some infants, especially those who are premature, have similar pulmonary symptoms without an increase in subarachnoid fluid, the association of the two conditions may have no significance.

Blood Vessels

ANATOMY.—The major branches of the vessels supplying the cortex of the brain lie directly on the brain surface in the arachnoid membrane. They follow the major fissures and sulci and give rise to many short branches extending at right angles outward onto the surface of the convolutions, the two sides of a convolution being supplied from different vessels. All of the arteries arise from the circle of Willis at the base of the brain, and the blood supply comes from below upward. The venous flow is in two directions: the superior cerebral veins that drain the upper part of the cerebral hemispheres empty in groups into the superior sagittal sinus, and the inferior cerebral veins that drain the lower portions empty into the inferior sagittal, cavernous, petrosal and transverse sinuses. The two central veins that drain the internal parts of the cerebrum converge to form the internal cerebral vein, commonly known as the vein of Galen. It is only about 1 cm long and empties into the anterior end of the straight sinus.

HEMORRHAGE.—Hemorrhage into the spinal or cranial cavity or the substance of the spinal cord or brain occurs more often during the delivery of premature than mature infants. In the older literature gross hemorrhages were reported to occur frequently, but now in a well-conducted obstetric service they are uncommon. In mature infants hemorrhage is most frequent under the dura or tentorium, while in premature infants it usually arises from the glial matrix vessels in the walls of the lateral ventricles. The frequency of the latter varies inversely with the birth weight.

Subdural hemorrhage results most frequently from an injury to the straight sinus caused by laceration of the tentorium near its junction with the falx or by rupture of the vein of Galen. In either case blood will be found at the base of the skull around the cerebellum and brain stem. With face and brow presentations, stretching of the falx by elongation of the vertex may tear bridging veins as they enter the superior sagittal sinus from the arachnoid membrane.

The diagnosis of a subdural hemorrhage over a cerebral hemisphere may be missed clinically until the formation of an organizing subdural hematoma causes pressure on the brain and enlargement of the head. The inner portion of the hematoma usually forms an organizing membrane with an abundant capillary network. This membrane, which may become partially calcified, lies on the surface of the brain unattached to the pia-arachnoid. The osmotic activity of the serum and free hemoglobin within it brings an increasing amount of fluid into the sac, which gradually develops. Ingraham and Matson found subdural hematomas most common in the 1st month of life, and in their study one quarter were directly related to known birth trauma. Later in the first year nontraumatic subdural hematomas may be found following infectious illnesses with dehydration. Klein found on later examination that many such infants were mentally retarded.

The possibility of bleeding into the cord substance, meninges and supporting structures of the cervical region is a cause of concern in breech deliveries. Yates found that if the cord and surrounding tissues were serially sectioned in the region of the eighth cervical vertebra following such deliveries, hemorrhage was present in nearly half of the newborn infants examined at autopsy. Hemorrhage was subdural, extradural or into the ligaments, joint spaces or adventitia of the vertebral artery and was accompanied by spinal cord or nerve root injury in one third of the cases.

In mature infants mechanical injury to the great vein of Galen and disruption of the straight or lateral sinuses secondary to laceration of the tentorium are the most common causes of gross intracranial hemorrhage. Blood is found especially around the cerebellum and brain stem and in the base of the skull and, if sufficiently extensive, may be responsible for interference with function of vital centers as a result of pressure on the medulla. At the Chicago Lying-in Hospital subdural hemorrhage has been very uncommon; when present it has been generally limited to the region of the sylvian fissure and has appeared to result from injury to the middle cerebral vein. The superior cerebral veins rarely may be torn as they enter the sagittal sinus and give rise to diffuse subdural hemorrhage. Subarachnoid bleeding is more common and a slight extravasation of red cells is frequently found in infants dying of anoxia.

By far the most frequent lethal form of hemorrhage is the intraventricular hemorrhage of very premature infants, which may be caused by trauma but more often seems to be a result of anoxia. Riggs and Rorke found it in 46% of liveborn infants under 1,500 gm birth weight, although this is a far higher figure than that given by most investigators. The peak incidence was in those born at 28 weeks' gestation (Fig. 24–2, A). Such hemorrhages arise in the region of the terminal veins of the subependymal glial matrix; the latter is a linear mass of very immature proliferating embryonic tissue that persists long after other areas of the brain have matured. It lies along the lateral wall of the lateral ventricles; in this area the veins are large and form the main branches of the vein of Galen. The devel-oping matrix contains few glial fibers, and the immediate juxtaposition of the lateral ventricle permits very prompt leakage of any local intracerebral hemorrhage into the lateral ventricle (Fig. 24–2, B). Towbin believed that slowing of the blood flow through the large vessels in an infant with anoxia and a failing circulation is conducive to venous thrombosis with subsequent venous infarction, but this has not been seen at the Chicago Lying-in Hospital and rarely at the Boston Hospital for Women. Among 88 brains with para- and intraventricular hemorrhage Larroche found venous thrombosis in 16 and venous dilatation proximal to the vessels in the affected area in 10. She emphasized that dilatation of vessels in the germinal matrix is an accompaniment and possible precursor of the hemorrhage. In some instances, what appears to be ischemic necrosis can be recognized in this area in the absence of hemorrhage. Only rarely does the infarctive necrosis spread to the more distal parts of the area drained by the veins in question.

In most cases in which there is massive intraventricular hemorrhage the entire ventricular system is filled with blood (see Fig. 8–11), and a large amount is also present in the subarachnoid space around the brain stem and cerebellum. It is most frequently seen in small premature infants with respiratory distress, who often have a history of sudden apnea on the 2d or 3d day of life. Riggs and Rorke reported cases with fresh bleeding from 3 days to more than a week after birth. The hemorrhage may be so massive that it produces a sudden drop in hematocrit. Such hemorrhage is not seen in stillborn fetuses, with very rare exceptions, and does not appear to be prenatally determined. We have not recognized paraventricular leukomalacia in conjunction with this lesion, although Larroche found 33 instances among the cases she studied by serial section. In occasional cases enlargement of the entire ventricular system may result from the massive bleeding, and when the infant survives for a period of time, the aqueduct may be blocked by the detritus of the blood clot.

ACUTE INFANTILE HEMIPLEGIA.—According to Carter and Gold, this diagnosis is a symptom state rather than a specific disease. As the name implies, it indicates the rapid onset of a state of hemiplegia in a previously healthy infant and has many of the attributes of a stroke in elderly patients. It may appear in infants with a history of trauma, status epilepticus, congenital heart disease with its potential for embolism or bacterial endocarditis, or it may result from infections, especially when associ-

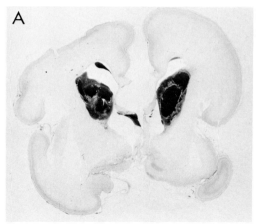 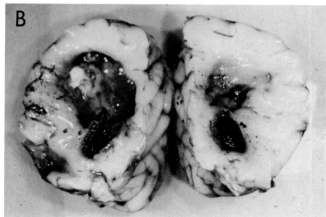

Fig. 24–2.—A, section of the brain of a premature infant dying a few days after birth with respiratory distress. There is hemorrhage into the lateral ventricles and germinal matrix of both cerebral hemispheres. (Courtesy Dr. P. Yakovlev.) B, section through the frontal lobes of a mature newborn infant with hemorrhage into the ventricles and cortical substance of the hemisphere.

ated with dehydration and venous thrombosis. When death follows the attack of hemiplegia, intracerebral hemorrhage is usually found at autopsy. In most cases, however, the infant survives and the cause is seldom satisfactorily explained.

THROMBOSIS.—Thrombosis of the dural sinuses with spread to the meningeal and cerebral veins, is seen chiefly in older infants. Local infections such as otitis media, mastoiditis or meningitis comprise the principal precursors; diarrhea, inanition and generalized sepsis account for the remainder. Dehydration, hemoconcentration and cardiac failure are responsible for sluggish flow through the sinuses, and thrombosis may occur without precipitating local factors. In such cases, according to Byers and Hass, the thrombi remain sterile. The thrombosis may involve the sagittal, straight or sigmoid sinus and often extends to the adjacent meningeal veins. Many hemorrhages are produced in the meninges and cortex, and there is often a remarkable proliferation of capillaries in the incompletely destroyed areas of the brain. The deep subcortical white matter and periventricular tissues are spared unless the vein of Galen is thrombosed. In 10% of the cases of Byers and Hass hydrocephalus was present. With the use of modern antibiotic and fluid therapy such lesions are rare.

MALFORMATIONS.—Aneurysms of the vessels of the circle of Willis are usually considered congenital in origin but rarely cause difficulty in early life and are never recognized at autopsy in the newborn unless they have produced symptoms. Newcomb and Munns reported two cases in infants under 3

weeks of age and found another in the literature who was under 6 months.

Diffuse angiomatosis and angiomatous increase in meningeal vessels were reported by Potter and by Holden (Fig. 24–3, A). In some of these cases the increased vascular bed had been responsible for cardiac enlargement and heart failure. The altered vasculature may be limited to the meninges or may involve other parts of the body.

Probably more common than either of these malformations is an arteriovenous fistula in the cerebral circulation. Stern *et al.* found 16 instances in his own material and in the literature. In such cases both the arterial and venous limbs are dilated and cardiac failure may be the presenting complaint. In one case reported by Silverman *et al.* the vein of Galen was greatly dilated. Much of the brain in the region of the fistula may be destroyed.

In the *Sturge-Kalischer-Weber syndrome* there is a diffuse capillary hemangiomatosis of the skin of the face in the general distribution of the trigeminal nerve, choroid coat of the retina, the meninges and the underlying brain. The vessels are small and blood flow is not appreciably increased. The affected eye is often enlarged (buphthalmos). Convulsions may occur in the first few weeks of life, but usually the only finding at this age is the hemangiomatous involvement of the face. Although the hemangiomatosis of the meninges and brain is present at birth and probably changes very little, the brain may become progressively destroyed by the increasing calcification of the brain parenchyma and the walls of the larger involved vessels. In

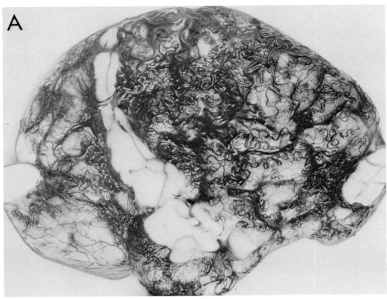

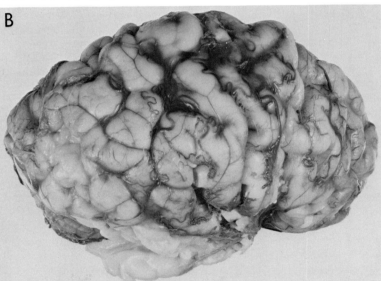

Fig. 24—3.—Diffuse angiomatosis of superficial cerebral vessels. **A,** severe generalized angiomatosis in which vessels covering the surface of both cerebral hemispheres and cerebellum are greatly increased in number and tortuosity. White areas are due to meningeal lacerations incurred during removal of the brain from the skull. Extreme cardiomegaly also present. **B,** mild angiomatosis of meningeal vessels frequently observed in infants with the hydropic form of erythroblastosis.

older individuals x-ray often shows characteristic parallel lines of calcification. The lines follow adjacent gyri and are caused by deposits of calcium close to the gyral surface (Fig. 24–4).

Mild telangiectasia of the cerebral veins has been observed at the Chicago Lying-in Hospital in sever-al hydropic stillborn fetuses with severe erythroblastosis and in one infant of a diabetic mother. These changes are overlooked unless the vessels are filled with blood, and there has been difficulty in photographing them because of the rapidity with which blood drains out of the skull after it is

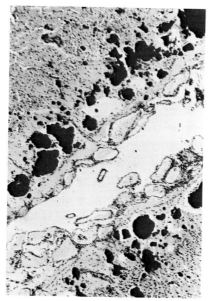

Fig. 24—4. — Sturge-Kalischer-Weber syndrome. A section of one sulcus and adjacent gyri with dilatation of the proliferated meningeal and cortical vessels. The black masses are calcific deposits in the superficial layers of the cortex.

opened (Fig. 24–3, B). They course circuitously over the surface of the brain instead of being distributed in the normal relation to the sulci. Chronic anoxia secondary to the severe anemia of the hydropic erythroblastotic infant may be the cause. Such infants usually have moderate cardiac hypertrophy.

Infection

The organisms causing *bacterial meningitis* in the newborn period are about equally divided between those that are gram-negative such as *Escherichia coli, Aerobacter aerogenes,* Klebsiella and Proteus, acquired in utero or in passage through the birth canal, and those that are gram-positive such as streptococci, staphylococci and pneumococci coming from air passages, umbilicus or skin after birth (Ziai and Haggerty; Groover *et al.*). In the series of Ziai and Haggerty, 30 of 39 infants had had unusually traumatic deliveries or were delivered from a breech position. Premature infants made up a large share of this group. Infants born with a meningocele or myelomeningocele covered by a thin, leaking sac soon acquire fatal meningitis.

The pathology of bacterial meningitis in the newborn does not differ from that in adults, and

because of the lack of specific symptoms the lesion may progress undetected so that the mortality rate is high. The prognosis for normal mental development following meningitis in the newborn period is poor (Ziai and Haggerty).

Like neonatal meningitis, *brain abscesses* in the newborn are often caused by enteric organisms. They seldom produce localizing signs although head enlargement, as in neonatal meningitis, is common (Munslow *et al.*). In about two thirds of the cases the cause is infection of the middle ear or myelomeningocele. Such abscesses are less well defined than in older individuals and are accompanied by more diffuse inflammation of the brain substance and more frequent involvement of the ventricles. Because of the latter, hydrocephalus is a common sequela. With infected myelomeningoceles, ventriculitis may antedate the involvement of the brain substance (Fig. 24–5).

Of the *viral infections* involving the brain in the newborn infant and in the 1st year of life, five are of especial importance. These are the viruses of herpes simplex, cytomegalic inclusion disease, rubella, Coxsackie and poliomyelitis.

Herpes type II virus infection in the newborn often produces brain lesions as part of a generalized involvement. Most often acquired in utero or in passage through an infected birth canal, it is the most common lethal virus infection of the newborn now encountered in North American obstetric practice. Grossly, the brain is not strikingly altered, although inflammation of the meninges may be visible over the pons, medulla and cerebellum (Wolf and Cowen). In these same regions the brain substance may have perivascular leukocytic infiltration,

Fig. 24—5. — Aqueduct of the midbrain in a 9-day-old infant with an infected myelomeningocele. The aqueduct lumen is filled with polymorphonuclear cells, and perivascular exudate is present in the periaqueductal tissues. The cerebral meninges were not affected.

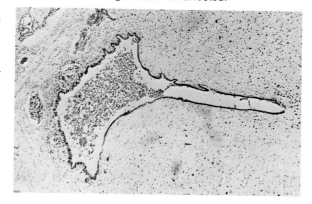

small hemorrhages and zones of focal necroses often containing microglia and macrophages. Typical intranuclear inclusions are present in nerve cells (see Fig. 9–12).

Cytomegalic inclusion disease, due to the salivary gland virus, is a generalized infection in the newborn that is usually acquired early in fetal life and often affects the brain. The brain destruction may be massive, because of the chronicity of the infection. Grossly, the meninges may be opaque, with focal areas of necrosis and scarring. The lateral ventricles of the cerebrum are often surrounded by areas of necrosis. Calcification of such zones is responsible for the semidiagnostic x-ray picture of a sharp zone of calcification outlining cerebral ventricles (Fig. 24–6). As in other parts of the body, the virus elicits only a minor inflammatory reaction, and necrosis is the chief tissue alteration. Because the virus is ordinarily already present when the brain is being formed, microgyria, porencephaly, cerebellar dysplasia and other abnormalities of gyration and lamination of the cortex may be produced (Wolf and Cowen). The ependymal and subependymal layers are particularly susceptible to the virus, and typical inclusions may be found here as well as in other parts of the brain substance. The ependymal layer may be replaced by glial nodules.

Fig. 24–6.—Roentgenogram of microcephalic skull of an infant with cytomegalic inclusion disease with calcium outlining the dilated ventricles *(arrows).* (Courtesy Dr. E. B. D. Neuhauser.)

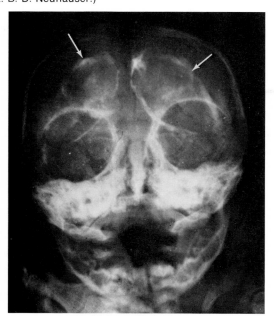

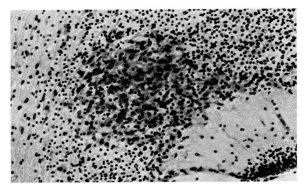

Fig. 24–7.—Cerebellar cortex of an infant dying with generalized Coxsackie infection. The internal granular layer shows a zone of local destruction and infiltration of large mononuclear cells.

Rubella virus most often produces lesions as part of the congenital rubella syndrome, in which most of the changes take place antenatally. The blood vessels, especially the small arteries, are damaged and exhibit endothelial proliferation, necrosis of the vessel walls and perivascular glioses (Rorke and Spiro; Desmond *et al.*). Focal ischemic necrosis in the subpial and periventricular white matter and the deeper layers of the cortex is followed by infiltration with histiocytes and glial cells. Myelinization of the centrum ovale and basal ganglia may be delayed.

Coxsackie virus, when responsible for a generalized infection in the newborn, may also involve the brain. It causes focal granulomas consisting of microglia, macrophages and astrocytes in the cerebellum, brain stem and meninges (Fig. 24–7). Both nursery epidemics and prenatal infection have been described.

Eastern equine encephalitis may occur but is rare since most infants are protected from the insect vector. In epidemic years, however, as many as 20% of cases may be in infants under 1 year of age (Farber *et al.*). During the acute stage of the disease the brain is swollen and edematous, and polymorphonuclear cells infiltrate meninges and areas around blood vessels. Thrombosis of small vessels is frequent. Infants who survive the first few days have marked destruction of neuronal elements, and mononuclear cells replace the polymorphonuclear cells in the lesions in the brain.

Poliomyelitis, like herpes infections, is most often acquired by the fetus as it passes through the birth canal. As in older individuals, the lesions are predominantly in the spinal cord, and anterior horn nerve cells exhibit pyknosis, ballooning, karyorrhexis and destruction. Lymphocytes and polymorphonuclear cells are present around the vessels in the anterior horn early in the disease but later are replaced by glial cells and macrophages. The glial net may be destroyed in the immediate vicinity of the anterior horns, and meninges may be mildly infiltrated with cells.

Among nonbacterial, nonviral infections in the newborn infant and the 1st year of life, which although generalized especially affect the brain, two are especially important. The first is *congenital neurosyphilis*. This rarely produces symptoms in the neonatal period but the meninges show vasculitis with many polymorphonuclear cells, plasma cells and organisms.

Severe infiltration around the basilar portions of the brain may lead to blockage of cerebrospinal fluid with resultant hydrocephalus. In the brain parenchyma the reaction is both vascular and perivascular, with swollen proliferated endothelial cells lining the small vessels and with proliferating glial cells and an infiltration of plasma cells in the surrounding tissue. Porencephaly and microgyria may result from these changes.

The second is *toxoplasmosis*. When acquired transplacentally the presenting symptoms include seizures, failure to thrive, microcephalus and microphthalmia. The organisms produce elevated yellow granulomatous plaques with necrotic centers in superficial portions of the cerebral hemispheres and zones of destruction in the white matter and periventricular tissues. The necrotic areas may become calcified and can be demonstrated by x-ray in about half of the cases. The meninges are thickened and the aqueduct often becomes obstructed, so hydrocephalus is common. In the brain stem and cerebellum the lesions are often less necrotizing and consist of local glial proliferation with only minor tissue destruction. In such areas the organisms are most easily found in pseudocysts (see Fig. 9–22), while vegetative forms are usually limited to areas bordering the cerebral necrosis. When congenital, the disease is frequently fatal.

Chagas' disease, due to American trypanosomiasis, is a rare cause of widespread inflammation which in the newborn may involve the brain and meninges in the region of blood vessels. Inflammation in the meninges is more acute than in the cerebral lesions. Both may be accompanied by local necrosis. Organisms may be present in the larger lesions (see Fig. 9–21).

Perivascularly distributed migrating primitive glial cells originating in the subependymal mantle layer in the region of the basal ganglia occasionally

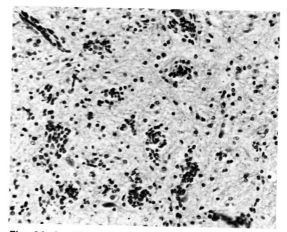

Fig. 24–8.—Photomicrograph of region of the basal ganglia in the cerebellum showing collections of primitive cells resembling medulloblasts. These are nonpathologic.

give rise to a suspicion of encephalitis in newborn premature infants. The uniformity of appearance of such cells and their similarity to the cells in the area of their origin are helpful in distinguishing this normal state of the developing brain from true encephalitis. Immature cells may be seen occasionally in small focal collections in the roof of the fourth ventricle and the region of the basal ganglia of the cerebellum (Fig. 24–8) of newborn infants, especially those who are premature; these cells have the appearance of the medulloblasts seen in medulloblastomas. They have no clinical significance and are not seen in older infants.

Kernicterus

Deposit of bile pigment in the brain is called kernicterus. Any area may be affected but especially involved are the hippocampus of the cortex, the thalamus, caudate nucleus, subthalamic nucleus of the basal ganglia, the roof nuclei of the pons, the dentate nucleus, nucleus fastigius, flocculus and vermis of the cerebellum and the roof nuclei and inferior olives of the medulla (Fig. 24–9). Pigment is often limited to the nerve cells, although in severe cases it may also be deposited in the glial cells and interstitial spaces. In the early stages of the process only minor changes can be seen in the cytoplasm of the affected nerve cells. In paraffin-embedded material much of the pigment is removed by the fat solvents used in tissue preparations. Then only a faint reddish-orange flush may be seen in the nerve cell bodies. Frozen sectioned material stained with

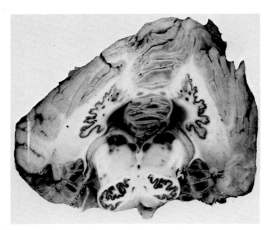

Fig. 24–9.—Kernicterus. Special filter renders yellow areas black. Characteristic distribution of pigment in brain stem and cerebellum.

toluidine blue and mounted in glycerin shows typical intra- and extracellular crystals of bilirubin in severe cases. It is unusual for kernicterus to be identified even on gross examination before 24 hours of life and is almost never seen in stillborn fetuses because of the ability of the placenta to remove bilirubin. By 24 hours sufficient time has elapsed for the bilirubin levels in the serum to have reached toxic levels.

After the first 36–48 hours of life degenerative changes begin in the nucleus and cytoplasm of the nerve or glial cells in severely damaged brains (Haymaker *et al.*). These consist of pyknosis of nuclei and cytolysis of cell bodies (Fig. 24–10). Damaged nerve cells gradually disappear in the first few weeks, followed by reparative gliosis. In severely damaged infants some myelin tracts are lost, especially those in the basal ganglia. In survivors with choreoathetosis the subthalamic nucleus (corpus Luysii) and hippocampus show striking nerve cell loss and gliosis (Greenfield).

Kernicterus results from the direct toxic action of bilirubin on the cells. Because indirect (nonconjugated) bilirubin binds to protein and is soluble in lipid, it crosses the blood brain and cellular membrane barriers with ease. Conjugated bilirubin, being water soluble, does not have these properties so does not cross these barriers at low concentrations. Because of the delay in the synthesis of the conjugating enzyme after birth, kernicterus is a disease almost exclusively of the newborn or of those unable to make conjugating enzyme (Crigler-Najjar syndrome). While in North America erythroblastosis due to maternal immunization to the Rh factor is the chief cause of kernicterus, mild

kernicterus may be due to immunization to A or B blood groups or may rarely develop as a result of sepsis, hemorrhage, diarrhea or intestinal obstruction, especially in premature infants (Zuelzer and Mudgett).

In ethnic groups other than those of North America enzyme deficiencies such as those of glucose-6-phosphate dehydrogenase and pyruvate kinase, which are related to the maintenance of the red cell membrane, or hemoglobin structural abnormalities may be the cause of high bilirubin levels. Most of these factors act to increase the rate of blood destruction or to decrease liver function, thus increasing the serum bilirubin level. Iatrogenic causes such as excess vitamin K administration or therapeutic administration of sulfonamides, which affect enzyme activity or the protein-binding capacity of bilirubin may increase the bilirubin level and produce kernicterus.

The presence of bilirubin is not limited to the brain but has been demonstrated in other tissues such as the kidney, pancreas and testis, but here no evidence of permanent damage has been demonstrated (Bernstein and Landing).

Among the Chinese high bilirubin levels occur in a large proportion of newborn infants without obvious cause; this may be a genetic predisposition to a slower than optimal production of the enzymes involved in bilirubin conjugation (Lee *et al.*).

Any infant with any degree of jaundice is a po-

Fig. 24–10.—Kernicterus. Hippocampus from an infant dying in the first few days of life with severe kernicterus. The larger neurons have shrunken dark nuclei and increased granular cytoplasm that has a reddish hue in sections stained with hematoxylin and eosin. No glial reaction is present.

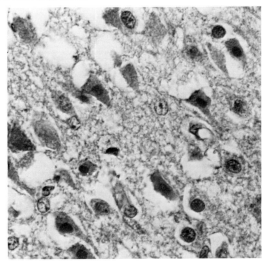

tential candidate for brain damage, and should be carefully observed. Bilirubin levels should be determined frequently until there is definite evidence of decline, so that treatment (ordinarily exchange transfusion) may be initiated before damage occurs. Levels below 20 mg per 100 ml have rarely been found to produce clinical damage except in anoxic premature infants weighing under 1,500 gm, in whom typical nuclear staining has been seen at levels as low as 10 mg per 100 ml (Stern and Denton).

Before exchange transfusions became the standard treatment of erythroblastosis, almost all infants who died of the disease more than 36 hours after birth had kernicterus. According to Lucey *et al.,* application of ultraviolet light to the skin causes a breakdown in the bilirubin molecule and makes a valuable therapeutic adjunct to exchange transfusion in the treatment of high bilirubin levels in the newborn.

Cerebral Palsy

In 1962 Eastman and co-workers published data from examination of birth records of 753 patients with cerebral palsy treated in a number of clinics. They examined without identification the birth records of the palsied patient and of the next-born infant who left the same maternity facility alive. They found that about 10% of the patients with cerebral palsy had had some identifiable postnatal event such as meningitis, acute infantile hemiplegia, encephalitis or obvious birth trauma to account for their neurologic symptoms. When the other 90% were compared to control infants, it was evident that there was an excess of mothers with histories of stillbirths, spontaneous abortions or premature infants (by a factor of 20 times for those under 1,500 gm), malformations, erythroblastosis (nearly all of these had dyskinetic rather than spastic cerebral palsy), twins (especially when one twin was stillborn), midforceps, breech deliveries, nonelective cesarean section (for disproportion, placenta previa, etc.) and the need for supplemental oxygen. This study showed a possible cause for hypoxia in an overwhelming majority of histories. Three quarters of the infants had no signs in the neonatal period indicative of their future difficulty, although the presence of such signs was nevertheless high in comparison to the control group.

The lesions that can be recognized in the early postnatal period and are thought to result from anoxia and be the precursors of cerebral palsy are neuronal damage, subependymal matrix hemorrhage and infarction and paraventricular leukomalacia (Banker and La Roche). (See Chapter 7.)

Most infants with cerebral and intraventricular hemorrhage die very soon after the initial episode occurs. Those that survive for a few days show beginning necrosis followed by infiltration of macrophages by 4 days of age and liquefaction and peripheral organization of the necrotic zone by 8 days (Greenfield). The macrophages in the loose glial scars may persist for 8 or more months. If the damage is severe and the area of necrosis is large, cystic spaces may form in the subcortical white matter. When less severe, damage may be limited to the axis cylinders and myelin sheaths, although such damage is usually accompanied by intense gliosis.

In the late stages of severe anoxic damage the brains of affected children have irregular gyral patterns with well-preserved neuronal ribbons of cortical cells but a loss of both white and gray matter deep in the sulci, which is responsible for narrow gyral stalks (ulegyria). These areas tend to be most common in the cerebral hemispheres in border zones between areas supplied by different arteries but may also be present in less striking form in the cerebellar hemispheres.

The basal ganglia, especially the corpus striatum and thalamus, may have an increase in the myelinated elements *(état marbré)* in addition to the gliosis and loss of neurons.

Hereditary Metabolic Defects Affecting the Brain

There are several congenital metabolic defects that cause severe, identifiable central nervous system lesions in the 1st year. The most important is *infantile amaurotic idiocy (Tay-Sachs disease),* which is one of a group of similar syndromes including early juvenile (Jansky-Bielschowsky), late juvenile (Spielmeyer-Vogt) and adult (Kufs) forms. Tay-Sachs disease may begin as early as at 2–3 months but most often begins at about 6 months of age with weakness, apathy, gradual loss of vision and evidence of mental deterioration. Despite severe generalized flaccidity, the deep reflexes are extremely active, and any sound produces arching of the back, flexion of the arms and extension of the legs (Fig. 24–11, A). Ophthalmic examination reveals macular degeneration and a bright red spot surrounded by a gray-white zone of necrotic and edematous retina in the region of the fovea of each eye. This red spot is found otherwise only in Niemann-Pick disease. Some optic atrophy is also pres-

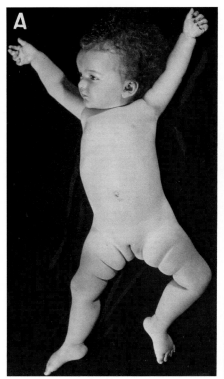
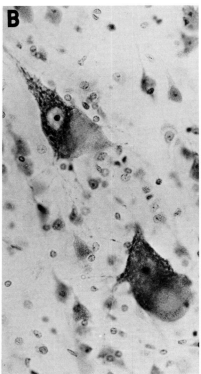

Fig. 24—11.—Infantile amaurotic idiocy (Tay-Sachs disease). **A,** infant aged 5 months with generalized spasticity and increased reflexes; position assumed when startled. **B,** ganglion cells in brain showing characteristic large pale peripheral swellings responsible for an increase in cellular size. Similar cells were present in the spinal cord. (Tissue courtesy Dr. Richard Richter.)

ent. The disease is progressive, and death usually occurs within 18 months.

In early stages there is edema of the meninges and a decrease in brain weight. Later, the cortical ribbon (neuron-containing portion of the cerebral cortex) is firm and leathery, but with neuronal damage and demyelinization it may become flabby and translucent (Rothstein and Welt). The sulci are often widened and the cerebellum is small and firm. The ventricles are dilated due to loss of brain substance. Formalin-fixed cortex may impart a grating feeling on cutting.

Biopsy early in the course of the disease reveals enlarged granular and vacuolated neurons with a decreased amount of Nissl substance and a nucleus displaced into the perikaryon (Fig. 24–11, B). There is little gliosis and no phagocytosis. Special stains reveal fat in neurons and macrophages in the cortex and white matter. Periodic acid-Schiff (PAS), Luxol-fast blue and stains for metachromasia are faintly positive in neuronal cells but more strongly positive in macrophages (Korey and Terry). Ultra-

structural studies show the cytoplasm of the neuronal cells crowded with laminated structures (Terry and Weiss). The macrophages contain dense bodies with a high lipid content. There is also a wallerian type of degeneration of the myelin sheaths. Gliosis begins in the molecular layer of the cortex and progresses inward. In the late stages many astrocytes are present in the white matter (Volk). Changes similar to those in neuronal cells of the brain are present in the retina, spinal ganglia and intramuscular plexus of the bowel. Unlike the disorders discussed below, this condition ordinarily has no involvement of extraneural parenchyma. The material stored in the neurons is a-acetyl neuraminic acid.

Hurler's disease, which causes alteration and degeneration of neuronal elements throughout the body, ordinarily does not show neurologic symptoms until after the 1st year, although occasionally they are present shortly after birth (Magee). The changes in the brain include a reduction in gray matter, an increase in white matter and some degree of hydrocephalus (Green). The meninges are thickened and infiltrated with macrophages similar to those found in other parts of the body. The cortical areas have neurons with swollen cell bodies and displacement of the nucleus into the axon hillock. Nissl substance is decreased and concentrated around the nucleus. Such cells are PAS positive, metachromatic and have a slight sudanophilia (Jervis; Diezel). As the disease progresses, nuclei degenerate and many neuronal cells are lost. The subcortical white matter contains swollen macrophages without lipid in perivascular areas. The changes in the basal ganglia, pons, medulla and spinal cord are much like those in the cortex but the cerebellum is little affected. Most patients with Hurler's disease are mentally retarded and only a few have normal mentality.

In *Neimann-Pick disease* clinical signs of brain damage may be absent in early life even though the brain is anatomically abnormal. Rarely, specific changes have been recognized in the fetus (Bume). The brain is usually underweight, the gyri small and the sulci deep. The cortex, except in the youngest infants, is softer than normal but the white matter is firm despite decreases in myelinization (Crocker and Farber). The ganglion cells, like those in Hurler's disease, are ballooned and often vacuolated with a loss of Nissl substance and displacement of nuclei. In older infants loss of neuronal cells, gliosis and demyelinization become more prominent. The pons, medulla and the Purkinje cells of the cerebellum are involved even in the very young (Crocker and Farber).

Foam cells typical of Niemann-Pick disease (see Fig. 10–15) can be found in the meninges, choroid plexus and perivascular spaces. The autonomic ganglia are involved in all age groups. In routinely prepared sections of the cerebral cortex Niemann-Pick disease may be indistinguishable from Tay-Sachs disease.

Gaucher's disease, infantile form, is the only form of the disorder in which the central nervous system is affected. Deterioration may begin any time in the 1st year and progress to death in 3–8 months. Increased reflexes, opisthotonos, blindness and decerebrate states may be present before death. The basal ganglia are small, and a linear band composed largely of Gaucher cells may be present below the cortical neuronal ribbon, most noticeable in the depths of the sulci. Unlike the other disorders in this group, the lesions are diffuse but focal in character. The ganglion cells in affected areas are ballooned and decreased in number (Banker *et al.*). The cortex, especially around the blood vessels, is

infiltrated with multinucleated, angular Gaucher cells with typically crinkled cytoplasm. These cells stain as do Gaucher's cells elsewhere; they are PAS positive, Sudan black positive and metachromatic with toluidine blue. The neurons of the hippocampus, thalamus, globus pallidus, medulla and pons may be swollen but nuclei are not displaced; they are often degenerated, and neuronophagia can be recognized. The Purkinje and cortical layers of the cerebellum are spared, although efferent tracts of the dentate nucleus and other cerebellar basal ganglia may have some demyelinization.

Generalized gangliosidosis (neurovisceral lipidosis), like Hurler's and Niemann-Pick diseases, is a combined neurovisceral disorder. The material stored in the neurons in the brain is a monosialoganglioside, while that in the viscera is probably a mucopolysaccharide, keratin sulfate (Suzuki). As in other diseases of this group, neurons are swollen but there is little destruction of the cortex (Fig. 24–12). The affected neuronal cells of the brain generally contain lipid but are only weakly PAS positive. Metachromasia can be demonstrated in the neuronal cells by special fixation. Astrocytes, some of which are filled with lipid, are present in increased numbers in the white matter (Landing *et al.*).

Infantile spinal atrophy (infantile muscular atrophy, Werdnig-Hoffmann disease) is a progressive, autosomal recessive disorder of a uniformly lethal nature, no surviving offspring of those affected having been recorded (Brandt). Although it is be-

Fig. 24–12.—Generalized gangliosidosis. Portion of cortex of infant dying at 6 weeks of age. Neurons have swollen pale cytoplasm with dispersion of the Nissl substance.

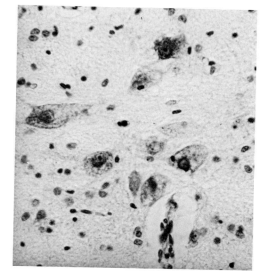

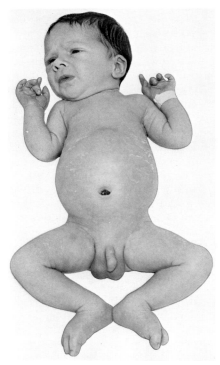

Fig. 24–13.—Infantile spinal atrophy. Infant aged 5 days with arms and legs in characteristic position.

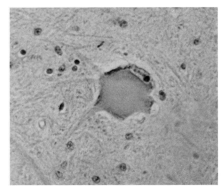

Fig. 24–14.—Infantile spinal atrophy. Photomicrograph showing a swollen degenerating anterior horn cell.

nervated fibers are composed of microfibers (Fig. 24–16). In older infants the muscle cells are absent and are replaced by fat.

Amyotonia congenita (Oppenheim's disease) was formerly used as a designation for all infants with symptoms of Werdnig-Hoffmann disease present at birth. Although most such infants have spinal cord

Fig. 24–15.—Infantile spinal atrophy. Spinal cord from thoracic level showing a decrease in number of anterior horn cells. Same infant as in Fig. 24–13.

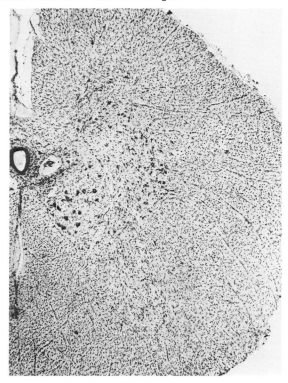

lieved to be caused by a metabolic defect, the exact defect has not been identified. Three clinical groups are recognized according to whether symptoms are first noticeable at birth, in infancy or during the 2d year of life (Byers and Banker). The chief symptom is loss of muscle power, especially in the proximal portions of the limbs, although all muscles except the diaphragm may be affected (Fig. 24–13). Muscle weakness is caused by degeneration of nuclei in the spinal cord. Death results from feeding difficulties and pneumonia after an average duration of 10 months.

The essential lesions are found in the cerebellum, cranial nerve nuclei and cells of the anterior horn of the spinal cord. In these areas the changes consist of a swelling of the cell body (Fig. 24–14) and dislocation of the Nissl substance and nucleus to the periphery, with final disruption and disappearance of the cell (Fig. 24–15). There is little glial response, and no abnormal storage material has been identified. The cortex is normal and no mental derangement is present. Atrophy of the peripheral nerves results in motor unit atrophy of the muscles. The muscle cells are affected fascicle by fascicle rather than individually, and in the young the de-

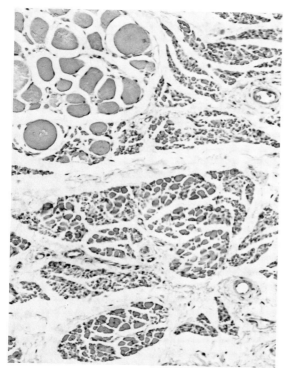

Fig. 24–16.—Infantile spinal atrophy. Skeletal muscle composed of fascicles of microfibers intermixed with fascicles of fibers of normal size.

changes, they are absent in a few and the term is now used only for the latter infants. The cause of the degenerative changes in the muscles is unknown. The prognosis is better than when the spinal cord is involved, and many affected individuals survive into adult life.

Cerebral Degeneration in Infancy

Since the etiology of the leukodystrophies is obscure, classification continues to be uncertain and debatable. Four of the best-defined conditions that have been recognized in the 1st year of life are discussed below.

The first, *sudanophilic cerebral sclerosis* (Schilder's disease) may occur as a sporadic or familial disease (Greenfield) that rarely begins in infancy, although symptoms may occur in the 1st year of life. The course of the disease is slow but with steady progression to blindness and dementia. In cases of many months' duration there may be loss of brain substance and cortical atrophy. The white matter is soft and opaque except at the cortical-subcortical junction, where a layer of axons and

myelin (arcuate fibers) is characteristically preserved. Almost any part of the centrum ovale, particularly the region of the occipital radiation, as well as cerebellum and brain stem can be affected. Microscopically the lesion consists of loss of myelin sheaths and to a lesser extent of axons. Lipid stains reveal large amounts of neutral fat in perivascular macrophages. The number of astrocytes may also be increased in cases with extensive myelin loss.

The term *Krabbe's diffuse globoid sclerosis* was originally restricted to cases beginning in early infancy but more recently has been broadened to include all cases of diffuse sclerosis in which tumor-like collections of macrophages and epithelioid cells are crowded around small blood vessels. Nearly half of the recorded cases are familial. Symptoms in Krabbe's original cases and those of others subsequently reported began in the first months of life, with death occurring in 3–10 months. Changes in the brain consist of loss of myelin, characteristic globoid cells and glial scarring. The cortical tracts in the pons and medulla as well as the white matter of the cortex may be lost. The globoid cells and some of the astrocytes and microglia are only faintly subanophilic but are PAS positive (Norman *et al.*).

Alexander's disease, which usually begins in early life, is characterized by retarded development, macrocephaly and internal hydrocephalus. It is mentioned here because of the absence of normal myelinization, which has been thought by some to be due to failure of myelinization rather than destruction. The brain shows areas without myelin but also without sudanophilia. There is a marked diffuse overgrowth of atypical astrocytes that contain eosinophilic masses thought to be mucoprotein. Similar material is found in extracellular

Fig. 24–17.—Section from a basal ganglion of a newborn infant with iron-calcium-phosphate deposits around a blood vessel. No other brain abnormalities were recognized.

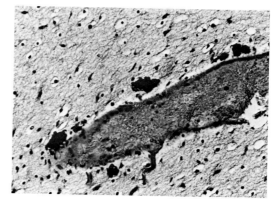

spaces around blood vessels. The deposits, which have a characteristic rod and fiber appearance, are called Rosenthal fibers and may be connected to the astrocytes.

Small deposits of calcium unaccompanied by other pathologic findings and unassociated with any clinical abnormality are fairly common in the newborn brain (Fig. 24–17). However, there is a familial disorder of infancy and childhood known as *Fahr's disease* (perivascular calcification) in which calcium in larger amounts and associated with tissue necrosis is found around capillaries and arteries of the basal ganglia (Melchior *et al.;* Babbit *et al.*). The areas chiefly affected are the putamen, globus pallidus and basal ganglia of the cerebellum. The calcifications can easily be demonstrated by x-ray, and similar deposits are occasionally seen in the eyegrounds. Affected individuals are spastic and have some degree of mental deficiency.

Mongolism (Down's Syndrome)

Mongolism has been the subject of a more voluminous literature than almost any other malformation because affected infants rarely die in the newborn period and offer a social problem not encountered when malformations are incompatible with an extrauterine existence. The exact incidence is unknown, although recent data based on chromosomal analysis indicate that the sporadic form due to anomalies of disjunction, which give rise to an extra chromosome #21, is about 1:700 births; about 90% of mongols fall into the disjunction pattern. Mosaics exist in which lesser degrees of malformation occur. In addition to this trisomy form of mongolism, there are the hereditary and sporadic translocation forms that make up the other 10% and have many of the same abnormalities as the nondisjunctive variety.

The increased frequency of mongolism in the offspring of older women has been related to the increased duration of the dictyotene (resting) stage with an attendant decrease in numbers of chromosome threads in older ova. It is postulated that a decreased frequency of sexual intercourse in older women permits a longer period between ovulation and fertilization, a potent source of chromosomal and other congenital anomalies in certain animal species.

Mongolism is usually found in only one of several siblings if of trisomy origin. Monozygotic twins with either trisomy or a translocation defect will both be mongols (Fig. 24–18). Usually only one of dizygotic twins is affected in the case of the trisomy

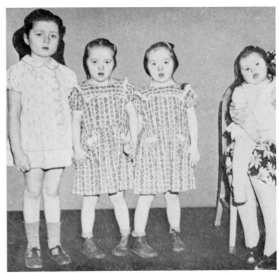

Fig. 24–18.—Mongolian idiocy in three siblings. Identical female mongolian twins aged 7 were firstborn; normal female 5 years 8 months was secondborn *(left),* and mongolian girl aged 1 year 9 months *(right)* was third born. (Courtesy Dr. Douglas N. Buchanan.)

form, but with a parental carrier of a translocation defect both twins might be affected more frequently. Carrier families may have more than one sibling affected, which would be rare in the trisomy form.

Affected individuals range from complete imbeciles to low grade morons, but all are incapable of caring for themselves. Some of the less severely affected may have a mosaic pattern or translocation variant instead of the usual chromosomal defects. Several physical abnormalities usually accompany the mental inadequacy although none is individually diagnostic and any one may occur in otherwise normal individuals with normal chromosomal complements.

The facial expression first draws attention to the child and singles it out from the other occupants of a nursery. The line of the palpebral fissures is unusually flat or slanted upward at the outer canthus. A fold curves over the inner canthus, often hiding the caruncle from view (Fig. 24–19, A). A shallow epicanthic fold may be seen occasionally in normal newborn infants but rarely reaches the prominence observed in mongolian idiots. These children are unusually quiet and placid but, when disturbed, facial grimaces cause characteristic folds in the forehead and at the sides of the nose and mouth (Fig. 24–19, B).

The head is brachycephalic, and large deposits of

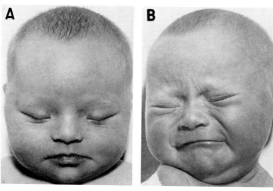

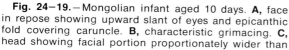

Fig. 24–19.—Mongolian infant aged 10 days. **A,** face in repose showing upward slant of eyes and epicanthic fold covering caruncle. **B,** characteristic grimacing. **C,** head showing facial portion proportionately wider than

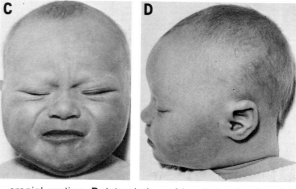

cranial portion. **D,** lateral view of head showing brachycephaiy, fat pad at back of neck, and ear with characteristic shape of helix.

fat in the cheeks ordinarily cause the face to be considerably broader than the upper part of the head (Fig. 24–19, C). There is a prominent fat pad on the back of the neck (Fig. 24–19, D). The upper jaw is smaller than the lower one and moderate prognathism is common. The mouth is small, and although the tongue is not enlarged, it often protrudes through the parted lips. The nose is flat and broad. There is an exaggeration of the iris pattern that has not been described in other conditions, although it is seen on rare occasions in normal individuals. The iris shows white stellate and linear markings that often assume the shape of a horseshoe, with the open side directed away from the pupil (Brushfield spots) (Fig. 24–20). They are present at birth and often become somewhat more

Fig. 24–20.—Eye of mongolian infant with characteristic white flecks in the iris. Child aged 6 months.

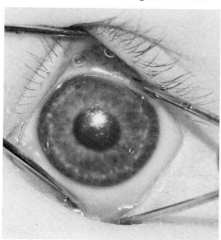

prominent as the child grows older. Nystagmus and imbalance of the ocular muscles are often present in the older child but can rarely be diagnosed in the newborn because of the normal lack of coordination at this time. Cataracts may occur in older children.

The shape of the ears is remarkably constant. The upper part of the helix is turned down more than usual over the anterior surface and its lower margin is flat and forms a right angle with the vertical diameter of the ear (Fig. 24–19, D).

The hands generally show two characteristic features. The second phalangeal bone of the fourth finger is hypoplastic, resulting in a short finger with the distal phalanx directed medially (Fig. 24–21, A). The palm is square and a single straight line parallel to the insertion of the fingers crosses it (simian crease) and replaces the two curved lines normally present (Fig. 24–21, B). Both of these changes may be hereditary in normal individuals and are not necessarily indicative of mongolism.

The feet often show some abnormality in the size or position of individual digits, and very commonly the great toe is held in such a position that it is widely separated from the second toe. A shallow cleft in the soft tissue of the ball of the foot often extends down from the space between the first and second toes.

The entire body is hypotonic and the joints are hyperextensible. Extreme dryness of the skin may cause cracks and fissures of the hands and feet.

Many mongolian idiots do not survive the 1st year of life, although death is unusual during the neonatal period. Cardiac malformations are responsible for most of the early deaths; different varieties have been described, but the most common is a persistent atrioventricular ostium (see Fig. 14–35).

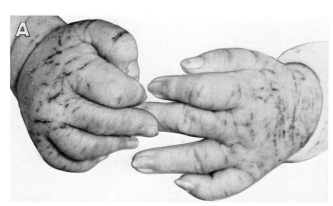

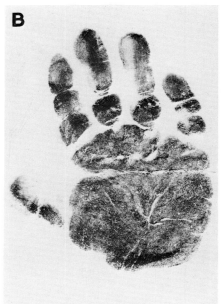

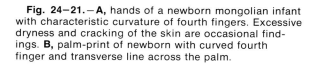

Fig. 24–21.—**A,** hands of a newborn mongolian infant with characteristic curvature of fourth fingers. Excessive dryness and cracking of the skin are occasional findings. **B,** palm-print of newborn with curved fourth finger and transverse line across the palm.

This malformation is largely limited to mongolian idiots and at times has been designated "the mongol heart."

The frequency with which cardiac abnormalities are observed varies with the age at death. In the first 3 years Berg *et al.* found an incidence of about 70%, while after 3 years it dropped to 19%. They emphasized the existence of a mongolian type of heart disease in which atrioventricularis communis, ostium primum, atrial septal defect and mitral and tricuspid atresias were several times more frequent in mongols than in a control population with congenital heart disease. Conversely, pulmonary stenosis and persistent truncus arteriosus were far less common than in other children with congenital heart disease. At the Chicago Lying-in Hospital the cardiac lesion was limited to an atrioventricularis communis and this was found exclusively in mongols. Intestinal malformations, although not common, are of interest because they consist largely of duodenal atresia and megacolon.

The brain may be slightly below average size and weight at birth but is proportionately larger then than in older affected children. The anterior portion of the brain is less well developed than the posterior or lateral areas (Crome). The cortical pattern may be simplified, the sulci shallow and the convolutions broad. The cortex is thin, the number of nerve cells is reduced, fibers are small and myelin is deficient. The blood vessels may be thickened and sclerotic. The cerebellum and brain stem are small in comparison to the cerebrum. However, there are no established pathologic findings that explain the neurologic and mental deficits (Penrose and Smith).

Few mongols have all the characteristics described, but the majority show at least several. The facial appearance combined with the shape of the head is the most important diagnostic feature; other individual findings may be present or absent. It has been thought that the more numerous the individual abnormalities, the lower the potential for mental development.

Dysfunction of the Autonomic Nervous System

Familial dysautonomia (Riley-Day syndrome) is a congenital disturbance in the physiology of the autonomic nervous system with symptoms usually present immediately after birth. It may be readily diagnosed in its typical form, but when atypical it is probably often missed. Conditions essential to the diagnosis, according to McKendrick, are Jewish ancestry, reduced tear secretion, excessive sweating, feeding difficulty, cold hands and feet, postural hypotension, poor motor coordination, corneal anesthesia, relative indifference to pain and emotional lability. The fact that this condition begins at birth is an important point in differentiating it from other states presenting some of these symptoms, e.g., fibrocystic disease of the pancreas, congenital absence of lacrimal glands, cerebral palsy, pink disease, pheochromocytoma and childhood schizophrenia. Excessive sweating and reduced lacrimal secretion are also characteristic of the Chediak-Higashi syndrome (see Chapter 28). Many children with dysautonomia die in infancy of respiratory infections, but the disease is not necessarily fatal, and physical and psychologic disturbances make rearing of the child difficult. It has not been described in adults. It is thought to be primarily a dysfunction of the autonomic nervous system. Pathologic changes have been described recently by Aguayo *et al.* who found a decreased number of unmyelinated nerve fibers in the sural nerve in comparison to a control; the numbers of myelinated fibers were normal except for the largest myelinated elements. They also found shortened internodal lengths, which suggested an arrest in maturation.

Badr El-Din described an unusual syndrome of *intrauterine convulsions* occurring in nine children of three related families, which he thought indicated inheritance of a recessive trait. Generalized rigidity, physical and mental retardation. reflex myoclonus and repeated episodes of clonic and tonic seizures were the outstanding symptoms. The most unusual aspect was that the convulsions had occurred in utero in three children from one family who died in status epilepticus at less than 16 months. From tetanic movements of the fetus after the 5th month of pregnancy, the mother was able to predict which children would be affected.

Tumors

Brain tumors are rare in infants under 1 year of age but, of those that do occur, medulloblastomas are more common and astrocytomas less common than in older children. Only 17 of 313 brain tumors in children under 12 years of age occurred in the 1st year of life in the series of Ingraham and Matson. Combining these 17 cases with 13 reported by Raskind gives the following distribution: medulloblastoma 10, papilloma of the choroid 8, astrocytoma 4, "glioma" 6 and miscellaneous 2.

Medulloblastomas, the most frequent of the tumors observed in very early life, often arise near the midline of the inferior surface of the cerebellum. They may fill the fourth ventricle and cause hydrocephalus and may metastasize widely by way of the spinal fluid. Microscopically, they consist of small cells with scanty cytoplasm and elongated nuclei. In some areas the cells resemble neuroblasts, although rosettes are not found. Since the cells infiltrate readily, tumor boundaries are not easily defined.

Papillomas of the choroid, the next most common tumors in this age group, usually occupy the lateral ventricle and ordinarily form large papillary masses. Such tumors secrete an excessive amount of spinal fluid and the ventricles are frequently dilated despite the absence of obstruction. Microscopically they are composed of papillary masses of columnar cells arranged in a pattern resembling normal choroid plexus but with larger, more crowded and more anaplastic cells. They do not usually invade the brain substance.

Astrocytomas, in this age group as in older children, are most frequently located in the lateral lobes of the cerebellum. They are relatively well circumscribed and in the very young are often cystic. They are composed of fibrillary astrocytes in tumors of lesser malignancy, which fortunately are the most common form seen in younger children. Occasionally a tumor may occupy only one wall of a cystic cavity. Astrocytomas (gliomas) of the brain stem, which are seen more often in older children, differ in that they are diffusely invasive.

The *unclassified gliomas* of early life may be found in either cerebrum or cerebellum. They are usually soft and bulky, actively invasive and seldom amenable to surgery.

Ingraham and Matson found no *craniopharyngiomas* or *teratomas* of the brain in infants under the age of 1 year. However, remnants of the neurenteric canal, which passes from the blastopore lip to the primitive gut in early embryonic life, may be found as small masses of squamous epithelium at any level along its tract from the cranial region to the sacrum. These growing cell collections may be continuous with the skin surface or may be isolated cystic structures. In the brain they are most frequent in the cerebellar region although they may lie along the falx, in the cerebellum or within the fourth ventricle. Similar structures may be found in the lumbosacral region as dermal sinuses. Craniopharyngiomas arise from the pituitary anlage in the nasopharynx, not from the neurenteric canal. They are usually attached to the roof of the mouth and may distend the buccal cavity (see Fig. 12–34), but they may extend into the cranium or, rarely, may be limited to the cranial vault. In the last instance they may produce symptoms associated with the pituitary gland or the optic chiasm or they may compress the fourth ventricle. They are generally cystic and have a somewhat variable pattern but

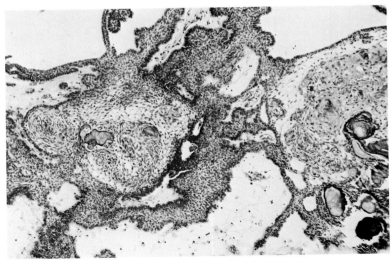

Fig. 24-22.—Craniopharyngioma showing multiple small cavities, adamantinomatous differentiation of cells, calcification and cornification.

always contain some areas resembling adamantinomatous tissue (Fig. 24-22).

Malformations with Head of Normal Size and Configuration

The gyri of the cerebral hemispheres are produced as a result of unequal growth of the white and gray substance, the superficial parts increasing more rapidly than the central core. The hemispheres in early fetal life are smooth and—except for the sylvian fissure, which appears during the 3d month—do not begin to appear until the 5th month. The largest develop first and others follow in a fairly regular order. The form and direction of the principal gyri and sulci are outlined during the 6th month, and by the time of birth all of the main ones are present, although a few smaller sulci appear later.

ABNORMAL CONVOLUTIONS.—In rare instances the convolutional development of the cerebrum is inhibited and only the major fissures are present.

Greenfield included the synonyms agyria and lissencephaly under the general term pachygyria, while Crome used the terms agyria and lissencephaly in which the gyri are totally absent as extreme examples of pachygyria. The pachygyric brain has two essential features, a reduction in the number of secondary gyri and an increased thickness of the gray matter in involved areas. The architecture of the gray and white matter is altered and the ventricles are enlarged. The brain mass is smaller than normal.

Moderate and local reduction in the number of sulci, at times associated with an increase in the brain substance, is called macrogyria. Decrease in size of gyri, usually associated with an increase in number, is called microgyria. All abnormalities in formation of gyri may be found in heads of normal size but are more often present with congenital hydrocephalus. This is especially true of microgyria (see Fig. 24-52).

Mental retardation is often associated with abnormality in size and number of gyri. A remarkable variation in size of gyri, some being several times the width of the others, was seen at the Chicago Lying-in Hospital in an infant with severe osteogenesis imperfecta who survived only a few minutes after birth.

TUBEROUS SCLEROSIS.—The convolutions of the brain in this disease are often of irregular size, some being larger and paler than others and of a cartilaginous consistency. This is due to the presence in the cortex of lesions that may be found in any part of the brain. They are a few millimeters to several centimeters in diameter and, because of their firmness, bulge above the surface when the brain is sectioned (Fig. 24-23).

Similar areas may be present in the spinal cord. Such lesions are composed of a dense fibrous matrix in which are embedded numerous large polyhedral cells thought to be atypical glia or ganglion cells (Fig. 24-24). Myelin sheaths are absent in these sclerotic areas. The diagnosis is rarely made in the newborn period unless the lesions in the brain are accompanied by rhabdomyomas of the heart that are responsible for death.

Thibault and Manuelidis reported a case of tuberous sclerosis with multiple cardiac rhabdomyomas in a premature (33-week) infant, and Globus

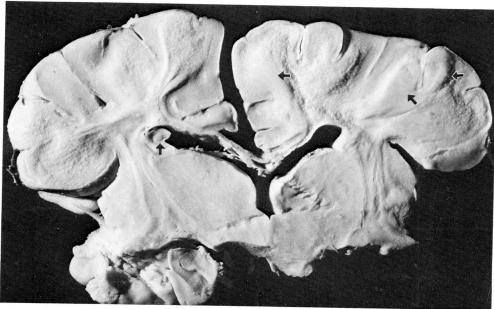

Fig. 24–23.—Tuberous sclerosis. Cross section of cerebral hemispheres in which there are several areas of cortical involvement. The largest (indicated by *arrows*) are visible as smooth masses that bulge slightly above the cut surface. A small nodule protrudes into the lateral portion of the left ventricle. Infant aged 22 days. (Courtesy Dr. Richard Richter.)

Fig. 24–24.—Tuberous sclerosis. **A,** subependymal nodule protruding into the lateral ventricle. Darker lateral portions are more cellular and appear to be more rapidly growing than the larger central area. **B,** abnormal cells and fibers from the same area. From brain shown in Figure 24–23. (Courtesy Dr. Richard Richter.)

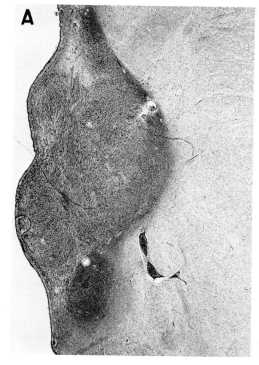

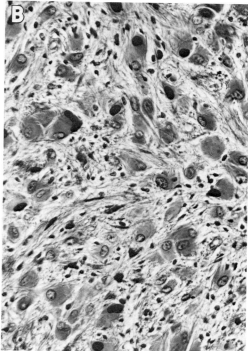

and Selinsky described an infant with tuberous sclerosis without other abnormalities who died soon after the onset of convulsions at 4 days of age. Although the lesions of tuberous sclerosis originate in intrauterine life, they continue to grow after normal growth processes have ceased and may not produce symptoms for many years.

A great variety of malformations may accompany tuberous sclerosis, but the most common are rhabdomyomas of the heart (see Fig. 12–37), cysts or adenomas of the kidneys (see Fig. 22–41, D) and areas of vitiligo in the skin. Sebaceous adenomas distributed in a butterfly pattern over the nose and cheeks are especially common in older children. Retinal lesions consisting of slightly elevated mulberrylike masses about twice the size of the optic disk and of a glistening yellow-white color are often an important aid to diagnosis and may be the only lesions visible in early infancy. At other times convulsions are the first sign of the disease, or there may be no symptoms except a reduction in muscle tone and delay in holding up the head and sitting. Mental deficiency is invariably present as the child grows older. Some investigators believe that tuberous sclerosis is an early manifestation of neurofibromatosis. It appears to be definitely hereditary.

SCHIZENCEPHALY.—This term was used by Yakovlev and Wadsworth to indicate a condition in which brain tissue is absent in localized, symmetrically bilateral areas with consequent local approximation of ependyma and leptomeninges. The brain may be of normal size or hydrocephalic. They believed that this was invariably a developmental anomaly resulting from agenesis of the cerebral mantle in the early stages of development and regarded it as separate from the encephaloclastic porencephalides.

HYDRANENCEPHALY.—This malformation, once a medical curiosity demonstrated only at autopsy, has come to be recognized with increasing frequency, and a sufficiently characteristic group of clinical findings has been described to permit its diagnosis during life. It consists of a great reduction in the amount of brain substance in a head that is of normal size at birth (Fig. 24–25). The cerebellum and medulla may be relatively normal and the cerebral hemispheres extremely rudimentary, often fused and containing a small single cerebral ventricle; or the cerebellum and medulla may be hypoplastic and the cerebral hemispheres completely lacking (Fig. 24–26). The space normally occupied by the cerebral hemispheres is filled with cerebrospinal fluid. The leptomeninges lie close to the dura under the calvarium, and the choroid plexus often floats

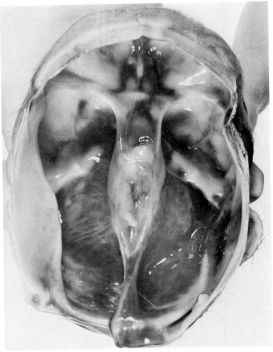

Fig. 24–25.—Hydranencephaly. Base of skull viewed from above after removal of the calvarium. Calvarium was of normal size but was filled only with fluid; the falx cerebri, tentorium cerebelli and brain substance, except for rudimentary medulla and cerebellum, were absent. The only existing brain tissue is still in situ as a small mass covered by a membrane between the posterior cranial fossae.

in fluid at the base of the skull. Circulation of fluid may be normal, or the outlets of the ventricles may be closed. In either case the head is usually of normal size at birth.

Hamby *et al.* reported seven cases diagnosed before death. Most of the infants were normal in appearance and behavior until 2–12 weeks after birth, when the head began to enlarge. The rapidity and degree of enlargement were not related to presence or absence of a block in the circulation of cerebrospinal fluid. Coincident with enlargement of the head the infants became hyperirritable and had convulsions. Percussion of the head gave a tympanitic note, and electroencephalography revealed a complete absence of electrical activity in all leads. These as well as other investigators have shown that transillumination of the head is of most value in establishing a diagnosis. When a strong beam of light is applied to the occiput, the entire cranium is transilluminated and the glow is transmitted through the pupils.

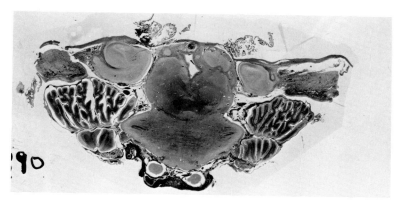

Fig. 24–26.—Hydranencephaly. Cross section of entire midbrain, pons and cerebellum. The choroid plexus lay in a large, fluid-filled cranial cavity.

This malformation is not incompatible with life, having been reported in children as old as 3½ years, but mental age remains at the newborn level. The adrenals may be hypoplastic and resemble those associated with anencephalus.

There is no sharp line of demarcation between hydranencephaly and external hydrocephalus with hypoplasia of the cerebral hemispheres (see Fig. 24–53). However, it should not be confused with severe internal hydrocephalus, in which the cerebral hemispheres are dilated and thinned out by an accumulation of fluid within the ventricles.

PORENCEPHALY.—Asymmetrical absence of part of a cerebral hemisphere may result in the ependymal lining of the ventricle being brought into con-

tact with the meninges or in the interposition of a cystic cavity between ependyma and meninges. Whether the defect is a developmental abnormality or whether it is secondary to destruction of brain tissue has been argued, but it seems reasonable to believe that at least part of these asymmetrical defects are a result of a destructive process. One of the few instances observed at the Chicago Lying-in Hospital involved the lower part of the anterior central and inferior frontal gyri in a stillborn fetus. The adjacent wall of the hemisphere gradually became thinned, and for a space of about 1 cm the slightly distorted left ventricle was separated from the dura only by ependyma and pia-arachnoid. In a newborn infant observed by Dr. S. M. Rabson a cav-

Fig. 24–27.—Porencephaly. Lateral ventricle is in local contact with the meninges. Numerous hemosiderin-containing macrophages are present in the ventricular

cavity and overlying meninges. Abnormally dilated vascular channels and interstitial hemorrhage are present in the adjacent brain tissue. (Courtesy Dr. S. M. Rabson.)

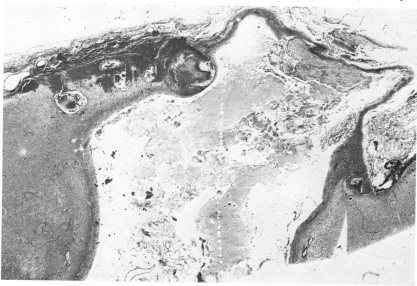

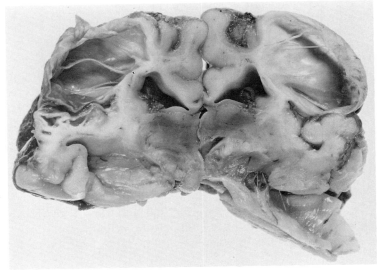

Fig. 24–28.—False porencephaly. Transverse section through both anterior cerebral hemispheres showing multiple cavities of varying size. (Specimen courtesy Dr. Philip Graff.)

ity was present, the exterior wall of which was covered by a thin layer of brain tissue; beneath this were numerous pigment-filled macrophages. Abnormally large blood vessels were present in the adjacent brain tissue (Fig. 24–27). This cavity was probably a result of abnormal development with secondary bleeding into it during intrauterine life. In older individuals it is sometimes difficult to be certain whether cystic cavities are congenital or secondary to areas of postnatal hemorrhage. Symptoms depend on the location of the involved area, and occasionally no symptoms are produced.

FALSE PORENCEPHALY.—Multiple cystic cavities, often somewhat symmetrically located, may be present anywhere in the cerebral hemispheres. They are not in contact with the ventricles or the meningeal space (Fig. 24–28). The cause is unknown.

ARACHNOID CYSTS.—Anderson and Landing described cysts of the arachnoid in young infants which lay in the substance of the pia-arachnoid and were not the result of trauma or hemorrhage. As with subdural membranes, they were apparently capable of acting as osmometers.

Malformations with Head of Abnormal Size or Configuration

MICROCEPHALUS.—This condition may be visible at birth or may not be noticed until later when it becomes evident that the calvarium is not growing at the same rate as the facial portion of the skull (Fig. 24–29). The cerebral hemispheres are most affected, being smaller than normal, although

otherwise they may be grossly and microscopically indistinguishable from those of a normal brain. The skull size is proportionate to that of the brain except rarely when increase in intrameningeal fluid enlarges the head to a normal or greater than normal size. Often the spinal cord also is hypoplastic. The facial expression is generally abnormal and suggests that mental retardation will be severe. The cause in most cases is unknown, although the condition is occasionally inherited and is that reported most frequently when an abnormality follows roentgen therapy given during pregnancy. A few cases have also been observed following rubella in the first few months of pregnancy. Infants with

Fig. 24–29.—Microcephalic idiot aged 6 days.

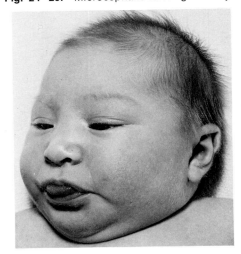

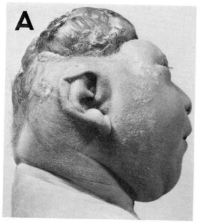

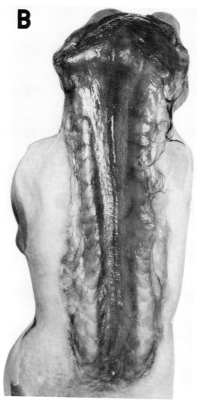

Fig. 24–30.—Anencephalus. **A,** basal portion of occipital bone and hypoplastic cerebellum present. Calvarium absent, and rudimentary cerebral hemispheres composed of blood vessels with small intervening masses of brain tissue. **B,** lack of closure of the entire neural groove with resulting complete craniospinal rachischisis. Note extension of hairline to midthoracic level.

cytomegalic inclusion disease who survive and continue to excrete virus may develop microcephalus.

ANENCEPHALUS.—Although many other terms have been used for this malformation, anencephalus is the simplest and best known. The abnormality involves the derivatives of the most anterior portion of the neural tube and the structures that encase it. The cranial vault is invariably absent and the cerebral hemispheres are completely missing or are reduced to small masses attached to the base of the skull (Fig. 24–30, A). Frontal bones are not present above the supraorbital ridge, and the parietal bones either are entirely absent or consist only of a narrow ridge. The anterior cranial fossae are foreshortened, the sella turcica is flattened and the hypophysis can rarely be identified grossly. The degree of posterior extension varies. At times the greater part of the occipital bone is present, but more often all of the squamous portion is missing, the foramen magnum does not exist and the spinal canal is partially or completely open (Fig. 24–30, B). The cerebral hemispheres consist of soft, red-purple, formless masses a few millimeters to a few centimeters thick lying on the exposed base of the skull. These masses are composed largely of thin-walled vascular channels distended with blood and separated by small irregular masses of brain tissue (Fig. 24–31). Irregular papillary structures resembling choroid plexus are prominent. The surface is often covered with a thin layer of squamous epithelium.

The rest of the brain and spinal cord may be composed of tissue similar to that making up the cerebral hemispheres, or they may be more completely formed. The cerebellum occasionally appears fairly normal, and in such cases an infant may live for several days. Rarely, a portion of cerebellar tissue may be herniated into the medulla (Fig. 24–32). The defect is always continuous, and closure of the cervical or thoracic spine with an opening at a lower level is unknown as an accompaniment of anencephalus.

The absence of the vault of the skull gives the face a characteristic appearance. The eyes bulge forward because of the foreshortening of the anterior cranial fossae and the shallowness of the orbital fossae. The ears are unusually thick and protrude from the sides of the head. When the defect

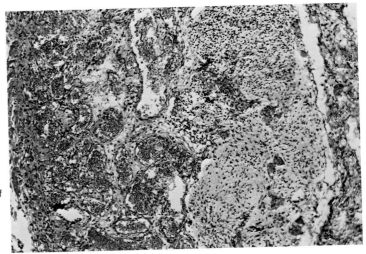

Fig. 24–31.—Anencephalus. Tissue from base of skull of an anencephalic monster showing numerous vascular channels intermixed with small areas of glial cells. Choroid plexus (not shown) was greatly increased in size.

extends into the spine, the trunk is short, the neck is absent and the anterior surfaces of the face and chest are on an almost continuous plane. The chin often lies low over the sternum. Because of the spinal deformity the length of the thoracic cavity is reduced, the heart and lungs are hypoplastic. If the upper part of the spine is normal, the neck is present and the thoracic cavity has a normal volume.

Fig. 24–32.—Anencephalus. Portion of the cerebellum herniated into the medulla.

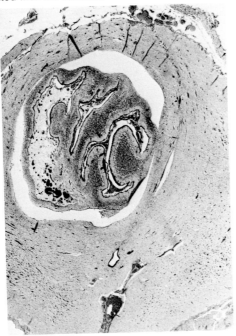

Anencephalus may be a result of the local action of an agent interfering with normal closure of the anterior portion of the neural tube, or it may be part of a generalized disturbance causing a widespread derangement in the development of the entire embryo. In the first instance the rest of the body is normal; in the latter, multiple anomalies are present.

In several experimental animal modules, studies on early embryos show that rupture of the forebrain vesicle is a forerunner of the development of anencephalus (Craig). Adherence to the amnion has been observed in human abortuses (see Fig. 3–54).

Except for clubfoot, which is frequently associated with anencephalus, skeletal defects are uncommon. If present, they most often involve the maxillary arch, palate or upper extremities. The palatine raphe in anencephalic monsters is always higher than the lateral palatine processes, and although it is closed, a deep depression extends the length of the hard palate (Fig. 24–33). Rarely, an actual cleft is present, usually associated with harelip and cleft of the maxilla. The bones of the upper extremities may be abnormal in shape or reduced in number. Absence of the radius and thumb with clubbing of the hand is among the defects most often found. Accessory digits are never present. This is interesting in view of the fact that they are so often associated with the cyclops defect, another anomaly related to severe malformation of the anterior part of the neural tube.

The viscera may show any type of malformation or may be normal except for specific changes secondary to the cerebral disturbance. The lungs and

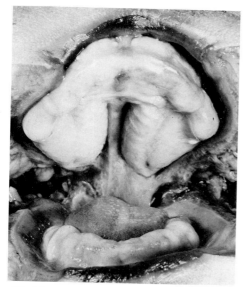

Fig. 24–33.—Hard palate of anencephalic monster. Abnormality caused by incomplete downgrowth of the central palatine process. No communication between buccal and nasal cavities.

glands of internal secretion have characteristic changes directly related to the anencephalus. When the thoracic cavity is compressed, the lungs are reduced in size and the bronchi and bronchioles are disproportionately numerous in relation to the extent of alveolar development. Alveoli may be partially undifferentiated and cuboidal cells may still form continuous coverings of some primitive air spaces, a condition that never exists in the normal fetus at term. The hypoplasia of the lungs is such that their state of development approximates that of lungs of the same weight in a smaller fetus.

Interstitial hemorrhage, most striking in the interlobular connective tissue and around the large bronchi, is consistently present. The thymus is increased in weight and anteroposterior diameter. The cortex is unusually wide and prominent owing to the high concentration of lymphocytes. The thyroid is composed of large acini well filled with colloid. The adrenal glands, although always present, are invariably extremely small. The combined weight is generally less than 1 gm, the fetal zone is rudimentary and the cortex resembles the definitive form normally found in much older children (see Fig. 16–21). The pituitary gland often cannot be seen grossly, although the anterior portion can often be identified microscopically in the hemangiomatous mass or within the substance of the occipital bone at the base of the skull. The cells are

usually narrow cords between greatly distended blood-filled sinusoids. Absence or hypoplasia of the diencephalic centers, the source of the pituitary hormone-releasing factors, is the probable cause of the small adrenal glands. Early in fetal life the adrenal glands appear to be normal (see Fig. 16–22).

The malformation is found predominantly in females, especially when the defect is limited to the neural tube and bony encasement. Among autopsies at the Chicago Lying-in Hospital females made up about 90% of this group. When defects involve other parts of the body as well, the preponderance of females is not quite so high. In both sexes the gonads and genital organs are normal.

Maternal hydramnios often accompanies anencephalus. It has been thought that the excess of fluid might be due to the open state of the skull and spinal cord—that cerebrospinal fluid might be formed in excessive amounts and add directly to the quantity of fluid surrounding the fetus. Since the normal fetus swallows and probably inhales fluid, which is subsequently removed through the maternal circulation, it has also been postulated that the abnormality of the brain interferes with normal deglutition and respiration and that failure of these functions is responsible for the hydramnios.

An alternative explanation is that the absence of the pituitary stalk and posterior pituitary gland gives rise to diabetes insipidus with the production of an excess of dilute urine because of lack of secretion of antidiuretic hormone. This pituitary deficiency may have some role in the delayed onset of labor that is commonly associated with anencephalus.

Prenatal x-ray examination of the uterine contents usually reveals the cranial abnormality. Postnatal x-rays disclose typical changes in the skull and spine (Fig. 24–34).

CYCLOPS.—This malformation has been of much interest to embryologists, not only because it presents a striking deviation from the normal mode of human development, but because of the frequency with which it is observed in other mammals and the ease with which it can be produced experimentally in lower forms of life. Interest has centered particularly on the eyes, but of equal importance and possibly fundamental to its occurrence is the associated abnormality of the brain.

The malformation has been observed in one member of a pair of twins and in one member of a double monster. Ballantyne found it in three members of a litter of eight pigs, an animal in which it seems to be particularly common. He stated that in

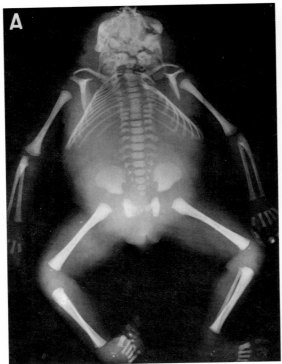
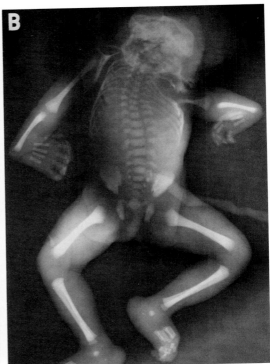
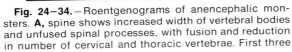

Fig. 24–34.—Roentgenograms of anencephalic monsters. **A,** spine shows increased width of vertebral bodies and unfused spinal processes, with fusion and reduction in number of cervical and thoracic vertebrae. First three ribs on left are hypoplastic and partially fused. Right talipes equinovarus, left calcaneovalgus. **B,** abnormality of upper ribs on left, absence of upper part of left humerus, bilateral absence of radius with clubbing of the hands.

many animals it ranks first in frequency, replacing anencephalus, which is the most common malformation of the nervous system observed in the human fetus. It has been found in human embryos of only a few millimeters.

Cyclops, and the accompanying arrhinencephaly, are among the malformations most consistently associated with D trisomy. Yakovlev suggested that the anomaly results from lack of proper induction of the brain vesicle material by the foregut, which also is deficient in substance. Most of the abnormal parts lie near the anterior neuropore. There is general failure of the forebrain to divide into two halves (halotelencephaly), and since the eyes are an outgrowth of the forebrain, they too take part in the failure of division. The failure of formation of the frontonasal and nasal processes follows.

The cyclops deformity consists of a single orbital fossa with globes absent or rudimentary, or with better-formed globes varying from a single structure impossible to differentiate grossly from the eye of a normal individual through all degrees of doubling to one consisting of two closely adjacent eyeballs that are fairly complete but of reduced size (Fig. 24–35). A single diamond-shaped palpebral fissure is present and the lids are rudimentary or absent. The nose is invariably abnormal; although occasionally it is completely absent, it is more often a tubular appendage with a single cavity lined by mucus-secreting cells placed above the centrally located eye. It ends blindly where it attaches to the skull and has no communication with the pharynx.

The skull is ordinarily somewhat small. A disproportionately large share of the base is occupied by the middle fossae, and both anterior and posterior fossae are diminished in size (Fig. 24–36, A). The small anterior fossa is undivided and contains a single opening through which the optic nerve passes. Several bones are usually missing; these include the ethmoid, presphenoid, inferior turbinates, nasal, lacrimal and premaxillaries. Since the bony portion of the nose is absent, the superior maxillae and vomers are approximated. The palate is closed, although abnormally high, and the philtrum of the lip is absent.

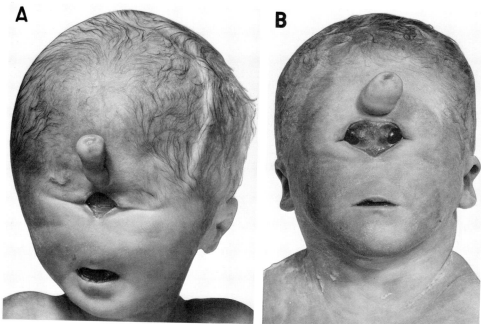

Fig. 24–35.—Cyclops. **A,** centrally placed, diamond-shape orbital opening with no evidence of a globe. Superiorly placed nasal proboscis contains a central cavity that ends blindly at the surface of the head. **B,** centrally placed orbit contains fused globe with double retina, lens, iris and pupil.

The brain has an almost constant pattern in which the cerebral hemispheres are fused into a single mass with a single open ventricle (Fig. 24–36, B). The hemispheral substance is reduced to one third or less the normal volume. The entire ventral olfactory apparatus is missing, including olfactory tracts and bulbs. Neither the corpus callosum nor septum pellucidum are present, and the margin of the ventricle is confluent with a thin membrane that balloons outward and lies immediately under

Fig. 24–36.—Cyclops. **A,** base of skull with a single extremely small anterior cranial fossa. **B,** sagittal section of head showing abnormality of bones of the face and skull, fusion and reduction in size of cerebral hemispheres and absence of corpus callosum.

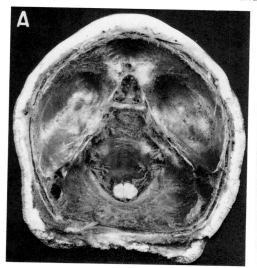
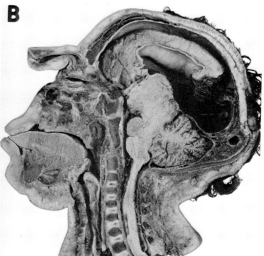

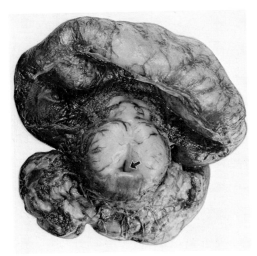

Fig. 24–37.—Cyclops. Brain viewed from above. Cerebral hemispheres are hypoplastic and fused. Interior of the lateral hemispheres is exposed, showing great increase in vascularity. *Arrow* points to opening of aqueduct of Sylvius.

the dura mater. The sac thus formed is filled with fluid. When the head is opened and the membrane removed, the interior of the fused lateral ventricle is visible at the base of the skull, and the corpora quadrigemina surrounding the opening of the third ventricle can be identified as a prominent protuberance (Fig. 24–37). Convolutions are poorly developed and the number of blood vessels on the surface of the brain and lining the ventricles is increased. The spinal cord and the portions of the brain below the cerebral hemispheres appear grossly normal except for a reduction in size similar to that of the forepart of the brain, but occasionally the cerebellum is also defective. The optic nerve is usually

single or absent and the first, third and sixth nerves are absent or hypoplastic.

The microscopic appearance of the eyes varies greatly. In those that are most completely differentiated the various parts of the globes are present and have a fairly normal pattern (Fig. 24–38). In most cases the retina shows rosettes and an abnormal proliferation of tissue which produces a pattern resembling that found in retinoblastomas.

CEBOCEPHALUS.—This malformation is closely related to the cyclops deformity, but the orbits are not fused, and the nose, although abnormal, is located beneath the rudimentary eyes (Fig. 24–39, A). The malformation of the brain is much the same in the two conditions. The optic nerve is single (Fig. 24–39, B), the olfactory nerves, corpus callosum and septum pellucidum are ordinarily absent and the anterior cranial fossae are shallow (Fig. 24–39, C). The cerebral hemispheres are fused but sometimes slightly demarcated by a median sulcus (Fig. 24–40). The posterior portion of the calvarium is filled with fluid contained within the meninges, which are attached to the edge of the fused ventricle.

The orbital cavities are small but separate. The bones in the central portion of the face that contribute to the formation of the nose are small or absent, and the interior of the nose is usually closed and contains no normal structures. The external nose may be completely absent, may consist of nothing but a single small aperture like the opening of a sinus tract or may be a fleshy proboscis similar to that found above the fused eye of the typical cyclops. Occasionally there is associated harelip, often combined with a cleft of the maxilla. The absence of the frontonasal process is responsible for a true median cleft (Fig. 24–41).

Unlike true cyclops, cebocephalus is compatible

Fig. 24–38.—Partially duplicated cyclopian eye. There are two optic nerves and two lenses (not shown). In the middle zone the retina is abnormally proliferated and contains many rosettes similar to those found in retinoblastomas.

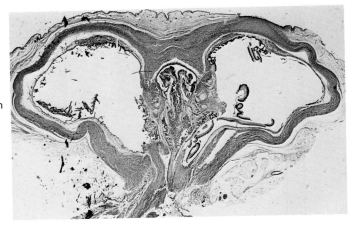

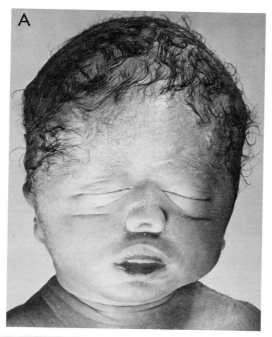

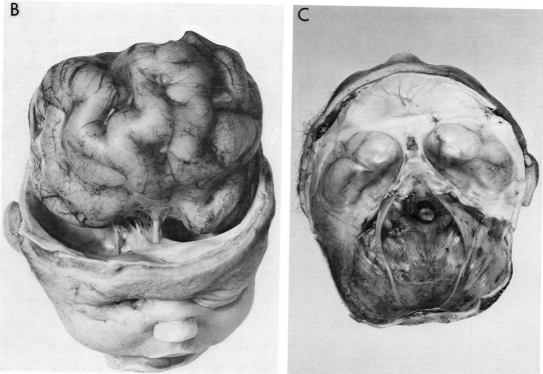

Fig. 24–39. — Cebocephalus. **A,** face showing microphthalmia and suborbital proboscis with single opening. **B,** fused cerebral hemispheres and single optic nerve. **C,** base of skull with small, single anterior cranial fossa.

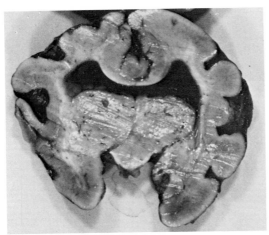

Fig. 24—40.—Cross-section of brain of infant with cebocephalus showing fused frontal lobes and a single ventricle. Note irregularity of gyri.

with continued survival (Fig. 24–42). Like cyclops, it is often associated with an extra chromosome, number 13–15.

CYCLOPS HYPOGNATHUS.—This is another modification of the cyclops deformity. It is the same as the

typical cyclops except for additional abnormalities caused by distorted development of the branchial arches. The proboscis of the typical cyclops is lacking, the ears are abnormally low, the mandible is rudimentary, the buccal cavity is only 1 cm or so in diameter and the orifice only 2 or 3 mm (Fig. 24–43). The development of the lower part of the face is similar to that found in the rare malformation known as synotia (see Figs. 25–54 and 25–55).

Except for polydactyly, malformations of other parts of the skeleton are rare in infants with cyclops and cebocephalus, although two siblings with cebocephalus associated with an unusual form of chondrodystrophy were observed at the Chicago Lying-in Hospital (see Fig. 25–9). Of 15 infants with some degree of cyclops or cebocephalus observed in that hospital, six had an accessory digit in the ulnar side of each hand and one had a duplication of the thumbs. Malformations of the viscera are common.

HYDROCEPHALUS.—This condition is characterized by an abnormal accumulation of fluid in the cranial vault. In internal hydrocephalus the fluid is within the ventricles; in external hydrocephalus it is between the brain and the dura mater, and in the combined form it is present in both locations

Fig. 24—41.—Cebocephalus. **Left,** bilateral microphthalmia, single nostril, median cleft of lip and maxilla. **Right,** view of interior of mouth showing highly arched palate similar to that found in anencephalus, central nostril and cleft of maxilla.

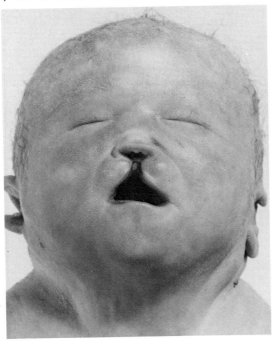

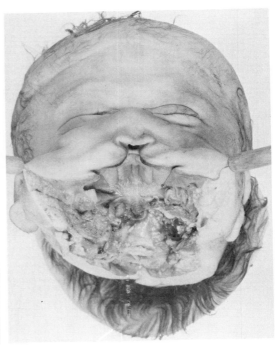

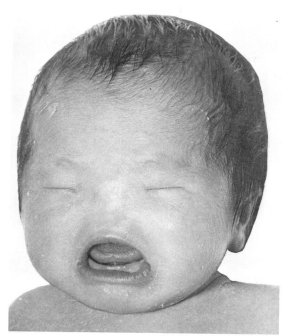

Fig. 24–42.—Cebocephalus with microphthalmia and absence of nose. Age 8 months.

(Fig. 24–44). Cerebrospinal fluid is normally secreted by the choroid plexuses. Fluid from the lateral ventricles passes through the foramina of Monro into the third ventricle and from there through the aqueduct of Sylvius into the fourth ventricle. It flows into the cisterna magna through the foramina of Luschka and Magendie, from where it passes into the subarachnoid space covering the brain and spinal cord. Approximately four fifths of the fluid is absorbed into the circulation through the arachnoid villi of the cerebral meninges, the remaining one fifth through the spinal meninges.

The presence of an excessive amount of fluid might be expected to result from (1) excessive production by the choroid plexuses, (2) interference with escape from the ventricular system or the cisterns or (3) failure of absorption by arachnoid villi.

The first cause, which is rare, is best exemplified by papillomas of the choroid plexus. The third is even more rare and has seldom been recognized. According to Russell, at least 99% of the cases of hydrocephalus found at all ages are caused by obstruction to the passage of cerebrospinal fluid into the subarachnoid space. In the fetus and newborn most obstructions result from malformations; in older infants and adults they may also be due to malformations but more often appear to be secondary to (1) the formation of adhesions about the base of the brain as a result of meningitis, hemorrhage or other chronic irritative or destructive process, (2) obstructions of the aqueduct from bacterial ventriculitis or organization of massive intraventricular hemorrhage, (3) sinus thrombosis or thrombophlebitis or (4) pressure from a neoplasm.

Hydrocephalus has been divided into two clinical types that are related to the ability of ventricular fluid to enter the spinal canal. If dye injected into the ventricular system appears in the spinal canal, it indicates a free passage of cerebrospinal fluid out of the brain into the surrounding cisterns and an absence of obstruction in the ventricular system. This is called communicating hydrocephalus, and the fluid accumulates in the ventricles because it cannot escape from the cisterna magna into the cerebral subarachnoid space. If dye does not appear in the cerebrospinal fluid, the obstruction must be located in the ventricular system. This is noncommunicating hydrocephalus, and the fluid accumulates because of an obstruction at or above the lower end of the fourth ventricle.

Hydrocephalus is seldom present at birth except with spina bifida. Our material supports Russell's statement that an *Arnold-Chiari defect* is almost invariably found when a meningomyelocele exists. She believed that the Arnold-Chiari defect interferes with the passage of fluid into the subarachnoid space and is directly responsible for dilatation of the ventricular system and therefore for the hydrocephalus associated with spina bifida. This malformation consists of a downward displacement of the cerebellum and medulla. The tentorium is low, almost at the edge of the foramen magnum, which greatly compromises the size of the posterior fossa (Cameron). The foramen magnum in the Arnold-Chiari malformation is not enlarged but the cerebellum and medulla are forced down into the spinal canal by the lack of space in the posterior fossa (Figs. 24–45 and 24–46).

If the spinal defect is not covered by a sac but lies open to the exterior, or if a fistulous opening is adjacent to the sac, cerebrospinal fluid may escape to the exterior and hydrocephalus may be prevented. It also seems possible that in some instances the wall of the sac acts as a mechanism for absorption of the cerebrospinal fluid into the bloodstream, because occasionally hydrocephalus is slight in the presence of the Arnold-Chiari malformation even though the spinal defect is covered by a sac. In

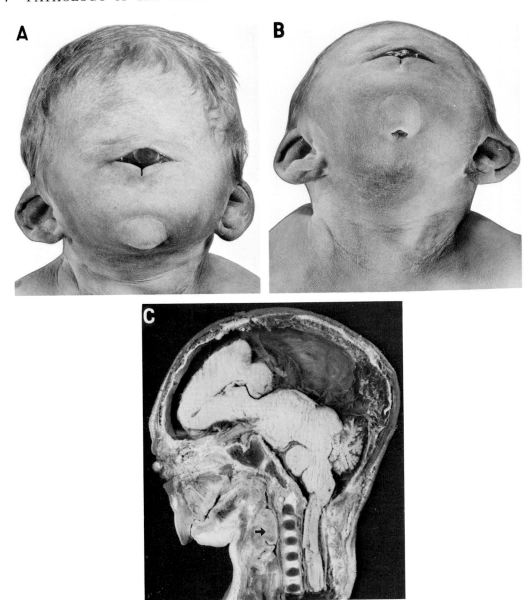

Fig. 24–43.—Cyclops hypognathus. Single central orbit almost perfectly formed, nose absent, buccal orifice and mandible rudimentary, ears unusually low. **A,** front view of face. **B,** head tilted backward to show buccal orifice. **C,** sagittal section through another head showing a malformation similar to A except for partial duplication of the globes. *Arrow* indicates position of the tongue. Note similarity of the brain to that shown in Figure 24–36.

some instances removal of the sac and closure of the spinal defect is stated to be followed by the development or aggravation of hydrocephalus. Actually, the enlargement of the head is ordinarily unrelated to the operation, instead being the result of a continued increase in hydrocephalus that was unrecognized at birth because the skull was not then enlarged. Hydrocephalus may also exist even though free drainage of fluid to the exterior is possible because of the absence of a sac. Cameron found that the aqueduct is narrowed in half of the cases and is the seat of glial reaction and forking or

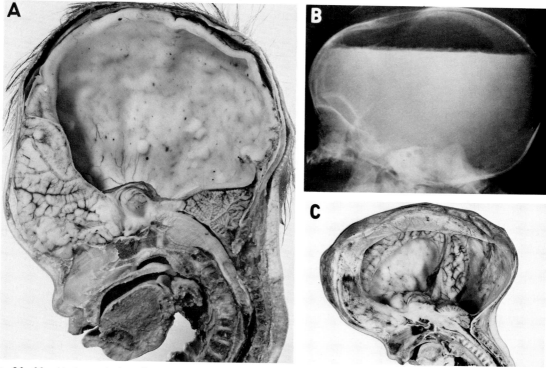

Fig. 24—44.—Hydrocephalus. **A,** internal hydrocephalus caused by Arnold-Chiari defect associated with lumbar meningocele. Aqueduct of Sylvius is patent although not visible. The extreme distention of the ventricles is associated with marked thinning of the cerebral cortex. Infant aged 2 hours. **B,** external hydrocephalus associated with extreme hypoplasia of the brain. X-ray made following withdrawal of small amount of fluid and introduction of air. (Courtesy Dr. Ralph Platou.) **C,** combined internal and external hydrocephalus. Infant aged 16 hours.

stenosis in a smaller number. In such cases associated noncommunicating hydrocephalus must be produced by compression of the ventricular system, most often in the region of the aqueduct of Sylvius.

In the brains of some infants with the Arnold-Chiari defect there is evidence of an architectonic disturbance in the arrangement of the neural and glial elements so that inappropriate elements are found in juxtaposition in the vermis and in the roof of the fourth ventricle, and atypical collections of glial cells are present in the cortex of the cerebellar uvula and nodule. Because of the hypoplasia of the falx and increased intraventricular pressure the gyri on the medial surfaces of the cerebral hemispheres become interdigitated. As in all congenital hydrocephalus, microgyria is common and nodules of mixed gray and white matter may be present on the internal surfaces of the lateral ventricles.

In the cervical region the nerve roots of the spinal cord run cephalad; in the thorax they again resume their normal direction. Hydromyelia is common, being present in most affected newborns.

According to Russell, only about half of all simple meningoceles have an associated Arnold-Chiari defect, and spina bifida occulta is almost never accompanied by this defect.

In the newborn, hydrocephalus other than that caused by the Arnold-Chiari defect is principally of the noncommunicating type and is a result of stenosis of the aqueduct of Sylvius or of septum formation at the caudal end of the aqueduct or at the lower end of the fourth ventricle in the region of the foramina of Luschka and Magendie. This is the Dandy-Walker syndrome, which may be associated with anomalies of the vermis, absence of the corpus callosum and abnormal collections of glial cells in the cerebellum (D'Agostino *et al.*). If hydrocephalus is visible at birth in the absence of a spinal defect, it is most often due to one of these abnormalities.

In the fetus and newborn the Arnold-Chiari defect is easily identified by proper dissection, but it

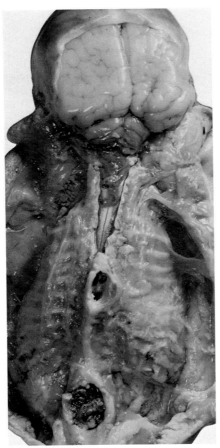

Fig. 24—45.—Arnold-Chiari defect associated with internal hydrocephalus and thoracic and lumbar meningoceles. A tonguelike prolongation of the cerebellum extends into the spinal canal and overlies the upper part of the spinal cord. Infant aged 2 days.

is often difficult to be certain whether any part of the ventricular system is obstructed. If the fetus dies before birth, the brain quickly degenerates, and even in liveborn infants the normally high water content makes the brain soft and difficult to handle. This is further aggravated by the frequency with which the hydrocephalic head is mechanically collapsed to facilitate delivery.

The anatomic changes associated with an abnormal accumulation of fluid in the head are variable. The following descriptions are of changes found in the newborn and are somewhat different from those produced by hydrocephalus originating after the sutures of the skull have closed. While the sutures are open, the skull can enlarge more rapidly and

attain a greater size than when the process begins at an older age.

In the newborn the skull may not be enlarged even though the ventricles are distended by fluid (Fig. 24–47, A). At times the enlargement is slight and is manifested principally by a moderate widening of the sutures and an abnormal bulging of the forehead over the region of the anterior fontanel (Fig. 24–47, B). At other times the size of the head is greatly increased. The enlargement may be symmetrical or may extend principally anteriorly or posteriorly (Fig. 24–48).

When the head is enlarged, the sutures are widened and the bones of the calvarium are increased in surface area. All margins of the parietal bones and the upper margins of the frontal and occipital bones are irregular and appear frayed where they merge gradually with the pericranium (Fig. 24–49, A). The bones may be so thin that they seem to be little more than a moderately stiffened membrane,

Fig. 24—46.—Arnold-Chiari defect. Sagittal section showing elongation of the lower part of the cerebellum that overlies posterior surface of the medulla and spinal cord, and elongation of the fourth ventricle.

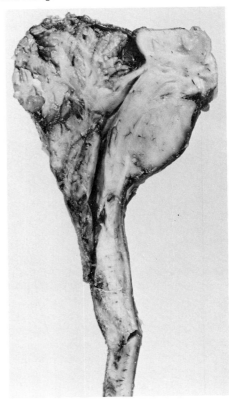

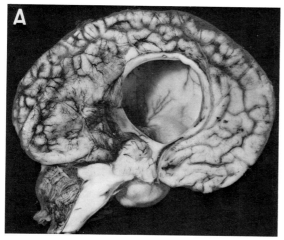

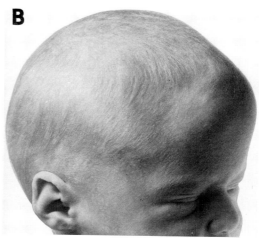

Fig. 24–47.—Internal hydrocephalus. **A,** severe dilatation of lateral ventricles in newborn infant without enlargement of the head. **B,** slight protrusion of brain through abnormally large anterior fontanel. Head otherwise not enlarged.

or they may be thicker and have irregular inner ridges separating small round or oval defects covered only by the pericranial membrane (Fig. 24–49, B). These defects are called *lückenschädel*, or cranial fenestrations, and are found commonly with hydrocephalus or sometimes with spina bifida in the absence of hydrocephalus. The base of the skull is increased in any or all diameters and the normal irregularities in the base are accentuated by the increase in pressure (Fig. 24–50).

If the child survives after birth, the fenestrations of the skull become greatly enlarged and much of the brain may be covered only by membrane (Fig. 24–51).

The changes in the brain are most conspicuous in the cerebral hemispheres. As the fluid accumulates, the cerebral cortex becomes progressively thinner. Despite this, the amount of brain tissue may be considerably greater than normal and the brain without fluid may weigh much more than the average. The convolutions are often greatly increased in number and decreased in size (microgyria) (Fig.

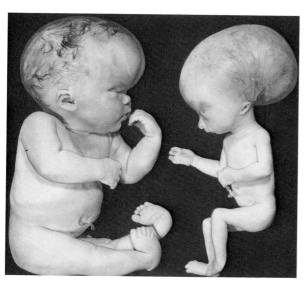

Fig. 24–48.—Internal hydrocephalus in two stillborn infants. The infant on the left has an Arnold-Chiari defect, lumbar spina bifida and commonly associated arthrogryposis of the knees and clubbing of the feet. The infant on the right has atretic aqueduct of Sylvius.

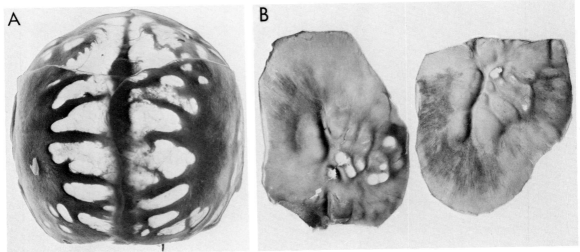

Fig. 24—49.—Skull bones in hydrocephalus. **A,** frontal and parietal bones of newborn infant; bone growth unable to keep pace with enlarging head. **B,** frontal bones showing ridges on internal surface with intervening fenestrations covered only by pericranial membrane.

24–52). The microscopic structure is usually not appreciably altered except as a result of the mechanical changes.

The aqueduct of Sylvius varies in size and shape at different levels and is always smaller in the newborn than in the adult. Rarely, obstruction of the aqueduct is visible only as a reduction in the size of the lumen but is seen more often as a "forking" deformity, described by Russell and others. Most cases described as atresia are actually a forking of the aqueduct and consist of a division of the channel into dorsal and ventral portions by normal brain tissue. The dorsal channel is usually considerably branched and the ventral channel is a narrow slit. They may communicate with the ventricles individually, may unite with each other or may dwindle out and be lost in the brain substance. A familial sex-linked noncommunicating hydrocephalus due to stenosis of the aqueduct without either gliosis or forking has been recognized (Edwards *et al.*).

External hydrocephalus is a rare condition that has not been encountered at the Chicago Lying-in Hospital except in two siblings who also had an

Fig. 24—50.—Base of skull of hydrocephalic stillborn infant showing generalized increase in size that is proportionately greatest in the posterior fossae. All irregularities in elevation are exaggerated by the increased pressure.

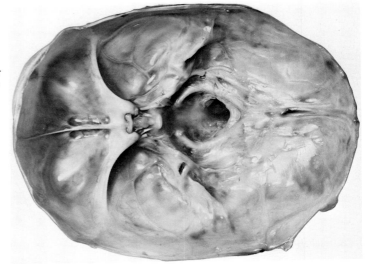

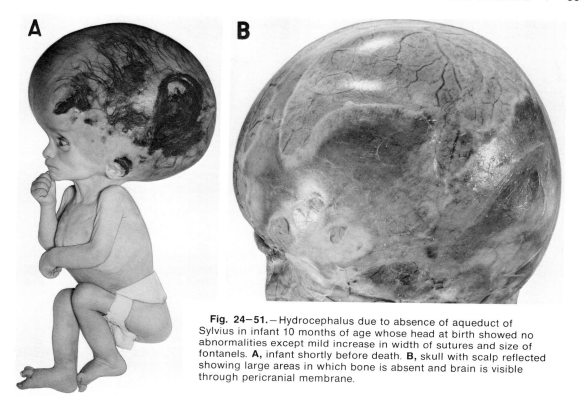

Fig. 24–51.—Hydrocephalus due to absence of aqueduct of Sylvius in infant 10 months of age whose head at birth showed no abnormalities except mild increase in width of sutures and size of fontanels. **A,** infant shortly before death. **B,** skull with scalp reflected showing large areas in which bone is absent and brain is visible through pericranial membrane.

unusual form of chondrodystrophy and cebocephalus (Fig. 24–53). It is associated with hypoplasia of the cerebral hemispheres, and although the choroid plexuses are able to secrete fluid, the arachnoid villi are either absent or nonfunctioning. In the living child it can be differentiated from internal hydrocephalus by x-ray examination. Extreme forms present as hydranencephaly.

Combined internal and external hydrocephalus may be due either to partial interference with passage of fluid from the fourth ventricle into the cerebral subarachnoid space or to a fistulous opening between the ventricular system and the subarachnoid space. Either must be associated with an abnormality of the absorbing mechanism of the arachnoid villi which interferes with the complete removal of fluid from this area.

Other malformations of the brain may be associated with hydrocephalus. One infant at the Chicago Lying-in Hospital had a severe enlargement of the head accompanied by fusion of the cerebral hemispheres (Fig. 24–54). The total amount of brain substance was increased and lay in the base of the skull. The interior of the lateral ventricles made a single cavity, the margins of which were attached to a thin membrane that extended over the inner surface of the calvarium under the dura. The inner surface was continuous with the ependyma, the outer surface with the pia-arachnoid. The corpus callosum and septum pellucidum were absent. The eyes were normal. The brain malformation was similar to that found in cyclopian monsters except that in the latter the head is rarely enlarged.

CEREBELLAR HYPOPLASIA.—This is much less common than reduction in size of the cerebral hemispheres, although it may appear as an isolated malformation (Fig. 24–55) in which the cerebellum is surrounded by a fluid-filled space. The cerebellum may be normal in shape except for a uniform reduction in size.

MEGALOCEPHALY WITH ACHONDROPLASIA.—Achondroplastic dwarfs frequently appear to have large heads and are often thought to have mild hydrocephalus. Of 10 infants with typical achondroplasia examined at autopsy at the Chicago Lying-in Hospital only one had hydrocephalus. In two the brain weight was considerably in excess of the normal, and in the others it was at the upper limits of normal. Dennis *et al.* called attention to the megalocephaly that may be associated with

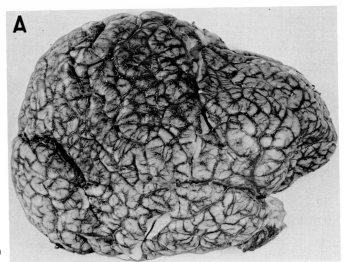

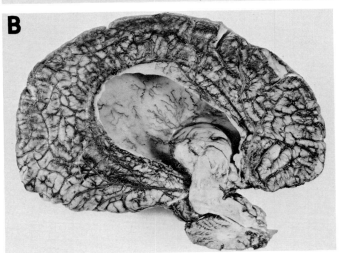

Fig. 24–52.—Hydrocephalus with marked increase in size of head at birth caused by Arnold-Chiari defect. Note extreme microgyrai. **A,** external surface of the left cerebral hemisphere. **B,** sagittal section through brain.

Fig. 24–53.—External hydrocephalus with absence of corpus callosum, fusion of rudimentary hemispheres and single optic nerve in a child with an unusual form of chondrodystrophy (see Fig. 25–9). This has features common to both cebocephalus and hydranencephaly. A sibling had identical malformations.

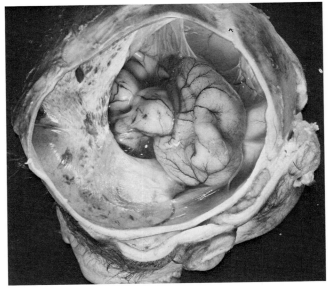

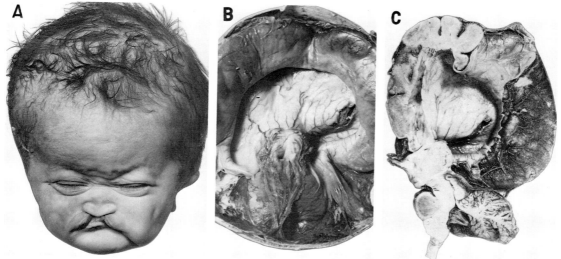

Fig. 24–54.—Hydrocephalus with malformation of the brain similar to that of cyclopian monsters. **A,** external view of the head. Bilateral harelip and cleft palate also present. **B,** brain lying in base of skull showing fusion of cerebral hemispheres. Membranes lying under the calvarium within which the fluid was contained were continuous with the brain at the margin of the ventricle and were severed at the outer edge of the visible portion of the brain. **C,** sagittal section of the brain with more of the membrane removed to show extreme vascularity of pia-arachnoid. Part remains attached to anterior margin of the brain. Internal surface is continuous with ependyma lining the ventricle, the outer surface with pia-arachnoid.

Fig. 24–55.—Cerebellar hypoplasia with normal-sized cerebral hemispheres. Brain stem has been cut and pulled forward to expose fluid-filled posterior fossa.

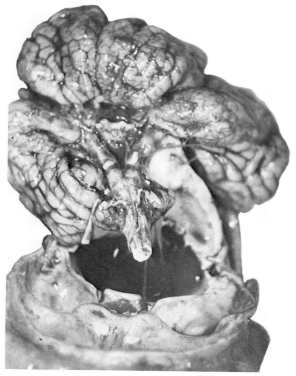

achondroplasia, which they believed was generally responsible for the large head even though a few of their cases also had a slight degree of hydrocephalus. They found the cerebellum small in comparison to the cerebrum. Some had paraplegia resulting from compression of the upper cervical cord by abnormal vertebral pedicles.

CRANIUM BIFIDUM.—Defects of the skull vary from small fenestrations that do not modify the normal contour of the head to those large enough to permit extrusion of most of the brain to the exterior. Those producing visible disturbances in contour are most often in the midline at the base of the skull and involve the squamous portion of the occipital bone. The occipital arch may be absent and the defect may be confluent with the foramen magnum (Fig. 24–56), or the arch may be present and the defect located entirely within the squamous part of the bone. The dura is invariably herniated through the opening. If the opening is small, the brain may be uninvolved (meningocele) (Fig. 24–57, A), but if it is larger, part of the brain as well as meninges are present in the sac (meningoencephalocele) (Fig. 24–57, B). Occasionally the calvarium is very small and most of the brain is outside the skull (Fig. 24–57, C).

Other parts of the skull are much less frequently affected. A defect in the upper part of the parietal bones may be responsible for a meningocele (Fig.

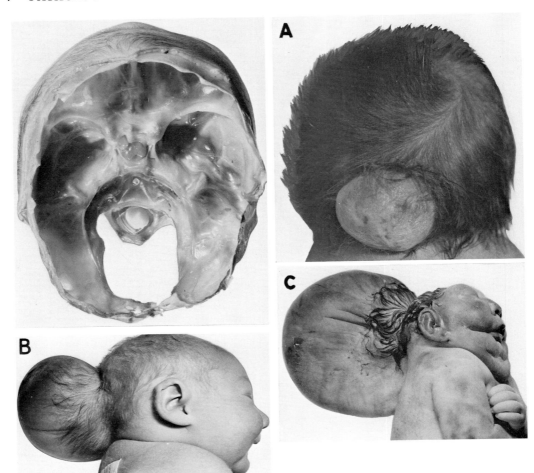

Fig. 24–56 (top left).—Cranium bifidum. Base of skull showing large defect of occipital bone confluent with foramen magnum. Associated with meningoencephalocele.

Fig. 24–57.—**A,** small meningocele of occipital region.

B, meningoencephalocele of occipital region. Bony defect was above foramen magnum and not confluent with it. **C,** encephalocele with most of the brain in the sac. Parietal bones closely applied to the base of the skull.

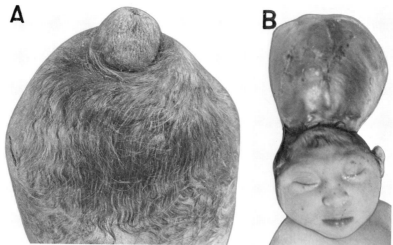

Fig. 24–58.—A, small interparietal meningocele. **B,** interparietal meningoencephalocele with almost all of both cerebral hemispheres contained in the sac. (Courtesy Dr. Waldyr Tostes.)

Fig. 24–59.—Frontal meningocele caused by defect between nasal and frontal bones. **A,** external view. **B,** sagittal section cut slightly to right of midline through the brain substance.

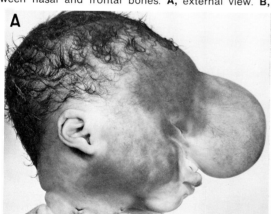

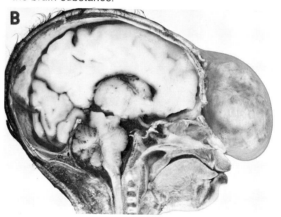

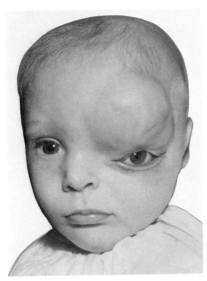

Fig. 24–60. — Supraorbital meningoencephalocele. Mass protrudes under skin through a small defect in the frontal bone.

24–58, A) or meningoencephalocele (Fig. 24–58, B) at the vertex. With anterior defects the opening is usually in the midline between the nasal and the frontal bone, and the sac seldom contains brain tissue (Fig. 24–59). Rarely, a lateral meningoencephalocele may be produced by a bony defect in the supraorbital portion of a frontal bone (Fig. 24–60). Browder and de Veer reported a case of rhinoencephalocele in which the ventral olfactory apparatus was absent and the anterior encephalocele communicated with both ventricles.

Ingraham and Matson gave the distribution of 247 meningoenceloceles as follows:

Occipital	139
Frontal	71
Parietal	27
Nasal	9
Nasopharyngeal	1

Encephalomyelocele. — Occasionally an abnormal opening in the occipital bone is accompanied by absence of the lamina and spinal processes of the vertebrae in the cervical and upper dorsal region or throughout most of the spinal column (Fig. 24–61). Brain, spinal cord and meninges may all be present in the sac. The amount of fluid in the ventricular system as well as external to the brain is usually increased.

Iniencephalus. — Like anencephalus, this is incompatible with extrauterine life. It is rarer than anencephalus and hydrocephalus but may be found in embryos or fetuses delivered at any stage of gestation. The name is derived from the fact that the neck, or inion, is the part principally involved. The malformation consists of a defect of the squamous part of the occipital bone, which produces a greatly enlarged foramen magnum, and of absence of the laminae and spines of the cervical, dorsal and sometimes lumbar vertebrae. The vertebrae, especially those of the cervical region, are reduced in number, irregularly fused and abnormal in shape. The spine is extremely lordotic and the neck hyperextended, so that the face looks skyward and the vertex is directed posteriorly. The open part of the skull is directed anteriorly against the posterior surface of the open spinal column, and consequently the brain and much of the spinal cord occupy a single cavity (Fig. 24–62).

The upper thoracic and cervical arches are bent laterally and forward increasingly from below upward (Gilmour). The brain is occasionally hydrocephalic with an absent corpus callosum and incompletely formed ventricles. In such cases the aqueduct is not usually identifiable and the cerebellar hemispheres are widely separated.

The spinal cord is usually abnormally short and defective. The entire mass composed of brain and spinal cord is ordinarily covered by skin, and only

Fig. 24–61. — Encephalomyelocele. Defect of occipital bone and failure of fusion of lamina of vertebrae. The greater part of the hydrocephalic brain and spinal cord are in the sac. This may be considered a mild form of iniencephalus.

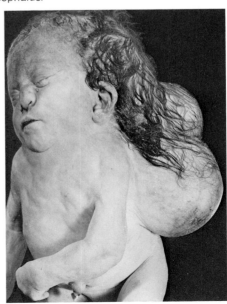

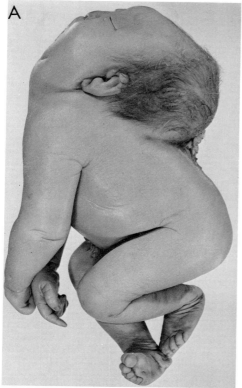

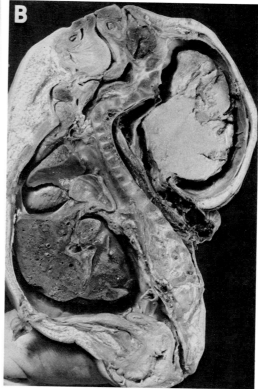

Fig. 24–62.—Iniencephalus due to confluence of cranial and spinal cavities. **A,** exterior view. **B,** sagittal section showing relation of cavity of skull to spinal canal. The brain is cut slightly to the right of the midline.

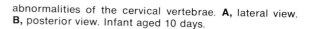

Fig. 24–63.—Klippel-Feil syndrome manifested by shortness and reduced mobility of the neck. Caused by abnormalities of the cervical vertebrae. **A,** lateral view. **B,** posterior view. Infant aged 10 days.

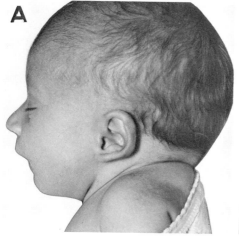

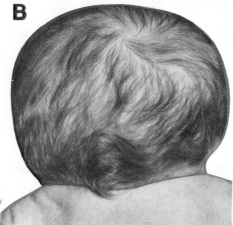

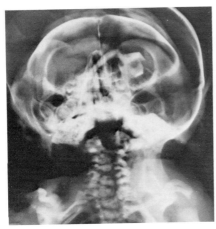
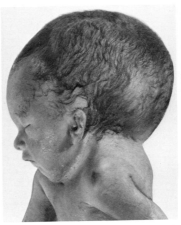
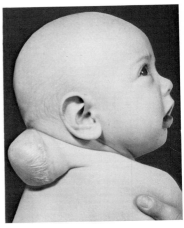

Fig. 24–64 (left).—Defective cervical vertebrae in newborn infant with Klippel-Feil syndrome. Postmortem roentgenogram. Brain has been removed.

Fig. 24–65 (center).—Intermediate stage between iniencephalus and Klippel-Feil syndrome.

Fig. 24–66 (right).—Cervical meningocele. Later successfully removed. (Courtesy Dr. Rustin McIntosh.)

rarely is the lower portion of the spinal canal open to the exterior. The skin of the face passes directly onto that of the chest and there is no indication of a neck. Malformations of the viscera are often associated and include umbilical or diaphragmatic hernias and transposition of the great vessels.

KLIPPEL-FEIL SYNDROME.—Iniencephalus is a great exaggeration of the much milder and more common defect known as the Klippel-Feil syndrome (Fig. 24–63). This consists of a shortening of the neck as a result of abnormalities of the cervical vertebrae. The vertebrae are reduced in number, often fused and irregular in shape and are bifid posteriorly as a result of defective formation of the dorsal rami (Fig. 24–64). The cranium and brain are normal. Intermediate stages are seen in which the head seems to be sunk deeply into the upper part of the trunk, and in these cases the squamous portion of the occipital bone as well as the vertebrae are defective (Fig. 24–65). The face is still directed anteriorly although the head cannot be rotated because of the vertebral anomalies. The trunk also is often abnormal with high scapulas, fusion of ribs and kyphosis or scoliosis (Gilmour). A minority are mentally deficient and spastic.

The principal difference between the abnormalities that range from the Klippel-Feil syndrome to iniencephalus and those included in the encephalomyelocele group is that the brain and cord in the former are confined in the bony skeleton and in the latter lie in a sac partially outside the bony framework of the head and spine.

Malformations Principally Involving the Spinal Cord

SPINA BIFIDA.—Absence of dorsal portions of the vertebrae is one of the most common malformations visible externally. Any part of the spinal column may be involved, although disturbances in the cervical region (Fig. 24–66) are rarer than those in the lower dorsal, lumbar or sacral portions. The involved vertebrae are usually continuous, although occasionally not, and separate openings may be present in dorsal and lumbar regions (see Fig. 24–45).

Spinal defects appear to be of two types and to result from two different causes. In one the abnormality is primary in the vertebrae; in the other it is primary in the neural tube.

The simplest form of primary bony disturbance is spina bifida occulta. The dorsal rami of one or more vertebrae, usually in the lower lumbar region, fail to fuse and the spinal canal remains open. It is covered by normal muscles and is invisible from the exterior except for a small tuft of hair, angioma or dilated venous channels overlying the defect. The spinal cord and nerves are usually normal. With more severe defects more vertebrae are involved, the meninges herniate through the opening and a sac is produced. A small sac (Fig. 24–67, A) is generally covered by normal skin and contains no nerve fibers (meningocele); a larger sac (Fig. 24–67, B) usually contains spinal cord and nerve trunks (meningomyelocele). Occasionally the larger sacs are covered by normal skin but many are covered

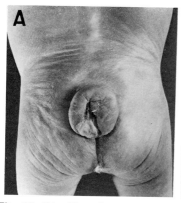

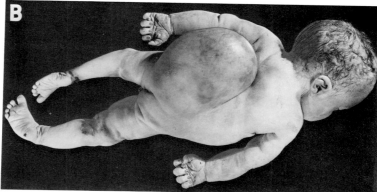

Fig. 24–67.—Closed meningocele of the lower spine. **A,** meningocele associated with small defect of the lower lumbar vertebrae. **B,** large myelomeningocele associated with a defect of lumbar and lower thoracic vertebrae. Bilateral clubfeet resulting from abnormality of the spinal cord.

only by a thin membrane which, if torn, often leads to meningitis.

Spinal abnormalities that result from failure of normal closure of the neural tube are not covered by a sac and are associated with more severe skeletal disturbances than those of the first group. The involved vertebrae always seem widened because of the flattening of the bodies and the lateral portions of the dorsal rami (Fig. 24–68). With small defects the spine may be otherwise normal (Fig. 24–69, A),

Fig. 24–68 (left).—Thoracic spina bifida associated with meningocele. Cleared specimen showing position of the dorsal rami.

Fig. 24–69 (right).—Spina bifida due to primary failure of closure of neural tube; no sac present. **A,** small lumbar defect. **B,** defect of thoracic and lumbar vertebrae associated with severe kyphosis.

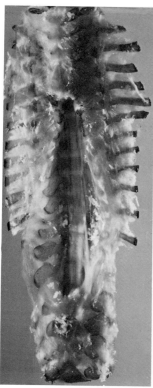

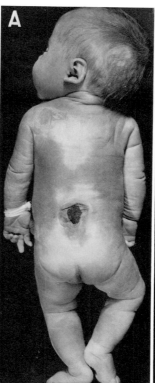

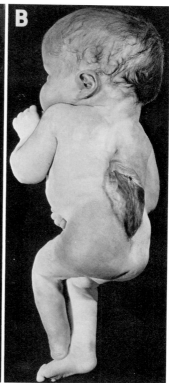

but with larger defects it is severely kyphotic (Fig. 24–69, B). Severe scoliosis, often associated with anomalous formation of other vertebrae and the ribs, is also common. The spinal cord is always abnormal. It is flattened over the surface of the exposed vertebrae, and nerve cells can rarely be identified.

In spina bifida, either with or without a sac, when the spinal cord is involved sphincter control is lost and the lower limbs are the site of trophic disturbances. The feet are clubbed, the legs small and the muscles hypoplastic; the knees are fixed in extension and the hips in flexion. The appearance resembles that often found in arthrogryposis (Fig. 24–70) (see also Fig. 26–6). In some cases of spina bifida with neurologic deficits a lipoma may be present in the region of the cauda equina (Dubrovitz et al.).

A spinal defect can be diagnosed before birth if the fetus is in a favorable position for x-ray examination. In a lateral view the absence of the spinous processes and the kyphosis can be seen; in an anteroposterior view the widening of the vertebral bodies may be visible.

DIASTEMATOMYELIA.—In this condition some part of the spinal cord is divided longitudinally into two portions by bone, fibrous tissue or cartilage. This transfixes the spinal cord and partially divides the neural canal anteroposteriorly in the midline, most often in the lower thoracic or lumbar region. It may be associated with spina bifida or meningocele or with a local hairy patch or nevus. The vertebral column grows more rapidly than the spinal cord, and fixation of the latter puts undue tension on the cord and nerve roots, resulting in incontinence, paresis, disparity in size of lower limbs, trophic changes and even paralysis. Since this abnormality arises, as does the congenital dermal sinus (see below), as a result of failure of the embryonic neurenteric canal to be obliterated, it may be connected to an esophageal or gastrointestinal duplication by a continuous tube or a fibrous or musculofibrous band that passes through the body of a vertebra. An intradural cyst is often associated.

CONGENITAL DERMAL SINUS.—This condition frequently goes unrecognized even when it gives rise to symptoms. It consists of a congenital sinus tract only 1–2 mm in diameter that extends from the

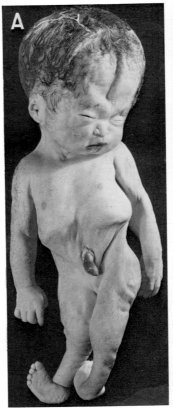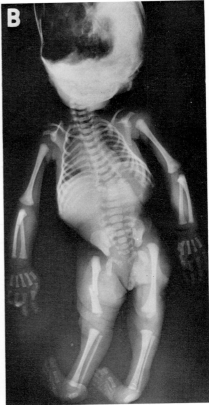

Fig. 24–70.—Large spinal defect without meningocele and with moderate kyphosis. Associated hydrocephalus, arthrogryposis and clubfoot. **A,** external view. **B,** roentgenogram showing widening of sacral, lumbar and lowest thoracic vertebrae.

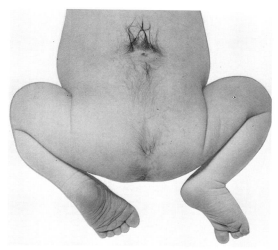

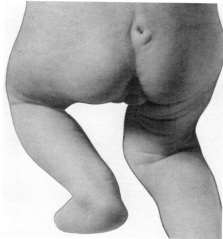

Fig. 24–71 (left).—Dermal sinus. Small opening leads to sinus tract that communicates with spinal canal in the lumbar region. It is surrounded by long dark hair.

Fig. 24–72 (right).—Pilonidal sinus. An invagination of the skin is present over the lower end of the sacrum. There is usually no communication with the spinal canal.

surface of the body downward between the bodies of two lumbar vertebrae into the spinal canal. It may penetrate the dura or end blindly at its outer surface. The point of attachment may be directly under the opening in the skin or it may ascend for several centimeters within the spinal canal. Hemangiomas and lipomas of the meninges have been reported at the place where the sinus enters the spinal canal.

The external opening may be easily visible or there may be a simple depression resembling a dimple. It is often surrounded by long hairs (Fig. 24–71). The tract leading to the spine is lined by squamous epithelium.

The communication between the meninges and the body surface permits entrance of bacteria into the spinal canal, leading to meningitis. In any child who has repeated attacks of meningitis a dermal sinus should be suspected.

PILONIDAL SINUS.—These sinuses are located lower on the back than are dermal sinuses. Although they may extend through the soft tissues to the sacrum, they rarely penetrate the spinal canal. The opening to the outside of the body is often larger and the canal wider (Fig. 24–72) than in a dermal sinus. Like the dermal sinuses, they are lined by squamous epithelium. Debris accumulating in the depths of a sinus is often responsible for local infection that can be cured only by excision of the tract. They almost never cause meningitis.

A dermal and a pilonidal sinus may be present simultaneously.

REFERENCES

Aguayo, A. J., Nair, C. P. V., and Bray, G. M.: Peripheral nerve abnormalities in Riley-Day syndrome, Arch. Neurol. 24:106, 1971.

Anderson, F. M., and Landing, B. H.: Cerebral arachnoid cysts in infants, J. Pediatr. 69:88, 1966.

Anderson, J. M., Milner, R. D. G., and Stritch, S.: Pathologic changes in nervous system in severe neonatal hypoglycemia, Lancet 2:372, 1966.

Babbit, D. P., Tang, T., Dobbs, J., and Berk, R.: Idiopathic familial cerebrovascular ferrocalcinosis (Fahr's disease) and review of differential diagnosis of intracranial calcification in children, Am. J. Roentgenol. 105:352, 1969.

Badr El-Din, M. K.: Familial convulsive disorder with unusual onset during intrauterine life, J. Pediatr. 56:655, 1960.

Ballantyne, J. W.: *Manual of Antenatal Pathology and Hygiene—The Embryo* (Edinburgh: William Green and Sons, 1904).

Banker, B. Q., and Larroche, J. C.: Periventricular leukomalacia of infancy, Arch. Neurol. 7:386, 1962.

Banker, B. Q., Miller, J. Q., and Crocker, A. C.: The Cerebral Pathology of Infantile Gaucher's Disease, in Aronson, S. M., and Volk, B. W. (eds.): *Cerebral Sphingolipidoses* (New York: Academic Press, 1962), p. 73.

Berg, J. M., Crome, L., and Frane, N. E.: Congenital cardiac malformation in mongolism, Br. Heart J. 22:331, 1960.

Bernstein, J., and Landing, B. H.: Extraneural lesions with neonatal hyperbilirubinemia and kernicterus, Am. J. Pathol. 40:371, 1962.

Brandt, S.: *Werdnig-Hoffmann's Infantile Progressive Muscular Atrophy* (Copenhagen: Einer Munksgaard, 1950).

Browder, J., and de Veer, J. A.: Rhino-encephalocoele, Arch. Pathol. 18:646, 1934.

Bume, J. C.: Niemann-Pick's disease in a fetus, J. Pathol. Bacteriol. 66:473, 1953.

Byers, R. K., and Banker, B. Q.: Infantile muscular atrophy, Arch. Neurol. 5:140, 1960.

Byers, R. K., and Hass, G. M.: Thrombosis of dural venous sinuses in infancy and childhood, Am. J. Dis. Child. 45: 1161, 1933.

Cameron, A. H.: Malformations of the neurospinal axis, urogenital tract, and foregut in spina bifida attributable to disturbances of the blastopore, J. Pathol. Bacteriol. 173:213, 1957.

Cameron, A. H.: The Arnold-Chiari and other neuroanatomical malformations associated with spina bifida, J. Pathol. Bacteriol. 73:195, 1957.

Carter, S., and Gold, A. P.: Acute infantile hemiplegia, Pediatr. Clin. North Am. 14:850, 1967.

Cohen, J., and Sledge, C. B.: Diastematomyelia, Am. J. Dis. Child. 100:257, 1960.

Craig, J. M.: Observations on the mechanisms of development of congenital anomalies in the rat produced by anti-rat kidney sera, Biol. Neonate 13:361, 1968.

Crocker, A. C., and Farber, S.: Neimann-Pick's disease—a review of 18 patients, Medicine 37:1, 1958.

Crome, L.: Pachygyria, J. Pathol. Bacteriol. 71:335, 1956.

Crome, L.: The Pathology of Down's Syndrome, in Hilliard, L. T., and Kirman, B. H. (eds.): *Mental Deficiency* (London: J. & A. Churchill, Ltd., 1965).

Crosse, V. M., Meyer, T. C., and Gerrard, J. W.: Kernicterus and prematurity, Arch. Dis. Child. 30:501, 1955.

D'Agostino, A. M., Kernohan, J. W., and Brown, J. R.: The Dandy-Walker syndrome, J. Neuropathol. Exp. Neurol. 22:450, 1963.

Daniel, P. M., and Stritch, S. J.: Arnold-Chiari malformation, J. Neuropathol. Exp. Neurol. 17:250, 1958.

Dennis, J. P., Rosenberg, H. S., and Alvord, E. C., Jr.: Megalencephaly, internal hydrocephalus and other neurological aspects of achondroplasia, Brain 84:425, 1961.

Desmond, M., *et al.*: Congenital rubella encephalitis, J. Pediatr. 71:311, 1967.

Diezel, P. B.: Histochemische Untersuchungen an primaren. Lipoidosen, Virchows Arch. Pathol. Anat. 326:118, 1954.

Dubrovitz, V., Lorber, J., and Zachary, R. B.: Lipoma of cauda equina, Arch. Dis. Child. 40:207, 1965.

Dyer, N., Raye, J., Guterbelet, R., Faxelius, G., Swanstrom, S., Brill, A., and Stahlman, M.: Timing of intracranial hemorrhage in newborn infants, Pediatr. Res. 6: 61, 1972.

Eastman, N. J., Kohl, S. G., and Maisel, J. E.: The obstetrical background of 753 cases of cerebral palsy, Obstet. Gynec. Survey 17:459, 1962.

Edwards, J. H., Norman, R. M., and Roberts, J. M.: Sex linked hydrocephalus—report of a family with 15 affected members, Arch. Dis. Child. 36:481, 1961.

Erskine, C. A.: An analysis of the Klippel-Feil syndrome, Arch. Pathol. 41:269, 1946.

Farber, S., *et al.*: Encephalitis in infants and children carried by virus of eastern variety of equine encephalitis, J.A.M.A. 114:1725, 1940.

Fenechel, G. M., and Engel, W. K.: Histochemistry of muscle in infantile spinal atrophy, Neurology 13:1059, 1967.

Gilmour, J. R.: The essential identity of the Klippel-Feil syndrome and iniencephaly, J. Pathol. Bacteriol. 53: 117, 1941.

Globus, J. H., and Selinsky, H.: Tuberous sclerosis in the infant, Am. J. Dis. Child. 50:954, 1935.

Green, M. A.: Gargoylism (lipochondrodystrophy), J. Neuropathol. Exp. Neurol. 7:30, 1948.

Greenfield, J. G.: *Neuropathology* (London: Edward Arnold [Publishers], Ltd., 1958).

Groover, R. V., Sutherland, J. M., and Landing, B. H.: Purulent meningitis of newborn infants, N. Engl. J. Med. 264:1115, 1961.

Hamby, W. B., Krauss, R. F., and Beswick, W. F.: Hydranencephaly: Clinical diagnosis, Pediatrics 6:371, 1950.

Haymaker, W., *et al.*: *Pathology of Kernicterus and Posticteric Encephalopathy* (Springfield, Ill.: Charles C Thomas, no date given).

Holden, K. R.: Diffuse neonatal hemangiomatosis, Pediatrics 46:411, 1970.

Ingraham, F., and Matson, D. D.: Subdural hematoma in infancy, Adv. Pediatr. 4:231, 1949.

Ingraham, F. D., and Matson, D. D.: *Neurosurgery of Infancy and Childhood* (Springfield, Ill.: Charles C Thomas, 1954).

Jervis, G. A.: Gargoylism (lipochondrodystrophy), Arch. Neurol. Psychiatr. 63:681, 1950.

Klein, M. R.: Subdural hematoma in infancy, Arch. Fr. Pediatr. 21:425, 1964.

Korey, S. R., and Terry, R. D.: Studies in Tay-Sachs disease. I. B. Chemical and pathological descriptions, J. Neuropathol. Exp. Neurol. 22:10, 1963.

Landing, B. H., *et al.*: Familial neurovisceral lipidoses, Am. J. Dis. Child. 108:503, 1964.

Lanman, J. Y., Partment, Y., Vuberg, S., and Lund, J.: Extracortical cerebrospinal fluid in normal human fetus, Pediatrics 21:403, 1958.

Larroche, J. C.: Hemorrhagies cerebrales intraventriculaires chez la premature, Biol. Neonate 7:26, 1964.

Lee, K. H., Young, K. R., and Young, C. Y.: Neonatal jaundice in Chinese newborn, J. Obstet. Gynaecol. Br. Commonw. 77:561, 1970.

Lucey, J., Ferreiro, M., and Hewitt, J.: Prevention of hyperbilirubinemia in prematurity by phototherapy, Pediatrics 41:1047, 1968.

Magee, K. R.: Leptomeningeal changes associated with lipochondrodystrophy (gargoylism), Arch. Neurol. Psychiatr. 63:282, 1950.

McKendrick, T.: Familial dysautonomia, Arch. Dis. Child. 33:464, 1956.

Melchior, J. C., Benda, C. E., and Yakovlev, P. I.: Familial idiopathic cerebral calcification in childhood, Am. J. Dis. Child. 100:787, 1960.

Munslow, R. A., Stovall, V. S., Price, R. D., and Kohler, C.: Brain abscess in infants, J. Pediatr. 51:74, 1957.

Newcomb, A. L., and Munns, G. F.: Rupture of aneurysm of the circle of Willis in the newborn, Pediatrics 3:769, 1949.

Norman, R. M., Oppenheimer, D. R., and Turguey, A. H.: Histological and chemical findings in Krabbe's leukodystrophy, J. Neurol. Neurosurg. Psychiatr. 24:223, 1961.

Penrose, L. S., and Smith, G. F.: *Down's Anomaly* (London: J. & A. Churchill, Ltd., 1969).

Poser, C. M.: The differential diagnosis of diffuse sclerosis in children, Am. J. Dis. Child. 100:380, 1960.

Potter, E. L.: Diffuse angiectasis of cerebral meninges of the newborn infant, Arch. Pathol. 46:87, 1948.

Potter, E. L., and Rosenbaum, W.: Association of mild external hydrocephalus with death in the early days of life, Am. J. Obstet. Gynecol. 45:822, 1943.

Potter, E. L., and Rosenbaum, W.: Normal amount of cerebrospinal fluid within the skull at birth, Am. J. Obstet. Gynecol. 45:701, 1943.

Raskind, R.: Brain tumors in early infancy – probably congenital in origin, J. Pediatr. 65:727, 1964.

Riggs, W. E., and Rorke, L. B.: Studies of Neonatal Brain Pathology, in *Fifth International Congress of Neuropathology,* International Conference Series #100 (Amsterdam: Excerpta Medica, 1965), p. 753.

Rorke, L. B., and Spiro, A. J.: Cerebral lesions in congenital rubella syndrome, J. Pediatr. 70:243, 1967.

Rothstein, J. L., and Welt, S.: Infantile amaurotic familial idiocy, Am. J. Dis. Child. 62:801, 1941.

Russell, D. S.: Observations on the Pathology of Hydrocephalus, Medical Research Council spec. rep. series #265 (London: His Majesty's Stationery Office, 1949).

Scammon, R. E.: A Summary of the Anatomy of the Infant and Child, in *Abt's Pediatrics* (Philadelphia: W. B. Saunders Co., 1925), Vol. 1, p. 318.

Sherwin, R. M., and Berthong, M.: Alexander's disease with sudanophilic leukodystrophy, Arch. Pathol. 89: 321, 1970.

Silverman, B. K., *et al.*: Congestive failure in the newborn caused by cerebral A-V fistula, Am. J. Dis. Child. 89: 539, 1955.

Stern, L., and Denton, R. L.: Kernicterus in small premature infants, Pediatrics 35:483, 1965.

Stern, L., Ramos, A. D., and Wigglesworth, F. W.: Congestive heart failure secondary to cerebral arteriovenous aneurysm in the newborn infant, Am. J. Dis. Child. 115:581, 1968.

Suzuki, K.: Clinical pathology of Gm1-gangliosidosis (generalized gangliosidosis), J. Neuropathol. Exp. Neurol. 28:25, 1969.

Terry, R. D., and Weiss, M.: Studies in Tay-Sachs disease. II. Ultrastructure of cerebrum, J. Neuropathol. Exp. Neurol. 22:18, 1963.

Thibault, J. N., and Manuelidis, E. E.: Tuberous sclerosis in premature infant, Neurology 20:139, 1970.

Towbin, A.: Central nervous system damage in the human fetus and newborn infant, Am. J. Dis. Child. 11: 529, 1970.

Towbin, A.: Spinal cord and brain stem injury at birth, Arch. Pathol. 77:620, 1964.

Towbin, A.: Cerebral intraventricular hemorrhage and subependymal matrix infarction in the fetus and premature infant, Am. J. Pathol. 52:121, 1968.

Volk, B. W.: *Tay-Sachs Disease* (New York: Grune & Stratton, 1964).

Wolf, A., and Cowen, D.: Perinatal infections of the central nervous system, J. Neuropathol. Exp. Neurol. 18: 191, 1959.

Yakovlev, P. I.: Pathoarchitectonic studies of cerebral malformation. III. Arrhinencephalitides (holotelencephalus), J. Neuropathol. Exp. Neurol. 18:22, 1959.

Yakovlev, P. I., and Wadsworth, R. C.: Schizencephalies; a study of congenital clefts in the cerebral mantle, J. Neuropathol. Exp. Neurol. 5:169, 1946.

Yates, P. O.: Birth trauma to the vertebral arteries, Arch. Dis. Child. 34:436, 1959.

Ziai, M., and Haggerty, R. J.: Neonatal meningitis, N. Engl. J. Med. 259:314, 1958.

Zuelzer, W. W., and Mudgett, R. T.: Kernicterus, Pediatrics 6:452, 1950.

25

Skeleton

Development

THE GREATER PART of the skeleton develops from multiple areas of condensed mesenchyme which gradually become converted into cartilage. At varying intervals during antenatal and postnatal life centers of ossification appear within the cartilage and spread peripherally until most or all of the cartilage has been transformed into bone. In a few places, especially the skull, mesenchyme is converted directly into bone. The bones so produced are known as membranous bones, in contrast to the cartilaginous bones that make up most of the skeleton. In mature bone it is impossible histologically to differentiate one from the other.

In all bones growth proceeds in two directions — in length, or surface area, and in thickness. Increase in thickness of a flat bone or in circumference of a long bone results from periosteal proliferation with loss of nuclei and conversion of the persisting acellular matrix into osseous tissue. At the ends of the bones growth takes place by penetration of capillaries and osteoblasts into cartilage (Fig. 25-1). The cells of the proximal zone of the cartilage align themselves in pairs parallel to the long axis of the bone. The cells nearest the metaphysis swell, the matrix in the cell columns loses its density and little resistance is offered the capillaries that grow into these vesicular cellular spaces. The deposit of calcium in the part of the cartilage where active invasion is going on produces a zone of provisional calcification. Destruction of cells leaves slender, delicate columns of cartilage that form the groundwork for the development of bone. The cartilaginous trabeculae are surrounded by osteoblasts that first produce the noncalcified bone known as osteoid tissue. With further development some of the bony trabeculae disappear and the rest grow and produce a latticed pattern with connective and hematopoietic tissues in the intervening spaces. This pattern is characteristic of

Fig. 25-1.—Normal osteochondral junction at lower end of femur in mature newborn infant. Note regular linear arrangement of cartilage cells and smooth plane between cartilage and bone.

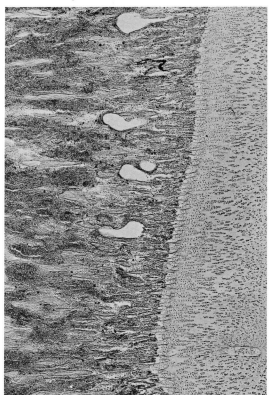

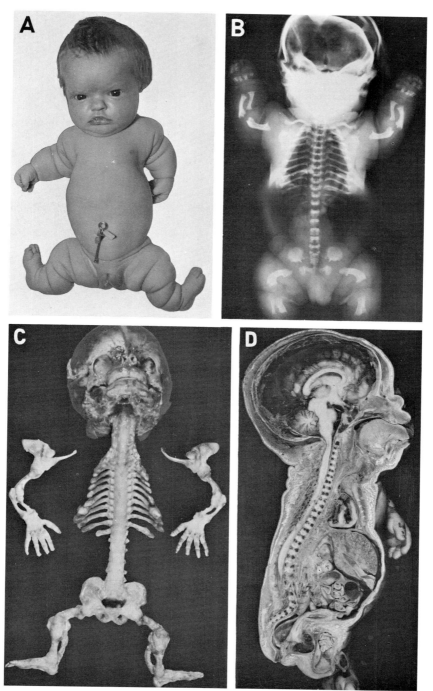

Fig. 25–2.—Achondroplasia. **A,** typical shortening of arms and legs. Infant aged 2 days. **B,** roentgenogram showing generalized shortening of the extremities and exaggerated curvature of humerus and femur. Bony portions of vertebrae are shorter than the intervening cartilaginous disks. Infant aged 1 day. **C,** skeleton showing similar changes. **D,** sagittal section of premature infant. Lumbar curve is exaggerated, causing decrease in anteroposterior diameter of the pelvis, volume of thoracic cavity is characteristically reduced and nasal bones are hypoplastic. Several loops of bowel are present in a large inguinal hernia.

cancellous bone. In compact bone, growth proceeds until the intervening spaces are largely replaced by osseous tissue.

The entire skeleton, except for the membranous bones of the skull, is present first in cartilage before any bone is formed. Osseous tissue appears first in the clavicle during the 7th week of gestation and soon thereafter in other areas (see Chapter 2).

Most disturbances in bone formation begin in intrauterine life. The general process by which bone is formed may be altered and the entire skeleton may be involved. The disturbance may rest primarily in an abnormality in the preparation of cartilage for conversion into bone, as in the chondrodystrophies, in an abnormality in the process by which cartilage is changed into definitive bone, as in osteogenesis imperfecta and osteopetrosis, or in excessive production of cartilage with a secondary disturbance in conversion to bone, as in chondromegaly. The anlage for any bone or group of bones may fail to appear. Abnormal division of the cartilage precursors of bone or the appearance of accessory centers of ossification may lead to branching, duplication or many other abnormalities of size and shape of individual bones. The majority of all disturbances in bone formation, both generalized and localized, are inherited.

Generalized Abnormalities

DWARFISM

Shortness of stature is most often caused by a generalized disturbance in bone formation that is present at birth and usually inherited (chondrodystrophy); less often it is a result of an inborn error of metabolism (hypophosphatasia, cystine storage disease) secondary to nutritional or endocrine inadequacies (scurvy, cretinism) or malformation of other organs (heart); or it may be caused by inadequate growth of histologically normal bone either as an isolated phenomenon (pituitary dwarfism) or in association with other abnormalities (de Lange syndrome, Silver syndrome, "bird-headed" dwarfism, progeria). Most affected individuals are already short at birth, but others, especially those with histologically normal bones, may be either of normal size or unusually small at birth; the latter have usually been designated as suffering from intrauterine growth retardation. The term chondrodystrophy has come to be used for the large group of diseases in which the normal preparation of cartilage for conversion to bone seems to be lacking. Cartilage cells fail to align themselves in palisades, and vascular penetration of cartilage is irregular. This ordinarily leads to retardation of longitudinal growth and is designated hypoplastic chondrodystrophy. The rare hyperplastic chondrodystrophy (chondromegaly) is the only member of the group in which total length of the bones is excessive; there is a great increase in amount of cartilage and although the zone of growth is more abnormal than in any other form, the diaphyses of the long bones are of approximately normal length.

With increasing clinical experience and more extensive radiologic and genetic investigation, an increasing number of syndromes are constantly being described. Unfortunately, pathologic studies are often inadequate and the basis for many of the syndromes described is clinical rather than histologic. Some attempt has been made to divide them into lethal and nonlethal varieties (Maroteaux; Lamy) but this does not seem meaningful because in almost all groups some individuals die soon after birth and some survive.

CHONDRODYSTROPHY. — *Achondroplasia (hypoplastic chondrodystrophy).* — Individuals with the classic form of this disease are easily recognized at birth by the presence of moderate enlargement of the head, a trunk of approximately normal length—usually with a small bell-shaped thorax, prominent abdomen and lumbar lordosis—and short extremities with a seemingly disproportionate increase in soft tissue volume (Figs. 25–2 and 25–3). Visceral malformations are rare.

The increase in head size is usually limited to the calvarium, giving an undue prominence to the forehead above a depressed glabella. Nasal passages are often narrowed and sinuses small. The anteroposterior diameter of the anterior cranial fossae is increased and the foramen magnum has two anterolateral protuberances and one posterior protuberance that decrease its diameter (Fig. 25–4). Rarely, they are large enough to reduce the foramen magnum to a narrow slit, and paraplegia resulting from compression of the cord has been described.

The brain may be of normal or excessive size (megalencephaly) (Dennis *et al.*), or, rarely, the lateral ventricles may be dilated, producing a mild internal hydrocephalus. No histologic changes in brain substance have been observed.

The trunk is usually of normal length; at birth the portion of the vertebral bodies visible on x-ray is unusually short, but this is compensated for by a proportionate increase in cartilage. The interpeduncular portions of the lumbar vertebrae are narrower than normal. The pelvis is small, particular-

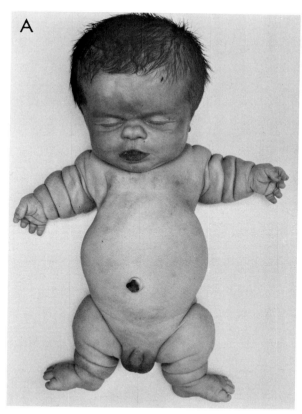

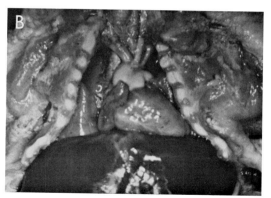

Fig. 25–3.—Achondroplasia. **A,** calvarium enlarged in relation to face, glabella depressed, limbs short, and soft tissue excessive. Thorax is small and abdomen protruberant. **B,** thorax small, as in A, with lower ribs flared to accommodate the liver. The excessive amounts of cartilage are visible on cut ribs.

ly in the anteroposterior diameter, and surviving females are unable to deliver an infant vaginally. Although the abdomen appears prominent, this is usually only in relation to the decreased size of the chest.

The ribs are often unusually short, giving a reduced volume that may be associated with pulmonary hypoplasia. The lower ribs flare out to accommodate the liver (see Fig. 25–3, B).

The long bones of upper and lower extremities are symmetrically short and moderately curved. Cartilaginous portions of the bones are increased in size. Soft tissues are excessive in relation to the length of the bones. The appearance suggests that they would be normal if attached to bones of normal length but are thrown into folds to accommodate them to the shorter bones.

The histologic structure of the bones presents a constant appearance. The shafts of the long bones are short. The diameter of the diaphysis is in striking contrast to the excessive width of the metaphysis next to the large masses of cartilage found at the ends of the bones. The osteochondral junction is severely abnormal. The epiphyseal cartilage is

normal, but cell proliferation in the endochondral growth zone is deficient and cartilage cells fail to align themselves in normal palisades. Capillaries grow irregularly into the cartilage, producing a jagged uneven plane between cartilage and osseous tissue (Fig. 25–5). Bone trabeculae, which are unusually large and well developed, may be found immediately adjacent to the cartilage, leaving no intervening zone of growth. Such bony masses may be present in the form of flat plates with one surface abutting directly on cartilage as well as extending into the diaphysis.

In the subperiosteal region the formation of bone appears to be more normal than in the region of the epiphyseal plate, and proliferation of perichondrial osteoblasts results in an increase of the diameter of the long bones, especially in the region of the metaphysis. In some instances parts of this rim of periosteal bone are turned inward at right angles to the longitudinal bone axis and interposed between the bone and cartilage at the periphery of the epiphyseal plate. All of the bone trabeculae are increased in size but reduced in number.

With extrauterine growth the bones become

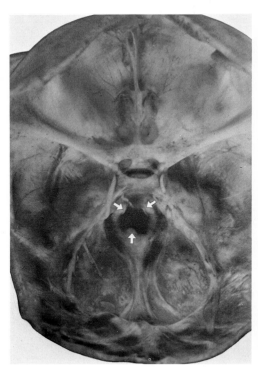

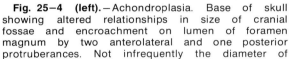

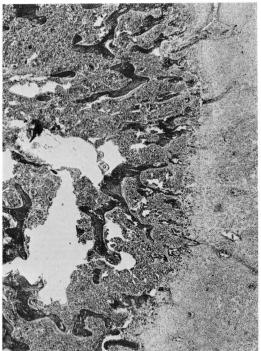

Fig. 25–4 (left).—Achondroplasia. Base of skull showing altered relationships in size of cranial fossae and encroachment on lumen of foramen magnum by two anterolateral and one posterior protruberances. Not infrequently the diameter of the foramen magnum is more greatly reduced.

Fig. 25–5 (right).—Achondroplasia. Osteochondral junction. Cartilage cells lack normal linear arrangement, the plane of capillary ingrowth is very irregular, and bony trabeculae are abnormally thick. Newborn infant.

straighter and the soft tissue appears less excessive but the extremities remain disproportionately short. The fingertips often reach only to the iliac crest. The joints in youth are exceptionally mobile, the hand and fingers can be bent back against the arm, and many positions impossible for a normal individual can be assumed with ease.

Visceral malformations, except for pulmonary hypoplasia, do not occur, although several achondroplastic infants born at the Chicago Lying-in Hospital had an abnormality in blood formation. All of the achondroplastic infants studied had moderate anemia with an excess of immature red cells in the circulating blood. Jaundice was not prominent, perhaps because of the short period of survival. Histologic examination revealed widespread moderate extramedullary erythropoiesis in all. With one exception the spleen and liver were not enlarged, and there was no reason to believe that these infants had a primary disturbance in formation or destruction of erythrocytes. In one instance of known maternal immunization to Rh in which the birth of an erythroblastic baby was anticipated,

a prenatal x-ray showed that the infant was an achondroplastic dwarf. This is the only case in which a malformation was observed in combination with erythroblastosis.

Achondroplasia is inherited through an autosomal dominant gene. However, it has one of the highest mutation rates of any known disease and most affected children have normal parents. In an investigation of achondroplastic dwarfs, Potter and Coverstone found about 40 living in the Chicago area, of whom four had one affected parent and none had both affected. They discovered one family consisting of normal parents, three normal children and three achondroplastic dwarfs and another family with normal parents, no normal children and five achondroplastic dwarfs. These two families seem to indicate the possibility of a recessive form of inheritance, but there were no known progenitors with the disease. The suggestion has been made that they were the result of a mutation occurring in a primitive germ cell still undergoing mitotic division, with the production of multiple defective definitive germ cells.

In 1970 Murdoch et al., in a study of 148 achondroplastic dwarfs in America, found 117 (79%) sporadic and 31 (21%) familial cases. Among 37 families in which one or both parents were dwarfs, all of 24 offspring survived when only one parent was affected, but seven of 16 died when both parents were affected.

This proportionately low mortality rate among infants born to affected parents is in contrast to the seemingly high rate when both parents are normal. All of 11 achondroplastic dwarfs examined at autopsy at the Chicago Lying-in Hospital had two normal parents. The only affected infant born in that hospital who survived had two achondroplastic parents. Autopsy findings were identical in all who died (all within 2 weeks of birth) except for slight differences in shape of the thorax and in relative shortening of the limbs. Histologic changes in bones were the same in all. The infant who survived seemed to have a lesser degree of involvement than did those who died at birth; the length of the extremities approximated that of the normal infant and the principal abnormality was a depressed glabella and prominent forehead (Fig. 25–6). Sitting was delayed, and severe kyphosis developed but subsequently disappeared. When last seen, at age 13 years, she was shorter than her parents.

Thanatophoric dwarfism. — An attempt has been made to differentiate a lethal form of achondroplasia under this designation (Maroteaux and Lamy), but the general description is the same as that ordinarily given for typical achondroplasia except for possible minor differences in ossification of the spine — decreased interpeduncular width with classic achondroplasia, increased width with the lethal variety.

There seems little to support the contention that there are two distinct forms of the disease. There are no reports of the histologic structure of the zones of growth in long bones of surviving infants, and the external and radiologic differences can be explained as variations in degree of involvement.

There is no way of determining the differences in mortality for those infants whose achondroplasia is caused by a mutation and those in whom it results from inheritance. Our own experience indicates that all those whose disease is caused by a gene mutation have a lethal form (11 cases), while those in whom it is inherited (one case) survive. However, this conclusion is negated by the fact that in about 80% of living achondroplastic dwarfs the condition was not inherited.

Asphyxiating thoracic dystrophy. — In this anomaly the ribs are short, horizontally placed and splayed at the ends. The chest is narrow, but the head and spine are normal; these features distinguish this form of chondrodystrophy from achondroplasia (Fig. 25–7). The limbs may be short in relation to the length of the spine but lack the increased metaphyseal width seen in achondroplasia. The changes in the pelvis are similar to those in achondroplasia.

Survival beyond early infancy is rare, but with continued survival the chest assumes a more normal shape and function (Langer); thus, death due to respiratory difficulty is rare after the 1st year. The process is inherited in an autosomal recessive manner.

The changes in asphyxiating dystrophy are fairly similar to those in the Ellis-van Creveld syndrome, but ectodermal changes and congenital heart disease are not present and polydactyly is less common.

Metatrophic dwarfism. — This disorder is usually recognized at birth because of the short ribs, long narrow trunk and short limbs. The metaphyseal areas are broadened and irregular, not only in the proximal long bones but also in the hands. Because of the deformities at the ends of the long bones motion may be restricted and there may be abduction of the shoulders, flexion of the elbows and knees and extension of the digits. Kyphoscoliosis of the lower thoracic and upper lumbar region may be recognized early and becomes progressively more severe. A characteristic feature is a fleshy caudal appendage.

On x-ray the vertebral bodies are decreased in height and have enlarged intervertebral spaces. The vertebrae, as seen in the anteroposterior view, contain two ossification centers, and on lateral view have a cuneiform appearance. This wedging of the anterior vertebrae is the cause of the kyphosis. The vertebral pedicles are normal. The proximal limb bones are short and thick with expanded, irregular, abnormally formed metaphyses, most marked at the proximal end of the femur. The metaphyseal areas remain deformed and are not appreciably remodeled by growth processes. The centers of ossification appear late in the vertebrae, long bones and distal tubular bones.

A few affected infants die of respiratory difficulties in early life. The process is probably inherited in an autosomal recessive manner (Maroteaux). Histologic structure of bones has not been described.

Diastrophic dwarfism. — As in other chondrodystrophies, the diastrophic dwarf has short limbs but, unlike classic achondroplasia, there are

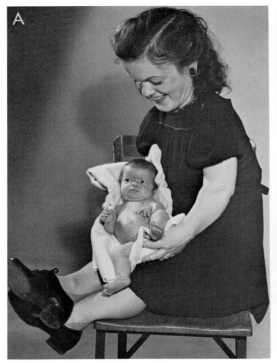

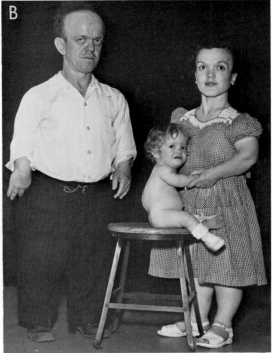

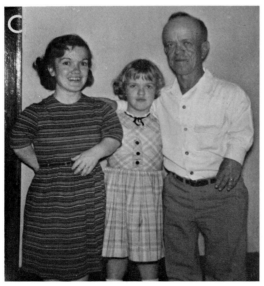

Fig. 25–6.—A, achondroplastic dwarf with daughter aged 10 days. **B,** parents with daughter at age 2 years 10 months. **C,** parents with daughter at age 13 years. The mother is 46 in. tall.

contractures of the knees and elbows, varus deformities of the feet, radial deviation of the hands and often a cleft palate sometimes associated with micrognathia. The proximal long bones and distal tubular bones are short, and the epiphyses are more irregular and abnormal than in achondroplasia, but the metaphyses are not conspicuously widened (Maroteaux and Lamy; Rubin). Scoliosis becomes prominent after weight bearing begins. There are often abnormal nodules in the ear pinnae. Some affected individuals are cryptorchid and mentally retarded (Dallaire and Fraser). Microscopic changes in the bones are similar to those in achondroplasia.

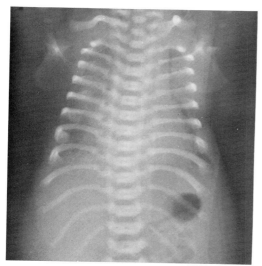

Fig. 25–7.—Asphyxiating chondrodystrophy. Roentgenogram. The ribs are short and the chest narrow in lateral dimensions. (Courtesy Dr. E. B. D. Neuhauser.)

A few affected infants die with respiratory trouble despite the characterization of the process as nonlethal. The shortened limbs and joint deformities are sufficiently conspicuous to call attention to the diagnosis at birth. Consanguinity has been recognized among the progenitors, and it is believed to be inherited in an autosomal recessive manner.

Spondylo-epiphyseal dysplasia (Morquio's disease).—This disorder, in which clinical symptoms in early stages are limited to the bones and joints, is one of the mucopolysaccharidoses. The disease may be recognized first by the presence of scoliosis and by roentgen studies, which reveal flattened vertebral bodies not unlike those seen in the early stages of Hurler's disease. Affected individuals are short due to the flattened vertebrae but the limbs are not reduced in length although there is some widening of the metaphyses. The ribs may be flared at birth and the sternum may be abnormally protuberant by 5 months of age. An enlarged head, elevated clavicles and a shortened neck, genu valgum with enlarged femoral condyles, and large flat feet with varus deformity have all been described as part of the syndrome. The diaphyses of the long bones have defective tubulation, metaphyses are widened and epiphyseal plates are irregular. In addition, there may be fragmentation of the epiphyses and an increase in the number of centers of ossification. In later childhood clouding of the corneas, hepatomegaly and deafness may appear. Mental retardation is occasionally present.

The abnormal material characteristic of this disease is keratin sulfate, which is present in the increased cartilage cells as alcian blue–positive material. Similar material is also present in vacuolated histiocytes beneath the perichondrium and sometimes in fibroblasts. Endochondral bone formation is faulty, and focal necrosis is found in both cartilage and bone in the zone of metaphyseal growth. Masses of cartilage lie between the zone of immature cartilage and the scanty new trabecular bone (Fig. 25–8). All of the articular cartilage and the bones of endochondral origin are affected. Reilly bodies (metachromatic masses) can be demonstrated in 65% of the peripheral polymorphonuclear leukocytes (Zellweger *et al.*). Small quantities of keratin sulfate can be demonstrated in the urine of affected individuals (McKusick). The disease is probably inherited in an autosomal recessive manner.

Chondrodystrophica calcificans congenita (stippled epiphyses, Conradi's disease).—Warkany suggested that two forms of stippled epiphyses occur. The first is a nonfamilial benign process found in otherwise normal individuals with the stippling tending to disappear by 3–4 years of age. It is far more common than the second form, which comprises only 10% of all cases and is a recessively

Fig. 25–8.—Morquio's disease. Photomicrograph showing masses of abnormal cartilage distal to the region of provisional growth. (Courtesy Dr. J. Cohen.)

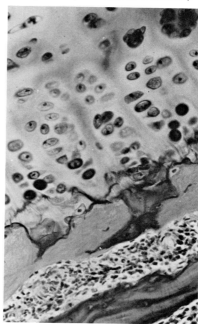

inherited disorder with consanguinity common among parents. This form can be recognized at birth because the stippled epiphyses are accompanied by shortened limbs, flexion deformities of the proximal portions of the extremities and short stubby hands. The head is of normal size, but craniosynostosis and hypertelorism have been described. Cataracts, syndactyly and polydactyly, erythematous scaly and ichthyotic skin lesions and meatal ulceration of the penis may be present. A mental defect has been found in nearly one half of affected individuals.

The epiphyses have irregular calcification around the secondary growth centers that can be demonstrated radiologically, and in severe cases irregular calcium deposits are found in the periarticular structures, metaphyses and some of the flat bones. The metaphyses are enlarged with irregular lines of ossification.

Pathologically, the disease is characterized by irregular degeneration and calcification of the provisional cartilage that precedes endochondral bone formation. Patchy areas of mucoid and cystic degeneration of the provisional and epiphyseal cartilage are accompanied by a loss of the cartilaginous ground substance. The vascularized cartilage canals of both epiphysis and provisional cartilage are broadened and the vessels are usually distended with blood (Yakovac). Calcified osteoid matrix is increased in the provisional zone of calcification. Any structures composed of cartilage (such as trachea or larynx) may be involved in the irregular degeneration and calcification.

One half of those affected with the familial severe form of the process die in the 1st year of life, often with pneumonia.

Chondroectodermal dysplasia (Ellis-van Creveld syndrome). — This chondrodystrophy is characterized by chondrodysplasia, especially of the more distal portions of the limb, ectodermal dysplasia, polydactyly and congenital heart disease (Ellis and van Creveld). When recognized at birth the ectodermal lesions are prominent; the infants have scanty hair, and the fingernails and toenails may be absent or small and concave, with longitudinal ridges and distal thickening (Weech). Teeth may be erupted at birth or may erupt prematurely, or there may be delay or failure of eruption. They are usually peg-shaped. The heart is malformed in nearly two thirds of the cases (Moore); the defects are of many varieties but septal defects, especially of the atrium, are especially common. In one third of the cases respiratory difficulty is associated with a

small thorax or with lobular emphysema due to absence of cartilage rings in the bronchi. Polydactyly is always present, and other malformations of many varieties have been described occasionally.

The long bones, especially the distal ones, are short and thick. The chief histologic defects appear to be a lack of proliferation with absence of maturation of cartilage cells and a paucity of active osteoblasts (Smith and Hand). There is no zone of provisional cartilage calcification.

The prognosis for those with congenital heart disease is poor, one half dying in the 1st year. The process is inherited in an autosomal recessive manner. It is a common form of dwarfism among the Pennsylvania Amish, among whom the cases originated from a single couple who immigrated to the United States in 1744 (McKusick).

Chondrodystrophy with cebocephalus. — A previously undescribed syndrome consisting of an unusual form of chondrodystrophy with associated cebocephalus and multiple cutaneous hemangiomas was observed in two siblings at the Chicago Lying-in Hospital (Fig. 25 – 9). Although one was male and the other female, the abnormalities were identical. The extremities were mildly shortened and the long bones slightly shortened, thickened and curved, the last most marked in ulnas and fibulas. Soft tissues seemed excessive for length of bones, as in achondroplasia. The skin was excessively hairy, and large intracutaneous hemangiomas were present in the extremities and trunk. The heads were small with a receding forehead and prognathism of the chin. The eyes were also small and the nose undeveloped. The brain was reduced in size, hemispheres were fused, corpus callosum was absent and there was a single optic nerve. A large amount of fluid surrounded the brain (see Fig. 24 – 53). The malformations of the heads were typical of those found in cebocephalus.

The osteochondral junctions were of great interest. In localized areas cartilage cells were arranged in palisades and showed the vacuolization and other changes that normally precede invasion by capillaries. In intervening areas the cartilage was almost devoid of cells, and palisading was absent; here capillary invasion was greatly retarded. As a result the cartilage masses projected considerable distances into the metaphysis of the bone (Fig. 25 – 9, C).

Chondromegaly. — This is an extremely rare disease. The few cases that have been described have usually been called hyperplastic chondrodystrophy. In most forms of chondrodystrophy, however, the

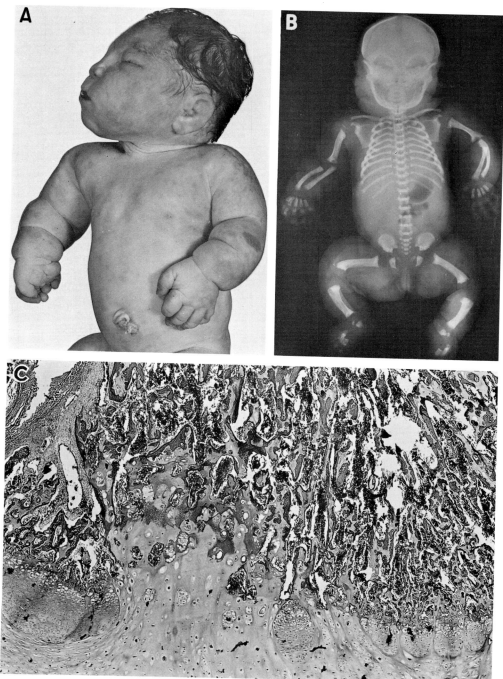

Fig. 25–9.—Chondrodystrophy with cebocephalus in infant aged 1 day. **A,** infant with microphthalmia, microcephalus and moderate shortening of the extremities. **B,** roentgenogram showing moderate shortening and bowing of the long bones. **C,** zone of growth at lower end of femur. Cartilage is composed of normal-appearing areas interspersed between acellular masses of matrix in which capillary invasion and conversion into bone is greatly retarded. Sibling identically affected. (For brain, see Fig. 24–53.)

disturbance appears to consist largely of an inhibition of the process by which cartilage is converted into bone, and the bones are consequently short. Also, there is no increase in the amount of cartilage and it seems excessive only because of the proportionately small amount of bone. In hyperplastic chondrodystrophy the primary disturbance seems to be an overproduction of cartilage with the abnormal conversion into bone being only secondary. Cartilage is present as large bulbous masses in all normal locations (Fig. 25–10). Its presence in the vertebrae increases the length of the spine, in the long bones the length of the extremities and in the phalanges the length of the fingers; in the coccyx it produces a tail-like appendage. The edges of the scapulas and the iliac crests are covered by a thick layer of cartilage. Because of the increase in amount of cartilage the joints are all greatly enlarged and the ends of the bones are widely flared to permit their attachment to the hypertrophied cartilage (Fig. 25–10, C).

One such infant observed at the Chicago Lying-in Hospital died as a result of difficulty encountered in delivery because of the excessive size. No malformations were present except in the bones. The bony trabeculae in the diaphyses were moderately increased in size but the striking changes were in the metaphyses. Large irregular peninsula-like masses of primitive cartilage with minimal evidence of palisading or preparation for conversion into bone greatly increased the width of the metaphyses. The peninsular pattern was produced by the irregular penetration of proliferating capillaries into the cartilage. The peninsulas were partially surrounded by osteoid tissue (Fig. 25–10, D).

NONCHONDRODYSTROPHIC DWARFS.—Many syndromes have been described in which dwarfism results from inadequate growth of bones. No histologic abnormalities have been described, and reduced stature is part of a general growth retardation. At birth some individuals are small and others are of normal size. Some are mentally retarded or have other associated malformations while a few appear to be miniature normal individuals.

Pituitary dwarfs.—Most individuals who are normal except for a symmetrical reduction in size fall in this group. At birth they may be small but are more often of normal size, with delay in growth first becoming apparent at a few months of age or sometimes not until childhood. The cause of the small size, when it is apparent in infancy, is usually an idiopathic disturbance in pituitary function, while when not noticeable until later, it is often caused by a pituitary tumor. Among 26 patients past the age of puberty reported by Martin and Wilkins seven cases were caused by tumors and 19 were idiopathic. Gonadotropic hormones were also often decreased.

In the idiopathic group there is a great preponderance of males. Several sibships have been described in which case distribution strongly suggests a genetic origin with inheritance by a recessive gene.

Russell-Silver dwarfs.—Both Russell and Silver have described children with severe intrauterine growth retardation who failed to grow at a normal rate after birth, often with one side lagging behind the other and producing hemiatrophy in addition to the generalized dwarfing. Additional features described by subsequent investigators include minute ear lobes, occlusion of ear canals, high palate sometimes accompanied by micrognathia, simian crease in the palm accompanied by in-curving of the little finger, enlargement of the clitoris, and *café au lait* spots in the skin (Holden; Szalay).

Seckel's "bird-headed" dwarfs.—Seckel described in detail two dwarfs with microcephalus and collected 13 more from the literature. All were of greatly reduced stature with small heads and mental retardation. Those described by Seckel weighed 1,715 and 1,960 gm, respectively, at birth after a gestation of 40 weeks, and postnatal growth continued to be slow. No visceral abnormalities were evident and bones were radiologically normal except for small size. The heads of such infants are usually telencephalic and the brain has a primitive appearance with no secondary gyral formation.

Progeria.—This rare condition is characterized by premature senescence both in general appearance and in the occurrence of arteriosclerosis, arthritis, coronary heart disease and cerebral hemorrhage as early as the 1st decade. Height may not exceed that of an average 4-year-old child when growth stops completely at 9–10 years. Warkany stressed the fact that most such individuals are unusually small at birth and that growth is abnormally slow even in infancy. The etiology is unknown.

Leprechaunism.—Donohue and Uchida, who first described this condition as "dysendocrinism," later gave it the name leprechaunism because of the facial appearance. The facial features are coarse, forehead hairy, eyes protruding, nose broad and flat, mouth large with protruding lips, and ears large and low-set. Birth weight is usually low for length of gestation and there is a marked subsequent retardation in growth. Hyperinsulinism with increase in islands of Langerhans and cystic hyper-

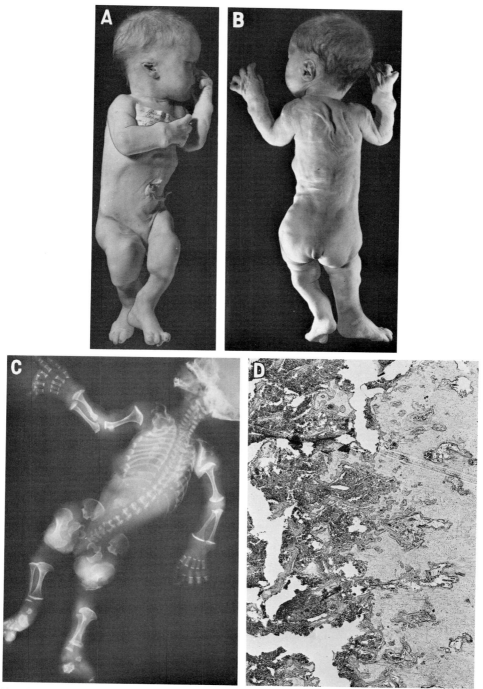

Fig. 25–10.—Chondromegaly (hyperplastic chondro-dystrophy) showing increase in diameter of all joints as a result of increase in volume of cartilage at ends of bones. Joints of phalanges as well as those of larger bones are involved. Excessive cartilage in the coccyx produces a tail-like appendage. **A,** front view. **B,** back view. **C,** roent-genogram. **D,** photomicrograph showing irregularity of the osteochondral junction. Large islands and penin-sula-like projections of cartilage extend into the meta-physis. Total length 65 cm at birth.

plasia of the ovaries have been recorded. The thymic and lymphoid atrophy, prominence of nipples and external genitalia and the absence of subcutaneous fat that have been described are probably a result of malnutrition rather than an integral part of the disease.

Cornelia de Lange's syndrome (typus amstelodamensis). — Affected infants are born prematurely and are small for length of gestation. The appearance even at birth is characteristic (McArthur and Edwards; Ptacek *et al.*; Schlesinger *et al.*; Verger *et al.*). The head is small with brachiocephaly, the forehead is covered with hair, the eyebrows are bushy and thick, the bridge of the nose is depressed and the nostrils face forward rather than downward. The upper lip is unusually long. The ears are placed low on the head, and the neck may be partially webbed. Extension of the elbows is restricted and the hands are small, often with deficient phalanges. The nipples are hypoplastic and set low on the body. The testes remain undescended. Visceral anomalies appear limited to hypoplasia of the pituitary, thyroid and adrenal glands. All affected infants are mentally retarded. In one case studied at the Boston Lying-in Hospital there were minor changes in the histology of the tongue, kidney and brain. De Lange's syndrome is inherited in an autosomal recessive manner and has been reported in several consanguinous families.

OSTEOGENESIS IMPERFECTA

This disease, also called osteopsathyrosis, fragilitas ossium and Lobstein's disease, is an inherited defect of mesoderm characterized by fragile bones, blue scleras and otosclerosis (Weber). Osteogenesis imperfecta appears in two main forms: *osteogenesis imperfecta congenita,* in which the fetus is severely affected and is born dead or survives only a few days, and *osteogenesis imperfecta tarda,* in which fractures are common in infancy (osteogenesis imperfecta tarda gravis) or in later life (osteogenesis imperfecta tarda levis) (McKusick). All are inherited by the same mendelian autosomal dominant gene, and both the congenital and tarda forms may appear in the same family. In the forms with late onset the bones may be radiologically normal and the increased fragility may first be recognized only after repeated fractures in adult life. Bone fragility is ordinarily the outstanding abnormality, but in affected families individual members may have any one or all three of the cardinal signs. Other less common features are precocious arcus senilis, laxity of ligaments, abnormal electrical reactions and feeble development of muscles, white patches in the nails, capillary fragility with macular bleeding, otosclerosis, unusual fineness of the hair and deficient dental enamel. In the severe forms, if the infant survives, the short stature and the broad thick diaphyses may be confused with achondroplasia. The thickening of the diaphyseal portion of the long bones results from compression and callus formation from multiple fractures. In the survivors there may be flaring and inward protrusion of the acetabulum. In the milder form, when compression from spontaneous fracture does not occur, the diaphysis is long and slender with a thin delicate cortex, while the metaphyseal cortex is of more normal thickness. Platybasia of the skull with resulting cerebellar disturbances and hydrocephalus, as well as calcification of the media of the pulmonary and cerebral arteries, have been observed in a few affected newborns (Rubin).

When the disease reaches its height in utero, the fetus dies before or during birth. Multiple fractures of long bones, ribs and clavicles are in various stages of healing, many being surrounded by a large mass of callus (Fig. 25 – 11, A, B, and C). The legs are always curved, owing partly to healing of fractured bone in poor alignment and partly to pressure of the uterine wall. Many fresh fractures are produced by the trauma of delivery. The calvarium is severely abnormal, often being a mosaic of innumerable wormian bones averaging 1 – 2 cm in diameter separated by narrow saw-toothed suture lines. Little calcium is present and the skull has the texture of a firm membrane (caput membranaceum). At other times bone in the calvarium may be limited to small central masses 1 – 2 cm in diameter in the center of each bone (Fig. 25 – 11, D). This extreme form of the disease is rare, having been observed only twice in over 100,000 deliveries at the Chicago Lying-in Hospital. The parents of both of these children were normal, and there was no family history of bony abnormality, blue scleras or deafness.

The characteristic bone changes seen microscopically are decreased size and number of the bony trabeculae of the diaphysis and an abnormal thinness of the cortex (Fig. 25 – 12). The cartilage at the ends of the bones ordinarily appears normal, and capillary invasion seems to progress normally. Though osteoid is laid down promptly by the osteoblasts that are present and matrix calcification is normal, a paucity of osteoblasts leads to a reduction in the total mass of trabeculae and cortical bone. There is also a failure of cross-binding of collagen fibers, since with silver impregnation the

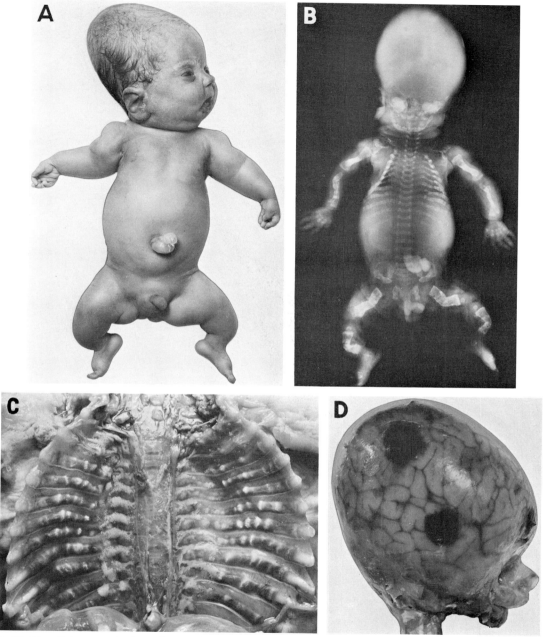

Fig. 25–11.—Osteogenesis imperfecta with extreme degree of bone involvement in infant aged 2 hours. Death from pulmonary hypoplasia. **A,** external surface of body. **B,** roentgenogram showing innumerable intrauterine fractures. Calvarium is composed almost entirely of membrane, and base of skull is poorly ossified. **C,** ribs showing large number of fractures and callus deposited around each. **D,** head with scalp and skin of face removed. Dark areas, which are bilaterally symmetrical, are the only bones present in the calvarium.

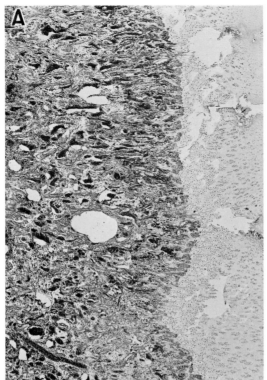
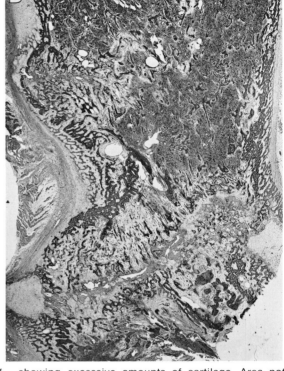

Fig. 25—12.—Osteogenesis imperfecta. **A,** zone of growth at lower end of femur. Cartilage appears normal, capillary invasion is progressing normally, but bony trabeculae are abnormally small. **B,** region of fracture showing excessive amounts of cartilage. Area not involved in healing process shows diminution in number and size of bony trabeculae. Mature stillborn fetus.

trabeculae show persistence of a reticulum pattern that normally disappears with aggregation of the reticulum fibers into coarser collagen bundles. An abnormal persistence of the metachromasia of the osteoid has also been described (Rubin). Callus formation may be excessive, and newly formed bone may become cystic. This process produces thin delicate bony trabeculae that surround a persistent cartilage matrix; in the metaphyses periosteal bone formation is also inhibited, with resulting thinning of the cortical layer in the diaphyses.

The blueness of the scleras is due to decreased thickness or increased transparency, which permits the underlying choroid to show through. In a family in which fragility of bones is present in some members, others may have only blue scleras or middle ear deafness (otosclerosis).

Another form of the disease that may be present at birth was observed in two siblings delivered at the Chicago Lying-in Hospital. The mother was less than 5 ft tall, had blue scleras and had had multiple fractures without production of apprecia-

ble deformity. A diagnosis of osteogenesis imperfecta was made several years before her first pregnancy. By different husbands she had two children, both of whom at birth exhibited bowing of the long bones with central areas of increased density in the middle of the shaft of each bone in the region of the lesser curvature (Fig. 25–13). The x-ray appearance of these areas resembled an exaggeration of the process described by Caffey, which he attributed to intrauterine pressure. At 15 months the x-ray appearance of the bones of the older sibling was only slightly changed from that found at birth. No fractures had occurred.

OSTEOPETROSIS (MARBLE BONES: ALBERS-SCHÖNBERG DISEASE)

Osteopetrosis is characterized by an abnormal density and brittleness of the bones and occurs both as a rapidly fatal autosomal recessive disease beginning in utero, with death usually occurring early in life from infection, and as a more benign autoso-

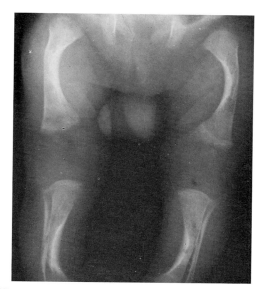

Fig. 25—13.—Osteogenesis imperfecta. One of two siblings with identical changes in x-ray appearance of bones of lower extremities consisting of zones of increased density on medial surfaces of femurs and tibias. Diagnosis of osteogenesis imperfecta had been made on the mother on the basis of blue scleras, middle ear deafness and multiple fractures. Infant aged 3 days.

mal dominant disease usually first manifested in later childhood or adult life (McKusick). Like most diseases with generalized skeletal changes, it varies greatly in time of onset and severity of symptoms. It has been diagnosed before birth in the recessive malignant form from the x-ray studies of the fetal skeleton made because of its known existence in other members of the family (Jenkinson *et al.*). It has also been diagnosed a few days after birth (infantile form, simple dominant), but in most instances several months or years elapse before the condition is suspected (simple dominant).

In the severe recessive form of the disease seen in the fetus and newborn the disturbance involves all bones (McCune and Bradley). When examined by x-ray, the long bones are found to have expanded and elongated metaphyses with a diffuse increase in density of the entire bone except the metaphysis (Fig. 25—14, A and B). The latter may have longitudinal and transverse linear striations. The skull bones are uniformly dense and lack the usual diploë. On cross-section both vertebrae and long bones show dense white cortical bone and sclerotic cancellous bone nearly replacing the marrow cavity. This cancellous bone is a diffuse mosaic of bone and persisting cartilage, sometimes called a chondro-osseous complex (Cohen). The cartilage at the

ends of the bones appears normal and most of the cells in the provisional zone of calcification are arranged in normal palisades. Capillary ingrowth proceeds as expected, producing a smooth flat plane between cartilage and metaphysis. Normally, much of the cartilaginous matrix temporarily persisting between the cellular spaces is destroyed by the invading capillaries, with only a portion remaining to form the trellis on which osteoid and osseous tissue are deposited. In this disease an abnormal amount of cartilaginous ground substance persists and is converted directly into bone without first forming intertrabecular spaces. As a result medullary spaces are abnormally small, and the amount of bone is excessive (Figs. 25—14, C and 25—15). Since mineralization is defective and the bones are chalky and unusually brittle, they break easily despite the seeming increase in density demonstrated on roentgen examination. Fractures often have sharp edges, in contrast to the usual greenstick fracture of the very young.

In the more mild dominant form with onset from birth to 13 years the presenting symptoms are often anemia and mental retardation. Hydrocephalus, subdural hematoma and increased intracranial pressure are common. Narrowing of the optic, auditory and other cranial nerve passages may lead to blindness, deafness and weakness of the facial and extraocular muscles.

In the adult a history of unusually brittle bones as a child may lead to the diagnosis.

Thyrocalcitonin, which has the capacity to block the action of the bone parathormone (Walker), is abnormally increased in the peripheral blood.

HYPOPHOSPHATASIA

Hypophosphatasia is an hereditary metabolic defect transmitted in an autosomal recessive manner. In this abnormality there is a marked decrease in the serum phosphatase, and decreased phosphatase levels have been demonstrated histochemically in osteoblasts and chondroblasts (Fraser). Serum calcium and urinary phosphoethanolamine are increased. As in other hereditary metabolic defects, the severity of the symptoms and body changes is related to the age at which the overt difficulties begin. When recognized in the newborn period, the majority of affected individuals die before reaching 1 year of age. They have poor bony support for the brain, large fontanelles and wide osteoid seams in the region of the cranial sutures; the latter close prematurely and cause synostosis, microcephalus and increased intracranial pressure. Since the ribs

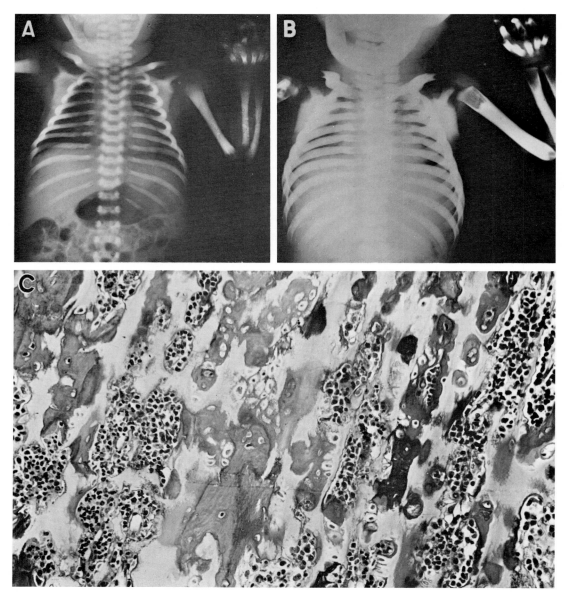

Fig. 25–14.—Osteopetrosis (marble bone disease). **A,** roentgenogram at age 2 months showing increased density of ribs. **B,** roentgenogram at 8 months. All bones show greatly increased density in all regions except terminal portions of the long bones. **C,** photomicrograph showing diffuse increase in bony tissue, absence of remodeling and reduction in size of marrow space. Age 2 years. (Courtesy Dr. C. H. Hatcher.)

grow poorly, at birth the costochondral junctions are displaced laterally and the volume of the thorax is greatly reduced. Consequently, respiratory distress may be extreme. The long bones are soft and subject to fracture, especially near the wrists and ankles, and repeated fractures eventually lead to decreased length. There is considerable widening of the metaphyses. The secondary growth centers are late in appearing and are poorly mineralized. The high serum calcium leads to anorexia, vomiting and failure to thrive (Barter). The high excretion of calcium causes nephrocalcinosis in early life in over half the cases. Calcium may be desposited in the collecting tubules of the kidney, chiefly in the

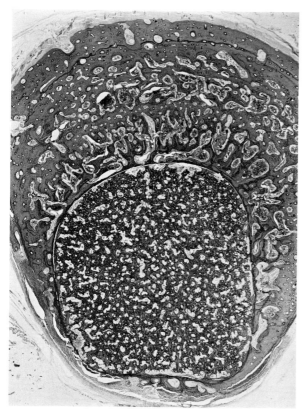

Fig. 25–15.—Osteopetrosis. Photomicrograph. Cross-section of long bone showing the marrow cavity filled with unremodeled epiphyseal endochondral bone. The cortical bone shows some degree of remodeling. (Courtesy Dr. J. Cohen.)

outer medulla, and in some of the cells of the proximal convoluted tubules (McCance *et al.*).

When the onset is from 6 to 16 months of age, failure to thrive, gastrointestinal problems, delayed eruption and premature loss of teeth and difficulties resulting from increased intracranial pressure are prominent symptoms. When the onset is still later, the presenting picture is often that of rickets. In long-term survivors a gradual amelioration of the signs and symptoms can be expected.

The most characteristic histologic findings are the persistence of broad uncalcified cartilaginous masses at the chondro-osseous junctions and of osteoid in the metaphysis and the trabeculae of the diaphysis of the long bones. Osteoblasts appear to be deficient. Because of the delay in the remodeling of the metaphyseal bone a broad band of spongiosa in the diaphysis may be surrounded by mature cortical bone.

FAMILIAL SEX-LINKED HYPOPHOSPHATEMIC RICKETS

In this disorder there is a diminished rate of reabsorption of phosphate by the kidney which is not corrected by vitamin D administration. Until the age of 6 months growth may be normal despite a lowered phosphate serum level. Bowing of the femurs, tibias and distal arm bones may become apparent in early infancy in about 20% of the cases. In the remainder the lesions are less severe and the process may not be recognized. The classic rachitic weight-bearing deformities of genu varum or valgum eventually develop.

As in rickets, the zone of proliferating cartilage is expanded and lacks calcification. The number of vessels in the provisional zone of calcification is increased (Winters *et al.*). The metaphyses contain an excess of osteoid. Remodeling of the cancellous bone is usually active, and osteoclasts fill the bays in the bony trabeculae.

IDIOPATHIC HYPERCALCEMIA OF INFANCY

This condition presents with symptoms of failure to thrive, repeated infections, vomiting, a characteristic elfin facies and increased radiologic density of the bones of the base of the skull, spine, pelvis and metaphyses of the long bones.

Benign and severe forms of this condition have been described as different entities, but enough intermediate cases have now been reported to make a separation seem unjustified. The mild form is transitory and has a good prognosis with no permanent disability; the severe form often results in renal damage and mental retardation. In England this process has been associated with vitamin D intoxication due to excess ingestion of fortified milk and other supplements.

The mildest cases appear to have only transient hypercalcemia; more severe cases have more prolonged hypercalcemia and retention of an abnormal amount of calcium. The face has been described as being characteristic and of aid in establishing the diagnosis. Epicanthic folds, a concomitant squint, retroussé nose, prominent upper lip, open mouth and slack lower lip with a receding chin are the features most commonly observed.

The incidence of this process has decreased with reduction in vitamin D supplements in infants' food. Suggestions have been made that the process is a metabolic defect in the ability of the body to deactivate vitamin D.

Autopsy has often failed to disclose calcification

of organs other than the kidneys, where small masses of calcium, which are adherent to the tubular basement membranes, project into the lumens of the proximal and distal convoluted and collecting tubules. At times the deposits in the collecting tubules may be large enough to be visible grossly on the cut surface of the kidney. In a few cases supravalvular aortic stenosis and calcification, peripheral pulmonary vascular stenosis or endocardial fibroelastosis have been associated with the process (Coleman).

In one case, study of the costochondral junction showed unusually wide, dense trabecular bone and persistence of cartilage in the provisional bone (Farber and Craig). In all cases the bony lesions eventually resolve. If death occurs, it is generally a result of renal failure.

INFANTILE CORTICAL HYPEROSTOSIS (CAFFEY'S DISEASE)

In this disease, which is characterized by rapid abnormal production of new subperiosteal bone, the onset is often preceded by systemic symptoms suggesting an infection. It is limited to young infants, almost always appearing before the age of 4 months. It has been reported as early as 10 days. Gerrard *et al.* pointed out that there are many familial cases and suggested that in some families there may be an autosomal dominant variety with variable expressivity and in others a recessive variety with several siblings involved but neither parent affected.

The first symptoms include irritability, refusal to eat, vomiting and fever. Firm tender swellings develop deep in the soft tissues (Fig. 25–16), and in a short time subperiosteal new bone can be detected on roentgenograms of the involved areas. The extent of the lesion varies, but it is often widespread and has been recognized in all parts of the skeleton except the phalanges, small bones of the tarsus and carpus, vertebrae and pelvis. The new bone symmetrically surrounds the shaft of the long bones and does not extend beyond the epiphyseal line (Fig. 25–17). Exacerbations and remissions are frequent, and with each exacerbation additional layers of new bone are laid down. The lines of demarcation between old and new bone gradually disappear, and as the shaft becomes progressively wider, the medullary cavity enlarges proportionately (Fig. 25–18). After varying lengths of time exacerbations no longer occur and the process begins to

Fig. 25–16 (left).—Infantile cortical hyperostosis. Typical facial appearance with involvement of both sides of the mandible. Infant aged 14 weeks.

(Courtesy Drs. Mary Sherman and David Hellyer.)
Fig. 25–17 (right).—Photomicrograph showing fibrotic subperiosteal new bone in an infant aged 10 days.

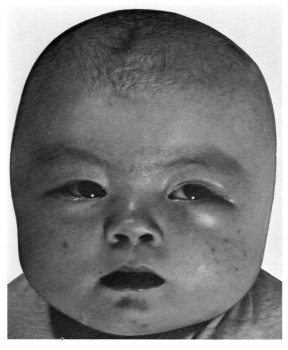

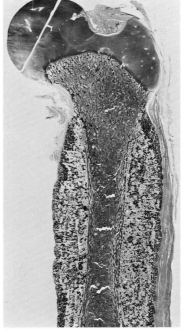

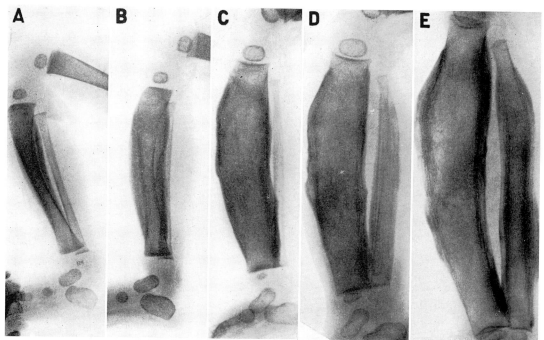

Fig. 25–18.—Infantile cortical hyperostosis. Roentgenogram of right leg. **A,** 2 weeks after onset of symptoms new bone surrounds three fourths of the tibial shaft. Other bones appear normal. **B,** 18 days later the new bone has doubled its thickness and begins to appear lamellated. Fibula and tibial metaphysis are not involved; lines indicating old cortex are still visible. **C,** 4 months after A, the old cortex has disappeared and the medullary cavity has expanded. New lamellations have been laid down and now extend from one epiphysis to the other. **D,** 6 months after A, the medullary cavity has expanded and absorbed some of the lamellae previously visible. The tibia appears osteoporotic and the fibula is now involved. **E,** 21 months after A, there is no further deposit of new bone. The metaphyses of the tibia and fibula are assuming a more normal appearance. (Courtesy Drs. Mary Sherman and David Hellyer.)

be reversed, the thickness of the bones becomes reduced and symptoms disappear. During the period of activity different bones show considerable variation in the stage of the process, some regressing while others are still progressing. The course is usually limited to a few months, although in one case under observation at Bobs Roberts Hospital it was still present 26 months after onset.

In the early stages, when fever and bone tenderness are present, there is some loss of cortical bone with acute inflammation in the periosteal area and occasional extension to the muscle (Eversole *et al.*) (Fig. 25–19). Osteoblastic and fibrous tissue reaction soon follows. In later stages the periosteum is thickened, edematous, unusually vascular and cellular. The superficial layer of new bone is composed of unorganized trabeculae with small marrow spaces filled with loose connective tissue containing many blood vessels. The old cortex is normal. In one case reported by Sherman and Hellyer the external surface of the periosteum blended into heavy fibrous tissue that surrounded the adjacent muscles and sent narrow fibrous cords to the skin. The muscles were small and showed definite degeneration and fibrosis associated with unusual proliferation of the intima of the local blood vessels.

Resolution of the process is usually complete by the age of 3 years. The cause is unknown and no therapy has been found to alter the course of the disease.

FIBROUS DYSPLASIA OF BONE

This disease has several variations, in all of which the fundamental lesion is a fibrous dysplasia of localized portions of one or several bones. It appears to be a congenital developmental defect without evidence of a genetic cause. As such it may be present at birth but may not become manifest until later in childhood (Jaffe).

The monostotic form usually affects children or young adults and is rare in infants. The bones most

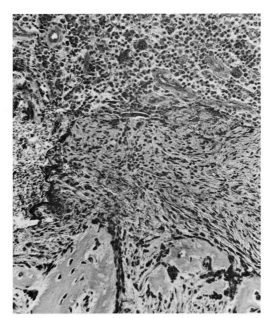

Fig. 25—19.—Infantile cortical hyperostosis. Photomicrograph showing an early lesion with inflammation, reactive fibrous tissue and new bone formation. (Courtesy Dr. J. Cohen.)

often involved are the ribs, tibia, femur, mandible and maxilla. The first sign may be a fracture, or there may be local swelling and tenderness. The child is usually otherwise normal. Histologically the marrow and osseous structures in sharply delineated areas are replaced by fibrous connective tissue. Affected areas tend to remain static and neither spread nor regress.

The only infant observed at the Chicago Lying-in Hospital with such a lesion was born with an abnormal curvature of the lower part of the left leg. X-ray examination revealed an expanded rarefied area in the tibia (Fig. 25–20). A fracture subsequently occurred and pseudarthrosis developed. At the age of 3 years this was still present, but after several operations the leg was stabilized and the child walked normally by the age of 6.

Polyostotic fibrous dysplasia is characterized by lesions in many bones, often by *café au lait* spots in the skin and occasionally by mental retardation. Portions of flat bones may be distended into tumor-like masses while the long bones may be curved, shortened and thickened. The blood calcium and phosphorus levels are normal but serum phosphatase is elevated. When the disease affects females, the endocrine system may be involved, and it may be associated with precocious osseous development and precocious puberty. This is known as the McCune-Albright syndrome.

Condon and Allen reported a condition of a multicentric nature involving the bones and soft tissues under the term *congenital generalized fibromatosis*. Characteristic punched-out lytic lesions occur in the metaphysis and diaphysis of the long bones as well as the vertebrae, scapulae, ribs and pelvis. X-ray examination reveals little evidence of sclerosis at the edges of the lesions. Ribs and vertebrae may be fractured. Circumscribed nodules composed principally of fibroblasts may be found in both viscera and bones (Fig. 25–21).

Jervis and Schein called attention to the fact that fibrous dysplasia of bone, like tuberous sclerosis and neurofibromatosis, is characterized by a curious combination of lesions in the skin, bones and nervous system and that any of the three may occur in incomplete or monosymptomatic forms. It is possible that all may be manifestations of inborn metabolic disturbances.

ENCHONDROMATOSIS (OLLIER'S DISEASE)

This process, though rarely recognized at birth, may be identified as early as 6 months of age. It consists of multiple cartilaginous tumors originating in the endochondral growth zone; the tumors grow with the remainder of the shaft and extend in a triangular fashion toward the diaphysis. Radiologically, they appear as rarefactions in the metaphysis and the end of the diaphysis, with expansion of the cortex around the tumor. The process is accompanied by shortening and bowing of the tumor-containing long bones and by distortion of the nearby joints. The tumors are usually unilateral and irregularly distributed. Histologically, they are often lobulated with marked variation in cellularity, organization, calcification and degeneration of cartilage (Fig. 25–22). In about one third of the cases the enchondromas degenerate into chondrosarcomas (Dahlin).

Unless sarcomas develop, the prognosis for life is excellent, although fractures or joint disability may be a handicap.

Some cases are complicated in later childhood by vascular anomalies, particularly angiomas, phlebectasias or hamartomas (Bean). When these are present, the condition is known as the *Maffucci-Kast syndrome.*

PRENATAL BOWING

Abnormal curvature of bone is usually symmetrical and frequently associated with partial absence or malformation of some part of the involved bones. The femur, tibia and fibula are more likely to be

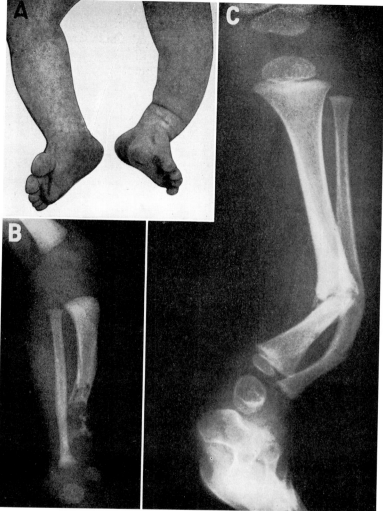

Fig. 25—20.—Localized fibrous dysplasia with pseudarthrosis. **A,** external surface of the left leg showing bowing present at birth. **B,** roentgenogram showing cystic area at lower end of diaphysis of the tibia at age 3 days. **C,** a fracture occurring soon after birth that persisted as a pseudarthrosis. Same infant at age 3 years.

affected than the bones of the arm. Bowing is occasionally observed in bones that appear otherwise normal, and in such instances the natural position assumed by the extremities often suggests that pressure exerted on the bones in utero was responsible for the changes in curvature.

Caffey described several cases of symmetrical bowing of the long bones of the extremities associated with x-ray evidence of thickening of the compact bone on the inside of the curve with consequent reduction in width of the marrow cavity. Cutaneous dimples were often present over the most prominent parts of the curves. The mothers were normal, the infants were otherwise normal and there was

no evidence of disturbed bone formation. Caffey believed that the condition resulted from pressure on impacted extremities before birth, but in renal agenesis, in which the amount of amniotic fluid is greatly reduced and the intrauterine position of the fetus would consequently be expected to remain more stationary, the legs are often bowed but show no other changes on x-ray examination. Two otherwise normal infants observed at the Chicago Lying-in Hospital with x-ray pictures similar to those reported by Caffey were in siblings whose mother had osteogenesis imperfecta (see Fig. 25–13).

In one previable fetus asymmetrical bowing of the tibias was associated with complete absence of

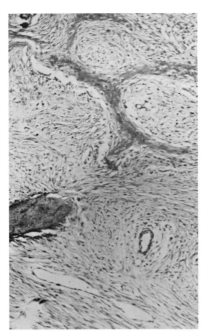

Fig. 25–21.—Fibrous dysplasia. Photomicrograph showing broad sheets of immature fibrous tissue, the individual cells of which are continuous with the osteoblasts in the narrow curved zones of osteoid tissue. (Courtesy Dr. G. Vawter.)

the marrow cavity in the area of abnormal curvature. This region was replaced by cancellous bone.

Hurler's disease, in which there is an abnormal storage of mucopolysaccharides, has generalized bone involvement consisting of shortening and thickening of long bones with decreased trabeculation. In *cystine storage disease* the bones may also be somewhat shortened and there are often wide zones of osteoid around the trabeculae. Since there are many associated abnormalities, these diseases are discussed in Chapter 10.

BACTERIAL INFECTIONS

OSTEOMYELITIS.—Since compound fractures are rare in infancy, most osteomyelitis in the 1st year of life is blood borne (White and Dennison). Staphylococci, streptococci and pneumococci are the most frequent causative organisms and, because they are present in the blood, can often be demonstrated in blood cultures (Einstein and Thomas). The source of staphylococci is most commonly infection of the skin or umbilicus, paronychia or breast abscesses, and of pneumococci and streptococci it is most often the respiratory tract.

The femur, humerus and maxilla are the bones most often affected (Dennison and MacPherson) and in many cases several bones are involved (Masse). Occasionally, particularly with staphylococci, soft tissue abscesses may be associated. The mortality rate for such generalized infections is high.

Fever, pain, redness, swelling and limitation of motion are the usual signs. The process is less destructive in young infants than in older children or adults. Because of the thinness and fragility of the cortex, the ischemic necrosis often found in the closed medullary cavity in adults is not present, and a true involucrum is seldom found (Fig. 25–23). Because of the abundant vascular connections to the epiphysis this and the adjacent joint space are more often involved than in adults. In older children, spread from the diaphysis to the epiphysis is less common because of the decrease in vascularity (Trueta).

The only infant with multiple foci of osteomyelitis observed at the Chicago Lying-in Hospital was a premature infant who had swelling of the right shoulder at 3 days of age. Before death at 9 days the lower end of the left tibia was also affected. Examination of the shoulder revealed inflammatory necrosis of the upper end of the humerus with extension into the joint cavity. The infant died in the preantibiotic era.

Fig. 25–22.—Enchondromatosis (Ollier's disease). Photomicrograph showing a large mass of irregularly arranged cartilage distorting the enchondral growth zone. (Courtesy Dr. J. Cohen.)

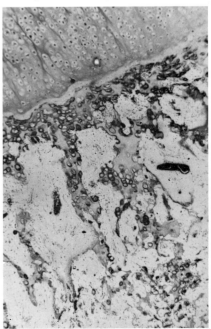

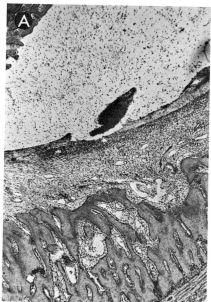
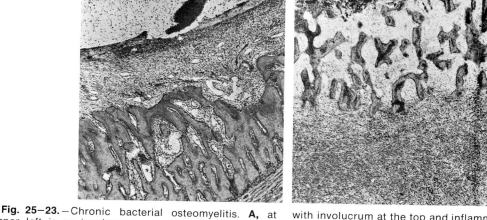

Fig. 25–23.—Chronic bacterial osteomyelitis. **A,** at upper left is an involucrum separated by an articular space and a layer of granulation tissue from a zone of subperiosteal new bone formation. **B,** a more acute lesion with involucrum at the top and inflammatory debris lying central to newly forming cortex, which is surrounded by acute inflammatory tissue lying immediately beneath the periosteum.

Tuberculous osteomyelitis in the 1st year of life is most often associated with miliary tuberculosis and, as such, the lesions are multiple. Although destructive processes are histologically similar to those in older infants, local destruction rarely progresses as far.

SYPHILIS.—The bone lesions observed in congenital syphilis are of several varieties; those present at any one time depend on the severity of the disease and the age of the infant. In the stillborn fetus or newborn infant with an advanced stage of the disease the disturbance is ordinarily an osteochondritis limited to the distal part of the metaphysis. The long bones of the extremities and the ribs are most severely involved. When a bone is split longitudinally, the junction of bone and cartilage is visible grossly as an irregular jagged line, and in severe cases a yellow layer 1–2 mm thick is interposed between bone and cartilage (Fig. 25–24). Histologic study of the milder cases shows an irregular ingrowth of capillaries with a corresponding irregularity of the provisional zone of calcification (Fig. 25–25, A). This produces the saw-toothed appearance that is visible grossly and on roentgenograms. Small groups of undestroyed cartilage cells may remain as isolated islands in the juxtaepiphyseal portion of the metaphysis. With more severe in-

Fig. 25–24.—Syphilitic osteochondritis. The osteochondral junction is an irregular saw-toothed line and the metaphysis is composed principally of fibrous connective tissue. Fetus stillborn at term. (Courtesy Dr. Aparecida Garcia.)

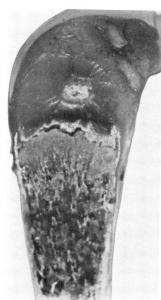

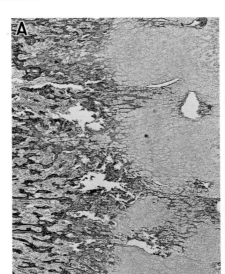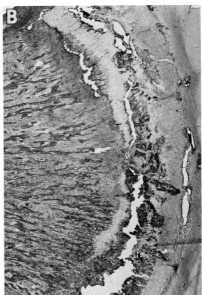

Fig. 25–25.—Syphilitic osteochondritis. Lower end of femur. **A,** provisional zone of calcification and capillary ingrowth are very irregular. Infant aged 2 days. **B,** zone of unchanged cartilage is present in the metaphysis, dis- tal to which there are capillaries and abnormal bone. Area proximal to the abnormal layer of cartilage is fi- brotic. Mature fetus stillborn at term.

volvement much of the distal metaphysis may be converted into dense connective tissue with only a few sparsely distributed bone spicules and capil- laries remaining. This zone of connective tissue is responsible for the thickened yellow line visible on gross inspection. X-ray examination sometimes reveals a duplication of the irregular epiphyseal line. This may be associated with two entirely dif- ferent histologic processes. In some instances a few capillaries penetrate the proximal portions of the cartilage and grow laterally, detaching a sheet of cartilage from the main mass at the end of the bone (Fig. 25–25, B). In other cases the metaphysis immediately adjacent to the cartilage contains very few bone spicules as a result of excessive destruc- tion and absorption, while a short distance proxi- mally there is a narrow zone in which they are unusually numerous and well calcified. As a result of thinning of the bone spicules in this area, epi- physeal separation may take place (Lichenstein).

In slightly older infants periostitis is the most common lesion, but it is never present at birth. A subperiosteal deposit of new osseous tissue encir- cles the shafts of the long bones (Fig. 25–26). It is not incorporated into the shaft, as is the new bone in cortical hyperostosis, but remains a distinct lay- er and disappears fairly promptly on treatment. In syphilitic osteomyelitis, areas of rarefaction are common at the ends of long bones (Fig. 25–27).

At the end of an extensive and well-documented study of the osseous lesions of congenital syphilis McLean concluded that the following types of le- sions, which can be identified by x-ray, warranted a diagnosis of congenital syphilis:

1. Well-defined saw-toothed metaphyses in well-calcified bones.
2. Deep zones (in the longitudinal axis) of submetaphys- eal rarefaction.
3. Multiple "separation of epiphyses" with or without impaction in bones that are not rachitic.
4. Bilateral symmetrical osteomyelitis of the proximal mesial aspects of the tibias.
5. Multiple circumscribed areas of osteomyelitis of the long bones, seen on roentgenograms as patchy areas of rarefaction.
6. Multiple longitudinal areas of rarefaction (osteomye- litis) in the shafts of the long bones, sometimes result- ing in fractures.
7. Destructive lesions at the mesial or lateral aspects of metaphyses (foci of rarefaction).
8. Multiple areas of cortical destruction, generally with- in 1 cm of the ends of the long bones.
9. Double zone of rarefaction at ends of long bones.
10. Localized periosteal cloaking occurring in more than one bone.

The bone lesions of congenital syphilis are a re- sult of chronic infection and are not unlike those of other chronic infections. Before birth, involvement is especially severe in the juxtaepiphyseal portion of the metaphysis and is due primarily to an irreg- ularity of growth and an excessive deposit of connective tissue. The metaphyseal fibrosis is part of the generalized proliferation of connective tissue that is responsible for the characteristic lesions of syphilis wherever they occur in the body. After birth other portions of bones become involved in both destructive and productive lesions. Within the shafts of the bones or in the metaphyses at the costochondral junctions, areas of rarefaction appear in which bone is replaced by connective tissue mildly infiltrated with leukocytes. In extensive involvement, fracture of the metaphysis with displacement and impaction of the terminal fragment and attached epiphysis into the shaft is not uncommon.

Although many of the changes that have been described in roentgenograms of infants with congenital syphilis are not limited to this disease and are not pathognomonic, a widespread disturbance characterized by a combination of destructive and productive lesions is found only in a chronic infectious process with bacteremia. Causative agents other than syphilis are extremely rare. However, there are two unusual generalized infections that may affect bone in the neonatal period. The first, which has been discussed previously, is rubella virus. The second is granuloma venereum (Scott *et*

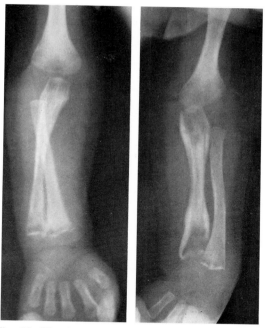

Fig. 25–27.—Syphilitic periostitis of right radius and areas of rarefaction caused by syphilitic osteomyelitis at ends of the bones.

al.), in which there is a fusiform enlargement of the long bones secondary to osteitis. Granulation tissue and microabscesses containing macrophages with ingested organisms (Donovan bodies) are present in the periosteum.

VITAMIN DEFICIENCIES

Because the fetus and young infant are growing rapidly, they are at particular hazard for the development of both scurvy (vitamin C deficiency) and rickets (vitamin D deficiency).

In *scurvy* the essential defect is a failure of fibroblasts and osteoblasts to produce intracellular matrix and osteoid. The most common lesions in young infants are in the diaphysis of the long bones, where increased fragility of capillary walls and decreased tensile strength of periosteal tissue cause subperiosteal hemorrhages (Fig. 25–28). Organization of the hemorrhage leads to the deposition of new periosteal bone outside the old cortical bone. Since the involved areas are tender and painful, the infant cries when handled. In infants with vitamin C deficiency, cartilage proliferates and matures normally in the process of endochondral new bone formation. Osteoblasts also proliferate normally but fail to produce the osteoid in which lime

Fig. 25–26.—Syphilitic periostitis. Photomicrograph showing a cross-section of shaft of a long bone with a new layer of cortical bone, beneath which is a large zone of granulation tissue.

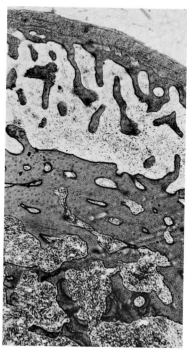

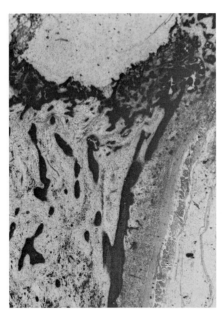

Fig. 25–28.—Scurvy. Periosteum is elevated from the cortical bone by recent hemorrhage. The marrow spaces are filled with fibrous tissue. There are many fractures of the thin trabeculae next to the epiphyseal plate.

salts are normally deposited for conversion to bone. The trabeculae of the spongiosa remain so thin and brittle that multiple infractions are caused by simple muscle pull. With attempts at repair the metaphyses become filled with sheets of osteoblasts and fibroblasts (Lichenstein). This process appears earliest and is most severe at the lateral borders of the metaphyses, where tendon and muscle strains are must acute. The metaphyses widen and the fibroblastic collections extend around the distal portions of the epiphyses. Some degree of healing is usually present. In young infants the lesions may often be most easily recognized at the costochondral junctions, where they are especially severe because of constant motion and strain.

Rickets may be found in young infants. At this age the most obvious gross deformities are often in the skull and ribs. Frontal bossing of the skull is common and costochondral junctions are enlarged. A groove at the level of the attachment of the diaphragm results from its pull on the ribs. The classic bow legs and pelvic deformities appear only with weight bearing when the child begins to walk.

The histology of the costochondral junction is characteristic. Inadequate absorption of calcium from the gut and low serum calcium result in inadequate calcification of mature cartilage and of os-

teoid in the spongiosa and cortical bone. Because of the lack of calcification, cartilage degeneration and capillary ingrowth are also impaired. Consequently, large masses of uncalcified or irregularly calcified mature cartilage persist in the metaphyseal zone and often spread laterally to cause widening of the metaphyses. Muscle pull causes the lines of cartilage to become distorted, and the small amount of new bone that is present is bordered by wide zones of osteoid. Infractions are often present.

In human beings it is rare for a single vitamin to be deficient, and changes resulting from both rickets and scurvy may be present in the same rib. Deficiency may be recognized frequently in infants dying of other causes, although in severe malnutrition, because growth ceases, the specific changes of rickets and scurvy may be suppressed.

Localized Abnormalities

HEAD

SKULL.—The calcium in the skull increases constantly during intrauterine life and the amount present at birth is ordinarily directly related to the gestational age at the time of delivery. Some investigators have postulated a variation in relation to the season of birth, the amount supposedly being greater in the skulls of infants born in the summer and fall than of those born in the winter and spring. However, attempts by these investigators to correlate an increase in birth trauma with poorer calcification of the skull have not been convincing.

Craniotabes.—Some infants are born with a definite deficiency of calcium that is demonstrable particularly in the upper portions of the parietal bones adjacent to the superior sagittal suture. The bones may be like celluloid so that when depressed they snap back, or the margins may be soft and merge gradually with the normal bone. This condition, while infrequent in mature infants, is more common and more severe in premature infants. It seldom appears to be associated with intracranial hemorrhage and the cause is unknown. The skull is usually normal by a few months of age.

Parietal foramina.—Small oval defects in the upper portions of the parietal bones, usually single and symmetrically placed on each side of the head, may be found sporadically or may be present in several members of a family. All defects are covered by two layers of pericranial membrane that are continuous with the normal covering of the bones. They have no clinical significance and often are not discovered until some other condition leads

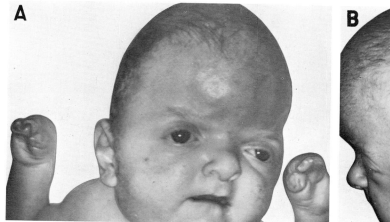

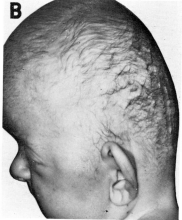

Fig. 25–29.—Acrocephalosyndactyly. The head is flattened posteriorly and protrudes anteriorly as a result of premature synostosis of the coronal sutures. The syndactyly involves all digits. **A,** front view. **B,** lateral view. (Courtesy Dr. Ralph V. Platou.)

to x-ray investigation of the skull. Multiple defects (cranial fenestrations) are rare except with spina bifida or hydrocephalus.

Premature synostoses of cranial sutures.—The shape of the head may be severely altered by the premature closure of one or more cranial sutures. The shape is determined by which sutures are involved, the limitation of growth being at right angles to the line of the involved sutures. The synostosis may already have taken place by the time of birth but abnormality of shape may not be noticeable until later. Whether the brain is affected depends on the extent of the involvement. If closure of sutures prevents enlargement of the brain, mental deterioration and blindness often follow. The two most commonly recognized conditions are acrocephaly (oxycephaly) caused by symmetrical closure of the coronal sutures (Fig. 25–29), which produces

a turret-shaped head, and scaphocephaly caused by closure of the sagittal suture, which produces a long narrow head with bulging forehead and occiput (Fig. 25–30). Irregular closure, called plagiocephaly, produces an irregularly shaped head.

Acrocephalosyndactyly (Apert's syndrome).—In this condition the parietal and occipital bones ascend steeply and the dome is turret-shaped as in all acrocephaly. The face is flattened, the expression becomes adenoid and the eyes protrude as the brain becomes compressed. The surface area of the base of the skull is diminished and the head often bulges where the frontal bosses normally appear. The absence of an occipital bulge is partly responsible for the characteristic appearance. The radius and ulna may be partially fused, and motion in hips, knees and elbows is often limited. A characteristic part of the syndrome is syndactyly of the fingers

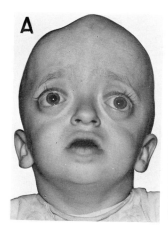

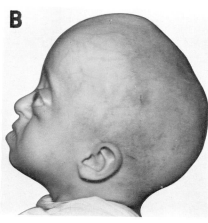

Fig. 25–30. —Scaphocephaly. The head is long and narrow and the occiput and forehead bulge as a result of premature synostosis of the sagittal suture. **A,** front view. **B,** lateral view. (Courtesy Dr. Douglas N. Buchanan.)

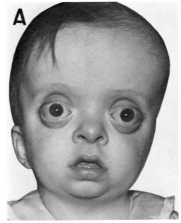 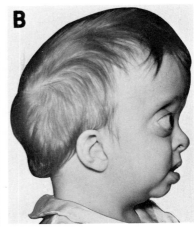

Fig. 25–31. — Craniofacial dysostosis (Crouzon's disease). Exophthalmos with coarsening of the features and prominent lower lip are features of this disease. **A,** front view. **B,** lateral view. (Courtesy Dr. Douglas N. Buchanan.)

and toes. The nails are usually fused into a single band (see Fig. 25–29, A). Visceral anomalies vary greatly but include esophageal atresia, pyloric stenosis, hydronephrosis, endocardial stenosis, hypoplasia of the pulmonary arteries, ventricular septal defect and partial transposition of the aorta. Mental impairment is occasionally present. Inheritance is autosomal dominant, but since few affected individuals marry, mutant genes must be responsible for many of the cases.

Craniofacial dysostosis (Crouzon's disease). — This hereditary premature synostosis, first described by Crouzon in 1912, consists of acrocephaly, a beak-shaped nose, hypoplastic maxilla, short upper lip with protruding lower lip, exophthalmos and external strabismus. The diagnosis is rarely made at birth but may become evident within a few weeks (Fig. 25–31). Convulsions, impairment of vision and mental deficiency are similar to those in the other forms of craniostenosis.

Platybasia. — This condition is a malformation of the base of the skull, sometimes also involving the upper cervical vertebrae. The posterior cerebral fossae are flattened and the space between the sella turcica and the descending part of the spinal canal is lengthened (Fig. 25–32). As a consequence the

Fig. 25–32. — Platybasia. **A,** infant shortly before death at 4 months. **B,** base of skull showing great increase in distance between anterior and posterior fossae. Before

the spinal cord can descend into the spinal canal it must run posteriorly for a distance of 1–2 cm.

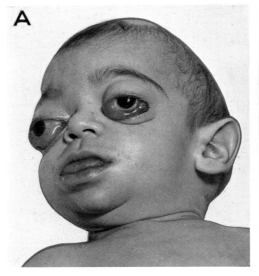 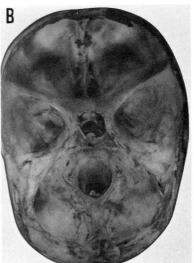

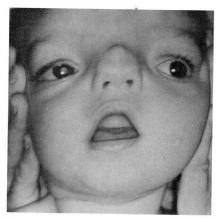

Fig. 25–33.—Hypertelorism. Abnormality of the sphenoid bone is responsible for retroussé nose and increased space between the eyes. (Courtesy Dr. Ralph V. Platou.)

medulla must extend posteriorly before it descends into the spinal canal. The upper cervical vertebrae are often fused to the base of the skull, and the medulla may be sharply bent over the odontoid process of the second cervical vertebra. The condition either may cause no symptoms for many years or may lead to symptoms of increased intracranial pressure, severe exophthalmos and early death.

Hypertelorism.—The diagnosis of typical hypertelorism is immediately evident on inspection of the infant. The disturbance results from an abnormality of development of the base of the skull, especially of the sphenoid bone, which leads to an abnormal increase in the space between the eyes. The head is characteristically broad and flat, the forehead prominent and the nose upturned (Fig. 25–33). Mental deficiency and ocular disturbances are common, although in mild cases they may be ab-

sent. In one instance observed at the Chicago Lying-in Hospital the condition was present in the mother, who was otherwise normal, as well as in the child. The anatomic peculiarities of the skull include a wide nasal aperture, broad cribriform plate, hypertrophy of the lesser wings and hypoplasia of the greater wings of the sphenoid and hypoplasia of the sella turcica.

Face.—Since a normal face requires a large number of closely integrated structures to develop normally, it is not strange that the face is a relatively frequent site of malformations. Certain abnormalities of the brain and sense organs may produce facial defects, but the most important structures related to malformation of the face are the frontonasal process and the first branchial arches.

The frontonasal process normally gives rise to the major portion of the forehead, the bridge of the nose and the philtrum of the upper lip. In embryonic life it grows downward between the orbits and the ingrowing maxillary processes derived from the first branchial arches. The nasal pits originate as two indentations on its inferior margin. The upper lip forms by fusion of the upper edges of the medial portions of the maxillary processes with the lower margins of the nasal pits, and the central margins fuse with the lateral margins of the most inferior part of the frontonasal process.

Clefts of soft tissues and bones.—Malformations resulting from failure of fusion of various portions of one or both maxillary processes to the frontonasal process are fairly common. They include facial fissures and unilateral or bilateral harelip or cleft palate.

An ectodermal invagination appears at about the 5th week of embryonic life that separates the lips from the bony portions of the upper and lower jaw. Because this separation begins before fusion of the

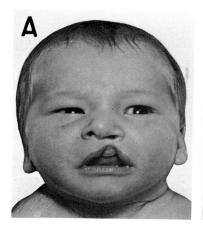

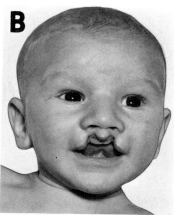

Fig. 25–34.—Harelip evidenced as a shallow notch in the lip without involvement of maxilla or palate. **A,** unilateral. **B,** bilateral.

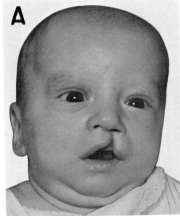
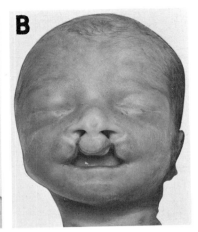

Fig. 25–35.—Harelip extending into nostril but without involvement of maxilla or palate. **A,** unilateral. **B,** bilateral.

maxilla and frontonasal process is complete, subsequent failure of fusion may involve the lip, the maxillary arch or both. It may be unilateral or bilateral.

A defect in these structures may be only a unilateral or bilateral shallow notch in the lip (Fig. 25–34), or it may extend into the nostril (Fig. 25–35). Frequently it also involves the bony portion of the maxilla. If bilateral, the portion of the maxilla that bears the incisor teeth is left unattached on both sides. As a result this portion projects upward and forward under the nose (Fig. 25–36). It produces more severe abnormality of the maxilla than a failure of fusion on only one side and is more difficult to repair satisfactorily.

Malformations of the palate are commonly associated with defects of the lip and maxilla but may be found as isolated defects. The hard palate is formed by the bilateral ingrowth of the palatine

shelves that arise from the maxillary processes. A small triangular anterior portion comes from the frontonasal process and contributes a small part to the final structure. As the palatine shelves approach the midline they fuse with each other and with the nasal septum. The posterior part that does not fuse with the nasal septum becomes the soft palate. Early in embryonic life the uvula is bifid, and in some instances this condition persists and is found at birth as a small cleft in the posterior part of the soft palate (Fig. 25–37, A).

If neither of the palatine shelves reaches the midline, a central defect is produced through which the nasal septum and turbinates are visible. The entire cavity of the nose then opens directly into the mouth (Fig. 25–37, B). If one side fuses with the nasal septum, the defect is lateral and only one side of the nose communicates with the mouth. At times only the anterior portion of one or both pala-

Fig. 25–36.—Harelip associated with cleft maxilla and palate. **A,** unilateral. **B,** bilateral.

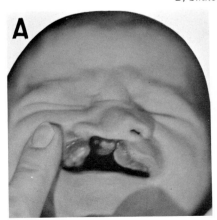
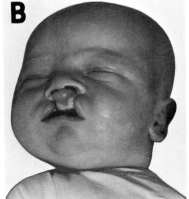

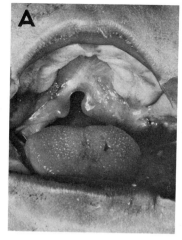
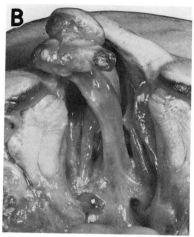
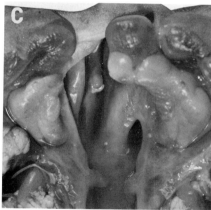
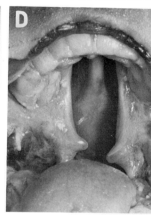

Fig. 25–37.—Cleft palate. **A,** cleft of the soft palate. **B,** complete bilateral harelip and cleft palate. The central palatine raphe with attached central portions of maxillary arch and lip are present centrally. Interior of the nose and turbinate bones are visible on both sides between the median raphe and lateral palatine processes. **C,** complete right harelip and cleft palate with partial left cleft palate. **D,** complete bilateral cleft palate without involvement of maxilla or lip.

tine processes reaches the midline, and the posterior portion remains open (Fig. 25–37, C). The converse is almost never true and the posterior portion seldom fuses to leave a defect in the anterior portion. It is also possible for the palate to be entirely open when the lip and maxilla are normal (Fig. 25–37, D). The maxilla and lip may be cleft although the palate is closed (Fig. 25–38, A), or the palate and lip may be completely cleft although the maxillary arch is partially or completely fused (Fig. 25–38, B).

When a complete cleft of the palate with intact lip and maxilla is accompanied by mandibular hypoplasia or backward displacement of mandibular condyles, the condition is known as the *Pierre-Robin syndrome* (Fig. 25–39). Glossoptosis may give rise to difficulty in swallowing or to suffocation.

Even though the palate is completely closed, it may be very highly arched. The location of the central palatine process remains as a narrow gutter in the roof of the mouth in anencephalic monsters. A high rounded arch is characteristic of achondroplasia, mongolism and some craniostenoses.

A central harelip and a central cleft of the maxilla occur only in association with cebocephalus, a condition in which the major portion of the frontonasal process is lacking. In this malformation the nose is ordinarily absent or rudimentary and the maxilla and upper lip are composed of the fused maxillary processes without interposition of the portion derived from the frontonasal process. Occasionally, however, maxillary processes fail to fuse and a central defect remains (see Fig. 24–41).

Facial clefts may involve only the skin or may extend deep into the underlying tissues. They may be found in several places but the majority are present in one of three locations. Failure of fusion of the lateral portions of the maxillary and mandibular processes is responsible for a cleft extending from one angle of the mouth directly back to the ear. If structures derived from the first branchial arch fail to fuse with those coming from the front-

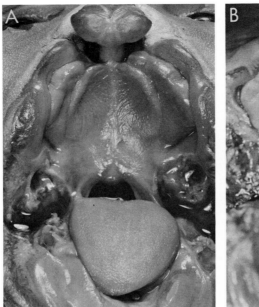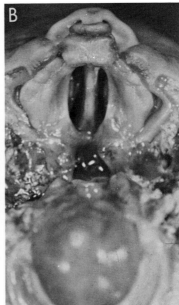

Fig. 25–38.—A, cleft of maxilla and lip with palate closed. B, bilateral harelip and complete bilateral cleft palate but with partial fusion of maxilla and frontonasal processes.

onasal process, a cleft will extend upward to the nose as in an ordinary harelip and will then run diagonally to the medial angle of the eye (Fig. 25–40, A). The outer wall of the nostril on the involved side will also be defective. A defect in such an area is often superficial, involving only the skin and subcutaneous tissues, and results from failure of closure of the nasolacrimal duct. A more common

facial cleft does not touch the nose but runs lateral to it and ends at the inner canthus (Fig. 25–41, A). In such instances the nares are completed by fusion of the medial and lateral portions of the nasal part of the frontonasal process without intervention of the maxillary processes. Clefts not related to normal lines of fusion are also occasionally present (Fig. 25–41, B). The third principal variety of cleft

Fig. 25–39.—Pierre-Robin syndrome. A, lateral view of head showing marked recession of lower jaw. B, cleft palate in same infant.

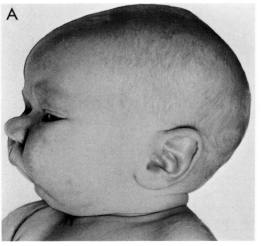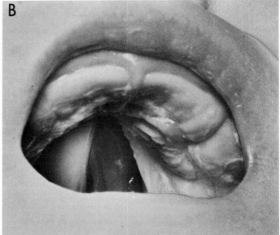

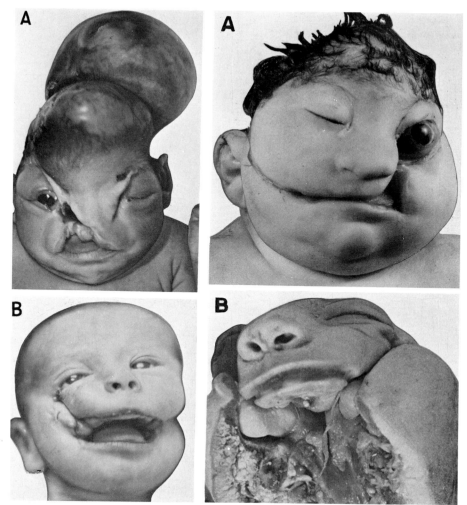

Fig. 25—40 (left). — Facial fissures. **A,** involvement of right lip and maxilla with extension into nostril and inner canthus. Another fissure extends from the outer canthus to the ear. Meningoencephalocele also present. **B,** bilateral fissures with macrostomia. One fissure extends to the outer canthus, the other to the ear. Both are associated with clefts in the lateral margins of the palate. Infant aged 3 weeks. (Courtesy Dr. Rustin McIntosh.)

Fig. 25—41 (right). — Facial fissures. **A,** involvement of the left maxilla, palate and lip with extension to the inner canthus without affecting the nose. Another fissure extends from the right angle of the mouth to a point above the ear and also communicates with the cleft of the palate. Calvarium absent. **B,** palate of infant with identical malformation except for reversal of right and left sides. (Courtesy Dr. Aparecida Garcia.)

extends from the lateral side of the mouth to the external canthus (Fig. 25–40, B) or the area slightly lateral to the eye. This defect is somewhat harder to explain embryologically but is also related to abnormal development of maxillary and mandibular tissues. When clefts reach the orbit, the lids of the involved side usually fail to develop and the eyeball is not covered.

Clefts of the mandible are among the rarest fa-

cial malformations. The mandible is formed by medial extensions and fusion of the lowermost of two parts that are produced by a splitting of the first branchial arches. Failure of normal growth of these two parts is responsible for the cleft. In one infant born at the Chicago Lying-in Hospital with such a malformation the tongue lay in the space between the two parts of the mandible. The lip was divided into two portions and the tip of the tongue

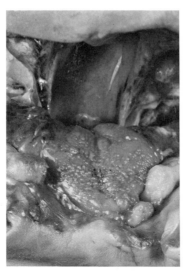

Fig. 25–42.—Mandibular cleft with tip of tongue attached to lip.

was attached to the edge of the skin between them (Fig. 25–42). In another case only the lateral rami had developed and although the lower lip was intact, the buccal orifice and mouth were abnormally small (Fig. 25–43).

Other less orderly disturbances in growth may give rise to bizarre malformations. Harelip, cleft palate and the facial clefts already described result

from a simple failure of fusion of two otherwise normal structures. Most of the other abnormalities consist of actual malformations of the parts involved, and exact duplicates are rarely found. One such example suggested precocious development of the maxillary processes with fusion to the frontonasal process before proper elaboration of that structure had taken place. The frontonasal process failed to grow down normally and the two maxillary processes were consequently drawn up to the region of the lower forehead. The nose was not present, the eyes were rudimentary and the brain and skull also were abnormal (Fig. 25–44). In another case, the head was attached to the placenta; skull, brain, eyes and nose were missing (Fig. 25–44, B).

Malformations of the brain are often present in association with abnormalities of the face other than those resulting from simple failure of fusion of adjacent parts. This finding suggests that in such instances the cause lies in actual mechanical injury in contrast to the simple reduction in rate of growth and failure of normal maturation that is responsible for the more common, frequently reproduced varieties of lesions.

Harelip and cleft palate may be inherited as a mendelian dominant character, or they may appear sporadically. According to Fogh-Andersen, two patterns of inheritance can be recognized: one in which the harelip is the primary anomaly, the other in which the palatal defect is primary and is found

Fig. 25–43.—Microstomia with nondevelopment of median portion of mandible. **A,** anterior view of face showing marked microstomia. **B,** sagittal section of head with tongue drawn slightly to the right to show abnormal development of the mandible with complete absence of bone in the midline.

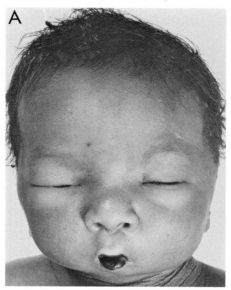

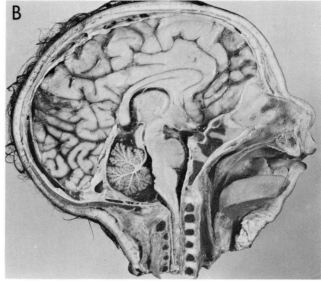

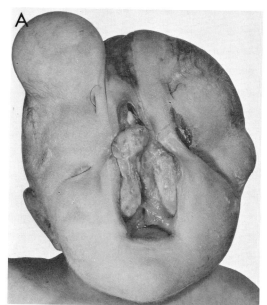 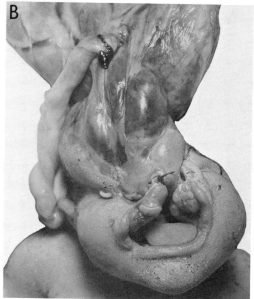

Fig. 25–44.—Malformations of the face. **A**, maxillary process drawn up to forehead; associated cleft palate. Anophthalmos and cerebral malformation. **B**, malformation associated with placental adhesion.

with or without a harelip. Cleft palate can be induced in experimental animals by a variety of antimetabolites or by other chemical agents such as cortisone. The frequency with which defects occur may be greatly modified by the genetic constitution of the animal. In some animals a deficient diet may be associated with an increase in such malformations. A well-known example of this was the occurrence of harelip in the offspring of the leopards in the London Zoo during a period when the parents were fed a diet containing no fresh meat.

The palate does not close in human beings until the 9th or 10th week of fetal life and may be affected by deleterious influences acting at a time too late to disturb most other parts of the body.

First arch syndrome.—Abnormalities of many varieties may follow a disturbance in development of the first branchial arch; McKenzie considered them an hereditary syndrome caused by a dominant gene or group of genes with variable specificity and only a moderate degree of penetrance. He believed that the penetrance of the gene depends on the nutritional state and diet of the mother during the first weeks of pregnancy and that when the gene is present only an "excellent" nutritional state can prevent its manifestation. The gene is thought to inhibit or prevent development of the stapedial artery with resultant inhibition of growth in the area supplied by the artery and its branches. Mc-

Kenzie included in this category (1) mandibulofacial dysostosis, (2) Pierre-Robin syndrome, (3) mandibular dysostosis, (4) deformities of the external and middle ear, (5) congenital deaf-mutism, (6) cleft lip and cleft palate, (7) hypertelorism and (8) congenital deafness and hypertelorism. Other authors have thought that these, like some other sporadic congenital anomalies, are a result of polygenic inheritance.

EYES.—*Development.*—The eye is derived from three sources. The parts concerned directly with visual function come from the neural tube and surface ectoderm; the parts forming the outer coats and accessory structures come from adjacent mesoderm. During the 3d week of embryonic life, while the ends of the neural tube are still open, the lateral surfaces of the widened anterior portions that will form the forebrain show depressions that deepen and are gradually cut off below the surface to form the optic vesicles. Subsequently the anterior part of each optic vesicle is invaginated into the posterior portion, which is attached to the brain, thus forming a double-walled cup. The invaginated inner part is converted into the sensory layer and the outer part into the pigment layer of the retina. The stalk by which the vesicle is attached to the brain forms a tract for the growth of the fibers of the optic nerve.

The lens makes its first appearance at about the

end of the 4th week. The ectoderm overlying the optic vesicle thickens, invaginates and is cut off from the surface ectoderm. It forms a thick-walled hollow sphere that pushes into the concavity of the optic vesicle. The anterior wall of the sphere becomes thinned, the posterior wall becomes thickened and the space between the two layers disappears. The cells of the posterior wall become considerably elongated and form the lens fibers.

Fibers continue to be laid down in the periphery of the lens throughout intrauterine life and for several years after birth. The inner portion, being the oldest, is more subject to adverse intrauterine conditions than are the outer, younger cells. Consequently, congenital cataracts most often involve the central portion of the lens.

As the lens grows it sinks deeper into the concavity of the optic cup. The mesenchymal cells adjacent to the periphery of the optic cup develop into the choroid coat, sclera and principal part of the cornea. The outer surface of the cornea is composed of a thin layer of epithelium derived from the superficial ectoderm where it closes over the lens vesicle.

The anterior chamber of the eye is a flattened cavity produced through rearrangement of the mesenchymal cells lying in front of the lens. The bulk of the tissue forms the anterior wall of the cavity and makes up the greater part of the cornea. A thin layer of cells temporarily persists as a posterior wall lying immediately in front of the lens. Delicate vascular loops extend radially into it from the iris and, with their connective tissue, form the pupillary membrane. Resorption of this membrane and its vessels takes place during the latter months of intrauterine life and is usually complete a few weeks before birth. Occasionally, portions of the membrane are still present in the newborn infant. Rarely, functional blood vessels are also present, but usually the blood vessels, if persistent, are atrophic cordlike structures without lumens. If parts or all of the membrane fail to resorb, the condition is known as a persistent pupillary membrane.

The blood supply to the eye comes from the ophthalmic artery, which enters the globe in the region of the optic stalk. In young embryos it is known as the hyaloid artery. It runs directly through the vitreous to the posterior surface of the lens, where it breaks up into several nutrient vessels. These vessels and the connective tissue holding them together are known as the tunica vasculosa lentis. During the latter part of fetal life the hyaloid artery and the posterior lental blood vessels normally degenerate and disappear; new branches arise from the ophthalmic artery that form the vascular supply of the retina. Rarely, part or all of the hyaloid artery and vascular tunic of the lens persists. This is known as a persistent tunica vasculosa lentis or, since considerable connective tissue is also present, as a persistent posterior vascular sheath of the lens.

The lids start to develop during the 7th week as folds of skin growing down over the cornea. They grow rapidly, meet and fuse by the 9th week and do not separate to permit opening of the lids until the 7th month.

The position of the eyes changes greatly during fetal life. They appear first on the lateral surfaces of the head and remain there until the 6th week. As the facial structures grow, the eyes gradually move toward the midline, and the optical axes begin to converge. By the 12th week the angle is only slightly greater than it is at birth.

Malformations of the globes.—Congenital defects of the eye are numerous and have been excellently described by Ida Mann in her book, *Developmental Abnormalities of the Eye.* Any part of the eye may be individually affected, or several structures may show related abnormalities.

Variation in number.—This is found only in severely malformed infants. Anophthalmos, the complete absence of an eyeball, is extremely rare as an isolated malformation. The lids and accessory structures may be present (Fig. 25–45) or they, as well as the globe, may be absent and the orbital fossa may be covered by an uninterrupted skin surface. A single abnormal eye is found in some cyclopian monsters (see Fig. 24–43), although the majority have two fused abnormal globes. Very rarely no global tissue is present. The presence of more than two eyes is evidence of some degree of duplication of the cephalic pole of the fetus. When three eyes are present, the nose and mouth are also duplicated (see Fig. 13–23, D), and when four eyes are present in a single head, the entire face is duplicated. When a single body exists, such duplication is usually on the anterolateral sides of the head; in Janus monsters, characterized by two bodies attached to a single head with the ventral surfaces facing each other, the faces are at right angles to the anteroposterior axis of the bodies (see Fig. 13–32).

Abnormalities of position.—These have been described under malformations of the face and nervous system; the most common varieties are hypertelorism (see Fig. 25–33), in which the forward shift of the eyes toward the midline is arrested so that they remain in a position normal for an 8–10-

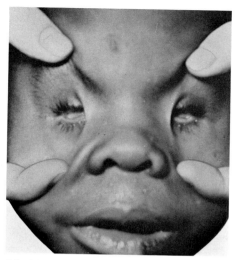

Fig. 25–45.—Anophthalmos. (Courtesy Drs. Lewis K. Sweet and John L. Parks.)

week fetus, and those in which the eyes are too close together, the ultimate form of this anomaly being the single median eye. Failure of orbital fossae to develop normally results in a forward displacement of the eyes called proptosis or exophthalmos. Mild degrees of this condition are present in oxycephaly, Crouzon's disease and platybasia. An anterior meningocele or meningoencephalocele, in which the meninges, or meninges and brain substance, are herniated through the sutures of the frontal bone, nasal processes of the maxilla or the ethmoid and lacrimal bone, may be responsible for either downward displacement, proptosis or anophthalmos (see Fig. 24–59).

Abnormalities of size.—These include varying degrees of microphthalmia and macrophthalmia. Microphthalmia may be unilateral or bilateral; when bilateral it is often associated with abnormalities of the nose, as in cebocephalus (see Figs. 24–39, 24–41 and 24–42). When unilateral, the involved eye may be normal except for size, but often a cataract, coloboma of the iris or choroid, persistent hyaloid artery or other abnormality is associated. In some microphthalmic eyes a cyst that is continuous with the vitreous chamber is present behind the eye or extends under the lower lid. In two cases of severe microphthalmia studied at the Chicago Lying-in Hospital no nerve fibers were present in the optic nerve and the visual cortex was missing from the brain.

Macrophthalmia is also known as megalophthalmos, buphthalmos, hydrophthalmos and congenital glaucoma. The eyeball is excessively large (the normal diameter is 17 mm at birth and 23 mm in adults). The front is more globular than normal, the anterior chamber deep, the cornea enlarged, the optic nerve cupped and the sclera often thin or unusually transparent, permitting the choroid to show through, which gives a bluish appearance.

The cause of enlargement of the globe is unknown, although the fact that it may be associated with arachnodactyly has led to the suggestion that an abnormality in calcium metabolism may be responsible both for the disturbances in bone growth and for a softening of the cornea sufficient to permit intraocular tension to cause an increase in size of the anterior chamber. Macrophthalmia caused by hydrophthalmos may be found at birth in association with a nevus flammeus involving the portion of the face adjacent to the affected eye and localized areas of calcification of the brain (Sturge-Weber syndrome).

The eyeball is ordinarily proportionately shorter in its anteroposterior diameter at birth than in adults. Growth is normally rapid during the first months after birth and the eye soon assumes the adult form. Myopia may result from failure of the diameters to change normally with growth or may be a consequence of an anteroposterior diameter that is unnaturally short at the time of birth.

Lids.—The lids may be absent and the eyeballs uncovered (ablepharon), the lids may be fused (ankyloblepharon), or skin may be continuous over the eyeballs without any indication of the formation of eyelids (cryptophthalmos). Lack of a covering for the eyeball is a result of persistence of the state that is normal in the first weeks of development; fusion of the lids represents persistence of a slightly later stage. All are rare except in association with other malformations of the face. Complete lack of lid development associated with a smooth layer of skin extending from forehead to cheek without a break is almost always accompanied by malformation of the globe. Ordinarily some vestige of the eye is present, although this may be reduced to a small mass of connective tissue. Extrinsic eye muscles may be present even though no portion of the globe can be identified.

The lids are usually small with microphthalmia, and although at times they are of normal size, they are often partially or completely fused. A vertical fissure of one or both lids (coloboma) may be found alone or with facial fissures. Eversion (ectropion) and inversion (entropion) are rare; the former has been described in infants with severe ichthyosis.

Epicanthus.—This is a cutaneous fold covering either the inner or, very rarely, the outer canthus.

It is normal in the Mongolian race, although in these individuals the fold covers only the upper part of the inner canthus and ends at the point of contact with the lower lid. A narrow epicanthic fold is seen occasionally in normal non-Oriental infants during the first few years of life. A more pronounced fold is seen in infants with various abnormalities. In mongolism it is usually wide and prominent but ordinarily ends at about the level of the lower lid. It is most pronounced in bilateral renal agenesis, in which a semicircular fold arising on the upper lid and ending on the cheek completely covers the inner canthus (see Fig. 22–13, A). An epicanthic fold associated with bilateral ptosis of the lids has been described as an hereditary trait.

Lacrimal glands.—The lacrimal apparatus may be absent, the duct may be an open sinus (facial fissure) or it may be occluded. The usual cause of occlusion is failure of resorption of a fold of mucous membrane that normally involutes before birth. Since few tears are shed in the early weeks of life, the occlusion may not be discovered for several months. Occlusion interferes with drainage, and this may be responsible for a local abscess.

Cornea.—Individual parts of the eye are often malformed. The cornea may be abnormally large, small or dome-shaped. It may be opaque in the presence of either microphthalmia or macrophthalmia. Localized opacities may form a peripheral ring known as arcus juvenilis. When a beam of light is thrown into the eye, the pupil appears red because of reflection of the color of the retinal blood vessels. Any interference with transmission of this red color gives the pupil a white or gray appearance. This may be caused by opacities of the lens or cornea or by detachment and fibrosis of the retina.

Dermoid tumors of the cornea vary in size. The smallest, a fibrofatty tumor 3–4 mm in diameter located at the limbus, involves only the surface, the rest of the cornea being normal (Fig. 25–46). In other cases the whole cornea may be replaced by fatty connective tissue. The cornea is thicker than normal, protrudes between the lids and is covered by skin and hairs.

Iris.—The iris is gray-blue immediately after birth in almost all infants of white parents, but some evidence of brown pigment may be visible in Negroes. The pattern of the iris is more homogeneous in young infants than in older individuals, although in some, especially mongolian idiots, a distinct pattern is present at birth. White punctate areas seem to be distinctive of mongolism (see Fig. 24–20). A segment of the iris may be absent (coloboma) or, very rarely, the entire iris is absent (aniridia). In albinos it is devoid of pigment and appears pink because the underlying blood vessels are visible.

The pupil may be eccentric because of abnormalities in the shape of the iris, or it may appear to be duplicated if defects exist in the substance of the iris.

Part or all of the pupillary membrane that is

Fig. 25–46.—Dermoid tumor located at the posterior portion of the limbus. Infant aged 3 days. **A,** gross appearance of dermoid tumor. **B,** photomicrograph of dermoid tumor composed of fat, connective tissue, hair follicles and sebaceous glands.

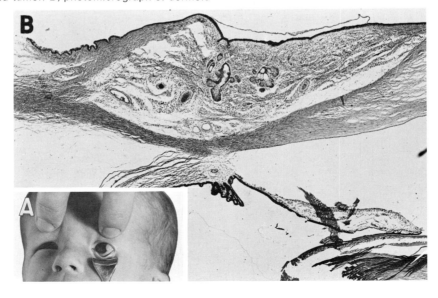

normally present in the young embryo may persist. Persistence of the entire membrane is rare, and the usual picture is one in which strands of tissue arising a short distance from the pupillary edge extend to the lens or across the pupil to the opposite margin. The fibers are usually white and opaque, although blood vessels are occasionally visible. Small fibers do not usually interfere with vision, although persistence of the entire membrane may cause a considerable reduction in visual acuity.

Lens.—The lens is rarely absent (aphakia) except with malformations of other parts of the eye. It may be abnormally small or excessively curved, or the margin may be irregular. Abnormality of position, called ectopia lentis, may occur as a single anomaly or with malformations of other parts of the eye or more remote parts of the body. Like macrophthalmia, it is often associated with arachnodactyly. Ectopia lentis has also been reported in association with a high degree of myopia.

Congenital cataracts are opacities of the lens that may be complete, zonular, dotted, anterior, polar and so on. They may be inherited or the result of some abnormality of intrauterine environment. Microphthalmia is frequently associated. Maternal rubella during the first 2 months of pregnancy may be responsible for cataracts, which are usually bilateral and often accompanied by microphthalmia. In such cases the embryonal nucleus of the lens is chiefly affected. The nuclear portion of the lens is amorphous and stains poorly, and the lens fibers making up the cortical zone are separated by vacuoles. Congenital cataracts may be seen as part of several syndromes including oxycephaly, Conradi's disease, Hollerman-Streif syndrome, Lowe's syndrome, Bonnevie-Ullrich syndrome and congenital hemolytic icterus (Cordes).

Persistence of the posterior vascular sheath of the lens is diagnosed by the presence of a white opaque mass behind the lens, giving much the same appearance clinically as a retinoblastoma. The eyes often also have a persistent pupillary membrane and are frequently somewhat smaller than normal. Vision is limited to perception of light.

Retina.—The retina is frequently abnormal if any other part of the eye is malformed, but it is also often the only site of involvement. In anencephalic monsters the ganglion cell layer is reduced in thickness, and only scattered ganglion cells are visible.

In Toxoplasma infections chorioretinitis is a constant finding although it usually cannot be seen until several months after birth even though the infection is acquired in utero. The early lesions may be mistaken for hemorrhages. As the chorioretinitis becomes more longstanding, yellow-white areas appear that may be bordered or studded with pigment. Although the lesions may appear in any part, they have an especial predilection for the region of the macula. Other eye lesions observed in congenital Toxoplasma infections include microphthalmia, enophthalmos and small masses of tissue in the vitreous. The latter are composed of granulation tissue that has grown into the vitreous from extensive areas of chorioretinitis. Evidence of hydrocephalus and cerebral calcification is usually found in conjunction with the eye disturbances and helps establish the diagnosis.

The infantile form of *amaurotic familial idiocy* is characterized by a cherry red spot in the center of the macula surrounded by a white area somewhat larger than the disk. The optic nerve is atrophic. Vacuoles are present in the ganglion cell layer of the retina as part of the disturbance in lipid metabolism.

Retrolental fibroplasia is the name given to the end-stage of a process found in premature infants subjected to prolonged high tissue–oxygen tension. In infants with marginal respiratory function, ambient oxygen tensions may be quite high and not cause difficulties because the tissue levels may be low or normal, but much lower tensions (any above 35%) may damage the retina of a premature infant, even one with good respiratory exchange. The earliest lesions are pigment deposition and fibrosis in the periphery of the retina (Gunderson *et al.*). Next comes retinal folding followed by an increase in fibrous tissue in the retrolental area, which gradually involves the retina and leads to its detachment (Fig. 25–47). Clouding of the cornea, cataract formation and microphthalmia are sequelae.

Petechial hemorrhages of the retina have been described as of frequent occurrence immediately after birth and have been reported in as many as 70% of all newborn infants. After vitamin K was discovered, it was stated that its administration would greatly reduce the frequency of such hemorrhage but this does not seem to have been the case. It is probable that petechial hemorrhages of the retina result from the general congestion and distention of cranial blood vessels that are almost always associated with vaginal delivery. They disappear promptly and do not interfere with retinal function. In older infants similar hemorrhages are considered pathognomonic of internal pachymeningitis.

Abnormal proliferation of the retina in the form

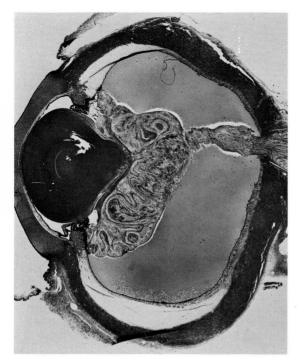

Fig. 25–47.—Retrolental fibroplasia. The retina is detached and is bound into a firm fibrous mass adherent to the posterior surface of the lens together with a mass of abnormally proliferated blood vessels. Infant weighed 1,100 gm at birth. Eye removed because of erroneous diagnosis of retinoblastoma at age 6 months.

of rosettes is almost constant in fused cyclopian eyes and is common with microphthalmia and other abnormalities. Rosettes have their origin in the unfolding of the external limiting membrane and outer nuclear layer.

Retinoblastoma.—Tumors of the eyes are almost never present at birth, but the fact that the majority of retinal gliomas occur in children under 3 years of age leads to the belief that they probably have their inception during intrauterine life. The histologic appearance is similar to that of the partially differentiated cells of the fetal retina (Fig. 25–48). The rosettes so commonly described are derived from early rods and cones and appear as a single-layered ring of cells resting against an inner basement membrane. At times the cells arrange themselves in layers 15–20 cells thick around blood vessels, the peripheral cells dying from lack of nourishment.

EARS.—*Development.*—The internal ear develops in the ectoderm on the lateral aspect of the anterior end of the neural groove as a placode which be-

comes invaginated to form a pit and subsequently a detached vesicle. The vesicle differentiates into the membranous labyrinth and forms the semicircular canals, ampulla, vestibule and cochlea. Condensation of mesenchyme around these structures produces a framework that is at first cartilage and later bone. The organ of Corti, the actual end-organ for the reception of sound, appears first during the 3d month as a thickening in the epithelium covering the floor of the cochlear duct.

The middle ear develops from the first pharyngeal pouch at the same time as the inner ear is being elaborated from the vesicle. The entoderm of the lateral end of the pouch comes in contact with the ectoderm at the bottom of the first gill furrow to form the eardrum. The lateral portion remains expanded to form the chamber of the middle ear, while the proximal portion becomes narrowed to form the eustachian tube. The ossicles develop from the mesenchyme of the primitive tympanic cavity. They become organized first in cartilage and extend between the inner ear and the eardrum, which marks the innermost portion of the external auditory meatus.

Malformations.—The range in size and shape of the ears is very wide at birth as well as in older individuals. The pointed pinna known as the satyr ear and the nodular thickening of the helix called

Fig. 25–48.—Retinoblastoma in infant aged 3 months.

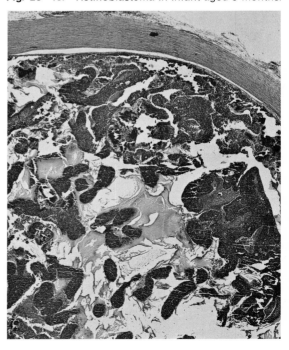

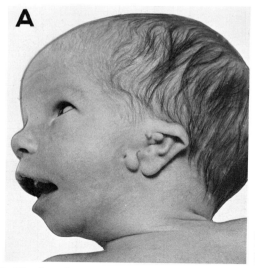 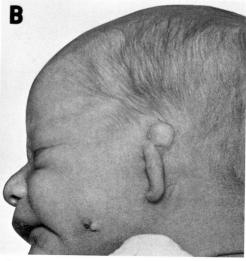

Fig. 25—49.—A, satyr ear associated with papillomas and an aural fistula caused by abnormal closure of the cleft between the first and second branchial arches. Same infant as in Fig. 25–46. **B,** hypoplasia of pinna with absence of external auditory meatus associated with a papilloma and aural fistula located midway between the ear and mouth.

the darwinian tubercle are among the more commonly occurring variants and are generally inherited. An exaggeration of the satyr ear with production of a definitely triangular pinna (Fig. 25–49, A) is often associated with deafness resulting from aplasia of the nuclei of the seventh and eighth nerves. Failure of the lobe to become separated from the side of the head is one of the most commonly observed malformations of the ears. It is more common in females than in males and is often found in all the females of a family. Ear pits, or congenital aural fistulas, are small, blind, epithelium-lined depressions extending usually not more than 2–3 mm into the subcutaneous connective tissue in front of the tragus or, more rarely, into the helix or other parts of the ear. They are more common in some races than others. They may rarely become infected but ordinarily produce no symptoms.

Irregular papillary or pedunculated masses of epithelium-covered connective tissue may be located immediately anterior to the tragus or on the cheek a greater distance from the ear. Usually present at some point on a direct line between the tragus and the angle of the mouth, they result from the aberrant growth of the aural portion of the first branchial arch and are not often found without other malformations of the external ear. They have been described under the terms persistent hillocks and polyotia. The latter term is undesirable since they are not accessory pinnas as the name would indicate.

More extensive digressions from the usual pattern may be found in otherwise normal infants or in infants with abnormalities. Large portions of the external ear may be missing, although complete absence seems to be even more rare than complete anophthalmos. When large portions of the external ear are absent, the middle ear is usually also defective and hearing is greatly impaired or completely absent (Fig. 25–49, B). There may also be aplasia of part or all of the nucleus of the facial nerve, leading to varying degrees of paralysis (Fig. 25–50).

The pinna of the ear, although normal in shape, may be abnormally large (macrotia) or small (microtia). Certain peculiarities that may appear sporadically may also be found as components of certain syndromes. Mongolian idiots often show a change in the upper part of the helix, the lower margin of the anteverted superior portion being straight across instead of having a curve following the outer margin (see Fig. 24–19). The ears of infants with renal agenesis are often excessively flat and large, the helix is without normal contours, the tragus may be missing and the position is usually lower and more horizontal than normal. An anteverted cup-shaped pinna was present in 20 otherwise normal individuals in six generations of a family studied at the Chicago Lying-in Hospital. Inheritance was autosomal dominant (Potter).

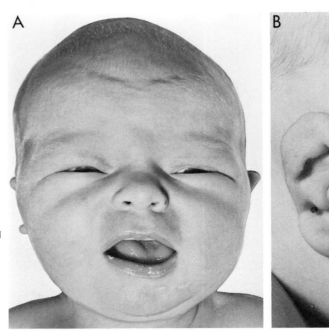

Fig. 25–50.—Malformation of external ear accompanied by deafness and right facial paralysis. **A,** face showing paralysis of the right side with mouth drawn to the left. **B,** malformed external ear and absent ear canal.

An abnormally low position of the ears is a result of arrested development. In the young embryo the anlagen of the external ears lie below the region that will develop into the mandible. They are horizontal and meet in the midline. With normal growth they move laterally and the axes shift through an angle of about 90 degrees. Development may be arrested at any stage. The rarest malformation, called synotia (see Fig. 25–55), is a result of complete lack of lateral shift of the ears so that they retain their horizontal position beneath the mandible. The mandible, buccal cavity, tongue and pharynx are always extremely hypoplastic. In certain cyclopian monsters the mandible and buccal cavity are similarly malformed. In such instances the position of the ears is usually less primitive and they seldom meet in the midline although they are abnormally low on the head and abnormal in shape.

Maternal rubella during the first 2 months of pregnancy is sometimes responsible for middle ear deafness in the child. It has been found most frequently when the mothers have had the disease slightly later than when it produces cataracts. It is often associated with the other disturbances in development characteristic of the rubella syndrome (see p. 125). Deafness is seldom discovered until the child is several months old.

Diseases.—Diseases of the ear are rarely recognized in the newborn period, although this may be in part because of the rarity with which ears are examined at autopsy. It has been suggested that Pituitrin or quinine administered to the pregnant woman (as in induction of labor) may cause injury of the infant's auditory nerve and be responsible for deafness, but the evidence to substantiate such a claim is meager.

Otitis media has been reported in infants a few days old. Amniotic fluid and meconium may be forced into the eustachian tube during delivery and may reach the drum. A sterile inflammation may be produced or, if the amniotic fluid is infected, the inflammation may be bacterial. It is also possible for infection to be secondary to infection in other parts of the body. If suppuration does not occur, the exudate may be gradually absorbed, leaving fibrous adhesions. It has been thought that this might prevent the formation of air cells and be responsible for a sclerotic mastoid.

NOSE.—The nose is subject to wide variation in size and shape but is seldom abnormal unless there are defects of contiguous structures. The most striking abnormalities are those found in association with cyclops or cebocephalus, in which cases it may be either absent or a fleshy proboscis with a central canal; it is usually located above the eye in infants with cyclops and below the eye in those with cebocephalus (see Figs. 24–35 and 24–39). In an anterior meningocele the herniation of meninges takes place between the frontal and nasal bones (see Fig. 24–59), and the nostrils may be the only part of the nose that can be identified externally. Duplication or splitting of the nose is usually associated with some degree of duplication of the eyes and/or mouth, and an infant with such a malformation is usually classed with the double monsters (see Fig. 13–23).

The most common malformation of the nose is found as part of the picture of cleft palate and harelip. A harelip is occasionally visible only as a notch in the upper lip, but more often it involves the maxilla and extends up into the nostril. When the palate is cleft, the floor of the nose is missing and one or both nasal cavities are continuous with the buccal cavity, the difference being dependent on whether one or both sides of the palate are involved (see Fig. 25–37).

Atresia of the nares has been reported as a result of occlusion of one or both nostrils by cartilage or membrane. Absence of the nasal bones is associated with absence of the bridge of the nose (Fig. 25–51). There is generally a depression between the eyes, and the nares are directed anteriorly. The nose fails to grow and remains a small hypoplastic structure, giving the face a bizarre appearance (Fig. 25–52).

The posterior part of the nose has been described as abnormally narrow in association with gargoylism, and as a consequence such infants are unusually susceptible to upper respiratory infections of which they may die. In achondroplasia, too, the bridge of the nose is poorly developed. A broad turned-up nose is one of the characteristic features of hypertelorism.

The nose is rarely the site of infection in the newborn period inasmuch as upper respiratory infections are not common until the child is several months old. Congenital syphilis sometimes produces excoriation and ulceration around the external nares. Healing may leave small radiating scars known as rhagades.

MOUTH.—The formation of the buccal cavity is primarily dependent on the splitting of each of the first branchial arches into the two parts that become the maxilla and mandible. The portions derived from each arch grow toward the midline, and the mandibular portions fuse without relation to other structures. The maxillary portions are dependent on the normal growth of the frontonasal process for transformation into their definitive form. The lining of the mouth cavity comes from the ectoderm of the oral plate.

Malformations.—The mouth is of greatly exaggerated width (macrostomia) and reaches almost from ear to ear only in association with other malformations. One infant observed at the Chicago Lying-in Hospital with an abnormally wide orifice, which extended laterally beyond the lip margins, had associated malformation of the ears and a dermoid tumor of the eye (see Fig. 25–49, A). The same unusual combination of anomalies was recorded by Gould and Pyle in *Medical Curiosities.*

The mouth orifice is sometimes unusually small (microstomia) as a genetically determined variant in certain family groups. In mongolism the mouth is almost always small. It may be greatly reduced in association with other facial malformations, especially those caused by maldevelopment of the first branchial arch (see Figs. 24–43 and 25–43). Complete absence is unknown unless all other structures relating to sense organs are also missing.

Moderate hypoplasia of the mandible with recession of the chin (micrognathia) may be hereditary but when more severe is usually sporadic (Fig. 25–

Fig. 25–51.—Absence of nasal bone and abnormality of septum. A, lateral view of head. The glabella is depressed and the nares are directed anteriorly. B, sagittal section through face and base of the skull.

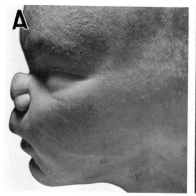
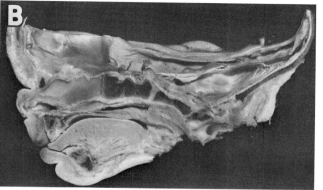

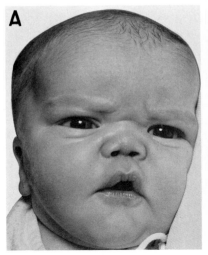

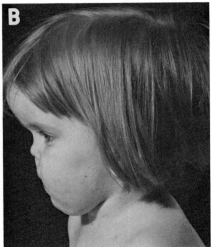

Fig. 25–52.—Characteristic facies produced by absence of nasal bone. **A,** infant aged 3 days showing depression of glabella and anterior direction of nares. **B,** same child at 2 years showing hypoplasia of the nose.

53). Subluxation of a mandible of normal size may give a similar appearance on superficial examination, and roentgen examination may be necessary to differentiate the two. Either condition is commonly associated with recession of the tongue (glossoptosis), which leads to cyanosis, respiratory disturbances and difficulty in feeding. When accompanied by a cleft palate, it is called the Pierre-Robin syndrome (see Fig. 25–39). Asphyxia or inability to nurse may be fatal unless it is possible to overcome the pharyngeal obstruction caused by the position of the tongue.

An extremely hypoplastic mandible is often associated with great reduction in size of the buccal cavity and is generally fatal. A miniature tongue and glottis are present low in the throat. The mandible is rarely more than 1 cm wide and a thin rim of mucous membrane surrounds a circular buccal

Fig. 25–53.—Hypoplasia of the mandible associated with glossoptosis leading to cyanosis, respiratory disturbances and difficulty in nursing. Palate normal.

Fig. 25–54.—Mandibular hypoplasia associated with microstomia and descensus of the ears. No communication between buccal cavity and pharynx. (Courtesy Dr. Aparecida Garcia.)

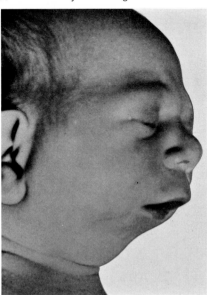

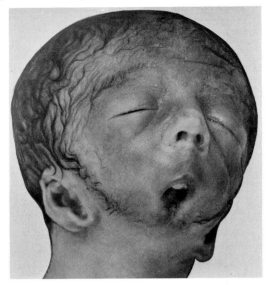

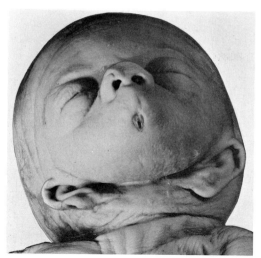

Fig. 25–55.–Extreme mandibular hypoplasia and microstomia associated with synotia. (Courtesy Dr. H. W. Edmonds.)

opening a few millimeters in diameter. The external appearance of the maxilla may be normal but the palatal portion is always hypoplastic.

This anomaly is usually associated with malformations of the ears since they arise in part from the inferior portion of the first branchial arch. The external ears are variable in configuration and are

set unusually low on the head, most often being at about the level of the maxilla (Fig. 25–54). Rarely they meet and fuse in the midline below the rudimentary mandible (Fig. 25–55). The parts of the face derived from the maxillary portion of the first branchial arch and the frontonasal process may be normal or abnormal. The cyclops deformity may be associated (see Fig. 24–43).

SPINE, PELVIS AND THORAX

SPINE.–Abnormalities of the spine associated with incomplete closure of the vertebral arches are described in Chapter 24 (Central Nervous System). Other malformations include a variation in total number and/or abnormal development of individual vertebrae. The spine is formed in early fetal life by pairing and fusing of the primitive segments that develop at the sides of the notochord. These masses extend posteriorly and each fuses with its mate of the opposite side. Interruption in this process produces many variations in form. Incomplete fusion of the two posterior portions leads to their separation by a vertical cleft. Hemivertebrae result from development of only one posterior segment. Segments may be incompletely separated, and partial or complete fusion of two or several vertebrae may result. Abnormalities are often multiple, and an intermixture of abnormal splitting, fusion and

Fig. 25–56 (left).–Absence of lower thoracic and upper lumbar vertebrae. Fetus stillborn at term.

Fig. 25–57 (right).–Absence of sacrum associated

with multiple anomalies of the vertebrae and ribs. **A,** iliac bones fused. The left arm lacks a radius and thumb. **B,** iliac bones connected by fibrous connective tissue.

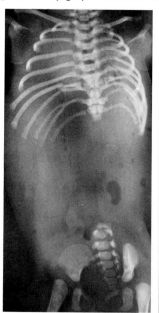
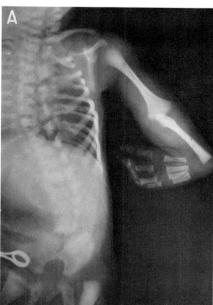
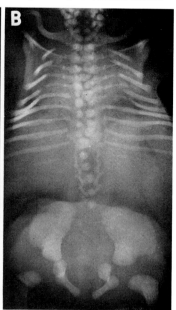

partial development is not uncommon. Hemivertebrae cause scoliosis unless compensated for by the presence of other vertebral anomalies.

One or several vertebrae may be absent. In anencephalus the missing vertebrae are most often cervical; in other cases they are most often lumbar or sacral (Sinclair *et al.*). Some investigators have found that a high percentage of such infants are the offspring of diabetic mothers (Banta and Nichols). This was not true at the Chicago Lying-in Hospital where two infants of nondiabetic mothers were observed who lacked all of the lower dorsal and most of the lumbar and sacral vertebrae. The lowermost dorsal vertebrae presented a rounded, closed lower surface and the spinal cord ended in the mid-dorsal region in each case (Fig. 25–56).

PELVIS.—Absence of the sacrum is found as a pelvic deformity in a few individuals who seem otherwise normal but is most common in association with other severe spinal defects. When the sacrum is absent, the wings of the ilia may be fused posteriorly or joined only by dense connective tissue (Fig. 25–57).

The pubic rami are separated or absent in association with ectropion of the bladder. The consequent anterolateral displacement of the pubic rami and eversion of the ischial bones change the direction of the acetabula, which face posteriorly instead of laterally; in extreme cases the direction of the legs and feet is the reverse of normal. In milder cases this malformation is responsible for a waddling gait when the child begins to walk.

RIBS.—Abnormalities of the ribs are usually secondary to malformations of the dorsal vertebrae. If part or all of a vertebra is absent, the related rib is generally missing. If two vertebrae are fused, two ribs may arise from a single process and divide into two parts a short distance from the spine. When severe scoliosis exists because of vertebral anomalies, some of the ribs on the concave side of the chest are often irregularly branched, fused or absent (Fig. 25–58). Branching of the distal portions occurs occasionally in otherwise normal individuals.

Rib abnormalities are common in generalized disturbances of bone formation. In osteogenesis imperfecta, multiple fractures often occur during intrauterine life. During the process of healing large masses of callus are produced and the ribs often look like strings of beads (see Fig. 25–11). In achondroplasia they are unusually short and are flared at the ends where joined by cartilage. The upper ribs may be especially short and the upper part of the chest may be greatly constricted. Short

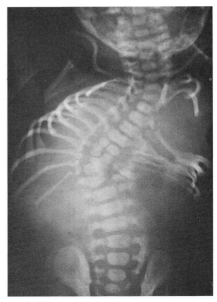

Fig. 25—58.—Abnormalities and reduction in number of ribs on the left side of the chest associated with scoliosis and kyphosis from hemivertebrae accompanying spina bifida. Bilateral talipes equinovarus.

ribs with a reduction in size of the thoracic cavity are also seen in asphyxiating thoracic dystrophy and hypophosphatasia.

The length of the ribs and the shape of the thorax may show marked variation in association with other abnormalities. In anencephalus with spina bifida the thorax is short and broadly flared. With large polycystic kidneys or any other condition causing a severe enlargement of the abdominal cavity the lower ribs are more widely expanded than normal. A diaphragmatic hernia causes a moderate increase in circumference of the entire chest.

Pressure of an arm against the chest wall during intrauterine life may produce a local depression (Fig. 25–59).

STERNUM.—Minor abnormalities in the shape of the sternum are encountered fairly frequently and consist largely of an unusual elevation or depression of some portion. An abnormal elevation most often involves the upper part and in older individuals is commonly known as a pigeon breast, whereas an unusual depression is found more often in the lower part and is known as a funnel chest (see Fig. 15–14). A pronounced depression may occur in infants with severe respiratory distress; whether it is responsible for symptoms or simply becomes exaggerated by labored respiration is not certain. Such severe depression is seldom observed with

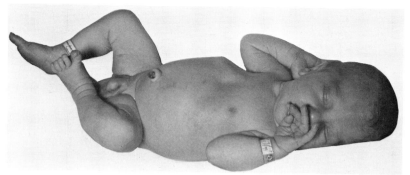

Fig. 25–59. — Infant with concavity of right side of chest into which the arm fits when it is drawn forward.

normal respiration. In at least some instances depression of the sternum is caused by a short central tendon of the diaphragm. According to Lester, depression of the sternum produces pulmonary and cardiac symptoms throughout life that can be overcome only by surgical intervention. Some doubt as to the curative value of the operation was expressed by Orazalesi and Cook as a result of pulmonary function studies.

Clefts of the sternum are occasionally present as isolated anomalies but are usually associated with other severe malformations of the chest. One infant born at the Chicago Lying-in Hospital who survived for several hours had a cleft of the sternum associated with a defect of the ribs and abdominal wall that exposed the heart, left lung and abdominal viscera to the exterior. Several instances of ectopia cordis have been reported in association with a cleft sternum. One infant observed by Parks and Sweet survived for 18 days with the heart outside the body as a result of a defective sternum (see Fig. 14–19).

SCAPULAS. — The scapulas are not often abnormal. Rarely, they are excessively large or small or extend outward at an angle from the chest. In Sprengel's deformity one or both scapulas are unusually high and the lower margin is turned toward the spine and is frequently attached to it by fibrous or cartilaginous tissue. The craniocaudal diameter is usually reduced and the transverse diameter increased. The arm cannot be raised above a right angle to the body. The condition may also be found as an isolated anomaly or in conjunction with the Klippel-Feil syndrome, torticollis or scoliosis.

CLAVICLES. — These bones are fractured more often than any others during delivery but they heal rapidly, usually without deformity. Absence of all or part of a clavicle, known as cleidodysostosis, is often accompanied by abnormalities of the skull.

CLEIDOCRANIAL DYSOSTOSIS. — This disturbance in ossification chiefly affects the skull and clavicles. The extent of involvement varies, infrequently being limited to the skull, most often affecting skull and clavicles and occasionally involving all bones. Characteristically, at birth the bones of the calvarium are soft, the sutures wide and fontanelles greatly enlarged. Ossification proceeds slowly and sutures may remain open until adolescence. The base of the skull and face are small in relation to the calvarium, the nasal and zygomatic bones may remain unossified and the eyes may have an antimongolian slant (Forlund). Clavicles are absent or rudimentary so that the clavicular strut action that holds the humeri away from the chest wall is lacking and shoulders droop and can be brought together in the midline. The metaphyses of the long bones may be widened and irregularly ossified, carpal and tarsal bones may have accessory centers of ossification and abnormalities of the vertebrae may later be responsible for scoliosis, lordosis or kyphosis.

EXTREMITIES

Malformations of the extremities are legion. They include abnormalities in size, shape, number and relationships of bones and abnormalities in size, number and attachment of muscles. They may be bilaterally symmetrical or asymmetrical and may involve upper or lower extremities or both. The stimuli responsible for division of the hand or foot plate into an excessive number of digits do not seem to be capable of affecting the more proximal parts of the appendicular skeleton, and the abnormalities of the upper and lower arm, the thigh and leg are largely confined to absence or reduced size of part or all of one or more bones; increase in number of these bones is unknown except in the fused extremities of double monsters. The hand and foot may show abnormal increase or decrease in number and size of bones. Extra digits are often associated with excessive size of the adjacent tarsal or carpal bones.

According to Birch-Jensen, all abnormalities of the appendicular skeleton may be divided into two major groups, those of endogenous and those of exogenous origin. Their differentiation consists primarily of the presence or absence of bones of abnormal size or shape. If whatever bones or portions of bones present are normal, the cause may be considered exogenous; if they are in any way abnormal or if there are soft tissue indications of an attempt to produce more distal portions, the cause is endogenous. According to Birch-Jensen, all bilaterally symmetrical abnormalities and those in which the abnormality consists of an excessive number of parts are endogenous. The principal exogenous malformations are those in which some part of the upper or lower extremity ends abruptly, usually with evidence of scarring at the terminal point. Such abnormalities are often multiple, different extremities being involved to a different degree. They are also frequently associated with linear depressions that completely encircle one or more digits or the forearm or leg, less often the upper arm or thigh (see Fig. 25–91). The digits may be irregularly fused, sometimes held together only at the tips and separate near their attachment to the hand (see

Fig. 25–81, C). Threadlike strands may attach the terminal portions to the amnion.

The cause of exogenous spontaneous amputations is unknown. Streeter, and others before him, thought that they were the end-result of local tissue degeneration that first produced encircling cicatrices and later caused complete separation of the part. Some earlier investigators thought that they were due to infection or abnormality of the amnion. The fact that it is occasionally possible to make out attachment of such abnormal extremities to the amnion at the time of delivery gives support to the idea of amniotic abnormality as an etiologic agent for this particular malformation.

Ainhum is a condition occurring in certain adult African natives in which an encircling depressed area develops around a digit, especially a toe, with the distal part gradually becoming amputated. Although the process resembles exogenous intrauterine amputations, ainhum is unknown in infancy and childhood and there is no apparent relation between the conditions.

Complete absence of all four extremities (amelia) is very rare, but we have seen one infant with such a deformity. The shoulder girdle and pelvis were disproportionately small but otherwise normal (Fig. 25–60). Only slightly less rare is phocomelia, a condition in which hands and feet are attached to the trunk by small, irregularly shaped bones (Fig. 25–61). In micromelia all segments of the extremities are present but are abnormally short (Fig. 25–

Fig. 25–60.—Amelia and hydrocephalus. **A,** front view. **B,** side view. **C,** roentgenogram. (Specimen courtesy Dr. Aaron Gunther.)

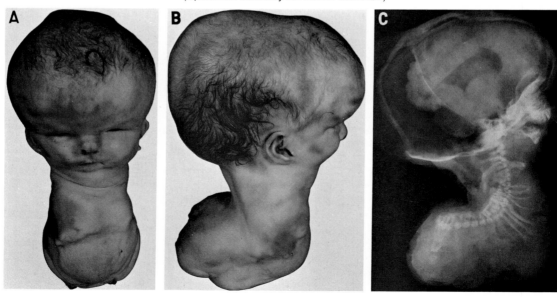

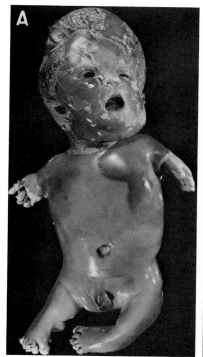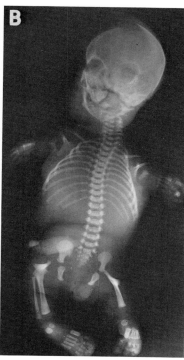

Fig. 25—61.—Phocomelia. **A,** external view. **B,** roentgenogram.

62). All gradations from this to only a slight short-ening of the long bones may be observed. Infants with only moderate reduction in bone length who belong in this group are easily differentiated from those with achondroplasia by the absence of other changes typical of that abnormality and, at autop-sy, by the presence of a zone of normally ossifying cartilage at the ends of the long bones. A few cases of hemimelia (Fig. 25–63) have been described, in which the distal portions of all extremities have been absent, although more often only a single ex-tremity is involved. A family in Brazil has been referred to many times in which two brothers and the four children of one had a malformation con-sisting of abrupt termination of both arms above the elbows and both legs below the knees.

Symmetrical absence of upper or lower extremi-ties may occur, with absence of the arms being less rare than absence of the legs (Fig. 25–64). In the museum of pathology in Rio de Janeiro is a wax model of a woman who appears to have been nor-mal except for the absence of legs; the feet are at-tached directly to the trunk.

Arms or legs may be symmetrically hypoplastic at birth even though all bones are present (Fig. 25–65). Such disturbances generally become more pronounced with increasing age of the child (Fig.

25–66) because growth is proportionately slower in the affected extremities after birth than it is before birth.

Maternally ingested thalidomide interferes with normal differentiation of the extremities, especially the upper ones. The disturbance may involve all four extremities and consists of an irregular absence and abnormal configuration of any or all bones (see page 172).

Fusion of the lower extremities is known as sym-podia or sirenomelia and is associated with a pro-found disturbance in the formation of the pelvis and genitourinary system. The single lower ex-tremity varies from one containing a normal num-ber of bones with fusion only of soft tissues to one in which bones are entirely absent and only a small tail-like appendage exists (Fig. 25–67). Most com-monly the femur is single or only partially divided, two or three bones are present below the knee and five or six digits are attached to the foot (Fig. 25–68). The position of the extremity is always re-versed and the kneecap is on the back, the leg bends anteriorly and the sole of the foot, if present, is di-rected anteriorly. The sacrum is usually absent, the iliac bones are fused and a single acetabulum is often present on the posterior aspect of the pelvis arising jointly from the fused ilia. The anus is

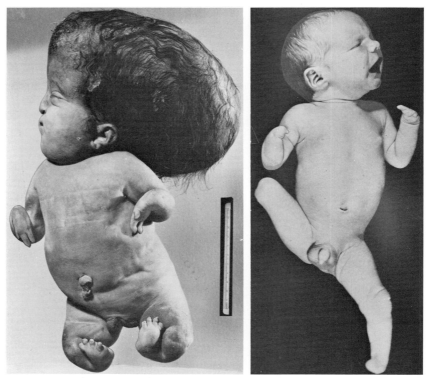

Fig. 25–62 (left).—Micromelia and hydrocephalus.
Fig. 25–63 (right).—Irregular form of hemimelia. Distal portions of all extremities missing.

Fig. 25–64.—**A,** congenital absence of both arms. **B,** congenital absence of both legs. (B, courtesy Drs. R. H. Barter and John L. Parks.)

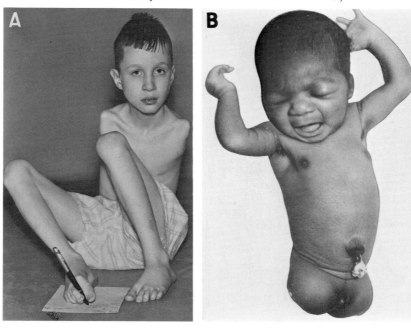

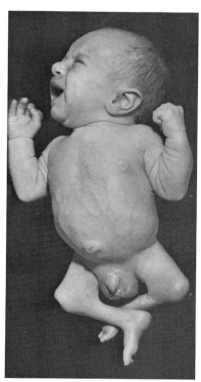

Fig. 25–65.—Hypoplasia of both lower extremities.

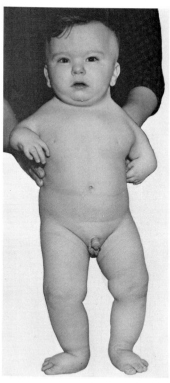

Fig. 25–66.—Hypoplasia of both upper extremities.

Fig. 25–67.—Sirenomelus showing fusion and varying degrees of hypoplasia of the lower extremities. In **A,** the structure extending posteriorly from the buttocks resembles a penis except for absence of a urethra.

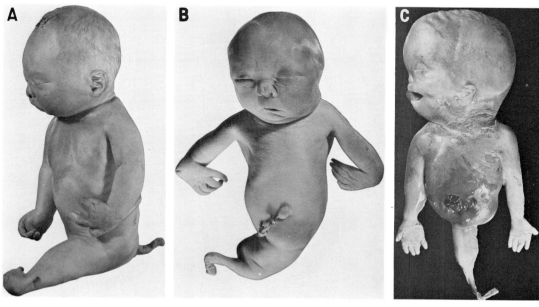

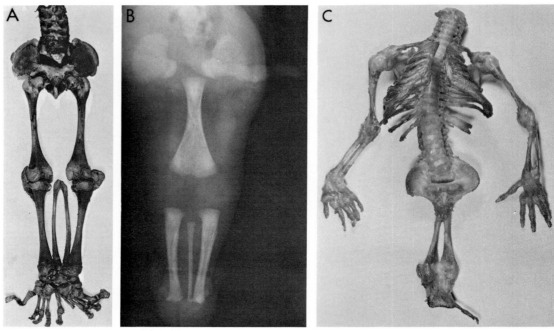

Fig. 25-68.—**A,** skeleton of sirenomelic monster with normal bones between hip and ankle. (Courtesy Drs. C. E. Proshek and F. L. Adair.) **B,** roentgenogram of infant shown in Fig. 25-67, A. **C,** skeleton showing abnormal sacrum and pelvis with partial fusion of femurs and fused upper portion of tibias. Remainder of lower extremities absent.

Fig. 25-69.—Sirenomelus of extreme degree. **A,** lower portion of abdomen and legs absent. Absence of kidneys responsible for changes in face, ears and hands. **B,** roentgenogram showing reduction in lumbar vertebrae and absence of pelvis. Three small bones distal to the spine are the only evidence of lower extremities. (Courtesy Prof. G. Sansone.)

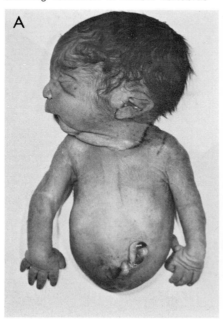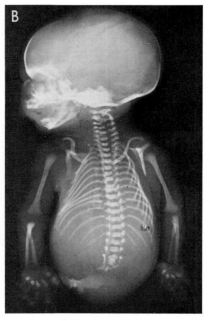

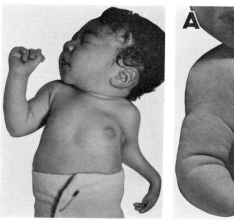
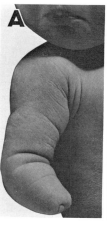
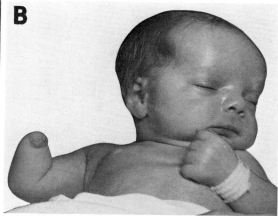

Fig. 25–70 (left).—Hypoplasia of left arm.
Fig. 25–71 (right).—Absence of distal portion of forearm and hand. **A,** exogenous amputation with dimple at end of stump. **B,** endogenous amputation with small nodules representing rudimentary digits at end of stump.

always imperforate, and kidneys, ureters, bladder and urethra are absent. Gonads are usually present but other genital organs are rarely found. In one infant delivered at the Chicago Lying-in Hospital a structure resembling a penis containing corpora cavernosa but no urethra arose from the posterior part of the body (see Fig. 25–67, A). It had no connection with any structure in the interior of the pelvis. Some sirenomeli show such a great reduction in the development of the lower extremities that they have no legs, but in such cases the lower part of the trunk is also abnormal and the malformation is incompatible with life (Fig. 25–69).

Unilateral symmetrical abnormalities of bones of both upper and lower extremities are almost unknown except in the mild degree designated hemi-

hypertrophy. Hemihypertrophy or hemiatrophy are uncommon in the newborn; when present the face and trunk as well as the extremities are usually involved. Associated malformations of brain and skin are common (see Fig. 27–15). A lesion in the central nervous system leading to hemiplegia may be associated with postnatal underdevelopment of the involved arm and leg, but at birth they are anatomically normal.

Absence of a bone or part of a bone is sometimes bilateral, but only one extremity is involved more frequently than when the number of bones is excessive. Absence of the thumb, for instance, is not often bilateral, whereas duplication of the thumb or little finger is frequently bilateral.

Abnormalities of both upper or lower extremities

Fig. 25–72 (left).—Unilateral absence of ulna and three lateral digits.
Fig. 25–73 (right).—Absence of radius and thumb.

When the radius is absent, the hand is almost always in varus position. For a roentgenogram of a similar malformation see Fig. 25–57, A.

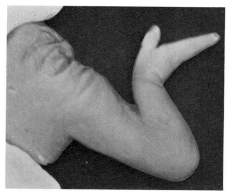
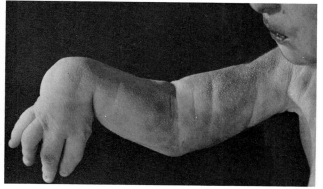

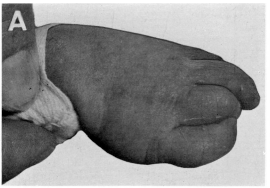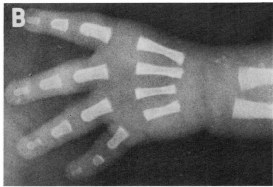

Fig. 25–74.—Thumb and first metacarpal bone absent with hand in normal position. Radius present. **A,** external view. **B,** roentgenogram.

include many disturbances involving a single extremity or affecting several extremities in a different manner. One entire arm may be hypoplastic (Fig. 25–70), or the humerus may be absent or shortened, or one or both condyles may fail to develop. The humerus, radius and ulna or any of the digits may terminate prematurely with the distal portion covered only by a fat pad (exogenous amputation) (Fig. 25–71, A); or rudiments of more distal portions may be present (endogenous amputation) (Fig. 25–71, B). When the radius or ulna is missing, the corresponding metacarpal and phalangeal bones are also absent. When the ulna is lacking, the only digits that ordinarily develop are the thumb and first finger (Fig. 25–72). When the radius is absent, the ulna is usually shorter and heav-

Fig. 25–75.—Malformation of the hand caused by shortening of metacarpal bones with hypoplasia of phalanges.

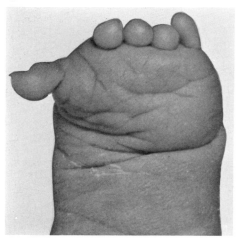

ier than normal and the thumb is ordinarily missing (Fig. 25–73). Regardless of the condition of the thumb, the hand is usually in a varus position if the radius is absent. The thumb is occasionally absent even when both bones are present in the forearm; the hand then is in a normal position (Fig. 25–74).

The bones of the hands may be the only site of abnormality. Any metacarpals or phalanges may be absent, short or abnormally long. Reduction in length of the middle phalanx of the fourth digit, producing a curve in the little finger, is an inherited characteristic in some families and is also commonly seen in mongolian idiots (Fig. 24–21) as well as in some chondrodystrophic dwarfs and cretins. All phalanges may fail to develop or be very rudimentary, and only a short abnormal palm may be present (Fig. 25–75). The phalanges are unusually long in arachnodactyly. In exogenous amputations the finger lengths are variable, multiple cicatrices are present and varying degrees of syndactyly are associated.

Excessive division of the terminal part of the limb buds is usually bilaterally symmetrical, in contrast with a reduction in number, which is often unilateral. Six or seven digits may be found on hands or feet or both. The duplication may begin with the metacarpals. Their number is rarely increased but either the hamate or the greater multangular bones may be considerably widened, and the proximal phalanx of the thumb or little finger may be completely duplicated or branched (Fig. 25–76). Branching may begin more distally; in its mildest form it consists only of an abnormal broadening of the terminal phalanx. Duplication most often involves the first or fifth digits with the inter-

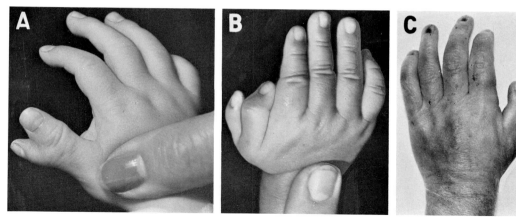

Fig. 25–76.—Duplication of thumb. **A,** duplication of distal phalanx. **B,** duplication of both phalanges. **C,** triplication of both phalanges of left thumb and duplication of those of the right (not shown).

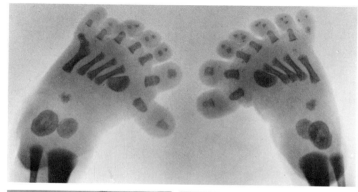

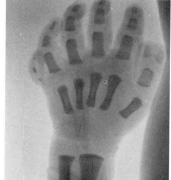 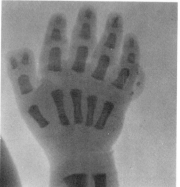

Fig. 25–77.—Bilateral symmetrical duplication of medial and lateral digits of hands and feet.

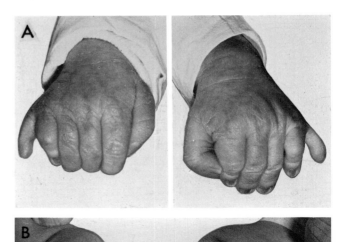

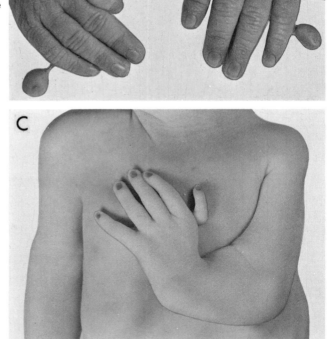

Fig. 25–78.—Bilateral duplication of fifth fingers. **A,** fingers containing bone. **B,** postminimi without bone. **C,** absence of bone in partially amputated thumb associated with clubbing of hand and hypoplasia of radius.

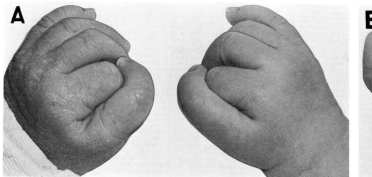
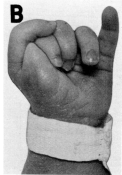

Fig. 25—79.—Elongation of thumbs with bony structure resembling that of the other digits. **A,** bilateral involvement with other digits normal. **B,** unilateral involvement similar to A, except for accompanying partial duplication.

vening digits rarely affected. Seven digits on all four extremities have been observed (Fig. 25–77); in the feet the abnormality began in the metatarsal bones, and all of the phalanges were separate and complete.

The little finger, in addition to being the common site of an actual bony duplication, often shows a milder disturbance in which a mass varying from a small round structure made up of fat and connective tissue to one considerably longer, containing bones and surmounted by fingernail at its distal end (Fig. 25–78), is attached by a small pedicle to the soft tissue covering the lateral surface of the proximal phalanx. These are known as postminimi and are especially common in Negro infants. This is true in Africa as well as in the United States. In Kampala, Uganda, facilities for removal of postminimi at the time of birth are available in the hospital delivery room (Potter). Many infants with cyclops or cebocephalus have an extra digit of varying length attached to the lateral aspect of each little finger.

The bony structure of the thumb may be similar to that of the other digits (Fig. 25–79, A). This gives a long slender thumb that is usually curved laterally over the other fingers. In one infant at the Chicago Lying-in Hospital it was accompanied by partial duplication of the thumb (Fig. 25–79, B).

Fanconi described multiple anomalies of the extremities (see Fig. 28–4) occurring with severe hypoplastic anemia, and similar cases have been observed by others. He postulated a mesodermal defect as the common etiologic factor responsible for both abnormalities.

A lobster-claw or split-hand deformity consists of an abnormal cleft between the central metacarpal or metatarsal bones with soft tissue fusion of the digits into two masses, one on either side of the cleft (Fig. 25–80). The third metacarpal or metatarsal and associated phalangeal bones are almost always absent. Other bones, especially those of the first digit, are also often missing. Such a deformity is even more common in the feet than in the hands (see Fig. 25–88).

Soft tissue anomalies may lead to fusion of any two (Fig. 25–81, A) or more digits, a condition

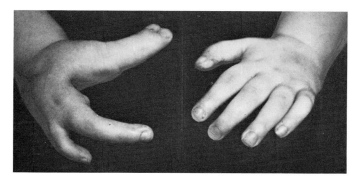

Fig. 25—80.—Absence of right thumb with syndactyly producing an atypical lobster-claw deformity. (Courtesy Dr. Ralph V. Platou.)

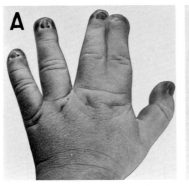 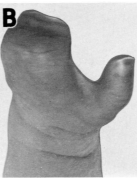 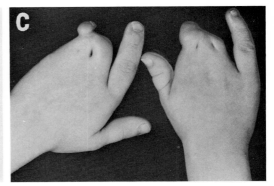

Fig. 25–81. — Syndactyly. **A,** fusion of first two fingers. **B,** fusion of all four fingers. Nails are fused into a continuous sheet. Head normal. **C,** exogenous syndactyly showing irregular fusion and abnormality of the digits.

known as syndactyly. Occasionally the fusion involves all of the digits with only the tips being recognizable as individual units, or the fusion may be more complete with the nails fused into a continuous band (Fig. 25–81, B). The latter may also be part of the acrocephalosyndactyly syndrome (see Fig. 25–29). Fusion of two fingers is often inherited as an autosomal dominant character. In another variety of syndactyly the distal parts of the digits are fused and often partially absent, while the more proximal parts remain separate (Fig. 25–81,

C). It is thought to be of exogenous origin and to be a secondary fusion caused by the binding together of digits that were originally separate (see also Fig. 27–39, A).

The lower extremities are subject to the same disturbances as those described for the upper extremities. Any of the long bones may be short (Fig. 25–82), or part or all of a bone may be missing (Fig. 25–83). If there is no fibula, the lateral digits are usually absent and a deep pit is present on the

Fig. 25–82. — Shortening of one otherwise normal femur. Newborn infant.

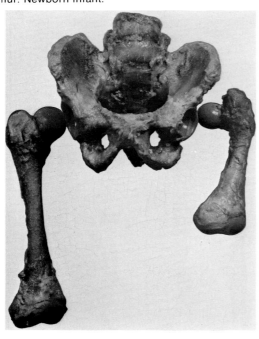

Fig. 25–83. — Absence of tibia with consequent shortening and bowing of the leg. Accompanying malformations of the vertebrae.

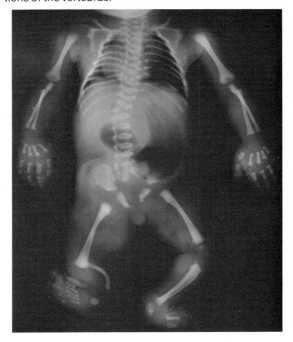

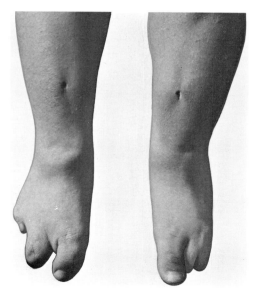

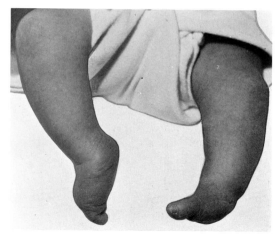

Fig. 25–85.—Bilateral absence of all digits of feet except great toes. Tibias and fibulas present.

Fig. 25–84.—Cutaneous pits associated with bilateral absence of fibula. Accompanying malformation and partial absence of digits. (Courtesy Dr. Mary Sherman.)

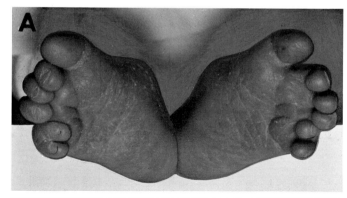

Fig. 25–86.—Bilateral duplication of fifth toes. **A,** bony malformations. **B,** postminimi containing no bone. Phalanges of great toe unusually broad.

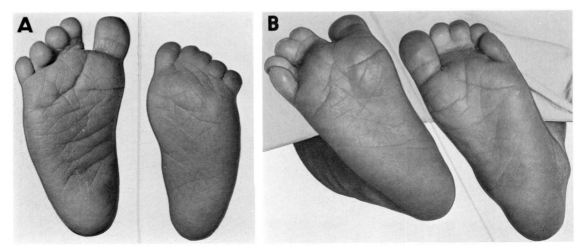

Fig. 25–87.—Syndactyly. **A,** unilateral fusion of three toes. **B,** bilateral symmetrical fusion of two toes.

Fig. 25–88.—Inherited dominant malformations of hands and feet. **A,** abnormality in the mother's hands is slight compared with that in the children. **B,** abnormality in the mother's feet *(right)* is almost as pronounced as that in her children. The striking difference in the hand abnormality indicates low expressivity of the responsible gene.

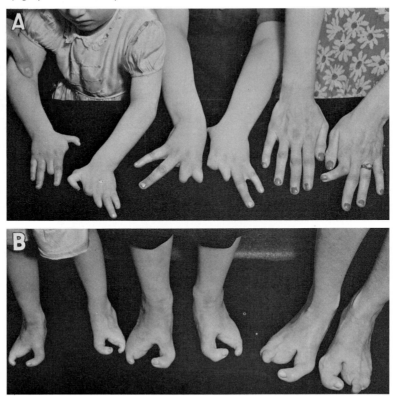

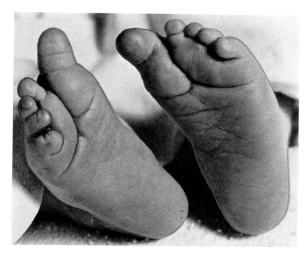

Fig. 25–89.—Abnormal cleft in feet of an otherwise normal infant. A similar defect has been described in association with mongolism.

anterior surface of the leg (Fig. 25–84). Lateral digits may be lacking even though the fibula is present (Fig. 25–85).

Duplication of digits is most often limited to the lateral side of the foot; the great toe is much less often involved than the thumb. Such digits may have a bony connection with the little toe or they may resemble postminimi (Fig. 25–86) of the hands. Rarely, first and fifth toes are both duplicated, and this may be combined with a similar condition of the fingers (see Fig. 25–77). Syndactyly may be unilateral or bilateral (Fig. 25–87) and may involve two or more toes.

The typical split-foot or lobster-claw deformity consists of a cleft in the foot extending into the metatarsal region with fusion of the digits into a single mass on either side of the separation. The metatarsal and phalangeal bones of the central digit are usually absent and others are often partially missing or otherwise abnormal. This defect, which is often accompanied by malformations of the hands, is inherited as an autosomal dominant character (Fig. 25–88).

A soft tissue cleft on the plantar surface of the foot, extending posteriorly from the space between the first and the second toes, has been described as a characteristic of mongolism, but similar or more severe abnormalities may be observed in otherwise normal infants (Fig. 25–89).

An unusually wide space between the great toe and the other digits has likewise been described as a characteristic of mongolism. This may also be

found in normal infants or in association with other malformations.

Individual toes are occasionally hypoplastic or in an abnormal position. Hammer toe is caused by an abnormally short flexor tendon. Superimposition of one toe on another is often caused by slight shortening of the corresponding metatarsal bone.

Exogenous amputations and cicatrices are similar to those involving the upper extremities. In a rare case observed at the Chicago Lying-in Hospital only the head of the right femur was normally developed and covered by soft tissues. Protruding from the lower end were two small uncovered bones, which had penetrated the abdominal wall (Fig. 25–90). Most often amputations are in a more distal part of an extremity (Fig. 25–91, A).

Fig. 25–90.—Intrauterine amputation of right leg with small bones protruding from the stump. They had penetrated the abdominal wall, producing a fistulous opening into the abdominal cavity which probably was responsible for loss of ascitic fluid and consequent gyrations of abdominal wall. Umbilical ring greatly distended. Same infant as shown in Fig. 22–60.

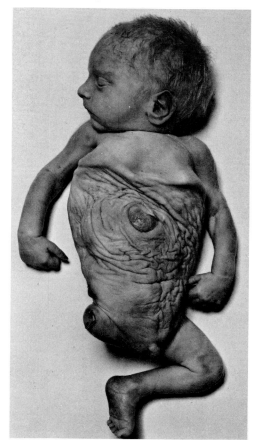

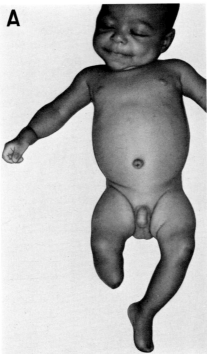

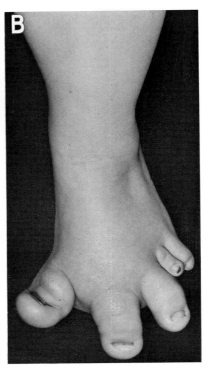

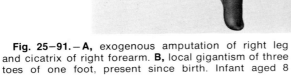

Fig. 25—91.—A, exogenous amputation of right leg and cicatrix of right forearm. **B,** local gigantism of three toes of one foot, present since birth. Infant aged 8 months. This is believed to be part of the syndrome of neurofibromatosis.

Local gigantism of the bones and soft tissues of one or more digits or of a hand or foot or even a larger part of an extremity is uncommon, but several cases have been observed (Fig. 25–91, B). This is believed to be part of the syndrome of neurofibromatosis. Irregular circumscribed areas of skin pigmentation are an almost constant feature and other evidence of the disease may be present although localized neurofibromas are rare in infants.

REFERENCES

Allensmith, M., and Lenz, E.: Chondrodystrophica congenita punctata (Conradi's disease), Am. J. Dis. Child. 100:109, 1960.

Banta, J. V., and Nichols, O.: Sacral agenesis, J. Bone Joint Surg. 51A:696, 1969.

Barter, F. C.: Hypophosphatasia, in Stanbury, J. B., *et al.* (ed.): *Metabolic Basis of Inherited Disorders* (New York: McGraw-Hill Book Co., 1966), p. 1015.

Bean, W. B.: Dyschondroplasia and hemangiomata (Maffucci's syndrome), Arch. Intern. Med. 95:767, 1955.

Birch-Jensen, A.: *Congenital Deformities of the Upper Extremities,* Vol. 19 of Opera ex Domo Biologiae Hereditariae Humanae Universitatis Hafniensis (Copenhagen: Ejnar Munksgaards Forlag, 1949).

Blank, C. E.: Apert's syndrome (a kind of acrocephalosyndactyly), Ann. Hum. Genet. 24:151, 1960.

Caffey, J.: Infantile cortical hyperostoses, J. Pediatr. 29:541, 1947.

Caffey, J.: Prenatal bowing and thickening of tubular bones, with multiple cutaneous dimples in arms and legs: Congenital syndrome of mechanical origin, Am. J. Dis. Child. 74:543, 1947.

Cohen, J.: Osteopetrosis, J. Bone Joint Surg. 33A:923, 1951.

Coleman, E. N.: Infantile hypercalcemia and cardiovascular lesions, Arch. Dis. Child. 40:53, 1965.

Condon, V. R., and Allen, R. P.: Congenital generalized fibromatosis, Roentgenology 76:444, 1961.

Cordes, F. C.: Developmental and Acquired Cataracts of Infancy and Childhood, in Liebman, S. D., and Gellis, S. S. (eds.): *The Pediatrician's Ophthalmology* (St. Louis: C. V. Mosby Co., 1966).

Dahlin, D. C.: *Bone Tumors* (2d ed.; Springfield, Ill.: Charles C Thomas, 1967).

Dallaire, L., and Fraser, F. C.: Diastrophic dwarfism, in *Birth Defects: Original Article Series,* Vol. IV (New York: The National Foundation-March of Dimes, 1969).

Dennis, J. P., Rosenberg, H. S., and Alvord, E. C., Jr.: Megalencephaly, internal hydrocephalus and other neurological aspects of achondroplasia, Brain 84:247, 1961.

Dennison, W. M., and MacPherson, D. A.: Hematogenous osteitis of infancy, Arch. Dis. Child. 27:375, 1952.

Einstein, R. A. J., and Thomas, C. G., Jr.: Osteomyelitis in infants, Am. J. Roentgenol. 55:299, 1946.

Ellis, R. W. B., and van Creveld, S.: A syndrome characterized by ectodermal dysplasia, polydactyly, chondrodysplasia and congenita morbus cordis, Arch. Dis. Child. 15:65, 1940.

Eversole, S. L., Jr., Holman, G., and Robinson, R.: Hitherto undescribed characteristics of the pathology of infantile cortical hyperostosis (Caffey's disease), Bull. Johns Hopkins Hosp. 101:80, 1957.

Farber, S., and Craig, J. M.: Clinicopathological conference, J. Pediatr. 51:461, 1957.

Fanconi, G.: Familiäre infantile pernizioaartige Anämie (perniziöses bluthild und Konstitution), in Jahrbuch der Kinderheilkunde, Vol. 117, p. 257, 1927.

Fogh-Andersen, P.: Inheritance of Harelip and Cleft Palate (Copenhagen: Nyt Nordisk Forlag, Arnold Busck, 1942).

Forland, M.: Cleidocranial dysostosis, Am. J. Med. 33:792, 1962.

Fraser, D.: Hypophosphatasia, Am. J. Med. 22:730, 1957.

Gerrard, J. W., et al.: Familial infantile cortical hyperostosis, J. Pediatr. 59:343, 1961.

Goldman, R.: Congenital malformation of vertebrae (hemivertebrae) with aplasia of corresponding ribs, associated with lateral meningocele, Arch. Pathol. 47:153, 1949.

Gould, G. M., and Pyle, W. L.: Anomalies and Curiosities of Medicine (Philadelphia: W. B. Saunders Co., 1901).

Gunderson, T., Liebman, S. D., and Podos, S. M.: Ocular Manifestations of Pediatric Systemic Diseases, in Liebman, S. D., and Gellis, S. S. (eds.): The Pediatrician's Ophthalmology (St. Louis: C. V. Mosby Co., 1966).

Hall, J. G., et al.: Two probable cases of homozygosity for the achondroplastic gene, Birth Defects 4:24, 1969.

Harper, R., et al.: Bird-headed dwarfs, J. Pediatr. 70:799, 1967.

Herdman, R. C., and Langer, M. O.: The thoracic asphyxiant dystrophy and renal disease, Am. J. Dis. Child. 116:192, 1968.

Holden, J. P.: Russell-Silver dwarf, Dev. Med. Child. Neurol. 9:457, 1967.

Jaffe, H. L.: Tumors and Tumerous Conditions of the Bones and Joints (Philadelphia: Lea & Febiger, 1958).

Jenkens, P.: Metatrophic dwarfism, Br. J. Radiol. 45:560, 1970.

Jenkinson, E. L., et al.: Prenatal diagnosis of osteopetrosis, Am. J. Roentgenol. Radium Ther. Nucl. Med. 49:455, 1943.

Jequier, J. C.: Asphyxiating thoracic dystrophy, Arch. Fr. Pediatr. 27:177, 1970.

Jervis, G. A., and Schein, H.: Polyostotic fibrous dysplasia (Albright's syndrome), Arch. Pathol. 51:640, 1951.

Keats, T. E., Ridderwold, H. O., and Michaelis, G. G.: Thanatophoric dwarfism, Am. J. Roentgenol. Radium Ther. Nucl. Med. 108:473, 1970.

Kernahan, D. A., and Stark, R. B.: New classification for cleft lip and cleft palate, Plast. Reconstr. Surg. 22:435, 1958.

Koylowski, K., Prokop, E., and Zybaczynski, J.: Thanatophoric dwarfism, Br. J. Radiol. 45:565, 1970.

Lamy, M.: Hereditary disorders of the bone—an overview, Birth Defects 4:8, 1969.

Langer, L. O.: The Thoracic Pelvic Phalangeal Dystrophy (Asphyxiating Thoracic Dystrophy), in Skeletal Dysplasias, Vol. V, Part IV, Birth Defects: Original Article Series (New York: The National Foundation-March of Dimes, 1968).

Lester, C. W.: Funnel chest and allied deformities of thoracic cage, J. Thorac. Surg. 19:507, 1950.

Lichenstein, L.: Diseases of the Bones and Joints (St. Louis: C. V. Mosby Co., 1970).

Lichenstein, L., and Jaffe, H. L.: Fibrous dysplasia of bone, Arch. Pathol. 33:777, 1942.

Lindsay, S., et al.: Gargoylism, Am. J. Dis. Child. 76:239, 1948.

Lorincz, A. E.: Hurler's syndrome in man and snorter dwarfism in cattle, Clin. Orthop. 33:104, 1964.

Mann, I.: Developmental Abnormalities of the Eye (2d ed.; Philadelphia: J. B. Lippincott Co., 1957).

Maroteaux, P.: Spondylo-epiphyseal Dysplasia and Metatropic Dwarfism, in Birth Defects: Original Article Series, Vol. IV (New York: The National Foundation-March of Dimes, 1969).

Maroteaux, P., and Lamy, M.: Le diagnostic des nanismes chondrodystrophiques chez nouveau-ne, Arch. Fr. Pediatr. 25:241, 1968.

Maroteaux, P., Lamy, M., and Robert, J. J.: Le nanismes thanatophore, Presse Med. 75:2519, 1967.

Martin, M. M., and Wilkins, L.: Pituitary dwarfism: diagnosis and treatment, J. Clin. Endocrinol. Metab. 18:679, 1958.

Masse, P.: Osteomyelitis in the newborn, Ann. Pediatr. 34:509, 1958.

McArthur, R. G., and Edwards, S. H.: De Lange syndrome: Report of 20 cases, Can. Med. Assoc. J. 96:1185, 1967.

McCance, R. A., et al.: Genetic, clinical, biochemical and pathological features of hypophosphatasia, Q. J. Med. 25:523, 1956.

McClean, F. C., and Bloom, W.: Calcification and ossification: Calcification in normal growing bone, Anat. Rec. 78:333, 1940.

McClean, S.: Osseous lesions of congenital syphilis, Am. J. Dis. Child. 41:1411, 1931.

McCune, D. J., and Bradley, C.: Osteopetrosis (marble bones) in an infant, Am. J. Dis. Child. 48:949, 1934.

McKenzie, J.: First arch syndrome, Arch. Dis. Child. 33:477, 1958.

McKusick, V. A.: Heritable Disorders of the Connective Tissue (St. Louis: C. V. Mosby Co., 1966).

McKusick, V. A., et al.: Seckel's bird-headed dwarfism, N. Engl. J. Med. 277:279, 1967.

Melnick, J. C.: Chondrodystrophia calcificans congenita, Am. J. Dis. Child. 110:218, 1965.

Moore, T. C.: Chondroectodermal dysplasia (Ellis-van Creveld syndrome) with bronchial malformation and neonatal tension lobar emphysema, J. Thorac. Cardiovasc. Surg. 4:61, 1963.

Murdoch, J. L., et al.: Achondroplasia: a genetic and statistical survey, Ann. Hum. Genet. 33:227, 1970.

Neimann, N., et al.: Dystrophe thoracique asphyxiante du nourisson, Pediatrie 18:387, 1963.

Orzalesi, M. M., and Cook, C. D.: Pulmonary function in children with pectus excavatus, J. Pediatr. 66:898, 1965.

Park, E. A., and Powers, G. F.: Acrocephaly and scaphocephaly with symmetrically distributed malformations of the extremities, Am. J. Dis. Child. 20:235, 1920.

Patterson, J. H., and Wolkins, W. L.: Leprechaunism in a male infant, J. Pediatr. 60:730, 1962.

Pines, B., and Lederer, M.: Osteopetrosis: Albers-Schönberg disease (marble bones), Am. J. Pathol. 23:755, 1947.

Pirnar, T., and Neuhauser, E. B. D.: Asphyxiating thoracic dystrophy of the newborn, Am. J. Roentgenol. 98: 358, 1966.

Potter, E. L.: Chondrodystrophy accompanying cebocephalus in siblings, An. Arrollo (Granada) 13:307, 1966.

Potter, E. L., and Coverstone, V. A.: Chondrodystrophy fetalis. Am. J. Obstet. Gynecol. 56:790, 1948.

Potter, E. L., and Nadelhoffer, L.: Familial lobsterclaw, J. Hered. 38:11, 1938.

Ptacek, L. J., et al.: Cornelia de Lange syndrome, J. Pediatr. 63:1000, 1963.

Rubin, P.: Dynamic Classification of Bone Dysplasias (Chicago: Year Book Medical Publishers, Inc., 1964).

Salmon, M. A., and Webb, J. N.: Dystrophic changes associated with leprechaunism, Arch. Dis. Child. 38:530, 1963.

Saxen, L., and Rapola, J.: Congenital Defects (New York: Holt, Rinehart, and Winston, 1969).

Schlesinger, B., et al.: Typus degenerativus amstelodamensis, Arch. Dis. Child. 38:349, 1963.

Scott, C. W., et al.: Neonatal granuloma venereum, Am. J. Dis. Child. 85:308, 1953.

Scott, R. B.: Congenital absence of the fibula, Am. J. Dis. Child. 61:1037, 1941.

Sherman, M., and Hellyer, D.: Infantile cortical hyperostosis: Review of literature and report of five cases, Am. J. Roentgenol. Radium Ther. Nucl. Med. 63:212, 1950.

Sinclair, J. G., Duren, N., and Rude, J. C.: Congenital lumbosacral defect, Arch. Surg. 43:473, 1941.

Smith, D. W.: Recognizable Patterns of Human Malformations (Philadelphia: W. B. Saunders Co., 1970).

Smith, H. L., and Hand, A. M.: Chondroectodermal dysplasia (Ellis-van Creveld syndrome), Pediatrics 21:298, 1958.

Szalay, G. C.: Intrauterine growth retardation vs. Silver's syndrome, J. Pediatr. 64:234, 1964.

Trueta, J.: The three types of acute hematogenous osteomyelitis, J. Bone Joint Surg. 41B:671, 1959.

Verger, P., Martin, C., and Martinerix, Y.: Typus amstelodamensis (C. de Lange), Arch. Fr. Pediatr. 22:91, 1965.

Walker, D. G.: In discussion, Birth Defects 4:308, 1969.

Warkany, J.: Congenital Malformations (Chicago: Year Book Medical Publishers, Inc., 1971).

Warkany, J., Beaudry, P. H., and Hornstein, S.: Attempted abortion with aminopterin; malformation of the child, Am. J. Dis. Child. 97:274, 1959.

Weber, M.: Osteogenesis imperfecta congenita, Arch. Pathol. 9:984, 1930.

Weech, A. A.: Hereditary ectodermal dysplasia (congenital ectodermal defect), Am. J. Dis. Child. 37:766, 1929.

White, M., and Dennison, W. M.: Acute hematogenous osteitis in childhood, J. Bone Joint Surg. 34B:608, 1952.

Wilson, D. W. C., Chrispin, A. R., and Carter, C. O.: Diastrophic dwarfism, Arch. Dis. Child. 44:48, 1969.

Winters, R. W., et al.: A genetic study of familial hypophosphatemia and vitamin D resistant rickets with review of the literature, Medicine 37:97, 1958.

Yakovac, W. C.: Calcareous chondropathies in the newborn infant, Arch. Pathol. 57:62, 1954.

Zellweger, H., and Taylor, B.: Genetic aspects of achondroplasia, Lancet 85:8, 1965.

Zellweger, H., et al.: Morquio-Ullrich's disease, J. Pediatr. 56:549, 1961.

26

Skeletal Muscles and Joints

GENERALIZED DISTURBANCES involving all muscles are rare in the newborn period, although such conditions as amyotonia congenita and myasthenia gravis are occasionally recognizable even in the first few days of life. Absence and abnormal location of muscles are most often secondary to other malformations. Positional abnormalities of the joints are frequently associated with some abnormality of regional muscles.

Abnormalities of Skeletal Muscles

INFANTILE SPINAL ATROPHY (WERDNIG-HOFFMANN DISEASE). — In this disease, which is characterized by extreme muscle weakness, the muscles atrophy because nerve fibers supplying them degenerate as a result of loss of cells in the spinal cord. Such muscle degeneration takes place fascicle by fascicle rather than by individual muscle cells as in muscular dystrophy (see Fig. 24 – 16). This disease is considered in detail in Chapter 24.

MUSCULAR DYSTROPHY. — The generalized progressive sex-linked form of muscular dystrophy (Duchenne type), which primarily involves muscles of the shoulder, pelvis and portions of the appendicular skeleton, is seldom recognized in the newborn period or in early infancy, probably because the young infant is not required to perform the antigravity muscular movements that are important for clinical diagnosis. It is only in the most severe cases with unusually early onset that the disease is life threatening. Only males are affected.

Two newborns (one the maternal uncle of the other) who had changes characteristic of muscular dystrophy in the intercostal and neck muscles as well as the limb muscles were examined at autopsy at the Boston Children's Hospital Medical Center.

Adams *et al.* thought that such early fatal cases might be a mutation from the more common Duchenne type of progressive muscular dystrophy. The muscles in this severe form of sex-linked dystrophy observed in the very young have the same general features as those found in the Duchenne type in older age groups. They consist of marked variation in size of muscle fibers within individual muscle bundles (Fig. 26–1, A. and B), in contrast to changes in infantile spinal atrophy, in which the variation is between muscle bundles, all fibers in a single fascicle being of similar size. In infantile muscular dystrophy there is also loss of cross-striations with homogenization and hyalinization of muscle cells and vacuolization, centripetal movement and degeneration of the nuclei. The substance of the muscle fibers is gradually lost, and fibers eventually disappear (Fig. 26–1, C). Ordinarily, there is little or no connective tissue proliferation around the affected muscles, and degeneration is seldom rapid enough to elicit a macrophage response.

A form of muscular dystrophy separable from the Duchenne type and its variants, which has an autosomal recessive form of inheritance, was reviewed by Zellweger *et al.* The affected infant may be weak at birth but may develop motor skills normally until the age of 2 years, when progressively increasing muscular weakness sets in; or contractures and joint fixation may be present at birth, giving the picture of arthrogryposis. Half of those affected die between early infancy and adolescence, the time of death depending on the severity and the course of the disease. Those surviving this period appear to have their disease stabilized with no further progression. Unlike the sex-linked Duchenne dystrophy, in which little fibrous tissue is laid down,

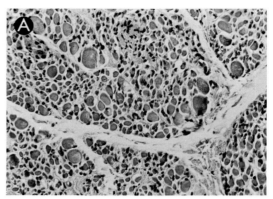

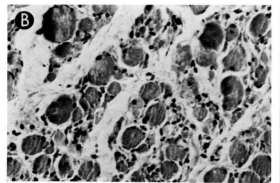

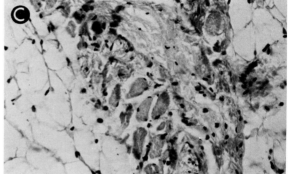

Fig. 26–1.—Muscular dystrophy. **A,** photomicrograph showing marked variation in size of individual muscle fibers in all fascicles. Infant dying within a few days of birth. (Courtesy Dr. G. Vawter.) **B,** portion of dystrophic muscle in a newborn infant presenting with signs of arthrogryposis. **C,** another peripheral muscle from same infant with almost complete loss of muscle fibers and replacement by fat.

this form has marked endomysial and perimysial fibrosis.

The more limited forms of muscular dystrophy involving only the shoulder girdle (fascio-scapular-humeral) or the ocular muscles produce no symptoms in the very young.

CENTRAL CORE DISEASE.—This is another disease in which weakness and hypotonia are present at birth or shortly thereafter. It was first described by Shy and Magee, who found weakness, reduced movement and delay in motor development to be the chief symptoms. The muscle fibers may be small, normal or increased in size. The identifying feature is the presence in the center of individual muscle fibers of an amorphous area in which refractility of cross-striations is diminished, argentophilia is increased and the usual oxidative and phosphoryl-ase activities are undemonstrable. It is inherited as an autosomal dominant character and, although it produces severe muscle weakness and delay in walking, it does not progress.

NEMALINE MYOPATHY.—This recently recognized muscle disorder, which also causes hypotonicity, is usually associated with feeding and respiratory difficulties secondary to weakness of the pharyngeal and intercostal muscles. In some instances it has been recognized at birth, in others not for several months. The muscles of the proximal joints of the limbs are most severely affected, and kypho-scoliosis may develop in older survivors. The disease is inherited as an autosomal dominant character with variable expression, so it may be seen in a parent as well as in the offspring. The symptoms are usually mild and nonprogressive, but fatalities in the first years of life have been recorded (Shafiq).

The severity of the muscle lesion is variable. In one autopsied case, although all of the muscles sampled showed some disturbance (Shafiq), the tongue and gastrocnemius muscles were especially abnormal. In general, a variation in fiber diameter is common, and some perimysial and endomysial proliferation of fibrous tissue is evident in areas of degeneration. Characteristic basophilic rods, 1×5 μ around the nucleus, are best seen by phase microscopy or Gomori's trichrome stain used on fresh frozen material. The presence of the stained "worms" gives rise to the appellation "nemaline." These masses are thought to result from degeneration of widened Z bands (Gonatas *et al.*). They give a positive test for tyrosine but are negative for tryptophan. Jenis *et al.* described a related disorder in which inclusions appear not only in the cytoplasm but also in the muscle cell nuclei. They differ from the rods in the cytoplasm in that they stain positively for tryptophan.

AMYOTONIA CONGENITA (OPPENHEIM'S DISEASE). — A few hypotonic infants with general symptoms of Werdnig-Hoffmann disease may be found with characteristic muscle changes but without the spinal cord changes to explain them. Such infants are unable to move their weak muscles against gravity but their cranial muscles are spared (Adams *et al.*). The cause of this disease is unknown. The prognosis is much better than when the spinal cord is involved, and there is usually a gradual improvement, although some muscle weakness, especially demonstrable on continued muscular effort, persists throughout life.

MYASTHENIA GRAVIS. — This muscle disorder may also produce hypotonia in infants and, like amyotonia congenita, has no demonstrable histopathology. Two varieties can be demonstrated in the newborn period — one a transient form transmitted prenatally by an affected mother, and the other a permanent form in which the mother is unaffected. Both are characterized by abnormal fatigability of skeletal muscle. In very young infants muscular movements are slow and infrequent, the sucking reflex is absent, the face is expressionless and strabismus is common. The cause is unknown, although in the transient form there may be a humoral block at the myoneural junction, while in the permanent form there may be an actual defect in which a deficiency of acetylcholine or an elevation of the sensitivity of motor end-plates partially blocks incoming nerve stimuli. In either case Prostigmin overcomes the defect and decreases the fatigability of the muscles. The response to this drug aids in establishing the diagnosis. Prostigmin may be used as replacement therapy, relieving the transient form or maintaining the permanently affected child for many years in a fairly normal state of health.

MYOTONIC DYSTROPHY. — In this disorder prolongation of muscle contraction or failure of relaxation after contraction has taken place are associated with muscle weakness and wasting. Relaxation improves with repetitive contractive movements. The condition may produce respiratory distress and

feeding difficulties in the neonatal period (Dodge *et al.*), or it may be first discovered in older infants in whom failure to meet physical performance standards becomes apparent. Cataracts, subluxation of the lens and testicular atrophy — features of the far more common disease in which the onset is late — are not seen in infancy and childhood, although there may be evidence of mental retardation. The disease is inherited as an autosomal dominant character with variable expressivity.

Pathologically, the muscle fibers are characteristically enlarged with nuclei centrally placed and often arranged in chains (Adams *et al.*). Other fibers may show degenerative changes such as vacuolation or fatty replacement.

CONGENITAL MYOTONIA (THOMSEN'S DISEASE). — This has some of the clinical features of myotonic dystrophy but the muscles often become greatly enlarged, and degenerative changes are absent. The eponym is justly deserved since Thomsen had the disorder himself and described and studied it in his own family. Its presence may be demonstrated in infancy by delay in sitting and standing, but really incapacitating difficulties, especially spasms, do not appear until adolescence or early adult life. The difficulty lies in initiating a new movement or in changing from one form of movement to another. Repetitive motion eases the difficulties.

All of the skeletal muscles are involved, and those of the thighs, forearms and shoulders become particularly large in older individuals. They are firm unless completely relaxed. Microscopically they show only hypertrophy and an increase in the number of microfibers.

GLYCOGEN STORAGE DISEASE TYPE II. — Although the principal symptoms of this disease are related to the heart, the skeletal muscles are usually as abnormal histologically as is cardiac muscle. Most severely affected are the tongue and diaphragm, but muscles of the neck, trunk and extremities may also be involved. Because of the characteristic histologic appearance, biopsy is of great help in establishing a diagnosis. The striated muscle fibers contain large glycogen deposits that may be demonstrated by appropriate fixation and staining technic but with the usual type of fixation appear as empty spaces (Fig. 26–2) (see Chapter 10).

INTRAMUSCULAR HEMORRHAGE. — Nontraumatic hemorrhage in individual muscle groups is rare, having been observed only once at the Chicago Lying-in Hospital. This was in an infant with severe erythroblastosis, all of whose muscles, including those of the tongue, diaphragm, abdominal wall and all extremities, contained diffusely scattered

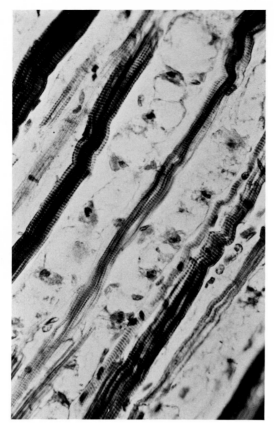

Fig. 26–2.—Glycogen storage disease type II. Pale areas between muscle fibers are caused by deposits of glycogen. Infant aged 5 months. (Courtesy Drs. Eleanor M. Humphreys and Katsuji Kato.)

small hemorrhages (Fig. 26–3). Normoblasts were present in the areas of hemorrhage because of the large numbers in the circulating blood, but there was no evidence of local erythropoiesis.

CALCINOSIS.—In this rare condition small masses of calcium are diffusely distributed in various parts of the body. Generally they are limited to the skin and subcutaneous tissues, in which case the condition is designated calcinosis circumscripta (Rothenstein and Welt). Less often, muscles and other parts of the body are also involved; this is called calcinosis universalis. Involvement of individual muscles is usually a result of injury. Those most commonly affected are the sternocleidomastoid, trapezius, erector spinae and triceps muscles.

The cause of generalized involvement is unknown. It occurs principally in young adults but is occasionally seen in small infants. An infant who was born at the Chicago Lying-in Hospital and was reported by Swanson *et al.* was found to have small hard nodules under the skin of the buttocks and thighs at about 2 weeks of age. X-ray examination revealed diffuse calcification of the soft tissues between the knees and buttocks, with moderate extension below the knees and over the lower abdomen (Fig. 26–4). After a short period of progression, calcification gradually diminished and had disappeared by the time the infant was 6 months old. Mineral metabolism appeared normal and no cause could be found. In this case most of the calcium seemed to be in the subcutaneous tissues, although muscles were also involved.

Calcium may be abnormally deposited in areas other than skeletal muscle during fetal life and in the newborn period. It is found most constantly and in greatest amounts on the surface of the intestine and peritoneum in meconium peritonitis. It is found occasionally in the endocardium and chordae tendineae in endocardial sclerosis, in the walls of the arteries, especially the coronaries, and in tumors, especially neuroblastomas. It has been reported in the brain in association with toxoplasmosis and cytomegalic inclusion disease and is occasionally present without known cause. It is deposited readily in areas of hemorrhage and, as a result, may be present in the meninges and adrenal glands of young infants. Necrosis of tissue, such as occurs after infarction in the heart or bowel wall, is commonly associated with calcium deposition.

FIBROPLASIA OSSIFICANS PROGRESSIVA (MYOSITIS OSSIFICANS).—The term fibroplasia ossificans given by McKusick is far more expressive of the nature of the disease than the older term myositis ossificans, because the process affects skin, fascia, ligaments and tendons as well as muscle. In many affected individuals (70%) there are associated malformations such as microdactyly, absence of the ear lobes or upper incisors, exostoses, hallux valgus and spina bifida (Adams *et al.*). Some have a family history of myositis or short thumbs. The condition is occasionally recognized at birth, but most cases come to medical attention in early childhood with a localized muscular swelling accompanied by mild edema, low grade fever and redness of the overlying skin (Nutt). The swelling subsides after a few days, and the indurated area becomes freely movable. The lesion gradually shrinks, hardens and finally forms a bony lump. Other areas are often subsequently involved in a similar manner. Microscopically the affected areas show a marked increase in highly cellular connective tissue in early stages, but cells are rapidly replaced by collagen and later by bone. Tendons, ligaments and fascia may be

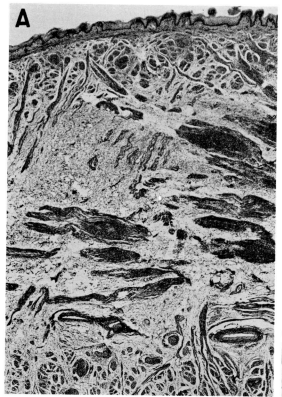

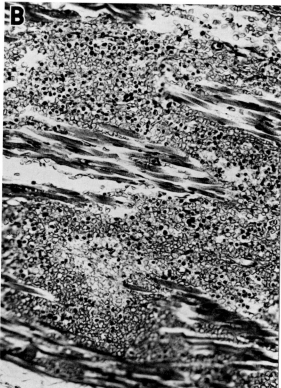

Fig. 26–3.—Intramuscular hemorrhage in erythroblastosis. **A,** tongue with hemorrhage in muscle bundles. **B,** gluteus maximus with hemorrhage in muscle bundles.

Fig. 26–4.—Calcinosis universalis showing diffusely distributed deposits of calcium in subcutaneous tissue and muscle. Infant aged 5 weeks; recovered by 6 months.

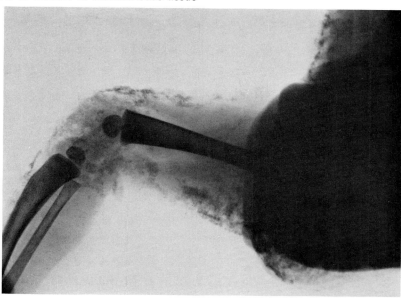

affected as well as muscles. The process may begin in any part of the body, and while the peripheral musculature is most often involved, the heart, diaphragm and other areas may be affected.

The shape of the bones of the thumb and great toe may also be altered owing to the presence of abnormal masses of calcium.

FIBROSIS.—In the newborn, muscular fibrosis is most common in the sternocleidomastoid muscle. A localized temporary or permanent swelling may appear in the central part of this muscle a few days or weeks after birth. Occasionally it is associated with torticollis, although usually the head is in a normal position. Histologic examination reveals separation and partial replacement of muscle cells by hyalinized connective tissue (Fig. 26–5). Trauma incurred during delivery has generally been considered the most probable cause; however, the possibility that a congenital malformation may be responsible has never been entirely excluded. Possibly, a combination of the two conditions is essential and a congenitally hypoplastic muscle is more susceptible to injury than a normal one.

HYPOPLASIA AND AGENESIS.—Severe hypoplasia and agenesis of various muscle groups have been reported as individual abnormalities or associated with other malformations. Muscles of the chest and abdomen are among those most commonly affected.

ARTHROGRYPOSIS.—This appears to be a symptom complex of variable etiology intimately associated with muscle weakness before birth and character-

Fig. 26–5.—Fibrosis of the sternocleidomastoid muscle associated with torticollis. Photomicrograph showing a small isolated, partially intact collection of muscle fibers surrounded by dense highly collagenous scar tissue.

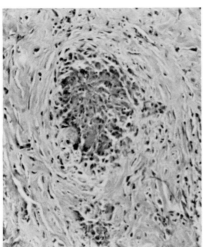

ized by stiffness or immobility of one or several joints. Stiffness results from fibrous contraction of the adjacent muscles and not from an intrinsic lesion of the joint itself. The muscle abnormality may rarely be primary, as in the severe recessive form of autosomal muscular dystrophy, or, more often, secondary to neural loss. The few infants with this form of muscular dystrophy who have contractures at birth fall into the arthrogryposis group. In the usual case of arthrogryposis contraction of flexor muscles is probably due to lack of extensor power responsible for flexion of the knees and elbows. Since in this form of dystrophy there is a tendency for endomysial and perimysial elements to be increased, fixation can be expected. The more peripheral muscles of the extremities are usually larger than the proximal ones, in contrast to those in which the disturbance is of neural origin.

In the more commonly encountered arthrogryposis of neural origin large segments of anterior horn cells are absent, and affected muscles are usually composed of microfibers (Katzeff). Malformations involving the central nervous system, such as hydrocephalus, spina bifida, absence of the sacrum or shortening of the cervical spine, may occasionally exhibit muscle abnormalities similar to arthrogryposis (Fig. 26–6).

Although nerve cells are absent and muscle cells are hypoplastic in infantile muscular atrophy, the absence of contractions in that disease is striking. The reasons for this must lie in the symmetrical involvement of flexors and extensors, the weakness of all of the muscles and the absence of fibrosis. In arthrogryposis, although the name indicates the presence of flexion deformities, the joints are fixed in extension with equal or greater frequency than in flexion. The area of involvement may consist of individual or asymmetrically distributed joints of the upper or lower extremities or may include both arms and/or legs. In most cases the hips are flexed, the knees extended and the feet are in the equinus position, or the shoulders are adducted, the elbows extended, the forearms pronated and the wrists flexed (Fig. 26–6). Hip dislocations are common. The affected extremities are either uniformly reduced in circumference with no demarcation at the knee or elbow and have an appearance that has been likened to a stuffed sausage, or the leg tapers from hip to ankle and the arm from shoulder to wrist as a result of the muscular wasting. The circumference of the involved legs or forearms is especially reduced regardless of whether fixation is in flexion or extension (Fig. 26–7). One child observed at the Chicago Lying-in Hospital had an associated

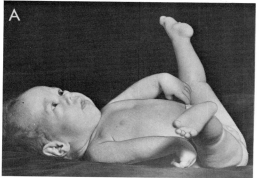
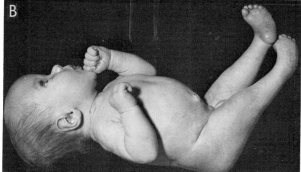

Fig. 26–6.—**A,** infant with arthrogryposis. Character-istic joint disturbances include fixation of elbows and knees in extension and hips in flexion. Position of the hands is similar to that observed in brachial plexus injury. **B,** infant with spina bifida. Fixation of the hips in flexion and knees in extension is similar to that found in arthrogryposis. Tapering of the legs with poor muscular development below the knees is also similar.

absence of hands and feet (Fig. 26–8). The condition of the joints remains fairly stationary throughout life. They may become slightly less rigid after prolonged treatment but never attain normal function.

In a child observed at the Boston Children's Hospital Medical Center with the picture of arthrogryposis, the immobility of the joints was secondary to marked fibrosis and atrophy of the muscles arising from the inflammatory destructive processes of dermatomyositis.

Abdominal muscle deficiency syndrome.—Severe hypoplasia or, less often, complete absence of some or all of the abdominal muscles, accompanied by megacystis, megaureter, hydronephrosis or renal dysplasia and cryptorchidism, is a well-recog-

Fig. 26–7.—Severe generalized arthrogryposis with knees flexed, elbows extended and hands and feet clubbed. **A,** age 3 days. **B,** age 21 months.

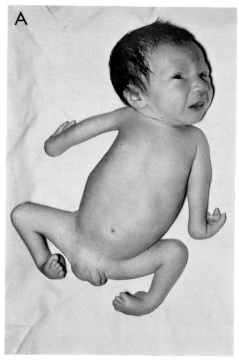
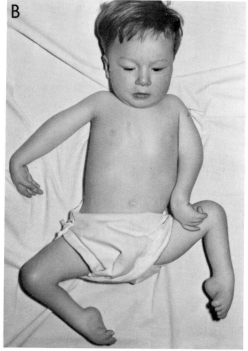

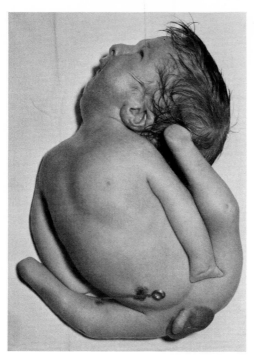

Fig. 26–8.—Infant with arthrogryposis and absence of digits involving all four extremities. Vertebrae normal but head dorsiflexed.

nized syndrome occurring almost exclusively in males (95% according to Welch). Williams and Burkholder believed it to be sex-linked, with the few females included in some series not having the true syndrome. It has been suggested that the absence of abdominal muscles is responsible for the enlargement of bladder and ureters, and vice versa, but since either may occur without the other, these explanations seem improbable.

In the typical case the infant at birth has an enlarged, lax abdomen with viscera easily palpable through the thin wall. The skin is usually only moderately wrinkled (Fig. 26–9), although the extreme wrinkling sometimes present (see Fig. 22–60, A) has been responsible for the imaginative designation *"prune-belly" syndrome*. The bladder and ureters are of excessive size and the urachus may be as large as the bladder (see Fig. 22–60, C) or normally closed. Part of the bladder musculature may also be missing. The testes are invariably undescended. The mesentery of the large bowel is unfixed to the posterior abdominal wall and the intestine is not properly rotated; volvulus is common. Malformations of the heart, central nervous system or bones are present in a small number of infants. Definite evidence of obstruction can seldom be found in the lower bladder or urethra to explain the bladder-ureteral hypertrophy, although phimosis is common and urethral occlusion is sometimes present.

The outlook for survival depends on the renal involvement, and the majority of affected individuals die in the first 3 months. However, survival to adult life has been reported.

Abnormalities of Joints

CONGENITAL WEBBING

NECK.—The most common site of congenital webbing, except for the digits, is the neck. Usually, only the skin is involved and, instead of following the normal contours of the neck and shoulders, the taut skin extends from a point immediately below the ear out toward the shoulder joint. It is invariably bilateral and, although sometimes found as an isolated abnormality, is often accompanied by other malformations. It has been observed in both males and females as part of a syndrome of dwarfism, hypogenitalism and edema of the lower extremities. In females this is known as Turner's syndrome and in males, or in females without hypogonadism, as the Bonnievie-Ullrich syndrome. At birth the webbing may not be well developed and may simply appear as an excessive amount of skin.

KNEES AND ELBOWS.—Webbing of the knees and elbows is variable, with the knees more frequently involved than the elbows. The only demonstrable abnormality may be in the skin, or the muscles may also be affected and their origins and insertions around the joints considerably altered. When the lower extremities are involved, the hips are usually abducted, and the deformity may be so pronounced that the heels are drawn up close to the buttocks. Such involvement of the lower extremities may be part of a widespread disturbance in development, as in one stillborn fetus delivered at the Chicago Lying-in Hospital (Fig. 26–10, A), or it may be the only demonstrable anomaly, as in an infant observed by Parks and Sweet (Fig. 26–10, B). No instance of isolated webbing of the elbows was found among the Chicago Lying-in Hospital autopsies, but mild webbing of both knees and elbows has been found in several abortuses.

LEGS.—A few cases have been reported in which the two legs have been bound together only by skin and connective tissue, but they are extremely rare. When the two legs are not separated, the developmental disturbance is ordinarily that of sirenome-

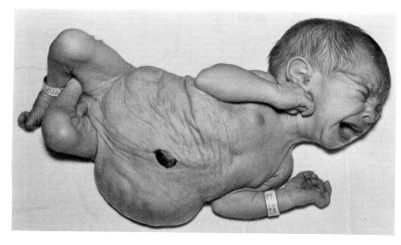

Fig. 26–9.—Absence of anterior abdominal muscles associated with hypoplastic right kidney and dilated persistent urachus attached to umbilicus. Intestines are in protuberant mass to the left of the umbilicus. Postoperative death at 9 weeks.

lus (see Fig. 25–68). Even when all bones are present, part of the muscles on the medial side of the legs is usually absent and the bones are generally defective.

DIGITS.—Syndactyly is considerably more common than any other form of webbing. Most often only two digits are involved and they are connected throughout their length by skin and connective tissue. If three or four digits are fused, the terminal phalanges may escape, or they too may be fused and may share a common nail (see Fig. 25–81). Associated muscular defects are more common

Fig. 26–10.—Webbed knees. **A,** stillborn fetus with multiple malformations. **B,** living infant, normal except for soft tissue deformity of the lower extremities. (B, courtesy Drs. John L. Parks and L. K. Sweet.)

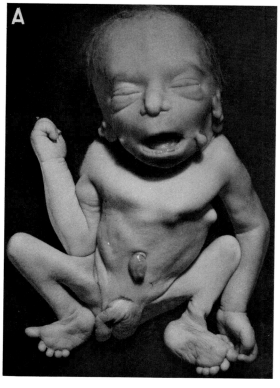

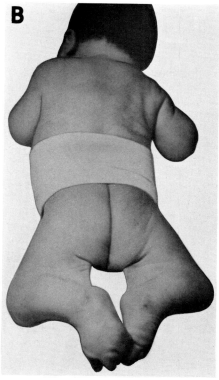

when multiple digits are involved than when only two are affected. In most instances the bones are normal, although in the well-recognized lobster-claw deformity the phalangeal and central metatarsal or metacarpal bones are missing and the remaining digits are united by soft tissues into two principal masses. Webbing of the flexor surfaces may infrequently be responsible for inability to extend the digits normally.

HIPS

DISLOCATION. — In most instances only a potential dislocation exists at birth, with symptoms not appearing until muscle spasm causes an actual displacement of the head of the femur. It is believed that in some instances a lack of tone in the joint capsule permits the pressure of the uterine wall against the flexed knees of the fetus to stretch the capsule and interfere with the normal relation of the head of the femur to the acetabulum. If the femoral head is not pressed into the acetabular cavity, the latter remains shallow, and ossification of the femoral head is delayed. Although intrauterine position may play a part in some cases, the fact that the incidence is seven times greater in females than in males (Badgley) and that several members of a family may be affected indicates that many may have a genetic basis.

Immediately after birth the affected joint may be excessively mobile. By the end of a month this disappears and the adductor and flexor muscles splint the leg in partial flexion and adduction. By 2 months of age the muscles, increasing in size and strength, begin to pull on the head of the femur, causing an upward displacement and malformation of the head and socket. The head of the femur is eventually forced into the concavity of the ilium, although this may not occur until weight is put on the femur when the child begins to walk.

Rarely, actual dislocation is present at birth. In such cases, or even when the dislocation occurs later, the affected leg is externally rotated and shortened, and the gluteal, inguinal and knee folds are higher on that side than on the other. The trochanter lies above Nelaton's line, the imaginary line from the anterior superior spine of the ilium to the tuberosity of the ischium. An early diagnosis is more difficult in bilateral than unilateral dislocation.

COXA VARA. — In this condition the neck of the femur is at approximately a right angle to the rest of the bone. It has been found rarely in the newborn period as a congenital malformation but most commonly appears later in infancy or childhood as a result of rickets, epiphyseal separation or other disease.

POSTERIOR ROTATION. — In almost all cases of exstrophy of the bladder the pubic symphysis is absent and the pubic rami are separated and directed laterally. This separation permits a backward rotation of the iliac bones, the acetabulum may be directed posteriorly and the legs seem to be attached so that, were they able to move forward, they would carry the rest of the body backward.

ELBOWS AND KNEES

Fixation of the elbows or the knees in extension is usually a result of arthrogryposis. Fixation in flexion is most often associated with absence of the radius or tibia. Less often it is a result of an abnormality of the upper end of one of these bones.

MEDIAL TORSION OF THE LEG. — This consists of a twist of the lower on the upper leg. The patella faces directly forward and the foot and ankle turn in. The tibia may be bowed.

GENU RECURVATUM. — Severe hyperextensibility of the knees occurs infrequently in otherwise normal infants and is most likely to be part of a widespread disturbance in muscular and skeletal development. When occurring as a single anomaly it is usually interpreted as being a result of intrauterine pressure, although such an explanation is always open to question. In one infant delivered at the Chicago Lying-in Hospital with unilateral involvement (Fig. 26–11), the knee became stabilized without treatment and appeared almost normal by the time of discharge at 10 days.

HANDS AND FEET

CLUBHAND. — Clubbing of the hand, which is ordinarily secondary to absence of the radius, consists of fixation in a varus position (see Figs. 25–57 and 25–73). The first metacarpal bone and the thumb are also usually absent, although this is not an essential part of the deformity.

CLUBFOOT (TALIPES). — The position of the feet varies greatly as a result of abnormal interrelationships of the tarsal and metatarsal bones (Fig. 26–12). Only rarely are the tibia and fibula involved. In the mildest form of clubbing, known as metatarsus varus, the tarsal bones are in approximately normal positions and the metatarsal bones are directed medially, giving an extreme curve to the outer border of the foot. The forefoot is supinated and the medial fibers of the plantar fascia are

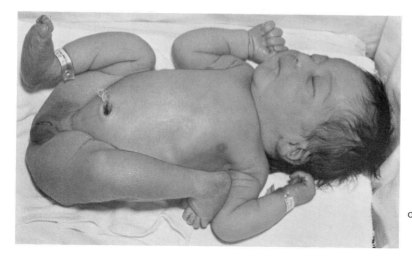

Fig. 26–11.—Genu recurvatum in otherwise normal infant.

contracted. Occasionally the posterior part of the foot is in a valgus position. If uncorrected, it produces a pigeon toe deformity as the child begins to walk and may predispose to the later production of hallux valgus.

In the most common form of true clubfoot the foot is in a varus position as a result of separation of the lateral and compression of the medial tarsal bones. When the forepart of the foot is pointed down and the heel is elevated, the condition is known as talipes equinus. The two are often present in combina-

tion, called equinovarus, in which the heel rolls inward at the ankle and the foot is in plantar flexion. The toes are directed down and toward the midline and the sole is posterior. Less common, and generally seen only in association with other skeletal defects, is the type known as calcaneovalgus. Here an anterolateral contracture tilts the foot up and out, with the dorsum against the outer surface of the leg.

Clubfoot may be inherited or may appear sporadically. In the latter cases intrauterine pressure has

Fig. 26–12.—Clubfoot. **A,** talipes varus, most common form. **B,** mild equinovarus. **C,** severe equinovarus.

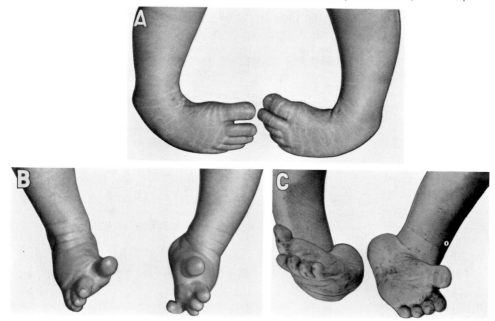

been considered a probable cause. This has been an especially attractive theory when one foot is in a calcaneovalgus position and the other fits over it in an equinovarus position, although clubfoot is seen occasionally in small abortuses that are contained in sacs filled with enough fluid to preclude the possibility of pressure being in any way responsible. This position of the feet is found almost constantly in association with renal agenesis. In this condition amniotic fluid is absent or greatly reduced in amount; tibias and fibulas are often slightly curved and the feet are clubbed as a result of fixation within the uterus (see Fig. 22–12).

Clubfoot is very common with lumbar spina bifida as a result of an abnormality of innervation. The constant association of clubbing of the foot in association with a congenital cicatrix encircling the lower leg is probably due to the same cause.

HAMMER TOE.—This anomaly, caused by a contracture of the extensor tendon, is seldom found at birth unless other malformations are present.

HALLUX VARUS.—This is an adducted great toe with a contracture between the first phalanx and the metatarsal bone. The toe can be pushed back into line but springs back when released. It is not present at birth and is always an acquired deformity.

Inflammation

Suppurative arthritis of the hip joint, associated with acute osteomyelitis of the intracapsular portion of the femur or ilium, may follow *Staphylococcus aureus* infection in other parts of the body in the premature or very young baby (Obletz). Disappearance of the femoral head may result. X-ray examination may show evidence of subluxation, and dislocation may follow if open drainage is not instituted. Occasionally the femoral head completely disappears. Other joints less frequently affected as a result of blood-borne infections in the 1st year of life include the knee, elbow and shoulder (Samilson).

REFERENCES

Adams, R. D., Denny-Brown, D., and Pearson, C. M.: *Diseases of Muscle* (New York: Paul B. Hoeber, Inc., 1962).
Badgley, C. E.: Etiology of congenital dislocation of the hip, J. Bone Joint Surg. 31A:341, 1949.
Banker, B. Q., Victor, M., and Adams, R. D.: Arthrogryposis multiplex due to congenital muscular dystrophy, Brain 80:319, 1957.
Chandler, F. A.: Muscular torticollis, J. Bone Joint Surg. 30A:566, 1948.
Conel, J. L.: Distribution of affected nerve cells in amyotonia congenita (second case), Arch. Pathol. 30:153, 1940.
Dodge, P. R., *et al.*: Myotonic dystrophy in infancy and childhood, Pediatrics 35:3, 1965.
Fenechel, G. M., and Engel, W. K.: Histochemistry of muscle in infantile spinal atrophy, Neurology 13:1059, 1967.
Fisher, R. L., *et al.*: Arthrogryposis multiplex congenita: Clinical investigation, J. Pediatr. 76:255, 1970.
Gonatas, N. K., Shy, G. M., and Godfrey, E. H.: Nemaline myopathy: Origin of nemaline structures, N. Engl. J. Med. 274:535, 1966.
Hudgson, P., *et al.*: Nemaline myopathy, Neurology 17:1125, 1967.
Jenis, C. H., Lindquist, R. R., and Lister, R. C.: New congenital myopathy with crystalline intranuclear inclusions, Arch. Neurol. 20:281, 1969.
Katzeff, M.: Arthrogryposis multiplex, Arch. Surg. 46:673, 1943.
Kibrick, S.: Myasthenia gravis, Pediatrics 14:365, 1954.
McKusick, V. A.: *Heritable Disorders of Connective Tissue* (3d ed.; St. Louis; C. V. Mosby Co., 1966).
Nutt, J. J.: Report of a case of myositis ossificans progressiva with bibliography, J. Bone Joint Surg. 5:344, 1923.
Obletz, B. E.: Acute suppurative arthritis of hip in neonatal period, J. Bone Joint Surg. 42A:23, 1960.
Rothenstein, J. L., and Welt, S.: Calcinosis universalis and calcinosis circumscripta in infancy and childhood, Am. J. Dis. Child. 52:368, 1936.
Samilson, R. L., Bersani, F. A., and Watkins, M. B.: Acute suppurative arthritis in infants and children. Importance of early diagnosis and surgical drainage, Pediatrics 21:798, 1958.
Shafiq, S. A.: Nemaline myopathy—report of a fatal case, with histochemical and electron microscopic studies, Brain 90:817, 1967.
Shy, G. M., and Magee, K. R.: A new congenital nonprogressive myopathy, Brain 79:619, 1956.
Silverman, F. N., and Huang, N.: Congenital absence of abdominal muscles, Am. J. Dis. Child. 80:91, 1950.
Swanson, W. W., Forster, W. G., and Iob, V.: Calcinosis circumscripta, Am. J. Dis. Child. 45:590, 1933.
Walters, G. V., and Williams, T. V.: Early onset myotonic dystrophy: Clinical and laboratory findings in 5 families and review of literature, Arch. Neurol. 17:187, 1967.
Welch, K. J.: Abdominal Musculature Deficiency Syndrome, in Mustard, W. T., *et al.* (eds.): *Pediatric Surgery* (Chicago: Year Book Medical Publishers, Inc., 1971), Vol. 2, p. 1191.
Williams, P. I., and Burkholder, G. V.: The prune belly syndrome, J. Urol. 98:244, 1967.
Zellweger, H., *et al.*: Severe congenital muscular dystrophy, Am. J. Dis. Child. 114:591, 1967.

27

Skin

AT THE END of the 1st month of development the embryo is covered by a single layer of cells derived from the non-neural portion of the ectodermal component of the embryonic disk. These cells gradually proliferate, and by the 4th month a superficial keratinized layer, an intermediate transitional zone and a basal germinative layer can be identified. In the early months the junction between epidermis and underlying dermal connective tissue is a smooth plane. As the epidermis thickens, the junction becomes irregular, and numerous shallow crypts are formed by connective tissue projections called dermal papillae that protrude into the epidermis.

The primordia of hair follicles and sebaceous glands appear during the 3d and 4th months. Hairs are not visible above the body surface until late in the 6th or early part of the 7th month. The first hairs are fine, are set close together and form a downy coat called lanugo. These hairs are mostly shed before or soon after birth and are replaced by coarser hairs that arise from new follicles.

Sebaceous glands develop simultaneously with hair follicles. They are actively secreting by the 7th month, and at the normal time of birth the fetus is usually irregularly coated with a thin layer of white cheesy material known as vernix caseosa. It is a mixture of sebum, desquamated squamous epithelium and lanugo. Although it is often described as a protection against the macerating effect of amniotic fluid, the skin is not harmed by exposure to amniotic fluid during the months before development of the sebaceous glands. It has been reported, but not confirmed, that vernix caseosa is excessive when the vitamin A content of the maternal diet is low.

Sweat glands begin to form slightly later than sebaceous glands. They appear first as solid cords of cells extending from the epidermis into the underlying connective tissue and begin to develop lumens during the 7th month, but there is no proof of secretion before birth.

Bullae and Moist Desquamation

MACERATION. — When death precedes birth, non-putrefactive tissue degeneration sets in immediately. Amniotic fluid does not normally contain bacteria, and the changes in the body of the fetus result from sterile cellular disintegration. The first changes in the skin appear within a few hours of death, after which the application of oblique pressure to the body surface will detach the epidermis. This is sometimes known as "skin-slipping." Fluid accumulates beneath the epidermis slightly later, and large bullae may develop (Fig. 27–1). Manipulation of the fetus during delivery is usually responsible for rupture, and much of the epidermis may be rubbed off, leaving parts of the body covered by the exposed bright red corium. Such separation of epidermis does not ordinarily occur until the last trimester of pregnancy. Before that time the epidermis is less well differentiated and more intimately associated with the underlying connective tissue.

On rare occasions bullae form before birth in the skin of an otherwise normal infant. Their rupture during delivery is responsible for the statement that maceration may occur in living infants. In general, such bullae have no pathologic significance, and healing is rapid. Maceration can ordinarily be considered proof of intrauterine death and generally indicates that death occurred prior to the onset of labor.

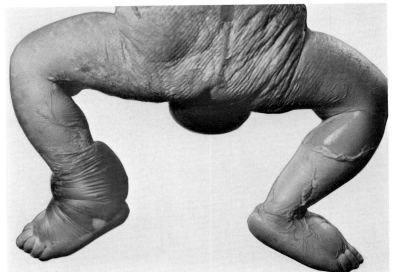

Fig. 27–1.—Maceration as a result of death 3 days before delivery. A large unruptured bullous accumulation of fluid is present over the left foot and ankle. Similar bullae on the right leg and the foot have been ruptured, causing partial denudation of the skin.

EPIDERMOLYSIS BULLOSA.—Two forms of epidermolysis bullosa are seen in children. The first, which is inherited as an autosomal dominant character (epidermolysis bullosa hereditaria lethalis), is present at birth or shortly thereafter and is usually fatal in the first weeks of life. The fundamental defect appears to be a poor attachment of the stratum granulosum to the basal layer of the epithelium (Lewis *et al.*), and minor traction on the skin surface consequently will cause separation of the superficial portion of the epidermis. Nikolsky's sign, i.e., the loosening of the epidermis by frictional rubbing of the skin, is positive, and bullae filled with clear or bloody fluid form in the damaged areas (Lamb and Halpert). As much as 60% of the body surface may be covered by bullae at one time. They are most common on the extremities but may occur on any area subject to pressure or trauma (Fig. 27–2). The rete pegs generally remain intact, and healing occurs without scarring or atrophy. Inflamma-

tion is not a primary feature of the disease although bullae may become secondarily infected (Fig. 27–3). In some cases the skin may show histologic evidence of parakeratosis, acanthosis or spongiosis. Atrophy of the epidermis and obliteration of the sebaceous and sweat ducts, looseness of the nails, ulcers of the buccal mucosa and histologic defects in the tooth enamel may also be present. Death results from fluid loss and the secondary infection that accompanies the massive involvement of the skin surface.

The second, less severe, form of epidermolysis bullosa has essentially the same basic underlying defect but the onset is later and the prognosis is better, survivors being common. In this form the skin may become atrophic with scars and epidermal cysts produced in the areas where bullae were previously located. Both dominant and recessive patterns of inheritance have been described.

One infant observed at the Chicago Lying-in

Fig. 27–2.—Epidermolysis bullosa. **A,** ruptured bullous lesion present on the wrist at birth. **B,** widespread infect-

ed lesions in the same infant, aged 23 days. Death at 28 days. (Courtesy Dr. Rustin McIntosh.)

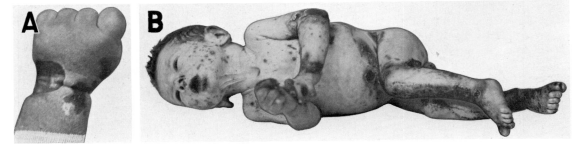

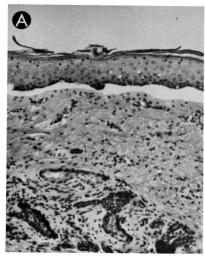 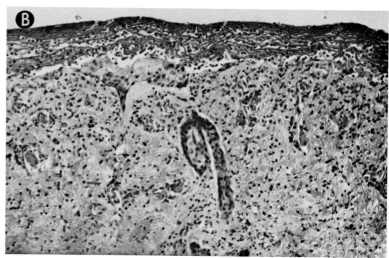

Fig. 27–3.—Epidermolysis bullosa. Photomicrographs. **A,** an area with loosening of the basilar epidermal layer and little inflammation. **B,** an area of secondary infection; note that fragments of basilar epithelium near sweat and sebaceous glands are intact. (Courtesy Dr. G. Vawter.)

Hospital (Fig. 27–4) with bullae present at birth was the 11th member of the family to be affected. The disorder had been inherited as a mendelian dominant character through four generations, with nine of the 11 being females.

RITTER'S DISEASE (EXFOLIATIVE DERMATITIS).— This form of exfoliation is entirely different from exfoliative dermatitis of adults. It begins in the early weeks of life with rapidly spreading lesions that generally appear first in the mouth or anal region as a bright red erythematous flush with a scalded appearance and a positive Nikolsky sign. Bullae form which, as they burst, leave a bright red, moist, raw skin surface (Fig. 27–5). In some

Fig. 27–4.—Epidermolysis bullosa in infant aged 4 days. Ten other members of the family were affected.

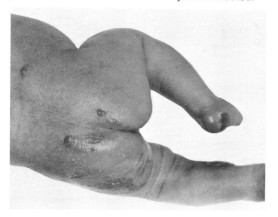

Fig. 27–5.—Exfoliative dermatitis (Ritter's disease) showing a characteristic lesion on the face as well as involvement of the chest, abdomen and arms. The epidermis is absent and the underlying corium is exposed. (Courtesy Dr. Ralph V. Platou.)

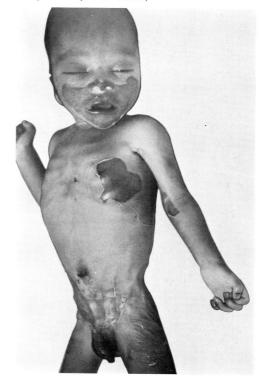

cases the first lesions resemble bullous impetigo. Skin cultures are positive for staphylococci. Histologically there is a marked dilatation of the blood vessels of the corium and hypodermis, with infiltration of polymorphonuclear leukocytes. All but the basal one to two cell layers of the granulosa are involved (Fig. 27–6). The disease yields to proper antibiotic therapy although mortality as high as 50% has been recorded (Barker *et al.*).

TOXIC EPIDERMAL NECROLYSIS.—This disease, which may occur in the first weeks of life, is also found throughout childhood. Associated with skin and enteric infections, it begins suddenly with skin tenderness, erythema, a scalded appearance and cleavage of the upper epidermal layers. The essential lesion is a limited necrosis of the superficial layers of the granulosa and cleavage of the upper layers of the epidermis, which produces vesiculobullous lesions with lamellar scaling and parakeratosis. There is no inflammation unless complications develop (Margileth) (Fig. 27–7).

The process often follows gastroenteritis, impeti-

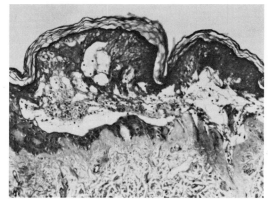

Fig. 27–7.—Toxic epidermal necrolysis. Photomicrograph showing necrosis of the superficial layers of the granulosa layer.

go, secondarily infected chickenpox or scabies. The general features of toxemia are not present, and recovery is usually prompt, though fatalities do occur when more than one half of the skin surface is involved. Cases with localized areas present at birth have been reported (Sweetman *et al.*). Corticoids are believed to aid in the prevention of spread of the lesions and the return of the skin to normal. The disease is considered to be a toxic reaction rather than a direct bacterial involvement.

A related syndrome is *acrodermatitis enteropathica* in which the presenting tetrad of symptoms consists of apathy, diarrhea, ano-oral dermatitis and alopecia. The skin lesions are vesiculobullous with crusting and scaling. Secondary inflammation appears during exacerbations of the original process; these exacerbations may be prevented by the use of diiodohydroxyquinoline (Margileth).

Seborrhea and Dry Desquamation

MILIARIA.—Sebaceous glands function actively during the last few weeks of intrauterine life. The secretion normally exudes from the glands but occasionally collects in the gland ducts, distending them so that they are visible at birth as discrete pinpoint elevations known as milia. They are most often visible on the forehead, cheeks and sides of the nose.

Sometimes, when the distention is greater, sebaceous masses 2–3 mm in diameter are found on the face, backs of the hands or feet and, less often, on other parts of the body. The sebum is sometimes hard and firm but is more often soft and creamy and superficially resembles pus. The lesions are often numerous and present in small groups; less

Fig. 27–6.—Ritter's disease. Photomicrogram showing an intense inflammatory infiltrate in the keratin layer and granulosa layers. The basalis is intact but there is an inflammatory exudate in the dermis. (Courtesy Dr. G. Vawter.)

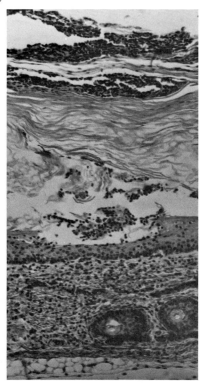

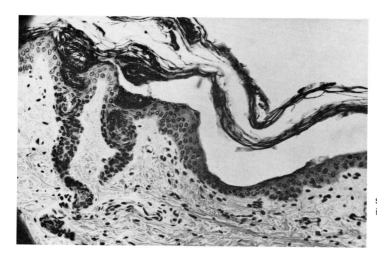

Fig. 27–8.—Miliaria. Photomicrograph showing a subkeratotic bulla without inflammation. (Courtesy Dr. G. Vawter.)

often they are single and widely scattered. They usually disappear without treatment in the 1st week of life. Occasionally the lesions are vesicular and also may be present in localized groups or widespread over the body (Fig. 27–8). This is known as *miliaria crystallina perifortis* (Fig. 27–9). The lesions generally disappear within a few days and do not recur.

SEBORRHEIC DERMATITIS.—This reaction of the skin to various causes is characterized by erythema, scaling and occasional vesiculation. The scalp is most often affected in young infants and, when located there, the disorder is often associated with incomplete removal of the vernix caseosa. The le-

sions are poorly defined yellow-red patches covered by waxy, easily removed scales. They often spread to cover the face and may extend onto the trunk and into the creases of the body. Scaling and lichenification are characteristic features of established lesions although they may not be present early.

In young infants or in those with recently evolved lesions, acanthosis, edema and occasional perivascular infiltration of leukocytes are characteristic. In older lesions hyperkeratosis is prominent except when infection is present. The rete pegs are long, uniform in depth and fairly broad, but over the edematous papillae there is little acanthosis. There is spongiosis of the basal layer of the

Fig. 27–9.—Miliaria crystallina perifortis consisting of 1–3 mm vesicles filled with clear fluid. Present at birth.

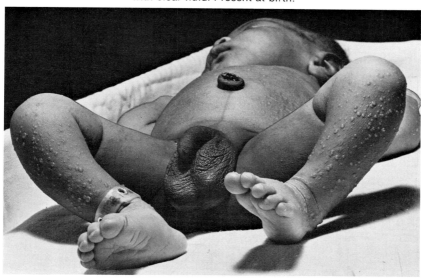

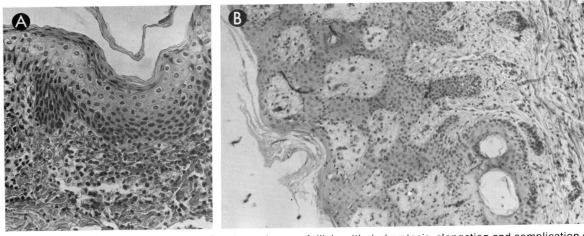

Fig. 27–10.—Seborrheic dermatitis. **A,** photomicrograph of skin showing dyskeratosis, acanthosis, intracellular edema and edema and infiltration of the dermis. **B,** photomicrograph of scalp showing plugging of a hair follicle with dyskeratosis, elongation and complication of the rete peg pattern and edema of the dermis. (Courtesy Dr. G. Vawter.)

epidermis, but the basement membrane is usually well defined. Nuclei are enlarged and hyperchromatic in the granular layer of the epidermis and in the endothelial cells of the capillaries in the corium. If the crusts become infected, the subjacent skin is infiltrated with monocytes and polymorphonuclear cells (Prose and Sedlis) (Fig. 27–10).

Seborrheic dermatitis is common with atopic eczema but may be found in a variety of other diseases. In some, such as Letterer-Siwe's disease and

Fig. 27–11.—Desquamative erythroderma (Leiner's disease). **A,** mild form in infant aged 6 weeks. (Courtesy Dr. Rustin McIntosh.) **B,** severe form in infant aged 2 weeks. (Courtesy Dr. Ralph V. Platou.) Both infants recovered.

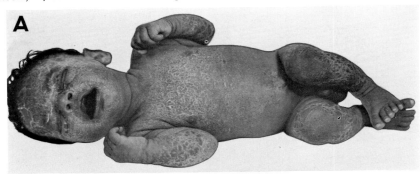

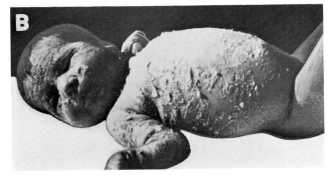

Hurler's syndrome, cells characteristic of these conditions that indicate the cause are also present. In many others, such as Aldrich's syndrome, sex-linked agammaglobulinemia, ataxia-telangiectasia and phenylketonuria, no identifying features are present, and the skin lesions can be distinguished from those of atopic eczema only by knowledge of the existence of the underlying disease (Rostenberg). In some of these the dermatitis is mild and self-limited, and the skin soon returns to normal, while in others the lesions are progressive, becoming more severe as the infant grows older.

DESQUAMATIVE ERYTHRODERMA (LEINER'S DISEASE). — Closely allied to seborrheic dermatitis, this disease often seems to be only a more severe form of the same condition. It is rare before the end of the 1st month, although it may appear soon after birth. The first evidence may be dry reddened areas on the buttocks and in the gluteal folds or on the scalp. Often, much of the body is erythematous and covered by gray-white branny or greasy scales a few millimeters to 1 cm or more in diameter (Fig. 27–11). Desquamation ordinarily begins in a short time and the skin slowly returns to normal. Histologically, it has much in common with seborrheic

dermatitis but with elongated rete pegs, parakeratosis and irregularity of the granular layer (Barker *et al.*). Infrequently, cracks and fissures appear between the scales and become secondarily infected. Associated constitutional symptoms include intermittent fever, diarrhea, generalized lymphadenopathy, edema and albuminuria. The condition may persist for weeks accompanied by symptoms of intestinal toxemia and pneumonia. The mortality rate is about 30%.

ICHTHYOSIFORM ERYTHRODERMA (ICHTHYOSIS). — The skin of the newborn normally shows varying degrees of keratinization. Removal of the vernix caseosa after delivery often simultaneously removes the superficial keratinized layer, but if this layer is unusually thick, desquamation may continue for several days.

As far as is now known, all forms of true ichthyosis are inherited abnormalities. The skin of the entire body is affected although mucous membranes are spared. The time of onset, severity and mode of inheritance vary. The most severe form is *ichthyosis congenita gravis,* or harlequin fetus (Fig. 27–12), which is inherited as a recessive characteristic and is present at birth. The skin is extremely

Fig. 27–12.—Ichthyosis congenita gravis. **A,** severe form of the disease incompatible with survival. The entire body is covered with thick horny plaques separated by fissures. There is marked ectropion of the eyes and mouth. **B,** photomicrograph of scalp showing marked hyperkeratosis of the surface with nonobstructive plugging of hair follicles and sweat ducts.

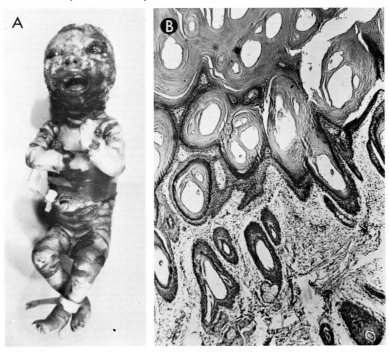

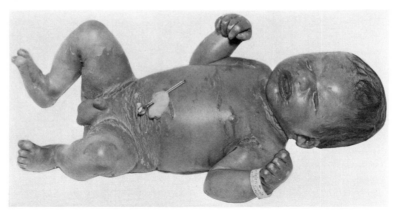

Fig. 27–13.—Ichthyosis congenita levis in an infant aged 2 days. Older affected sibling died in neonatal period. This child at age 10 years had thick, dry, easily cracked skin.

hyperkeratotic with large rigid plaques between which are fissures in whose bases the corium is visible. The hands may appear moist and weeping, with no apparent skin covering, and the nails may be unrecognizable. Ectropion of the eyes, nostrils and mouth are common. Difficulty in eating, breathing and controlling infection lead to early death. Other anomalies may also be present in the eyes such as corneal opacities, pigmentary retinitis and microphthalmia. The bones of the fingers and toes may be poorly developed.

The changes in the less severe congenital form *(ichthyosis congenita levis)* are somewhat similar but most affected patients survive early infancy (Fig. 27–13). A yet milder form has no abnormality at birth. The affected skin in all of these forms is characterized by severe hyperkeratosis, marked acanthosis and rete peg hyperplasia.

In *lamellar ichthyosis of the newborn,* or "collodion baby," the upper keratin layer of the skin forms a layer distinct from the usual stratum corneum; this superficial layer is thought to be derived from the epitrichium as it contains scattered parakeratotic nuclei (Nix *et al.;* Scott and Stone; Finlay and Pound). The epitrichium is a distinct covering layer seen in certain animals before birth and has been said to be present in human beings early in gestation. If this is true, the collodion membrane might be considered a persistence of a normal early structure (Emery and Gordon). The stratum corneum in lamellar ichthyosis may be thickened or normal, but the granulosa layer is often unusually thin. Some degree of inflammation is usually present in the corium. Changes may be similar to those found in other forms of ichthyosis but are considerably less disfiguring (Fig. 27–14). In most

Fig. 27–14.—Lamellar ichthyosis. Infant aged 3 days. At birth the entire body was encased in a parchmentlike covering with a few breaks in the region of the joints. Part of this layer had already disappeared when this photograph was taken, and most of the remainder had disappeared by 10 days. The infant also had bilateral clubfeet.

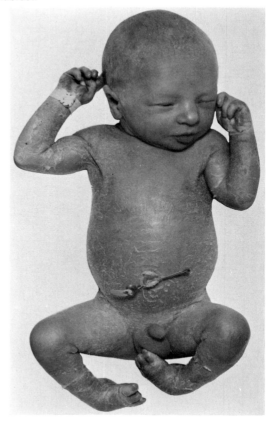

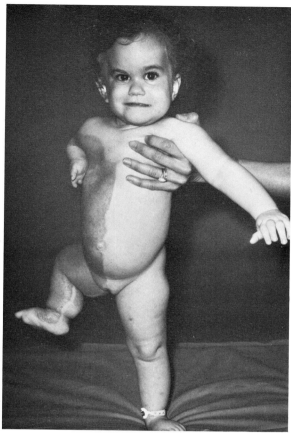

Fig. 27–15.—Infant with congenital unilateral psoriasis, hemiatrophy and ectromelia. (Courtesy Dr. C. S. Shear.)

cases the membrane soon desquamates, and nothing but a mild type of desquamating ichthyosis remains permanently. The disorder has an autosomal recessive pattern of inheritance.

Three other forms of ichthyosis were reported by Wells and Kerr. The first, which has a sex-linked recessive inheritance, occurs only in males. It appears in the first few months after birth with initial involvement of the antecubital and axillary areas. Large scaly portions of the skin are shed episodically. The histology is similar to the more severe forms of ichthyosis. The second and third forms are inherited as autosomal dominant characters. Symptoms in the second form, which begin at about 3 weeks of age, are considered a result of allergy. The skin has fine white scales, mild hyperkeratosis and follicular plugging. The third condition is the same but lacks the allergic component.

PSORIASIS WITH ECTROMELIA AND CENTRAL NERVOUS SYSTEM ANOMALIES.—Psoriasis is almost nev-

er seen in children, but in 1971 Shear et al. reported an infant in whom a diffuse unilateral involvement of the skin, present at birth, was associated with hemiatrophy of the involved side, ectromelia of upper and lower limbs and mental retardation (Fig. 27–15). Four similar cases were found in the literature. The histologic appearance of the skin was characteristic of psoriasis, with large scaling plaques, severe parakeratosis and elongation and clubbing of rete pegs. The diagnosis was confirmed by autoradiographic studies using tritiated thymidine. The index of proliferative activity obtained by this test is far higher in psoriasis than in other skin diseases. The mother and grandmother also had psoriasis but no other abnormalities.

Infectious and Papulovesicular Eruptions

DERMATITIS.—The skin of the newborn is highly susceptible to irritation, and eruptions of various sorts develop with little or no apparent provocation. They are most frequent in hot weather, when greater portions of the skin are often involved, than at other times of the year. Innumerable small papules may develop over the entire body within a few minutes after exposure to heat or at times without known cause (Fig. 27–16). They may be evanescent and disappear as rapidly as they come. Most eruptions are more prolonged and include macular, papular, vesicular and pustular lesions. The macular and papular lesions are often widespread but are commonly most severe in the folds of the skin, the axillae, groins and on the buttocks; when limited to these areas, they are called intertrigo (Fig. 27–17).

The perianal region and the area covered by the diaper are especially susceptible to erythema, excoriations and vesicular lesions. Irritation by feces and ammonia in the urine is responsible for most cases of dermatitis involving this area, although substances used in laundering or sterilizing diapers occasionally seem to be irritative.

ERYTHEMA TOXICUM NEONATORUM.—This common disorder affects as many as one third of all newborns (Freeman et al.), in whom erythematous macules, papules and pustules are simultaneously present. The lesions last 3–4 days and usually disappear with no sequelae, but in malnourished or neglected infants secondary infection may cause serious illness.

All lesions have the same basic histology, consisting of edema with intense eosinophilic infiltration with a few neutrophilic polymorphonuclear

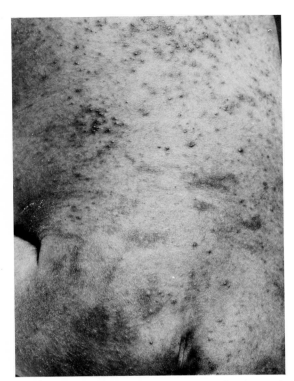

Fig. 27–16.—Diffusely disseminated fine papular eruption often found as a result of exposure to excessive heat. Infant aged 3 days.

and mononuclear cells. The macules are perivascular in distribution, the papules are centered on the hair follicles with acanthosis of the overlying epithelium (Freeman *et al.;* Luders), and pustules are related to the ducts of sweat and sebaceous glands.

Such lesions can be identified by the finding of eosinophils rather than polymorphonuclear neutrophils in smears of the lesions unless secondary infection has taken place. If large portions of the skin are rubbed off and secondary infection occurs, the usually benign process may be fatal. The cause of this disease is not known and, if uncomplicated, it is usually unaccompanied by other symptoms.

Drug dermatitis.—Many drugs taken by the mother are secreted in the milk and ingested by the infant. Bromides are those that most commonly cause a reaction in the infant's skin. The legs, the buttocks and at times other portions of the body are covered by nodular or discoid lesions 0.5–2 cm in diameter. They may be dry and smooth but more often are moist and crusted. If the drugs have been given during pregnancy, eruptions may be present on the infant's face or body at birth (Fig. 27–18).

Acne neonatorum.—This term is used to designate the comedones, papules and pustules found on the nose, cheeks and forehead of infants with oily skin. They usually disappear in a few days or weeks.

Impetigo.—In older infants and children impetigo is a distinct clinical entity usually caused by staphylococci or streptococci. Its early course is characterized by the presence of superficial vesicular lesions filled with seropurulent material. The lesions may be single or multiple and, although often only a few millimeters in diameter in the beginning, they spread rapidly and may soon reach a diameter of several centimeters. They often appear first on the face and then spread by autoinoculation to other exposed surfaces or eventually to all parts of the body. The disease is transmitted by direct contact.

Fig. 27–17.—Intertrigo. A fine papular eruption present in the axillae. It may be located anywhere that moist surfaces are approximated.

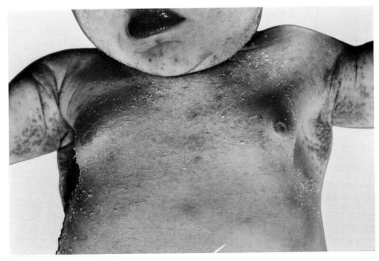

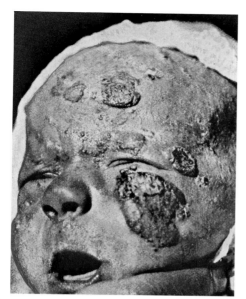

Fig. 27–18.—Bromoderma. The mother had taken bromides in the final month of pregnancy. (Courtesy Drs. S. William Becker and Maximilian E. Obermeyer.)

A similar condition is occasionally found in newborn infants and has been reported as present at birth (Fig. 27–19). It may become a grave problem by spreading through a nursery, but more often the small vesicles present in the newborn are self-limited, sterile and noncontagious. In the first few days of life it may be difficult to distinguish the infectious from the noninfectious lesions, but it is evident that the application of the term impetigo to all affected vesicles means that many noninfectious lesions will be included under this heading. The

Fig. 27–19.—Impetigo. Bullous lesions present in the groin. Contents slightly purulent.

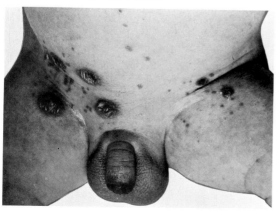

disease is not a sharply delineated entity in the newborn as it is in the older child.

ERYSIPELAS.—This disease is particularly severe when it occurs in newborn infants and may be rapidly fatal. It is practically unknown in well-conducted maternity hospitals but may be found wherever aseptic technic is not practiced during delivery or when the mother has a bacterial infection at the time of the infant's birth. It is caused by streptococci, which are most often introduced when the cord is cut or which gain entrance through fine abrasions in the skin after birth. The genital region is the most common starting point of the disease. The skin becomes reddened, swollen and hot. The margins often blend with the surrounding tissue and

Fig. 27–20.—Multiple cutaneous abscesses widespread over the entire body surface in an infant aged 3 months.

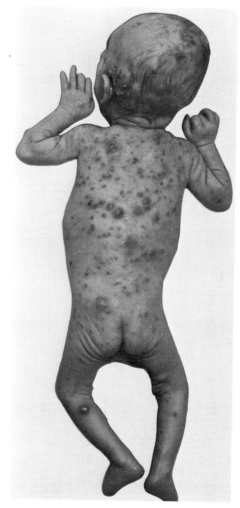

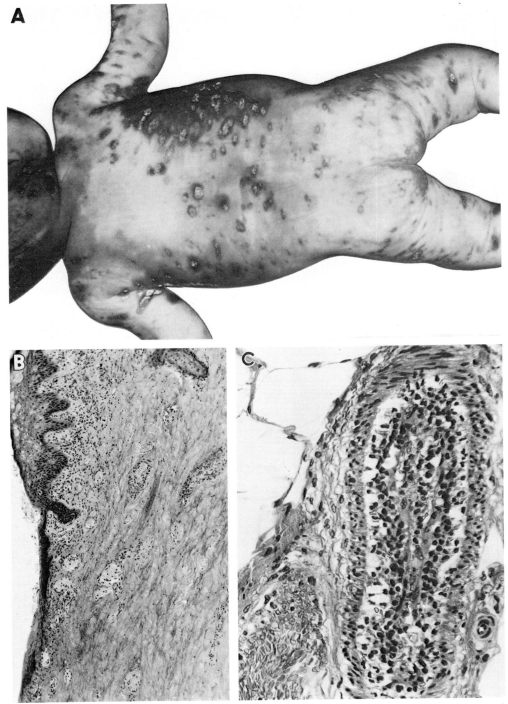

Fig. 27–21.—Gangrenous dermatitis. **A,** postmortem photograph of an infant who died of congenital heart disease at 3 weeks of age. The entire body was covered by punched-out, craterlike areas of skin necrosis. **B,** one of the skin lesions showing lack of cellular exudate and bacteria. **C,** terminal cutaneous vessel showing endarteritis responsible for the skin necrosis.

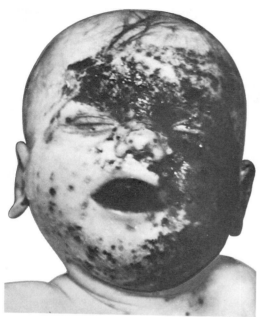

Fig. 27–22.—Eczema with secondary vaccinia. Infant aged 6 weeks with eczema who came in contact with a vaccinated older brother. (Courtesy Dr. Ralph V. Platou.)

are not sharply demarcated as they are in the adult. The lesion spreads rapidly, and the lower half of the body and occasionally the upper part are soon involved. Vesicles may appear, and in fatal cases areas of necrosis and gangrene may develop.

Fig. 27–23.—Syphilis. Characteristic desquamation with lesions (rhagades) at nose, mouth and inner angles

The child usually dies of septicemia unless vigorously treated in the early stages.

MULTIPLE CUTANEOUS ABSCESSES.—Multiple cutaneous abscesses may be found in neglected or malnourished infants. They can occur on any part of the body but are especially common on the back, buttocks and occiput (Fig. 27–20). They often appear in crops and may be palpable first as deep nodules, or they may be superficial red areas. They quickly soften and discharge large amounts of foul-smelling yellow-green pus. Adenitis, lymphangitis, ulcers and draining sinuses are frequent complications. *Staphylococcus pyogenes* is a common causative organism, although other bacteria have been isolated. Pilosebaceous follicles and sweat glands are the usual sites of entrance to the skin.

GANGRENOUS DERMATITIS.—This may occur in infants who are malnourished, ill or doing poorly for any reason. *Bacillus pyocyaneus,* pyogenic bacteria and other organisms have been isolated, and occasionally the lesions have seemed to be sterile. The initial lesions are nodular, vesicular or pustular. The centers become necrotic and slough, leaving punched-out craters. The craters are often very deep and occasionally are confluent and involve large parts of the body surface (Fig. 27–21). Leukocyte response at the margin of the craters is minimal. The back and buttocks are the most frequent sites of infection. Death may result from septicemia or a general state of toxicity.

GENERALIZED VACCINIA.—This rare condition may be found in infants or older individuals after vaccination or accidental inoculation of the skin by

of the eyes. **A,** infant who died at 3 days of age. **B,** infant aged 2 months who recovered.

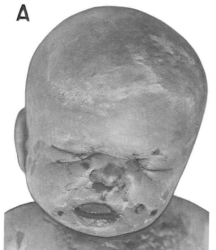

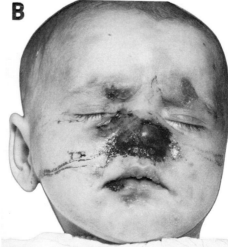

contact with a vaccinated person. It occurs only in those with eczema or other dermatitis. The eczema becomes exaggerated, and vesicles appear that become confluent and often hemorrhagic (Fig. 27–22). Healing ordinarily takes place without scarring.

SYPHILIS.—Skin lesions present at birth as a result of an intrauterine syphilitic infection are extremely variable but in general may be divided into diffuse and localized disturbances. The diffuse lesions have an especial predilection for the face, palms and soles. The skin in the affected areas has a coarse, shiny appearance varying in color from red-blue to brown. The surface is brittle and shiny, often cracked and covered by large thick scales.

Rhagades are seldom present at birth but often develop in the first few days of life. They are moist ulcerating lesions extending outward in a linear manner from the angles of the eyes, nose and mouth (Fig. 27–23). Those around the nose are especially severe because of irritation from the nasal discharge (snuffles) that is so often present.

Circumscribed lesions may be bullous or may be a mixture of macules, papules and pustules. The bullous variety is called syphilitic pemphigus, and bullae are frequently found on the palms and soles, where they are seldom found from other causes (Fig. 27–24). In syphilis the vesicles are filled with milky or definitely purulent material. When they rupture, moist and weeping surfaces are produced, which soon dry and become covered by crusts.

A maculopapular eruption may cover much of the body. The lesions are slightly elevated, round, flat and shiny and measure a few millimeters in diameter. They may enlarge and become confluent or may become vesicular and eventually pustular.

Moist flat papules several centimeters in diameter (condylomas) may be present in the genital and intragluteal regions.

Most of the skin lesions contain spirochetes and are highly infectious.

Edema and Induration

LOCALIZED EDEMA.—Some degree of edema is not unusual in the newborn infant. Mild edema, which is usually limited to the face, feet and legs below the knee, is most noticeable in the eyelids and on the dorsum of the feet. It is more common in premature than in term infants and may be present at birth or develop 1–2 days later. It usually soon disappears spontaneously. Water retention resulting from inadequate excretion by the immature kidneys is believed to be the most common cause.

MILROY'S DISEASE.—Milroy's disease is the name given a rare hereditary enlargement of the lower extremities that resembles severe edema. It is present at birth and is usually limited to the feet and legs. Both plantar and dorsal surfaces are involved, and the toes are small projections from the end of the thick puffy foot. True Milroy's disease is always familial, usually persistent and not associated with constitutional symptoms (Mason and Allen; Cooperstock). It appears to be due to mild lymphangiectasia of the involved areas and does not seem to be related to edema caused by water retention. The "edematous" areas do not ordinarily pit, and on pressure the tissue is soft and resilient.

TURNER'S SYNDROME.—Edema indistinguishable from that occurring in Milroy's disease is often

Fig. 27–24.—Syphilitic pemphigus. Bullae have lost their fluid and are now in the stage of desquamation. Infant aged 7 weeks. The most characteristic locations are hands and feet. **A,** hands. **B,** feet.

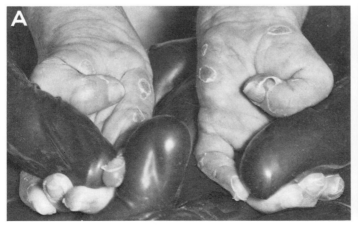
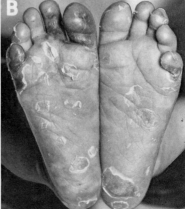

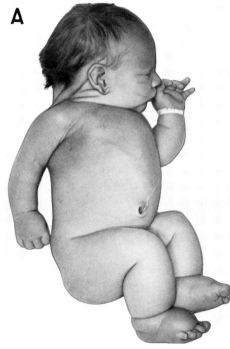

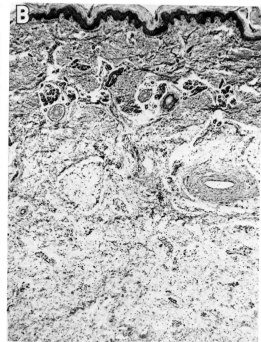

Fig. 27–25.—Turner's syndrome with edema of the lower extremities simulating that observed in Milroy's disease. The skin on the back of the neck is excessive. The heart was enlarged as a result of endomyocardial fibrosis and calcification (see Fig. 14–13, A). Ovaries were hypoplastic and contained few ova (see Fig. 23–2, A). Death at age 10 days. **A,** external view of infant. **B,** skin showing increase in thickness of layer of subcutaneous connective tissue without appreciable increase in lymphatic channels.

found without a hereditary background. It may appear as an isolated phenomenon in an otherwise normal infant but more often is part of Turner's syndrome in which it is accompanied by ovarian agenesis, pterygium colli and occasionally by other malformations (Fig. 27–25). One infant observed at the Chicago Lying-in Hospital who died at 10 days also had fibroelastosis of the heart and medullary sponge kidneys. The edema usually subsides within a few months and extremities are subsequently normal.

EDEMA WITH LYMPHANGIOMATOSIS.—Localized areas of edema that are much more severe than those already described may involve one or more extremities. The tissues are hard and pit easily, and the overlying skin is tense. The areas in the immediate vicinity of the joints are not involved, and deep creases are usually present at the ankle, knee, wrist or elbow. The joints cannot be flexed because of the excessive tissue volume. The lymphatics are dilated and increased in number. Although the disease is generally most conspicuous in one extremity, postmortem examination may re-

veal cystic dilatation of lymphatic channels in the muscles and subcutaneous connective tissue of the entire body.

GENERALIZED EDEMA.—Generalized edema of any degree may be present at birth. When severe it is often designated fetal hydrops, and affected infants are usually born dead or survive only a short time. Excessive fluid, which is present in the subcutaneous tissues, muscles and pleural and peritoneal cavities, exudes from any cut surface. Its accumulation in the connective tissue between muscle groups frequently gives the anterior abdominal wall a striking sandwich-like arrangement of thick layers of fluid-filled connective tissue separating thinner layers of muscle (Fig. 27–26).

Erythroblastosis is the most common (Fig. 27–27, A) but by no means the only cause of such edema. It is present in erythroblastotic fetuses only when the disease is very severe, and when due to this cause, the edema is invariably associated with profound abnormal erythropoiesis and extreme anemia. There is an accompanying deficiency of plasma proteins, the values for which may be as

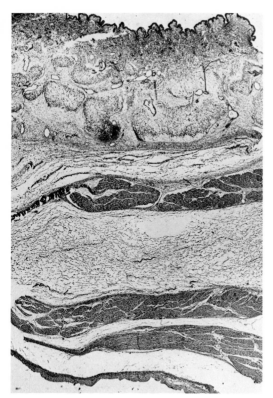

Fig. 27–26.—Anterior abdominal wall of an infant with erythroblastosis in whom the skin and individual muscle layers are widely separated by edematous connective tissue. A focus of erythropoiesis is visible in the dermis. For gross appearance of cut surface of the abdominal wall see Fig. 21–4.

low as 1.5–2 gm%. This appears to be largely responsible for the edema.

Similar edema is sometimes found in the children of Rh-positive women who have no evidence of immunization to any blood factor. It has been reported in infants with malformations of the heart or other organs and in children of women with toxemia, nephritis and other chronic diseases. The suggestion has been made that intrauterine cardiac failure might be a cause, but since it occurs in the absence of cardiac abnormalities, and since the most severe forms of cardiac malformations are seldom associated with edema, this explanation does not seem tenable. Over 20 hydropic fetuses with no evidence of erythroblastosis were observed at the Chicago Lying-in Hospital. All of the mothers tested were Rh positive, several were of the same AB blood group as the fetus and many were primigravidas. Malformations of various sorts were

present in six (Fig. 27–27, B), but in 14 there were no demonstrable abnormalities except edema (Potter). The cause of such edema is unknown.

SUBCUTANEOUS FAT NECROSIS (ADIPONECROSIS SUBCUTANEA NEONATORUM).—The considerable confusion that exists in the use of the terms sclerema, scleredema and scleroderma is due in part at least to the fact that these conditions have no clear-cut distinguishing features. All are uncommon in the United States and seem to be growing less frequent as the general care of the newborn improves. One condition, however, that can definitely be isolated from the group because of specific tissue changes is subcutaneous fat necrosis. This has been called sclerema neonatorum and scleroderma, but most authors describe other conditions under these terms.

Subcutaneous fat necrosis in most instances consists of sharply defined, nonelevated areas of subcutaneous induration that appear from a few days to a few weeks after birth in large, well-developed, otherwise healthy infants. The lesions may be single or multiple and, in order of frequency, are most common on the back, cheeks, arms, thighs, buttocks, calves of the legs and shoulders. They are woody in consistency and do not pit on pressure; the overlying skin is blue or violet. Softening, fluctuation and cyst formation are unusual complications. These areas ordinarily disappear in 3–4 months without treatment.

Obstetric trauma in the form of extreme pressure against hard underlying structures is believed to be the primary cause. It is related to the facts that the subcutaneous fat of the newborn is low in olein content and that, according to McIntosh et al., the melting point of the fat of the newborn is actually above the normal body temperature. The subcutaneous fat in the involved areas is altered in its physical aggregation but not in its chemical state, and no lipase capable of hydrolyzing body fat is present. Zeek and Madden described an important case in which both internal and external fat deposits were affected; thus, trauma as a sole cause of subcutaneous fat necrosis of the newborn seems unlikely.

Microscopic examination reveals normal epidermis and corium with characteristic changes in the fat cells of the subcutaneous tissue (Fig. 27–28). The fat cells contain doubly refractile crystals arranged in a sheaflike or rosette pattern. Multinucleated giant cells typical of a foreign body are irregularly distributed among them. Fibroblasts and lymphocytes are common around the periphery. Polymorphonuclear leukocytes are seldom present.

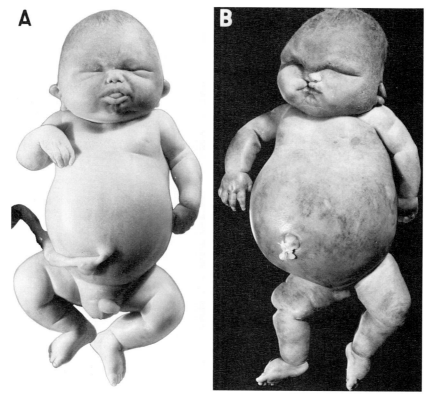

Fig. 27–27.—Generalized anasarca. **A,** fetus stillborn because of erythroblastosis. **B,** fetus without erythroblastosis but with multiple malformations.

SCLEREMA NEONATORUM (SCLEREMA ADIPOSUM).— This term is generally used for a widespread induration of the skin that begins between the 3d or 4th day and the 3d or 4th week after birth (Hughes and Hammond). It appears first on the legs or face and in a short time may involve all of the body surface except the palms, soles and scrotum. The affected areas are smooth, hard, dry and cold to the touch and whitish or waxy in appearance. They do not pit on pressure and the skin cannot be separated from the underlying tissues. The limbs may be inflexible as a result of induration and loss of elasticity. The temperature is often low, somnolence is conspicuous and tube feeding may be necessary. The prognosis is poor, with death occurring in 75% of cases in a short time. The condition is limited almost exclusively to premature infants and fortunately is rare in the United States.

The cause of the disease is unknown, and microscopic examination reveals no characteristic changes. Suggestions have been made that the fat contains a higher proportion of saturated fats and lesser amounts of oleic acid than normal (Horsefield and Yardley). It may accompany fatal pneumonia and other terminal states (Werwick *et al.*).

SCLEREDEMA.—This condition usually appears from the 2d to the 4th day following delivery and is similar to sclerema except for the added factor of edema. It may occur in malnourished or seemingly healthy premature or full-term infants and, like sclerema, most often begins in the legs. The affected areas are not circumscribed, are swollen and doughy in consistency and pit on pressure. The skin is pale, waxy and tense. The infant usually becomes apathetic and does not suck; the temperature is low and pulse and respiration are feeble. Death may occur in a few days, or recovery may finally take place after a protracted illness.

Microscopic examination reveals intense edema with mild nonspecific changes such as dilatation of vessels, edema and minimal inflammation in the skin, subcutaneous tissue and sometimes the underlying muscle. The cause is unknown, although cortisone is said to aid recovery in some cases.

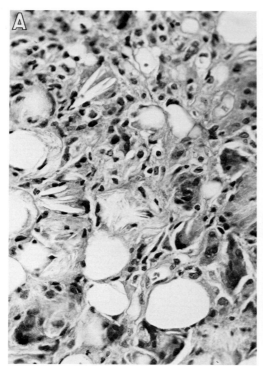
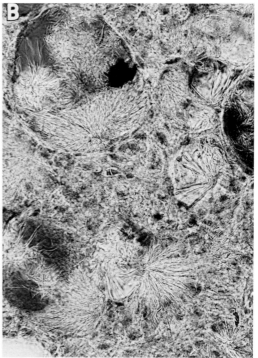

Fig. 27–28.—Subcutaneous fat necrosis. **A,** tissue fixed in formalin and stained with hematoxylin-eosin showing fat cells, spaces from which crystals have been dissolved, connective tissue and foreign body giant cells.

B, unstained tissue with doubly refractile crystals arranged in the form of rosettes and sheaves. Infant aged 4 weeks.

Icterus and Abnormalities of Pigmentation

ICTERUS.—Icterus is a yellow discoloration of the skin associated with an excess of bilirubin in the circulation. It generally appears in adults when the serum bilirubin value is above 1.6 mg per 100 ml, but infants may remain free from icterus despite a much higher level. Icterus is almost never present at birth even though, as in infants with a hemolytic anemia such as erythroblastosis, the bilirubin level in the circulation is high. Fetuses with severe erythroblastosis excrete large amounts of bilirubin in the urine, which discolors the placental surface, umbilical cord and vernix caseosa, giving a false impression of discoloration of the skin. Old meconium in the amniotic fluid may produce similar yellow discoloration. When the vernix caseosa is removed, the underlying skin is free from icterus, although in infants with a high level of serum bilirubin it becomes icteric almost immediately afterward. The sudden postnatal development of icterus is a result, at least in part, of loss of the placenta as

a means of removing bilirubin from the circulation. During intrauterine life a large share of the bilirubin is transferred to the mother's blood, and when this is no longer possible, bilirubin accumulates in the infant's body.

Icterus associated with atresia of the bile ducts does not generally develop until several days after birth. It persists throughout the few months that the infant survives unless the atresia is relieved surgically.

Less frequent causes of icterus are septicemia and intracranial or intra-abdominal hemorrhage.

ALBINISM.—This rare condition is associated with complete generalized absence of pigment in the skin, mucous membranes, hair and iris (Fig. 27–29). The iris appears pink because the blood vessels are visible through the translucent cornea. Photophobia and nystagmus are almost constant symptoms; otherwise, affected individuals are usually normal. The condition is believed to result from a faulty pigment-producing apparatus related to lack of some ferment needed for the elaboration of pigment, most probably an absence of tyrosinase in-

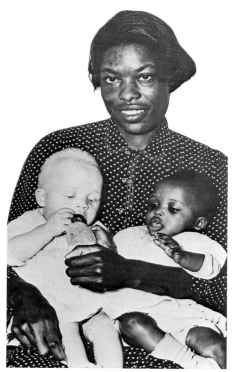

Fig. 27–29.—Albinism in one of dizygotic twins of Negro parents. (International News photo.)

side the melanocytes in the skin. It is inherited as a recessive character and is manifest only in a homozygous state.

PARTIAL ALBINISM.—This is usually inherited as a dominant character although the condition may be seen in children of normal parents. In one typical piebald child (Fig. 27–30) born at the Chicago Lying-in Hospital the parents and siblings were normal. The child was also normal except for the

presence of large irregular patches of skin devoid of pigment. A white forelock, which is often accompanied by mild white spotting of the skin, is also generally inherited as a dominant character. Males seem to be affected more often and transmission is often from father to son. Albinism of the eye alone is associated with albinism in the fundus, hypoplasia of the macula, nystagmus, head-nodding and amblyopia. It is ordinarily transmitted as a sex-linked recessive character, with maternal carriers transmitting it to sons.

INCONTINENTIA PIGMENTI (BLOCK-SULZBERGER SYNDROME).—This is an unusual family affliction that has been reported almost exclusively in females but without a definitely determined mode of inheritance. Before or shortly after birth multiple linearly distributed vesicles appear on the scalp, arms, legs or trunk. They involve the granular layer of the epithelium over areas infiltrated with eosinophils and lymphocytes. Some develop into bullae and others become pigmented and crusted before the end of the 1st week. Pigment is centered in the dendritic layer, and keratotic plugging of sweat glands is common. Lesions eventually heal, leaving affected areas permanently hyperpigmented.

URTICARIA PIGMENTOSA (MAST CELL DISEASE).—In this disease bullous or nodular lesions associated with focal or diffuse infiltration of mast cells in the skin appear in infants, usually before 6 months of age (Fig. 27–31). They may be preceded by a pink macular rash and fever; later, plaques may develop in the dermis. The lesions consist of masses of mast cells located on the upper part of the dermis with overlying epidermis normal except for increased melanin in the basal layers. The cells are often spindle shaped and their identity may not be appreciated without a Giemsa stain to demonstrate the presence of metachromatic granules. When discrete, the lesions usually disappear in childhood.

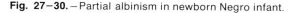

Fig. 27–30.—Partial albinism in newborn Negro infant.

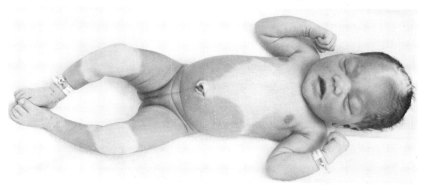

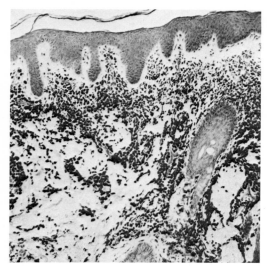

Fig. 27–31.—Urticaria pigmentosa. Photomicrograph showing the localized infiltration of mast cells which have a metachromatic reaction with thiazine dyes. (Courtesy Dr. G. Vawter.)

When diffuse, they may persist throughout life, the disease may be generalized and the liver, spleen and bone marrow may become involved. Leukemia may eventually develop (Ellis; Rider *et al.;* Waters and Lacson).

MONGOLIAN SPOTS.—These are gray-blue areas 1–3 cm in diameter, present in the midline over the sacrum in a large proportion of Oriental infants and occasionally in those of other races. In non-Orientals they are most common in the children of dark-skinned parents. The color comes from melanoblasts in the corium. The spots generally disappear during childhood.

PIGMENTED NEVI.—See page 186.

Malformations of the Skin and its Appendages

DERMATOLYSIS (LOOSE OR PENDULOUS SKIN).—This is a malformation of the skin that may be present at birth or may not be visible until later life. Often related to Recklinghausen's disease, it is characterized by hypertrophy or looseness of the skin. In most cases in which lax skin can be diagnosed at birth, the neck is the region of principal involvement. Rarely, the skin over the entire body at birth seems too loose for the underlying structures. The muscles and connective tissue seem shrunken, and it may be possible that fluid or actual tissue loss has taken place before birth. When the infant begins to gain weight, the laxness generally disappears. It is common in infants with renal agenesis and is sometimes associated with postmature birth. This condition is not inherited.

DERMATORRHEXIS (EHLERS-DANLOS SYNDROME).—In this condition both skin and joints are hyperextensible. The overelasticity of the skin has its origin in a decrease in the amount of elastic tissue and a thinning of the dermis. The staining properties of both the elastic tissue and the collagen are normal (Wechsler and Fisher). Capillaries, veins and arteries are increased in the dermis, and profuse hemorrhage may follow minor trauma because of the poor support provided by the connective tissue. Nodules and pseudotumors are present in the subcutaneous tissue because of herniation of subcutaneous fat through the thinned dermis. If not stretched beyond the elastic limit or the full stretch of the collagen bundles, the skin and joints return to normal positions when released. Later in life, because of the connective tissue defects, diaphragmatic hernia, visceral diverticulae, aortic aneurysm or megaesophagus may develop. Tissues are easily injured, and visceral hemorrhage and postpartum uterine hemorrhage have been described. Associated malformations include widely spaced prominent eyes and tetralogy of Fallot. The condition is transmitted in an autosomal dominant manner.

CUTIS LAXA.—This rare disease, also present at birth, has many features in common with the Ehlers-Danlos syndrome, but the joints are not involved. The skin, as the name implies, is loose and droops in folds, especially about the eyelids, where it leads to ectropion. It may be accompanied by pulmonary emphysema, dilatation and hypertrophy of the heart, and dilatation of the pulmonary artery with cardiac failure. Diverticulae may form early in the upper gastrointestinal tract (Goltz *et al.*). In contrast to the Ehlers-Danlos syndrome, the elastic tissue stains indistinctly and shows granular degeneration. The process is inherited as an autosomal recessive character, and a high degree of consanguinity among the parents has been reported.

HEREDITARY ECTODERMAL DYSPLASIA.—This involves the skin and appendages although the sweat glands may not be affected. In the *anhidrotic* form the sweat glands are absent or rudimentary, and both dermis and epidermis are abnormally thin. The scalp hair is soft and sparse, the eyebrows are absent, the eyelashes few, the internal nasal structures are dry and ozena is present; the teeth are hypoplastic, the nails are absent and the subcutaneous tissue is so sparse that the skin is easily picked up and folded on itself (Richards and Kaplan; Jespersen). By the age of 3 months the infant may resemble an old man. X-ray examination of the jaw may confirm the diagnosis by showing absence of tooth buds. The *hidrotic* form, in which the sweat glands are not affected, is inherited as an autosomal dominant character (Robinson *et al.*). Here, although the general findings are the same, the changes are less regular and there may be hyperkeratosis of palms and soles and hyperpigmentation of some parts of the body, especially the elbows, axillae and areolar area of the breasts.

FOCAL DERMAL HYPOPLASIA (GOLTZ SYNDROME). — This is an abnormality of the skin associated with a wide variety of malformations of other parts of the body (Goltz *et al.*; Holden and Akers). Some of the identifying skin changes may not be present at birth, but they include thinning of the dermis, hypo- and hyperpigmentation, telangiectasia, focal absence of skin appendages and herniation of the subcutaneous fat into the skin. The latter is secondary to the thinning of the dermis and the absence of the dermal elastic tissue. The nails are fissured, striated and atrophic. Associated anomalies may include those of bone — such as spina bifida, fused vertebrae, syndactyly and hypoplasia of the ribs — and those of the eye, such as microphthalmia, strabismus and coloboma. It is inherited as an autosomal recessive disorder.

CONGENITAL CUTANEOUS DYSTROPHY (ROTHMUND-THOMSON SYNDROME, POIKILODERMA CONGENITALE). — A recessively inherited disease in which skin lesions and congenital cataracts were outstanding symptoms was described over 100 years ago by Rothmund. Considerably later, Thomson observed similar skin lesions, usually in individuals with other abnormalities but without cataracts, and subsequent investigators have combined the two names to designate this disease. The skin lesions begin near the middle of the 1st year as a network of fine red lines separating areas of normal skin over part or all of the body. The red lines gradually widen, reducing the amount of normal skin. As the child grows older, the involved skin becomes irregularly atrophic, hyperkeratotic and pigmented. In about half of the patients cataracts begin suddenly at 4–6 years of age. They spread rapidly and involve the entire lens in a few days. The other abnormalities described have been variable and the majority have been present in only a few cases. They include alopecia, defective teeth and nails, minor skeletal malformations and hypergonadism.

GYRATE OR CONVOLUTED SKIN. — The skin in this congenital anomaly resembles the convolutions of the brain. The thick ridges separated by irregular linear depressions are caused by an overgrowth of underlying connective tissue. The skin over the vertex of the skull is most often involved, but the anomaly has been described in other areas. In a similar condition involving the anterior abdominal wall, known as the "prune-belly" syndrome (Williams and Burkholder), it is commonly associated with absence or hypoplasia of muscle of the anterior abdominal wall and often accompanied by megaloureter, megalocystis, a distended urachus and renal hypoplasia. In one such case observed at the Chicago Lying-in Hospital there was an accompanying intrauterine amputation, and pressure from protruding bones had produced a fistulous opening through the abdominal wall. It was thought possible that an excessive amount of fluid in the abdominal cavity had escaped and been responsible for the rugose appearance of the skin (see Fig. 25–90).

COCKAYNE SYNDROME. — This shares some features with the Rothmund-Thomson syndrome. Affected infants may develop photodermatitis as early as 6 months of age (Paddison *et al.*); in the skin the stratum spinosum may be thin, without formation of rete pegs but with an overlying hyperkeratotic and parakeratotic layer. Liquefactive degeneration may be present in the basal layer, and the dermis contains many chronic inflammatory cells. The papillae may be edematous, and the superficial vessels may show degenerative changes. Associated skeletal anomalies include small stature with kyphoscoliosis, long extremities with large hands and feet, and a thickened skull. Neural abnormalities include optic atrophy, retinal degeneration, partial deafness and mental retardation. Transmission of this syndrome is autosomal recessive.

LOCAL HYPOPLASIA OR ABSENCE OF SKIN. — Seemingly excavated areas of various sizes may be found on the surface of the body as a result of local absence of subcutaneous tissue and muscle. In some instances they are covered by a thin layer of abnormal skin that appears to be entirely unkeratinized (Fig. 27–32). At other times there is no skin covering (Fig. 27–33). They may be present on any part of the body and are always followed by scarring (Fig. 27–34). The most common site is the vertex of the head in the region of the hair swirl. There they are generally round, have sharp punched-out margins and measure 1–1.5 cm in diameter (Fig. 27–35). The lesion may be limited to the skin, but more often the subcutaneous tissues are also absent. Rarely, it extends through the skull, exposing the

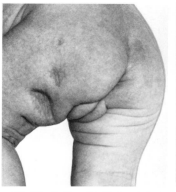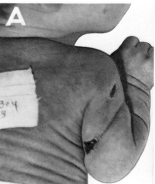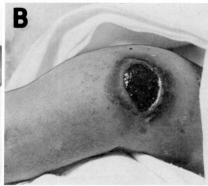

Fig. 27–32 (left).—Multiple defects of subcutaneous connective tissue and muscle covered by a thin transparent layer of epithelium. Infant aged 1 day.

Fig. 27–33 (right).—Multiple areas on body surface in which skin and connective tissue are lacking. Largest defects are on the right arm **(A)** and left knee **(B).**

brain (Fig. 27–36). When the skin alone is absent, the surface ordinarily heals, leaving a hairless scarred area. Infrequently the lesions spread and require skin grafting and even then are sometimes difficult to heal. In one form described by Bart *et al.*

Fig. 27–34.—Defect of skin of anterior body surface at level of the costal margin. **A,** infant aged 1 day. **B,** same child at age 22 months with scar in region of original skin defect. (Courtesy Dr. Rustin McIntosh.)

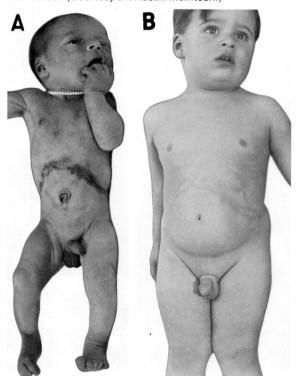

the process is inherited as an autosomal dominant character with complete penetrance. In Bart's case the lower extremities were involved and, besides the areas of absent skin, which had healed by 2 months after birth, there was an absence of toenails. Absence of the scalp may be found with 13 trisomy.

In the older literature such skin defects were frequently reported as being secondary to adhesions

Fig. 27–35.—Skin defect extending through the subcutaneous tissue, present at birth. The location at the vertex is the most common site of such an abnormality.

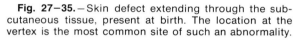

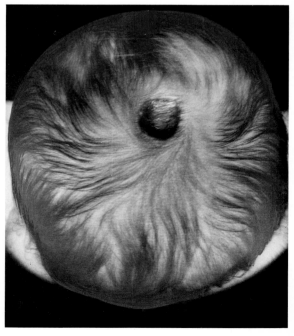

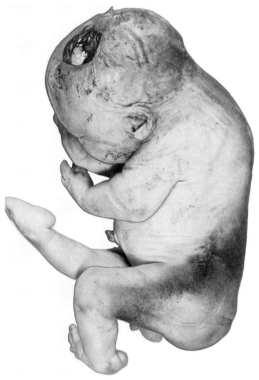

Fig. 27–36.—Defect in the parietal region extending through the skull and exposing the brain. The infant was delivered from a breech presentation, and the ecchymoses in the skin in the area where the cervical ring came in contact with the buttocks are well shown. Respiration never established. (Courtesy Dr. T. R. Brown.)

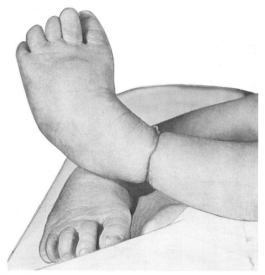

Fig. 27–37.—Unilateral cicatrix associated with bilateral clubfoot. Infant 3 days old.

between the amnion and the body surface caused by infection of the amnion. Growth of the fetus was believed to elongate the adhesions into bands called Simonart's ligaments. The defect was then explained as an evulsion of tissue at the point of attachment occurring during delivery. This explanation would seem untenable for many reasons. The edges of the lesions show no evidence of fragmented tissue that would represent the frayed edge of a torn adhesion. When adhesions between the amnion and a part of the fetus exist, the part of the fetus to which they are attached is usually drawn outward in a funnel-like projection or a definite papilloma.

CICATRICES.—Linear constrictions may encircle one or more extremities at any level but are most common on the forearm, leg or digits. The appearance in general is as if a thread had been tied so tightly around the affected part that it is hidden from sight by the bulging upward of tissue on both sides. When located on the leg, the foot is always clubbed (Fig. 27–37). When the digits are involved, the constricted areas are usually multiple, and parts of the phalanges may be abnormal or missing (Fig. 27–38). Their possible etiology and relation to exogenous amputations are discussed on page 596.

AMNIOTIC BANDS.—Connections between parts of the body of the fetus and amnion are rarely found at term, but they are not uncommon in fetuses aborted in the early months of pregnancy (Fig. 27–

Fig. 27–38.—Symbrachydactyly. Hands of infant 10 months of age showing multiple abnormalities of the digits including cicatrices and syndactyly.

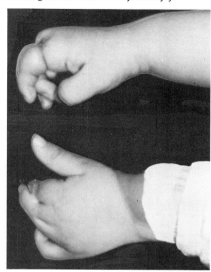

39). They may be fine threadlike strands extending between the fetus and an apparently normal amnion, or the amnion may be drawn up off the chorion in an elongated funnel-like shape with the apex attached to the body, head or ends of digits (see Fig. 3–54). During the first weeks of life the amnion closely surrounds the embryo, and it is possible that on rare occasions a local cellular abnormality exists that permits the amnion to adhere to the embryo. At that time the extremities protrude at right angles from the body and, together with the head, come into closer contact with the amnion than other parts of the body.

The umbilical cord may be twisted many times around the strands extending from fetus to amnion and may cause death by interference with circulation through the cord.

SKIN PITS. — These are similar to cicatrices except that only a single point is involved instead of a linear area. They are limited largely to the face and the anterior surface of the legs. Those on the face are most common immediately in front of the ear, although they may occur on the upper lip, chin or cheeks. Those related to the ear are often hereditary. They have no clinical significance.

Pits on the anterior surface of the leg are commonly associated with absence of the fibula (see Fig. 25–84). They have also been observed in association with prenatal bowing of the tibia. In the latter condition it has been suggested that pressure of the uterus against the legs is responsible for the change in shape and that pressure over the most protruberant part is sufficient to cause the pitting. This does not seem a satisfactory explanation.

Skin pits over the spine usually extend into the spinal canal and are known as dermal sinuses (see Fig. 24–71). Slightly larger pits located over the sacrum are called pilonidal sinuses and are rarely connected with the spine.

ALOPECIA. — Complete absence of hair follicles is rare as an isolated malformation. Absence or abnormalities of the teeth and nails are usually associated with it and are part of several syndromes described elsewhere. Sebaceous and sweat glands may also be absent but, if present, open directly onto the skin.

HYPERTRICHOSIS. — The presence of an excessive number of follicles from which coarse hairs arise is much more common than a lack of hair follicles. In the children of dark-skinned parents it is not rare to see dark hairs covering most of the forehead, sides of the face, shoulders, arms and back; except for length, they are similar to those on the head. They may be shed during infancy or persist throughout life.

MALFORMATIONS OF THE NAILS. — Congenital abnormalities of the nails include aplasia, hypoplasia, ridging and abnormalities in thickness and shape. All nails may be involved, or the disturbance may be limited to fingers or toes or occasionally to single digits. Many disturbances are inherited, usually as autosomal dominant characters. The genes responsible for such conditions are usually of low expressivity, and a considerable range in the degree of involvement is found in different members of the same family. Abnormalities of the teeth are sometimes associated (hereditary ectodermal dysplasia). Nails are fused into a single band in the syndactyly that is part of the *acrocephalosyndactyly syndrome* (see Fig. 25–29).

Fig. 27–39.—**A,** multiple cicatrices of digits with attachment of terminal portions to the amniotic sac. Fetus of 10 weeks' gestation. **B,** partial fusion and malformation of digits associated with amniotic adhesions in mature infant who was a sibling of the abortus whose hands are shown in **A.**

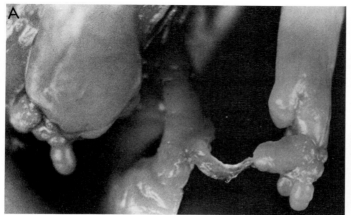
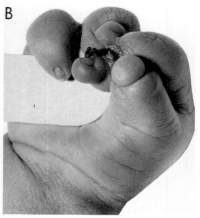

Nails, especially those of the thumb and index finger, are partially or entirely absent or thin and grooved in *osteonychodysplasia* (nail-patella syndrome); nails of the toes are seldom involved. Absence or hypoplasia of the patellas and partial fixation of the elbows are associated abnormalities. Since the condition is inherited as an autosomal dominant character with pleiotropic effects, many additional disturbances have been described, the most common of which are iliac horns and renal nephropathy.

PAPILLOMAS. — Papillomas may be found at birth as localized outgrowths of skin and connective tissue. They may be present on any part of the body but are most common on the side of the face in front of the ear, where they arise by anomalous growth of tissue surrounding the first branchial cleft (Fig. 27–40). The ear is also often abnormal in shape. In one infant observed at the Chicago Lying-in Hospital multiple papillomas resulted from adhesions attaching the skin to the amnion. The amnion enclosed only the upper half of the fetus and, where it encircled the waist, had caused papillomatous elevations of several areas (Fig. 27–41).

FIBROUS HAMARTOMA OF INFANCY. — Under this term Enzinger described poorly circumscribed, rapidly infiltrating tumors of the dermis and subcutaneous tissue, present at birth or appearing in the

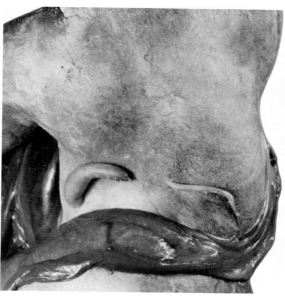

Fig. 27—41. — Papillomas of skin resulting from attachment of skin to edge of amniotic sac. An omphalocele was present, and the placenta was attached to the anterior abdominal wall. Half of the body developed outside the amniotic sac, and localized portions of skin were attached to the margin that encircled the waist.

1st year of life (average age 5½ months), which occurred almost exclusively in males. Most frequent in the region of the shoulder, axilla and upper arm, they consisted of loosely arranged cellular connective tissue and fat. Some lesions spread or recurred locally following removal, but distant metastases did not occur.

Fig. 27—40. — Papillomas of the skin located in the line where the maxillomandibular process closes to form the buccal cavity.

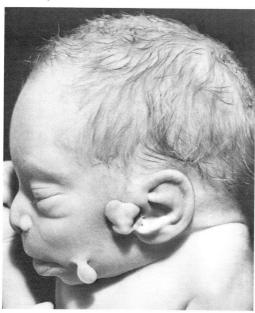

REFERENCES

Barker, L. P., Gross, P., and McCarthy, J. Y.: Erythrodermas of infancy, Arch. Dermatol. 77:201, 1958.

Bart, B. J., *et al.*: Congenital localized absence of skin and associated abnormalities resembling epidermolysis bullosa, Arch. Dermatol. 93:296, 1966.

Beare, M.: Toxic epidermal necrolysis, Arch. Dermatol. 86:638, 1962.

Becker, S. W., and Brunschwig, A.: Sinus preauricularis, Am. J. Surg. 24:174, 1934.

Bergenholtz, A., and Olsson, O.: Epidermolysis bullosa hereditaria letalis, Acta Derm. Venereol. 48:220, 1968.

Bloom, D., and Goodfried, M. S.: Lamellar ichthyosis of the newborn, Arch. Dermatol. 86:336, 1962.

Cockayne, E. A.: *Inherited Abnormalities of the Skin and Appendages* (New York: Oxford University Press, 1933).

Cooperstock, M.: Congenital enlargement of the extremities, Am. J. Dis. Child. 57:309, 1939.

Craig, J. M., Goldsmith, L., and Baden, H.: An abnormality of keratin in the harlequin fetus, Pediatrics 46:437, 1970.

Eagle, J. F., and Barrett, J. S.: Congenital deficiency of abdominal musculature with associated genito-urinary abnormalities, Pediatrics 6:721, 1950.

Ellis, J. M.: Urticaria pigmentosa, Arch. Pathol. 48:426, 1949.

Emery, J. L., and Gordon, R. R.: Persistence of foetal periderm and Zenker's degeneration of muscle in full term infant, J. Pathol. Bacteriol. 71:231, 1956.

Enzinger, F. M.: Fibrous hamartoma of infancy, Cancer 18:241, 1965.

Finlay, V. L., and Pound, J. P.: Collodion skin in neonate due to lamellar ichthyosis, Arch. Dis. Child. 27:438, 1952.

Fraser, J. E.: The pathology of congenital syphilis, Arch. Dermatol. Syph. 1:491, 1920.

Freeman, R. G., Spiller, R., and Knox, J. M.: Histopathology of erythema toxicum neonatorum, Arch. Dermatol. 82:586, 1960.

Freud, P., Rhodes, A. W., and Weisz, A.: Hereditary skin defect in newborn infant, J. Pediatr. 27:591, 1945.

Goltz, R. W., et al.: Cutaneous laxa, Arch. Dermatol. 92:373, 1965.

Goltz, R. W., et al.: Focal dermal hypoplasia, Am. J. Dis. Child. 86:708, 1962.

Hess, J. H., and Schultz, O. T.: Keratosis diffusa fetalis (ichthyosis congenita), Am. J. Dis. Child. 21:357, 1921.

Holden, J. D., and Akers, W. A.: Goltz syndrome: Focal dermal hypoplasia; combined mesodermal dysplasia, Am. J. Dis. Child. 114:292, 1967.

Horsefield, G. I., and Yardley, H. J.: Sclerema neonatorum, J. Invest. Dermatol. 44:326, 1965.

Hughes, W. E., and Hammond, M. L.: Sclerema neonatorum, J. Pediatr. 32:676, 1948.

Janssen, T. A. E., and de Lange, C.: Familial congenital hypertrichosis totalis (trichostasis), Acta Paediatr. Scand. 33:69, 1945.

Jespersen, H. G.: Hereditary ectodermal dysplasia of anhidrotic type. Report of 3 cases in boys aged 3–4 months, Acta Paediatr. Scand. 51:712, 1962.

Katzenellenbogen, I., and Loron, Z.: A contribution to Bloom's syndrome, Arch. Dermatol. 82:609, 1960.

Killum, R. E., Roy, T. L., and Brown, G. R.: Sclerema neonatorum, Arch. Dermatol. 58:372, 1968.

Klaus, S. W., and Winkelmann, R. K.: Course of urticaria pigmentosa in children, Arch. Dermatol. 86:68, 1962.

Lamb, J. H., and Halpert, B.: Epidermolysis bullosa of the newborn, Arch. Dermatol. Syph. 55:369, 1947.

Lantes, S. H., and Hoblenzer, P. J.: Solitary mast cell tumor, Am. J. Dis. Child. 99:60, 1969.

Lewis, I. C., Stevens, E. M., and Farquhar, J. W.: Epidermolysis bullosa in newborn, Arch. Dis. Child. 30:277, 1955.

Luders, D.: Histologic observation in erythema toxicum neonatorum, Pediatrics 26:219, 1960.

Lyell, A., Dick, H. M., and Alexander, J.: Outbreak of toxic epidermal necrolysis associated with staphylococcus, Lancet 1:789, 1969.

Margileth, A. M.: Acrodermatitis enteropathica; case report and review of the literature, Am. J. Dis. Child. 105:285, 1963.

Mason, P. D., and Allen, E. V.: Congenital lymphangiectasis (lymphedema)., Am. J. Dis. Child. 50:945, 1935.

McIntosh, J. F., Waugh, T. R., and Ross, S. G.: Sclerema neonatorum (subcutaneous fat necrosis), Am. J. Dis. Child. 55:112, 1938.

Miller, R. C., and Shapiro, L.: Bullous urticarial pigmentosa in infancy, Arch. Dermatol. 91:595, 1965.

Nix, T. E., Jr., Kloepfer, H. W., and Derbes, V. J.: Ichthyosis—lamellar exfoliative type, Dermatol. Trop. 2:142, 1963.

Paddison, R. M., Moosy, J., Dirkes, V. J., and Koepfer, H. W.: Cockayne's syndrome, Dermatol. Trop. 2:195, 1963.

Pers, M.: Congenital absence of skin: Pathogenesis and relation to ring construction, Acta Chir. Scand. 126:388, 1963.

Potter, E. L.: Universal edema of the fetus unassociated with erythroblastosis, Am. J. Obstet. Gynecol. 46:130, 1943.

Prose, P. H., and Sedlis, E.: Morphologic and histochemical studies of atopic eczema in infants and children, J. Invest. Dermatol. 34:149, 1960.

Richards, W., and Kaplan, J. M.: Anhidrotic ectodermal dysplasia, Am. J. Dis. Child. 117:597, 1969.

Rider, T. L., Stern, A. A., and Abbuhl, J. W.: Generalized mast cell disease and urticaria pigmentosa, Pediatrics 19:1203, 1957.

Robinson, G. C., Miller, J. R., and Bensimon, J. R.: Familial ectodermal dysplasia with sensorineural deafness and other anomalies, Pediatrics 30:797, 1962.

Rook, A., and Whimster, I.: Congenital cutaneous dystrophy (Thomson's type), Br. J. Dermatol. 61:197, 1949.

Rostenberg, A. J., and Solomon, L. M.: Infantile eczema and systemic disease, Arch. Dermatol. 98:41, 1968.

Rubin, L., and Becker, S. W.: Pigmentation in Block-Sulzberger syndrome (incontinentia pigmenti), Arch. Dermatol. 74:263, 1956.

Rudberg, S.: Cutis gyrata with unusual localization, Acta Paediatr. Scand. 27:67, 1939.

Scott, O. L. S., and Stone, D. G. H.: Lamellar degeneration of the newborn—"collodion baby," Br. J. Dermatol. 67:189, 1955.

Shear, C. S., et al.: Syndrome of unilateral ectromelia, psoriasis and nervous system anomalies, Birth Defects 7:197, 1971.

Silver, H. K.: Rothmund-Thomson syndrome: An oculocutaneous disorder, Am. J. Dis. Child. 111:182, 1966.

Sweetman, W. P., Barlow, A. J. E., and Dennis, R. G.: Intrapartum toxic epidermal necrolysis, Arch. Dis. Child. 37:517, 1964.

Thompson, C. J.: Pathology of fetal maceration, J. Obstet. Gynaecol. Br. Commonw. 34:40, 1927.

Waters, W. J., and Lacson, P. S.: Mast cell leukemia presenting as urticaria pigmentosa, Pediatrics 19:1033, 1957.

Wechsler, H. L., and Fisher, E. R.: Ehlers-Danlos syndrome, Arch. Pathol. 77:613, 1964.

Wells, R. S., and Kerr, C. B.: Genetic classification of ichthyosis, Arch. Dermatol. 92:1, 1965.

Werwick, W. J., Ruttenberg, H. D., and Quie, P. G.: Sclerema neonatorum—a sign not a disease, J.A.M.A. 184:680, 1963.

Williams, P. I., and Burkholder, G. V.: The prune belly syndrome, J. Urol. 98:244, 1967.

Zeek, P., and Madden, E. M.: Sclerema adiposum neonatorum of both internal and external adipose tissue, Arch. Pathol. 41:166, 1946.

28

Blood

Development

THE FIRST BLOOD CELLS appear either simultaneously with or slightly later than the first blood vessels in the yolk sac mesoderm of the presomite embryo of about 19 days. They are hemocytoblasts, many of which soon differentiate into hemoglobin-filled primitive megaloblasts while a few become histiocytes. A few hemocytoblasts are also formed in the body stalk, and some observers have reported an origin in the mesoderm of the embryo and in chorionic vessels apart from the body stalk. Cell development continues by mitosis of primitive cells, largely within the blood vessels. The first cells that can be identified as belonging to the erythrocyte series are known as primitive or primary erythroblasts. They have vesicular nuclei and abundant hemoglobin-filled cytoplasm and are much larger than the cells of the secondary or definitive series that appear slightly later. Only the cells of the definitive series are present in later fetal life and after birth. The terms megalobast and normoblast are also used for the nucleated cells of the primitive and definitive cell lines; when the nuclei disappear, the cells are known as megalocytes and normocytes (FIG. 28–1).

In embryos of 10–12 mm, erythroblasts of the definitive series appear for the first time in the yolk sac and the liver. Blood cell formation continues for only a short time in the yolk sac but constantly increases in the liver; this soon becomes the major source of red blood cells and remains so until near the end of fetal life. The cells, which come from free hemocytoblasts budded off the mesenchyme lining the sinusoids of the liver, are intravascular. Beginning at about the 70 mm stage and persisting through most of fetal life, small numbers of red cells are formed in the pulp and later in the sinuses of the spleen. They are also formed in the early

part of fetal life in small numbers in the loose connective tissue around blood vessels, in the connective tissue of the thymus and lymph nodes and sometimes in the intertubular connective tissue of the kidney.

According to Gilmour, definitive red cells are

Fig. 28–1.—Blood smear from normal fetus of 8 weeks' gestation measuring 3 cm in length and weighing 3.1 gm. Most of the nucleated cells are megaloblasts. Non-nucleated cells are an intermixture of megalocytes and normocytes. One megaloblast is in mitosis.

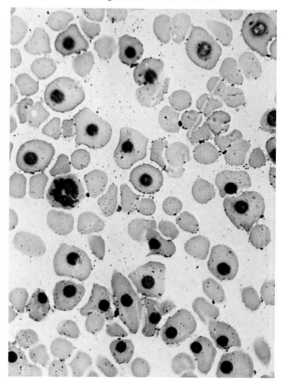

present in small numbers in the circulation of 28–35 mm embryos, are almost as numerous as the primitive cells in 48 mm embryos and are the only variety of red blood cell found in embryos of 65 mm or more.

The clavicle is the first cartilaginous mass in the body to become converted into bone and is the first site of marrow erythropoiesis. Blood formation begins here in the fetus of about 40 mm and spreads rapidly to other bones. Only late in fetal life is the marrow the major site of erythropoiesis.

Polymorphonuclear leukocytes are first formed at about the 20 mm stage in the liver, the connective tissue of the meninges, mesentery and stroma of lymph plexuses. They are subsequently formed in the parenchyma and portal areas of the liver, in the bone marrow and in small numbers in the adventitia of some arteries, in the septa of the thymus and in the spleen. All leukocyte formation is extravascular.

Lymphoid cells were identified by Matsumura and colleagues in the mesentery as early as the 8th week of gestation and about 1 week later in the thymus. At 10 weeks these cells were first seen in the peripheral circulation. The tonsils contained lymphocytes at 14 weeks but in the appendix or spleen they were not seen until 17 weeks. Gitlin pointed out that gamma globulin can be synthesized by 10 weeks before the appendix is populated with lymphoid cells, suggesting that humoral antibody-producing cells do not necessarily have to reside in the cecal area before they acquire activity, as appears to be true in some species.

One group of lymphocytes is believed to arise in bone marrow and reticular tissue and to disseminate to the rest of the body after having passed through the thymus. These cells, designated long-lived (T) lymphocytes, are concerned with cell-mediated immunity and hypersensitivity reactions. The lymphocytes concerned with gamma globulin production appear to populate the lymphoid structures without a sojourn in the thymus. In certain species the latter cells come from a portion of the lymphoid apparatus of the cecal area, but such an origin is not certain in man (Craddock *et al.;* Cooper *et al.*).

By the time of birth, erythropoiesis has largely disappeared from the liver, and within 4 or 5 days erythrocytes, granular leukocytes and platelets are normally formed only in the bone marrow. The lymphocytes of the blood come from the lymphoid tissues in the body—the malpighian corpuscles of the spleen, lymph nodes, tonsils and lymphoid follicles of the intestines. Germinal centers of lymph nodes and malpighian corpuscles are not present until after birth. The large cells at the periphery of the germinal centers are assumed to be the progenitors of lymphocytes in postnatal life.

Cells in many parts of the body that under normal conditions are not called upon to produce blood cells have hemopoietic potentialities and under abnormal stimuli readily respond to a demand for such cells. This is more true in fetal life than at any other time, and widespread hemopoiesis may be present at birth. It is ordinarily in the region of blood vessels, described by Maximow as the site of totipotential cells, that hemopoiesis is greatest. The excessive production of erythrocytes in severe cases of erythroblastosis is one of the best examples of response to abnormal stimuli. Congenital leukemia is a rare but striking example of abnormal leukocyte formation. Milder degrees of hemopoiesis may be found around the blood vessels in the pancreas, thymus, general connective tissue or other areas as a result of infection or from unknown cause.

The cellular constituents of the blood at the time of birth (umbilical cord blood) show little variation in relation to the weight of the fetus, and after the period of viability is reached (28–30 weeks and 1,000–2,000 gm), the blood of all infants is remarkably similar. The red cells are somewhat larger than those of adult blood, averaging $7-9$ μ in diameter, and appear to be more spherical than they are a little later. They are well filled with hemoglobin, which can be differentiated from that of the adult by its greater resistance to the denaturing effect of alkali or salicylate and lesser resistance to urea. Fetal hemoglobin is more nearly saturated at low oxygen tensions than is adult hemoglobin, and this facilitates transfer of oxygen from maternal to fetal blood. Walker and Turnbull gave values for fetal hemoglobin in the fetus and newborn infant that showed a gradual replacement of fetal hemoglobin by adult hemoglobin as gestation progresses, but in mature newborn infants as much as 70–80% of the hemoglobin is still of the fetal type.

The number of histologically immature red cells in the blood of a mature fetus is relatively small. About 1–2% are reticulocytes, and not more than 5% of all nucleated cells are red blood cells. In many newborn infants the peripheral blood contains no nucleated red cells. In a study made at the Chicago Lying-in Hospital 70% of 244 normal infants had no immature red blood cells on the 1st day of life and 99.6% had none on the 8th day.

Nucleated white blood cells often appear slightly less mature at birth than in later infancy. Most of the lymphocytes are large, easily distorted cells with pale nuclei and abundant cytoplasm. Granulocytes often have less well-defined lobules.

After birth the concentration of the blood cells and the hemoglobin vary slightly in relation to the time of interruption of blood flow from the placenta. When the cord is not clamped until after it stops pulsating, the infant obtains 50–100 ml of blood of which it is otherwise deprived. Concentration of blood cells in those infants receiving a large share of placental blood is moderately higher during the first few days of life than in those whose cord is cut immediately after delivery, but no difference can be demonstrated by the end of a month. The blood volume after birth is approximately 100 ml/kg of body weight; this varies a little, depending on how much placental blood the infant received.

In most of the 244 infants in whom studies were carried out at the Chicago Lying-in Hospital, the cord was clamped before pulsation had stopped or was stripped before clamping. In the first 24 hours the average hemoglobin content of the blood obtained by heel puncture was 20.7 gm. By the 8th day it had fallen to 18.4 gm. Erythrocytes on the 1st day averaged 6,190,000 cells and on the 8th day 5,470,000. Leukocytes varied from an average of 19,540 on the 1st day to 11,560 on the 8th day. On the 1st day polymorphonuclear leukocytes made up 70.9% of the white blood cells and on the 8th day only 49.2%. These figures with the normal variations are given in Table 28–1. The same study showed that the value for hemoglobin in cord blood

averages about 2 gm less than that for venous blood obtained by jugular puncture soon after birth, and the latter, in turn, is about 2 gm lower than in capillary blood obtained by heel puncture.

These figures for erythrocytes and hemoglobin are slightly higher than the averages given by Smith, who obtained his data by averaging several reports; his averages were 5,640,000 erythrocytes and 19.85 gm of hemoglobin on the 1st day of life. Venous blood invariably has a lower concentration of cells, and in Smith's data the erythrocytes averaged 4,800,000 and hemoglobin 17 gm in cord blood or venous blood obtained during the 1st day. Walker and Turnbull reported even lower levels at 40 weeks, with a mean of 16.5 gm and a range of 15–18.6 gm. They thought that a decrease in oxygen supply causes an increase in red blood cells, that the normal hemoglobin level of cord blood should be 14.8 gm with a red cell count of 4,000,000 and that the higher the level above this, the more depressed the oxygen supply must have been before birth.

The serum protein of the newborn is slightly less than that of the adult, the greatest difference being in the globulin fraction. The majority of healthy mature newborn infants have a total protein value between 5 and 6 gm%. The average (cord blood) for 30 such infants in the Chicago Lying-in Hospital laboratory was 5.6 gm%. Protein content rises progressively during intrauterine life, with the globulin fraction developing at a somewhat slower rate than the albumin fraction. Darrow and Carry reported total protein at birth in infants weighing over 2,500 gm as 5.6 gm with 3.7 gm albumin and 1.9 gm globulin. Average levels for premature infants were 4.9 gm total protein with 3.6 gm albumin and 1.3 gm globulin.

The youngest fetus whose protein values were determined at the Chicago Lying-in Hospital weighed 54 gm. Total proteins were 2.84 gm with albumin 2.39 and globulin 0.45 gm.

Icterus

Destruction of erythrocytes occurs normally by disintegration in the bloodstream followed by reticuloendothelial phagocytosis. The hemoglobin molecule is split into globin and hematin. The latter is further fragmented into iron, which is reused or stored, and bilirubin, which is excreted by the liver. The newly formed bilirubin is bound to the albumin and carried in the plasma, where it gives an indirect bilirubin reaction. In the liver indirect-reacting bilirubin is conjugated with glucuronic acid by the

TABLE 28–1.—BLOOD FINDINGS IN 244 NORMAL INFANTS (POTTER AND BERNSTEIN)

	MEAN	RANGE
Hemoglobin (gm)		
1st day	20.7	15.2 to 26.2
8th or 9th day	18.4	13.5 to 23.3
Hemoglobin variation		
1st to 8th day	2.6	+1.6 to −6.8
Erythrocytes (millions)		
1st day	6.19	4.33 to 8.05
8th day	5.47	3.93 to 7.01
Erythrocyte variation		
1st to 8th day	0.80	+0.58 to 2.18
Leukocytes (total)		
1st day	19,540	6,980 to 32,100
8th day	11,500	5,840 to 17,280
Percentage of polymorpho- nuclear leukocytes to total leukocytes		
1st day	70.9	53.7 to 88.1
8th day	49.2	27.9 to 70.5

action of glucuronyl transferase and uridine diphosphate-glucuronic acid dehydrogenase to form the more soluble bilirubin glucuronide. This enters the bile and is excreted into the intestinal tract, where it is changed to urobilinogen. This is eliminated in the feces or urine or is resorbed to be excreted in the bile again.

When excessive numbers of red blood cells are destroyed, the liver may be unable to conjugate the total amount of indirect-reacting bilirubin presented to it, and part will then accumulate in the serum. If some of the excess is satisfactorily conjugated, abnormally large amounts may be found in stools and urine. Urinary urobilinogen may also be increased when hepatic function is depressed even though the rate of cell destruction is normal.

If excretion of bilirubin is blocked beyond the point at which bilirubin glucuronide is formed, it may be regurgitated into the blood, where it will give a direct reaction. If none reaches the intestine, urobilinogen will be absent from feces and urine.

Jaundice may be a result of four different conditions: (1) excessive destruction of blood cells with the liver normally able to metabolize and excrete bilirubin, (2) excessive destruction with the liver unable to metabolize or eliminate all bilirubin, (3) normal rate of cell destruction with depressed liver function and (4) normal rate of cell destruction but interference with passage of bile into the intestinal tract.

When destruction of erythrocytes is excessive, some degree of bilirubinemia results; the bilirubin is largely indirect-reacting as long as the liver is able to eliminate all of the bilirubin it can conjugate. The liver cells contain excessive amounts of iron but no demonstrable bile, and canaliculi are not distended. Jaundice results from increase in indirect serum bilirubin. The feces and urine contain large amounts of bile pigment, and hemoglobinemia and hemoglobinuria may occur. The spleen and, to a lesser degree, the liver enlarge as a result of the increased activity of the reticuloendothelium. Compensatory erythropoiesis occurs first by excessive production of cells in normal locations (before birth principally in the liver, after birth principally in bone marrow) and, when the stimulus is greater, by production in abnormal areas (spleen, kidney and periarteriolar areas in any part of the body). Reticulocytes increase and nucleated forms appear in peripheral blood. When the liver is unable to excrete completely all conjugated bilirubin, it is reabsorbed into the blood, and direct-reacting serum bilirubin is elevated. Bile pigment is usually visible in hepatic cells, and the bile canaliculi are

often distended. Urobilinogen in the feces is decreased although excessive amounts may be present in the urine. This may occur with a normal liver if cell destruction is very great, in which case both direct- and indirect-reacting bilirubin are elevated, or with an abnormal liver even with a normal rate of cell destruction, in which case only direct-reacting serum bilirubin is abnormally high.

When the liver is properly able to conjugate and eliminate into bile ducts all products of cell destruction, there remains the necessity for elimination into the intestine. Obstruction at any level causes reabsorption and elevation of direct-reacting serum bilirubin. Atresia or absence of extrahepatic ducts is responsible for distention of the bile ducts in a progressively retrograde manner, with smaller and smaller radicles becoming distended as the process is of longer and longer duration. Distention of the bile canaliculi is a late feature. Acute early obstruction may be unassociated with impaired liver function, but if the obstruction is of significant duration, liver function soon begins to deteriorate. This may be due to an increase in secretion pressure or secondary to descending infection.

Varying numbers of infants become jaundiced during the 1st week of life. Jaundice appearing in the first 24 hours is almost always pathologic and is an indication that an abnormal state existing before birth has been responsible for excessive erythrocyte destruction or for interference with liver function and the inhibition of conjugation of indirect to direct bilirubin. Indirect-reacting bilirubin in such infants is always abnormally high before birth, as is evident from an increased amount in cord blood, and were it not for the existence of unknown factors that prevent the development of visible jaundice before birth, such a child would be jaundiced when born. What proportion of bilirubin may be eliminated through the placenta in either normal or abnormal states is not known, but unless the mother herself has hyperbilirubinemia from some cause unrelated to the fetus, the bilirubin level in the cord blood is always higher than in the maternal blood. There is no specific level in cord blood that can be considered the upper limit of normal nor one that forms a dividing line between infants in whom jaundice can be expected to appear in the first 24 hours and those who will not become jaundiced. Allen and Diamond considered a cord blood level of 7 mg per 100 ml an indication for exchange transfusion in erythroblastotic infants, and evidence suggests that this level is probably not reached normally.

When jaundice first appears after 24 hours, it

may also be pathologic; it may become rapidly progressive and produce permanent brain damage within a few days. Consequently, any child who has any visible degree of jaundice during the newborn period should be carefully studied immediately. The recognizable causes of jaundice in the neonatal period include erythroblastosis due to Rh, AB or other incompatibility; infections including various bacterial, parasitic and viral agents, especially cytomegalic inclusion, herpes simplex, Coxsackie B and possibly infectious hepatitis viruses; certain congenital diseases of the blood such as those characterized by abnormal hemoglobin or enzyme deficiencies related to the maintenance of cell membrane structure; intracranial and intra-abdominal hemorrhage; poisoning from certain substances including antibiotics and vitamin K; congenital or extrahepatic bile duct atresia or absence; and so on.

PHYSIOLOGIC JAUNDICE. — Mild jaundice for which a specific cause cannot be found appears in many infants who seem otherwise normal. This is generally designated "physiologic jaundice" or "icterus neonatorum." Its reported incidence depends to some extent on the care with which the infants are examined. As many as 75% of all newborns have been stated to have some degree of jaundice, but in not more than about 25% does it ordinarily become readily visible. The higher the level of bilirubin in cord blood, the greater the likelihood that jaundice will appear. A study conducted at the Chicago Lying-in Hospital on 274 seemingly normal infants gave a mean total cord blood bilirubin level of 3.1 mg per 100 ml for infants who did not become jaundiced and 4.4 mg per 100 ml for those who did. In nearly all infants the serum bilirubin level rises after birth regardless of whether or not jaundice appears. The bilirubin level at birth seems to be about the same in both premature and mature infants: it rises a few milligrams promptly in mature infants and normally begins to fall by the 4th or 5th day; a greater, more prolonged rise is common in premature infants, with the maximum often occurring toward the end of the 1st week.

Whether "physiologic" hyperbilirubinemia is a result of temporarily increased hemolysis or of inadequate liver function has been argued for many years; at present it appears that both have a role although the latter seems to be the more important. Since hemoglobin and erythrocyte levels are higher at birth than in later infancy, it has been assumed that these were high before birth because of relative hypoxia and that after birth, when no longer needed, the cells were destroyed. Mollison and Cutbush demonstrated, however, that polycy-themia is not by itself responsible for cell destruction. They found that when a normal newborn infant was transfused with adult cells, they were destroyed at the rate of 1% a day even in the period of greatest polycythemia. When placental blood was given, they were destroyed at 2% a day for the first 10 days and at 1% a day thereafter. The conclusion was drawn that the cell population of the newborn is more variable than that of the adult and that some intrinsic character of the cells is responsible for the slightly greater rate of cell destruction in the 1st week of life.

Decrease in erythrocytes, however, is proportionately slower than rise in bilirubin, and it seems likely that temporary inability of the newborn liver to convert indirect- to direct-reacting bilirubin is largely responsible for the transient elevation of serum bilirubin. Probably due to a deficiency of glucuronyl transferase, one of the enzymes responsible for conversion of indirect-reacting bilirubin to the direct-reacting form, it is more marked in premature than in mature infants. Thus, an increase in indirect-reacting serum bilirubin can result either from breakdown of cells at a more rapid rate than a normally functioning liver can dispose of the end-products or from an inadequately functioning liver in the presence of a normal rate of cell destruction. In the majority of newborn infants, so-called physiologic jaundice seems to be due to a combination of mild degrees of both increased cell destruction and liver inadequacy. Almost any condition affecting a newborn infant, however, may cause abnormal acceleration of blood destruction or inhibition of glucuronyl transferase activity.

In the early days of life the increase of serum bilirubin is largely of the indirect-reacting variety, but whenever more bilirubin is conjugated by the liver cells than can be eliminated through the bile ducts, it returns again to the blood as the direct-reacting form. Interference with movement through bile canaliculi may occur whenever extreme cell destruction presents such an excessive amount of bilirubin to the liver that, even though capable of conjugation it is not capable of eliminating all of it into bile canaliculi, or, once in the canaliculi, it cannot move into larger bile ducts with sufficient rapidity to prevent reabsorption. Such an increase rarely occurs before the end of the 1st week, is probably always pathologic and is rarely confused with physiologic jaundice. It may be a result of inability of bile to leave the liver because of atresia of extrahepatic ducts, inability to reach the hepatic duct because of absence of portal bile ducts or inability to reach portal ducts because of plugging of ductules or bile canaliculi. Damage to liver cells by anoxia, shock or sepsis may so impair their function that they are unable to secrete even a normal amount of bile into the canaliculi.

Anemia

Anemia is very common in early infancy, especially in premature infants, and often appears to be a result of physiologic rather than true pathologic disturbances. However, almost all conditions responsible for anemia in later infancy and childhood may occasionally cause symptoms in the first few weeks of life. Anemia in general can be divided into that due to inadequate production of erythrocytes or hemoglobin and that due to blood loss by hemorrhage or hemolysis. Anemia present at birth is almost always a result of intrauterine blood loss either from hemorrhage or from cell destruction by antibodies or infectious agents. Because the liver is the main source of blood cells before birth, the anemia caused by abnormalities of bone marrow responsible for inadequate blood formation does not appear until later. Also, the disturbances resulting from the presence of abnormal hemoglobin do not become manifest until after the time at which fetal hemoglobin normally disappears.

Anemia due to inadequate production of cells or hemoglobin includes the hypoplastic and aplastic varieties resulting from inadequate numbers or depression of activity of cell precursors in the marrow or from specific nutritional deficiencies. Anemia due to loss of red blood cells by hemorrhage may occur in an acute or chronic form either before or after birth. Hemolysis as a cause of anemia may result from hereditary abnormalities in cell form, hemoglobin or enzymes or from acquired abnormalities caused by toxic or infectious states or immune reactions.

Anemia from Antenatal Blood Loss

When blood loss occurs late in labor or during delivery, blood obtained from the umbilical cord or from the infant soon after birth may appear to be normal, but within a few hours readjustment of total blood volume makes anemia evident. This can be differentiated from more chronic anemia of intrauterine origin by lack of both hyperbilirubinemia and evidence of compensatory erythropoiesis in the form of an abnormal increase in reticulocytes or nucleated red blood cells in the circulation.

Any infant with blood loss may be in shock at the time of birth, and symptoms may simulate severe intrauterine anoxia. It must always be remembered that bleeding from the maternal vagina may be of fetal origin, and this possibility must always be considered when vaginal bleeding has occurred and the infant is in poor condition at birth. Even though anemia cannot be demonstrated at birth, the fall in hemoglobin level may be very rapid and may be apparent within an hour.

A similar situation may occur after birth in association with rupture of a subcapsular hematoma of the liver with bleeding into the abdominal cavity.

Hemorrhage from vasa previa.—The most clear-cut and best-documented loss of blood before birth is from rupture of a velamentous vessel located in the fetal membranes overlying the cervix. In a velamentous insertion of the umbilical cord one or more vessels course through the membranes for varying distances between the placenta and the umbilical cord. Even though they are more susceptible to damage than when embedded in Wharton's jelly, they are nevertheless injured very infrequently. On rare occasions the cord may arise in the membranes opposite the placenta and a vessel may cross the dilated cervix and be stretched to the point of rupture by the descending head; more often the vessel slips aside and the infant is delivered uneventfully.

Hemorrhage from vessels on the surface of the placenta.—Occasionally the amniotic fluid is bloody when the membranes are ruptured, or blood may be found, usually only in small amounts, between the amnion and the chorion. Ordinarily in such instances small injuries can be identified in vessels on the surface of the placenta. They are rarely of sufficient extent to be responsible for appreciable bleeding.

Hemorrhage from villi (fetal hemorrhage syndrome).—The total extent of the vessels within the villi is enormous. Even in terminal villi several vessels can be seen when a villus is viewed in cross-section. They are made up of only a single layer of endothelial cells, are surrounded by a small amount of mesoderm, and the outer surface of the villus is covered during the latter two thirds of pregnancy by a single layer of syncytial cells. It seems reasonable to assume that these thin-walled vessels within the villi may break and fetal blood escape into the maternal circulation; this assumption has been substantiated by several investigators.

By the use of differential agglutination or staining technics McLorey and Fish showed that small amounts of fetal blood may be lost into the maternal circulation at any time during pregnancy and that larger amounts pass into the maternal circulation at the time of a spontaneous or induced abortion as well as during delivery in later pregnancy. In guinea pigs, experimental obstruction of the umbilical vein results in a prompt and massive passage of blood out of the villi. No visible lesion of the placenta is necessary for this passage (Dancis *et al.*). Shiller described an infant in shock at birth whose placenta contained fetal red blood cells in intervillous spaces, and the maternal blood contained significant amounts of fetal hemoglobin soon after delivery. Fetal hemoglobin disappeared from maternal blood in a few weeks concomitantly with a rise in anti-A isoagglutinins.

In practically all placentas after midpregnancy small amounts of an homogeneous eosinophilic material are found on the surface of occasional villi. Sometimes this is on the surface of individual villi, sometimes several villi are embedded in a single mass, or occasionally the masses are large enough to be visible grossly and are designated infarcts. Such areas have been thought by some investigators to be the end-result of hemorrhage from villi, but no evidence has proved this contention.

Areas resembling thrombi are present in a few placentas; these also have been described as proof of fetal hemorrhage, but a study at the Chicago Lying-in Hospital showed them always to be composed of maternal and never of fetal blood. Such areas are located centrally within cotyledons, are roughly cuboidal, never contain villi and rarely exceed 1 cm in diameter (see Fig. 3–23). When 1,600 placentas were examined at the Chicago Lying-in Hospital, 56 such areas in which blood cells could still be typed were found. Maternal and infant bloods were also typed. In every one of 12 cases in which the mother and infant were of different blood groups the cells of the thrombus were of the same group as that of the mother.

Although some leakage of fetal red cells occurs throughout pregnancy, it is only at term or with operative interference for abortion that the size of a dose of Rh-positive cells is sufficient to induce immunization in an Rh-negative woman. Cesarean section and manual removal of the placenta following vaginal delivery should be avoided in Rh-negative women if at all possible because the procedure is almost certain to cause villous rupture.

TWIN TRANSFUSION SYNDROME. — In the monochorionic placentas of monovular twins, anastomoses between blood vessels of the portions belonging to the two fetuses are common. This ordinarily produces no disturbance and both twins maintain separate circulations, but infrequently a disproportion-

ate amount of blood may accumulate in one twin at the expense of the other. One of a pair of twins observed at the Chicago Lying-in Hospital at birth had a hemoglobin value of 8.5 gm with an erythrocyte count of 2.04 million, while the other had a hemoglobin level of over 20 gm. On the 2d day of life the hemoglobin of the latter twin was 25.8 gm and the erythrocyte count was 7.82 million. One portion of the placenta was extremely pale and contained little blood; the other was dark red-purple, and all villi were distended with blood.

ANEMIA FROM ANTENATAL BLOOD DESTRUCTION

ERYTHROBLASTOSIS FETALIS. — The principal cause of antenatal blood destruction is erythroblastosis. Cytomegalic inclusion disease and alpha thalassemia are rare causes. The hematologic findings are the same in all. Evidence of blood destruction varies, depending on the extent of the destruction and the ability of the fetus to compensate for blood loss. An increase in bilirubin in tissues and circulating blood and an increase in erythropoiesis constitute the two main findings substantiating a diagnosis of blood destruction. While the fetus is still in the uterus, bilirubin may become elevated when red cells are destroyed, but the greater part is transported across the placenta to the maternal circulation. The level is almost never more than 8–10 mg per 100 ml in cord blood although it may become two or three times as high as soon as the infant loses the placenta as a means of elimination. The greater part is indirect-reacting bilirubin because the increase in bilirubin results from a hemolytic process and because of the paucity of conjugating enzymes in the fetal liver.

When red blood cells are destroyed at an abnormally rapid rate before birth, erythropoiesis in the liver is increased. If the need becomes excessive and the liver cannot compensate, other potential sources of erythropoiesis are called into action. Maximow described totipotential cells in the immediate vicinity of small blood vessels, which he designated pericytes, that are capable of producing blood cells under stress. Abnormal erythropoiesis as a result of stimulation of such cells first becomes evident in the kidneys, especially in the connective tissue in the immediate vicinity of lobular blood vessels at the corticomedullary junction and in the spleen; later it may be found around the blood vessels in any organ or tissue.

The degree to which the spleen is involved is

variable. Sometimes the kidneys and other organs are the site of marked erythropoiesis at a time when the spleen contains only small numbers of immature red blood cells; or both the pulp and the sinuses may be filled with extremely immature cells (see Fig. 21–6). Before 28 weeks' gestation, even in severe erythroblastosis, the spleen, as well as all other organs, has a minimal increase in erythropoiesis.

A reduction in lymphoid tissue usually accompanies excessive erythropoiesis. The thymus is decreased in size, owing especially to a reduction in cortical lymphocytes, lymph nodes are small, malpighian corpuscles disappear from the spleen and lymphoid tissue in general is inconspicuous. On rare occasions Peyer's patches and solitary follicles in the intestine are replaced by areas of erythropoiesis (see Fig. 18–23, A). This reduction in lymphoid tissue, particularly in the thymus, is probably a response to adrenal cortical hormone secretion as a result of the stress associated with the anoxia accompanying severe blood destruction.

The extent to which potential centers of erythropoiesis are stimulated seems to be directly related to the degree of destruction of red blood cells. When the need for replacement is mild, only the liver and bone marrow become more active, the majority of cells are not released into the circulation until nuclei have been lost and the only evidence of increased activity is an increase in reticulocytes. As the need becomes greater and other potential areas of erythropoiesis become active, young cells may undergo mitosis even in the peripheral blood (Fig. 28–2, C). The proportionate number of immature cells in the circulating blood can be directly correlated with the extent of erythropoiesis in body tissues. The barrier that holds back nucleated red blood cells in the liver and bone marrow seems to be missing in erythropoietic centers in other tissues, and cells in such areas have free access to the circulation. In fact, the examination of such foci of erythropoiesis prompts speculation as to whether they are of aid in producing oxygen-carrying cells or whether the cells escape so prematurely into the peripheral circulation that only the number of nucleated forms is increased.

The infants who at birth have the lowest hemoglobin values and erythrocyte counts have also the most immature forms in greatest number in the peripheral blood. These extreme changes in the blood are generally accompanied by severe edema (fetal hydrops), and the infants almost never survive (see Fig. 27–27). Not only may hemoglobin be as low as 3–5 gm and the blood filled with extremely immature forms, but the total volume of circulating blood generally seems to be greatly reduced. We have often tried unsuccessfully to get sufficient blood for chemical determinations from the heart and peripheral vessels at autopsy; it seems as if all the fluid were in the tissues with little remaining in the blood vessels. It is in such infants, too, that evidence of antenatal biliary obstruction in the form of distended bile canaliculi is most common.

This extreme demand for replacement of red blood cells produces a truly remarkable picture in smears of peripheral blood. Nucleated cells in all stages of development are present (Fig. 28–2, A and B). Generally there are many large basophilic erythroblasts, a scattering of stem cells with finely granular chromatin and multiple nucleoli and occasional mitotic figures. Non-nucleated cells are extremely variable in size, with macrocytes and microcytes both present in large numbers. Phagocytes containing red blood cells are occasionally seen (Fig. 28–2, D).

Evidence of abnormal erythropoiesis can rarely be found before the fetus reaches 28 weeks of gestation, and it seems probable that blood destruction before this time is not great enough to stimulate increased blood formation. Consequently, it is assumed that most fetuses are not affected by maternal antibodies until fairly late in pregnancy, but in some instances, at least, there is contrary evidence in the placenta. In cases of severe erythroblastosis the cytotrophoblast covering the surface of the villi may persist until term, whereas normally it is lost before the end of the 1st trimester of pregnancy. This persistent growth and immaturity of the villous trophoblast is reflected in the maternal levels of placental lactogen and heat-stable alkaline phosphatase. When the destruction of blood cells is mild, the placenta may appear normal, but when it is severe, the placenta is always enlarged, the villi are bulbous and edematous and the vessels within individual villi are often increased in number and almost completely filled with immature red blood cells (see Figs. 3–27 to 3–29).

When blood destruction is severe, plasma protein is usually decreased and in severely hydropic infants may be as low as 2–2.5 mg per 100 ml. This failure of protein production may be because anemia has caused anoxic damage to the liver. It has also been suggested that heart failure as a result of severe anemia may be the cause of the edema; although this may contribute, the primary cause more often appears to be hypoproteinemia.

Since erythroblastosis is a hemolytic anemia

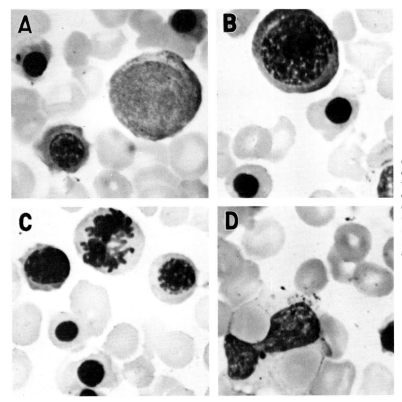

Fig. 28-2.—Immature red blood cells in peripheral blood in severe erythroblastosis. **A,** hemocytoblast, two normoblasts and late erythroblast. **B,** early basophilic erythroblast and two normoblasts. **C,** mitotic figure, two late erythroblasts and two normoblasts. **D,** histiocyte with two phagocytosed erythrocytes.

originating before birth as a result of destruction of fetal erythrocytes by isoantibodies transmitted through the placenta from maternal blood, it is characterized clinically by anemia, hyperbilirubinemia and erythroblastemia.

D (R_0) is the substance that most often produces antibodies responsible for erythroblastosis, although they may be produced as a response to any of the other Rh antigens such as C (R′), E (R″), c (H′), e (H″) and rarely to other related substances such as Kell, Duffy, Lutheran and so on.

Antibodies against A or B substances in group O women may also cause erythroblastosis, but then the disease is ordinarily mild. A range of 17–22% of incompatibility exists between the fetus and mother in the ABO system (Mollison and Cutbush; Stern *et al.*), but antibody formation sufficient to produce severe fetal anemia seldom occurs. Mollison and Cutbush believed kernicterus to be the only real threat to such infants, although Stern *et al.* reported four fatalities from hemolytic anemia caused by ABO incompatibility. At the Chicago Lying-in Hospital erythroblastosis due to D-immunization occurred in about 5% of Rh-negative white women and to A- or B-immunization in about 0.5% of group O white women. Among more than 400 women observed there before 1968 whose fetuses or infants were affected by Rh antibodies, all but six were immunized to D; four were immunized to c, and one each to C and E.

Immunization to Rh may be caused in an Rh-negative woman by transfusion of Rh-positive blood or by passage of Rh-positive fetal cells into the maternal circulation. Firstborn infants are almost never affected unless the mother has been transfused previously or has had an abortion, and it appears that fetal cells ordinarily do not enter the maternal circulation in sufficient numbers to cause fetal damage until the time of abortion or delivery. Separation of the chorionic vesicle or placenta opens maternal vessels which receive blood from traumatized placental vessels, and immunization follows that affects the child of the next pregnancy. Because of this, antibody formation may be almost completely prevented by the use of human anti-Rh gamma globulin (Rhogam), provided the Rh antiserum is given within 72 hours after delivery or abortion (Katz). Immunization to the Rh factor, once established, is permanent and each succeeding Rh-positive child is at risk.

Although in about 13% of pregnancies in white women the wife is Rh-negative and the husband Rh-positive, only a small minority terminate in clinically affected babies. If the father is blood type A or B and the mother type O, fetal cells, when they reach the mother's circulation, are rapidly coated with A or B isoantibody and removed from the circulation, so maternal immunization either does not take place against an accompanying Rh antigen or, if it does, is of minimal degree.

If the father is heterozygous for the Rh factor, only half of his children will be Rh-positive; thus, even if a mother is sensitized and has had affected children, the child of any subsequent pregnancy has a chance of being Rh-negative and unaffected. On the other hand, women with husbands homozygous for the Rh factor will continue to have affected infants. In some instances all infants may be mildly affected; in others the disease may become progressively severe in successive infants.

The severity of the process can be gauged to some extent by following the concentrations in the amniotic fluid of bile excreted in the urine in the latter half of pregnancy (Gudson *et al.*). Since in a nonaffected fetus the fetal serum bilirubin level will not exceed the renal threshold, bile will not appear in the amniotic fluid. With early demonstration and rising levels of bilirubin in amniotic fluid, intrauterine transfusion may be indicated and may save some otherwise doomed infants. There is some evidence that some of those who might die if left in utero until term will survive if they are delivered prematurely and receive prompt exchange transfusion after birth. However, what might be gained by early delivery must be balanced against the direct hazards of prematurity.

When fetal hydrops can be diagnosed by x-ray (a greatly thickened scalp is usually diagnostic), the prognosis is so poor that most experienced physicians will attempt neither intrauterine transfusion nor early delivery. Such fetuses almost invariably succumb regardless of treatment.

The outlook for the child of any pregnancy is more closely related to the outcome of the preceding pregnancy than to maternal antibody titer. Ordinarily, a high titer indicates that the child will be severely affected, but a low titer may be followed by the birth of either a mildly or a severely affected infant. A rising titer as a result of an anamnestic reaction sometimes occurs with an Rh-positive fetus. Consequently, antibody titers during pregnancy are not always of great prognostic significance (Potter).

Clinical and pathologic findings vary in relation to the severity of the hemolytic process and the extent of the erythropoietic response. In mildly affected infants the anemia may be minimal, and there may be little evidence in the form of nucleated red blood cells or reticulocytes that the disease exists. There may be nothing more on which to base a diagnosis than a positive Coombs test, mild early jaundice and mild indirect hyperbilirubinemia. The Coombs antiglobulin test indicates whether antibodies are attached to fetal cells and is almost invariably positive if antibodies are present in maternal blood and the infant is Rh-positive; thus it gives little additional information if these two facts are already known. Its greatest value is in the very severely affected child whose blood may seem to be Rh-negative because of the saturation of the Rh combining bonds with incomplete antibodies, inasmuch as cells with such antibodies have no bond to react with the ordinary anti-Rh serum. In such a case a positive Coombs test proves that the cells are actually Rh-positive and do have attached antibodies.

Increase in severity is indicated in the fetus by increased anemia, hyperbilirubinemia and erythroblastemia, the extent of the change indicating the severity of the disease process. In the most severe cases the fetus appears unable to compensate for the excessive intrauterine cell destruction and dies before birth. In slightly less severe cases the child may be born alive, often with generalized edema—so-called fetal hydrops—but may succumb immediately after birth. However, in some instances a child born with hemoglobin content of only 4 or 5 gm, a high bilirubin level and evidence of very extensive ectopic erythropoiesis may still survive. In such cases preparations made before birth for transfusion to be given immediately after delivery may save the life of an infant who may otherwise die.

In severely affected infants the bilirubin of cord blood is usually high and rises rapidly after birth since the avenue of escape into maternal blood is cut off. The skin becomes jaundiced within a few hours, for true jaundice is never present at birth although it may be simulated by pallor and staining of the skin with pigment present in the amniotic sac as a result of excessive excretion in fetal urine. Anemia gradually becomes more marked because formation of cells in ectopic areas of erythropoiesis ordinarily ceases after birth and cells continue to be destroyed by the action of the antibodies that entered the fetal blood before birth. The spleen may be enlarged to several times its normal size, although any weight in excess of 15 gm should always arouse suspicion of erythroblastosis. The liver is more mildly enlarged, rarely showing more than a 50% increase. Purpuric hemorrhages may be present in the skin (Fig. 28–3).

The treatment of erythroblastosis in the severely affected fetus who is not expected to survive without the development of fetal hydrops before the period of good viability, i. e., beyond the 37th week of gestation, is to supply the fetus in utero with Rh-negative red cells that will not be affected by maternal antibodies. These cells, by providing an adequate red cell mass, will not only supply enough oxygen-carrying cells, but will tend to suppress the infant's own hemopoietic apparatus and thus decrease the number of cells available for hemolysis.

The salvage rate of fetuses severely affected in the 3d trimester who require an intrauterine transfusion is about 30–40%, depending on the criteria used for case selection (Corston *et al.*).

After birth an exchange transfusion of Rh-negative cells of the same AB type as that of the infant fulfills three objectives: (1) to supply an effective oxygen-carrying mass of blood, (2) to replace sensitive Rh-positive cells by Rh-negative cells not subject to hemolysis by the circulating maternal anti-Rh antibodies and (3) most importantly, to reduce the level of circulating indirect bilirubin and thus prevent kernicterus. If indirect bilirubin is allowed to accumulate in the blood, the basal nuclei of the brain are damaged, the child becomes lethargic, opisthotonos develops and the child may die within a short time or survive with a permanent disabil-

Fig. 28–3.—Erythroblastosis. Purpuric hemorrhage that developed soon after birth under the skin of the face in infant who survived.

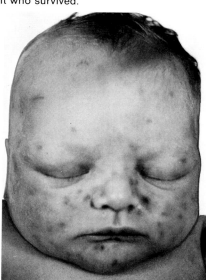

ity, most often characterized by choreo-athetosis. Such a disturbance in the brain rarely occurs unless the indirect bilirubin level rises above 20 mg per 100 ml in the first few days of life. If it reaches 30 mg per 100 ml, permanent damage may be anticipated.

When erythrocyte destruction continues after birth, the excessive production of bile is responsible for its accumulation in hepatic cells and bile canaliculi. The direct-reacting bilirubin in the serum rises, and stools may become acholic. When the child is treated with exchange transfusions this is rare, but when it does occur, recovery is normally spontaneous and rapid.

Findings at autopsy depend largely on when death occurs. When the child is of less than 28 weeks' gestational age, a diagnosis of erythroblastosis cannot be made on anatomic grounds since neither the spleen nor the liver are enlarged, bile pigment is not increased in the liver and hydrops is not present. Often there are no specific findings or, at most, only a slight increase in hemosiderin in the liver. The location and amount of erythropoiesis may not differ from those of a normal fetus of the same gestational age.

If death occurs in utero near term, maceration may mask changes in many organs, although enlargement of the spleen, liver and heart is usually evident. Anasarca is common and especially prominent in the face, producing swelling of the eyelids and protrusion of the tongue. The lungs retain an affinity for stains longer than other organs, and immature red cells can usually be identified in pulmonary capillaries and larger vessels (see Fig. 15–27). In some instances the fetus shows no edema, and the only demonstrable evidence of the disease is the presence of large immature cells, presumably hemocytoblasts, in the lungs (Potter).

If death occurs immediately after birth, extreme edema, ordinarily so severe as to be called fetal hydrops, is usually present (see Figs. 27–26 and 27–27). All subcutaneous tissues and muscles contain an excess of fluid at the expense of the fluid in the circulation, the total volume of blood within the fetus being reduced. Anemia is extreme, with blood hemoglobin as low as 2–3 gm. Great numbers of extremely immature red blood cells are present in the blood, with non-nucleated erythrocytes varying greatly in size (Fig. 28–2). The liver may weigh twice the normal amount and, histologically, usually shows more extreme erythropoiesis than is found from any other cause. Large amounts of iron are present in hepatic and Kupffer cells, and bile canaliculi are frequently distended (see Fig. 20–

24). The spleen is often four to six times the normal size, malpighian corpuscles are small or absent; sinusoids are large and prominent and may be empty or contain nucleated red blood cells. Marked erythropoiesis is present in the pulp (see Figs. 21–5 and 21–6). The heart is commonly somewhat enlarged and dilated although local erythropoiesis is usually not evident (see Fig. 21–4). Kidneys are not enlarged, but erythropoiesis in perivascular areas is usually striking (see Fig. 22–11). The adrenal glands are usually moderately enlarged, and the lipid content of the fetal portion of the cortex is usually increased. The vessels in the meninges may be unusually tortuous (see Fig. 24–3), the thymus is small, and all lymphoid tissue is hypoplastic.

The placenta is greatly enlarged and may weigh half or more than half as much as the fetus. Villi are enlarged, stroma is edematous and fetal vessels are often marginated and may contain many nucleated cells. Cytotrophoblast sometimes persists (see Fig. 3–29).

In a nonhydropic infant changes are rarely as severe, and with proper treatment the infant usually survives. If exchange transfusion is not given, however, death may occur in severe cases in the first day or two of life, the immediate cause most often being pulmonary hemorrhage. With death occurring after 36 hours of age, kernicterus is usually also present (see Fig. 24–9).

When death occurs more than 4 or 5 days after birth, erythropoiesis may have completely disappeared and histologic evidence of the disease may be lacking. Rarely, cirrhosis of the liver appears to be a sequel (see Fig. 20–25).

Surviving children who have been treated in such a way that circulating indirect bilirubin has not been elevated sufficiently to cause brain damage are normal, although a prolonged marrow depression may develop postnatally (Corston *et al.*). Those whose serum bilirubin level has been high for an appreciable length of time often exhibit blue or green discoloration of deciduous teeth when they are erupted (see Fig. 18–4), and choreo-athetosis, indicating brain damage, is common.

Differential diagnosis at the time of birth or in the early days of life includes intrauterine infection (syphilis, toxoplasmosis and viral infections, especially cytomegalic inclusion disease), nonspherocytic and other hemolytic anemias, alpha thalassemia, congenital malformations of the intra- and extrahepatic bile ducts and neoplasms of the liver. The hydropic form must be differentiated from extreme generalized edema of unknown cause.

Postnatal Anemias

Anemia demonstrable in the first few days of life has ordinarily originated before birth and is generally a continuation of the same process. Anemia caused by blood loss from the cord or placenta becomes more noticeable at 12–24 hours than it is at birth because of the dilution brought about by the readjustment of total blood volume. Loss of blood into the intracranial or body cavities or into a viscus as a result of injury at birth may also be responsible for early anemia.

Anemia from Inadequate Erythrocyte Production

Physiologic anemia of mature infants. — Anemia that is not due to prenatal disturbances or to hemorrhage occurring during or soon after birth is usually not manifested for several weeks. The high levels normally present before birth are usually readjusted downward during the first few weeks of life, and often by the 3d month the hemoglobin averages only about 11 gm and the red cell count only slightly over 4,000,000 per cu mm. The anemia is always hypochromic and the erythrocytes are usually small, averaging only 5–6 μ in diameter. These levels are often maintained until the latter part of the 1st year, when a gradual increase begins. Normal adult levels are frequently not attained until puberty.

Anemia of prematurity. — Premature infants are especially susceptible to anemia and often experience a more abrupt and more extensive decline in hemoglobin and number of red cells than do infants born at term (Gairdner *et al.*). The causes are probably the same as in more mature infants, with the added factors of an initially smaller blood volume and a more immature hemopoietic system. All premature infants are somewhat anemic, the degree being inversely proportional to the weight. Toward the end of the 3d month a gradual improvement begins, provided the infant is growing satisfactorily, and toward the end of the 1st year the erythrocyte count averages about the same as for mature infants. In premature as well as full-term infants the hemoglobin rise lags behind the rise in number of cells, and with a count of 5,000,000 cells per cu mm the hemoglobin value may be only 12–13 gm.

Iron deficiency anemia. — Iron deficiency anemia superimposed on the physiologic anemia of the mature or premature infant results in a greater fall or greater prolongation of low levels of hemoglobin and erythrocytes. The cells are small and deficient in hemoglobin. The lack of iron may be due to inadequate storage, loss or poor utilization. Inadequate intake, although a common cause in later infancy, does not ordinarily play a role in the first 3 months.

Anemia in the mother, although not associated with changes in the blood at birth, may be responsible, according to Diamond *et al.*, for anemia beginning at about the 3d month. This anemia, which is microcytic and hypochromic, is stated to be preventable by the administration of iron after birth. Twins are reported to be more susceptible than single infants.

HYPOPLASTIC ANEMIA.—In this condition anemia is not present at birth and, although sometimes manifest at 3 or 4 weeks of age, is generally not pronounced for 2 or 3 months. It is due to inability of bone marrow to produce an adequate number of erythrocytes, although other formed elements are normal. The red blood cell count may fall below 1,000,000 per cu mm, and the hemoglobin value is proportionately reduced since the anemia is normocytic and normochromic. Reticulocytes are not over 2%. The condition is often familial and is of unknown origin, although a disturbance in the intermediary metabolism of tryptophan has been reported. The prognosis is guarded, although a spontaneous cure may occur at any time, especially at about the time of puberty. Death may occur from intercurrent infection. Diagnosis is based on the presence of severe normocytic normochromic anemia without evidence of red cell regeneration or of abnormality of other elements of the blood. Pathologic changes that are specifically related to the disease consist only of hypoplasia of red cell precursors in the bone marrow. In long-term female survivors secondary sexual characteristics may fail to develop. Hemosiderosis may occur as a result of multiple transfusions, and cirrhosis has been seen as early as 8 years of age.

A similar type of congenital hypoplastic anemia has been observed in conjunction with dwarfism, with mental retardation, inverted nipples, webbed neck, widely spaced eyes, exophthalmos, wide fontanelles and skeletal and renal anomalies (Hughes; Minagi and Steinboch).

FAMILIAL HYPOPLASTIC ANEMIA WITH MULTIPLE CONGENITAL DEFECTS (FANCONI'S SYNDROME).—In 1927 Fanconi described three brothers between 5 and 7 years of age with aplastic anemia and multiple congenital anomalies. Since then many similar cases have been reported. The anemia is normocytic and normochromic with accompanying leuko-penia and thrombocytopenia. It is not manifested until weeks or months after birth, but in the preanemic stage the marrow may be hyperplastic with "megacytoid" cells (Smith). Later it is hypoplastic or aplastic. The most frequently associated abnormalities are pigmentation of the skin, especially the skin folds, and malformations of the bones of the extremities, especially absence or abnormality of the thumb and radius (Figs. 28–4 and 28–5). Other abnormalities that have been observed include syndactyly; dislocation of the hip; growth retardation; strabismus; microphthalmia; mental retardation; and malformations of the heart, kidneys or gonads.

The syndrome is caused by an autosomal recessive gene of variable penetrance. Because of this, the pancytopenia and hypoplasia of bone marrow may be found without other mesodermal abnormalities in some families. It is of interest that, according to Smith, leukemia is present in 8% of females with this syndrome. Dignan *et al.* found a small extra abnormal acrocentric chromosome in individuals with a similar phenotype but with an additional myeloid-leukemoid reaction.

SECONDARY HYPOPLASTIC ANEMIA.—Chemical agents, radiation injury and so on are rare causes

Fig. 28–4.—Fanconi's syndrome of hypoplastic anemia and multiple congenital defects. Infant aged 2 months at onset of anemia.

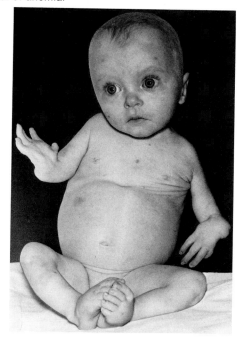

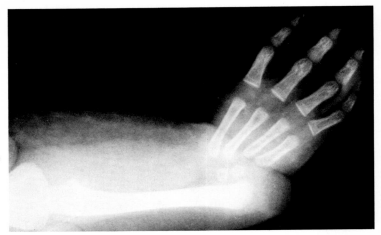

Fig. 28–5.—Roentgenogram of forearm of infant with Fanconi's syndrome. (Courtesy Dr. E. B. D. Neuhauser.)

of aplastic anemia in early infancy; the administration of certain antibiotics, especially Chloromycetin, has been followed by severe depression of the bone marrow. Some intrauterine infections have been reported to be responsible for aplastic anemia, but ordinarily anemia from such a cause is hemolytic rather than aplastic. Accompanying thrombocytopenia may be found in congenital viral infections such as rubella, herpes or cytomegalic inclusion disease, but in these instances capillary damage and peripheral platelet consumption are also increased.

PERNICIOUS ANEMIA. — This condition is extremely rare in infancy, but, according to Smith, has been reported with an onset as early as 4 months. Spurling *et al.* found that 26 of 29 cases reported in children began before the age of 2 years. It is caused by a genetically determined absence of the "intrinsic" factor in gastric secretions that is responsible for the failure of absorption of vitamin B_{12} in the terminal ileum. This leads to the development of megaloblastic anemia and degenerative lesions in the central nervous system. Atrophy of the papillae of the tongue and recurrent glossitis are constant symptoms. Diarrhea, weight loss, anorexia and vomiting are common. Hepatosplenomegaly and mild jaundice may be present. Mental retardation and neurologic disturbances have been observed but are rare in infants. The anemia is macrocytic and hyperchromic with few reticulocytes; neutropenia is responsible for relative lymphocytosis. The bone marrow contains erythrocyte precursors characteristic of megaloblastic anemia and abnormal granulocytes consisting of giant metamyelocytes, hypersegmented polymorphonuclear leukocytes

and atypical mitotic figures. Treatment with vitamin B_{12} or liver extract containing vitamin B_{12} is specific.

MEGALOBLASTIC ANEMIA. — In infants megaloblastic anemia due to folic acid deficiency is found most often in the latter half of the 1st year. Caused by dietary deficiencies, without treatment it may progress to a fatal outcome. Administration of folic acid effects a cure within a few weeks (Zuelzer and Ogden). The anemia is usually hyperchromic and macrocytic. Megaloblasts have been observed in the peripheral blood; since in their absence this condition may be indistinguishable from other macrocytic anemias, examination of the bone marrow may be essential to establish a diagnosis. Marrow smears show erythroid hyperplasia with many megaloblasts and hypersegmented polymorphonuclear leukocytes.

MACROCYTIC ANEMIA. — Other anemias that respond to folic acid or liver extract may be caused by a number of different conditions, especially those involving the gastrointestinal tract. They include acute infection associated with complete achlorhydria, acute or chronic infections that interfere with absorption of the liver extract principle, intestinal atresia with operation bypassing portions in which the liver extract principle is elaborated or absorbed, and cirrhosis of the liver, which is usually associated with other malformations.

The degree of anemia is variable, but the decrease in the number of red cells is proportionately greater than the reduction in hemoglobin. The red cells are large, containing relatively more than a normal amount of hemoglobin, and the color index is over 1.

Anemia with Abnormal Erythrocyte Configuration

Congenital spherocytosis (congenital hemolytic anemia, familial acholuric jaundice). — This diagnosis is made more often in later childhood than in infancy, but it may be established in the early days of life on the basis of jaundice, anemia, increased fragility of erythrocytes, reticulocytosis and normoblastemia (Shapiro et al.). The mean cell diameter and volume are less than normal and the mean cell thickness is greater than normal, but the cellular abnormalities are not usually sufficient to establish a diagnosis. About half of the infants aged less than 1 year when the diagnosis is made have neonatal jaundice, usually accompanied by erythroblastemia and progressive anemia (Burman). Kernicterus has been reported, and replacement transfusions are sometimes required.

Although the course of the disease is extremely variable, it is only when symptoms are severe that an early diagnosis can be made. Even when the general course is mild, crises occur during which the anemia accelerates and the jaundice deepens. Such crises are often preceded by fever, weakness and abdominal pain. The spleen is usually enlarged but has no specific histologic abnormality although the sinuses are often large and empty. The liver and, to a lesser extent, the kidneys and lymph nodes often show mild hemosiderosis. The bone marrow is hyperplastic but spherocytes are present only in peripheral blood. Increased fragility of erythrocytes can usually be demonstrated on the first examination but often becomes more marked later. Splenectomy is ordinarily considered the preferred treatment, but since young infants are more susceptible than older infants to infections, especially pneumococcic meningitis, following splenectomy, the procedure should be postponed for as long as possible.

The disease is inherited through an autosomal dominant gene and is usually present in other members of the family.

Anemia Associated with Abnormal Cell Constituents

Congenital nonspherocytic hemolytic anemia. — This macrocytic anemia in which hemolytic anemia, jaundice and hepatomegaly may be evident in the first 24 hours, may be confused with erythroblastosis. With increasing hyperbilirubinemia caused by progression of the anemia, exchange transfusion may be required to prevent kernicterus. Erythrocytes are normochromic and normocytic with Heinz bodies often present. The latter are small fragments of degenerated cell envelopes that a healthy spleen is normally able to remove but that may remain in the cells when the phagocytic activity of the spleen is poor or following splenectomy. The anemia is caused by a structural abnormality of red cell membranes in which a lack of stability results from an insufficient concentration of reduced glutathione. This concentration is dependent on a series of oxidative reduction reactions requiring the presence of specific enzymes; 10 different hereditary enzyme deficiencies have been identified as causes of cell hemolysis. The most important are glucose-6-phosphate dehydrogenase and pyruvate kinase. The former is inherited through a sex-linked (X) recessive gene, the latter through an autosomal recessive gene.

Thalassemia (Cooley's anemia, congenital hemolytic anemia, erythroblastic anemia). — This anemia is an hereditary metabolic abnormality in which fetal hemoglobin replaces the normal hemoglobin A in variable amounts in the postnatal state. This lack of normal hemoglobin has been related to the inability of the cells to form beta chains in relation to the alpha chains and hence to form hemoglobin A. There is no amino acid chain substitution as in sickle cell disease, and both fetal and adult hemoglobins are normal in make-up and configuration. Electron microscope studies have demonstrated changes in the red cell membrane, and phospholipid studies show chemical changes in the cells.

When first described by Cooley, the disease was thought to occur only in certain countries bordering on the Mediterranean basin, but it has since been described in many races.

Thalassemia minor, which is associated with the heterozygous state of a recessive gene, produces only mild anemia and a slight increase in reticulocytes and hypochromic abnormal non-nucleated erythrocytes in the peripheral blood. Hepatosplenomegaly, bone changes and a need for transfusion are unusual.

Thalassemia major is associated with the homozygous state but, because of the variable penetrance of the gene, the severity of the symptoms varies. Severe anemia is usually the outstanding symptom. It is not present at birth but develops in early infancy at the time that fetal hemoglobin normally disappears from the cells.

The affected homozygous child is pale and often slightly icteric, with progressing splenomegaly followed slightly later by moderate hepatomegaly. The anemia may be rapidly fatal without transfusions. The red blood cells are hypochromic with considerable variation in size; the majority are microcytes, but some are very large, measuring as much as 12–15 μ in diameter. Concentration of hemoglobin at the margin and in the center of the cells gives a "target cell" appearance. Nucleated red blood cells, stippling, polychromatophilia, Howell-Jolly bodies and an increase in reticulocytes are demonstrable in smears of peripheral blood.

Temporary support may be obtained from transfusions but survival beyond the 2d decade is rare. Children with this condition tend to resemble one another in moderate stunting of growth, mongoloid appearance with mild slanting of the eyes and prominent epicanthic folds and generalized changes in bone.

The earliest bone changes, which occur during the latter part of the 1st year, consist of widening of the medullary spaces, thinning of cortices and decrease in size of the bony trabeculae. The phalanges of the hands may be first affected and may appear rectangular instead of tubular. Somewhat later, the diploic spaces of the membranous bones become widened, and radiating bony trabeculae traversing this space have a characteristic hair-on-end appearance on x-ray examination.

Postmortem changes are not striking. The spleen is always greatly enlarged but may show no changes except abnormal erythropoiesis, some increase in fibrous trabeculae and occasional infarcts. Hemosiderosis is generally marked in the liver and sometimes in other organs. Bone marrow is hypercellular as a result of increase in erythrocyte precursors and may contain foam cells. The latter may also be seen in the spleen.

ALPHA THALASSEMIA. — Since this defect is a failure to form alpha chains of hemoglobin, the hemoglobin for the most part consists of tetrads of four gamma chains (Bart's hemoglobin) with a small percentage of beta chain tetramers. Affected individuals, and those who are homozygous for this abnormality, are usually of Chinese or Malayan extraction and are stillborn with massive fetal hydrops (Eng; Pearson *et al.*). Bart's hemoglobin is a poor oxygen carrier and releases oxygen to peripheral tissues less efficiently than normal hemoglobin. This may account for the severe edema of these fetuses. The pathologic changes are similar to those of a hydropic fetus whose hydrops is caused by Rh incompatibility. The placenta is often larger than

the fetus and has the same immaturity and increased villus budding of a placenta from an infant with severe erythroblastosis due to Rh incompatibility. The mothers often have the same hydramnios and toxemia that is sometimes found in association with high titers of Rh antibodies and severely hydropic erythroblastotic infants. Two such fetuses of Chinese extraction have been seen at the Boston Hospital for Women.

In the heterozygous state the infant is normal and the small amount of Bart's hemoglobin disappears from the circulation in the first months of life.

SICKLE CELL DISEASE. — Occurring almost exclusively among Negroes, this inherited defect in the synthesis of hemoglobin — the substitution of a single amino acid, valine, for glutamine in otherwise normal adult hemoglobin, with the production of hemoglobin S — causes erythrocytes to assume a crescentic or elongated filamentous shape under certain conditions of lowered oxygen tension. Although the defect is manifested in both heterozygous and homozygous states, the former is associated with no clinical symptoms and is known as the "sickling trait"; the latter is associated with persistent hemolytic anemia punctuated by painful crises during which the anemia is accentuated and is known as "sickle cell disease." Symptoms begin to appear in about the 2d and 3d month of life in 30–50% of affected children, at about the time that fetal hemoglobin disappears and is replaced by abnormal hemoglobin S. The first evidence of the disease may be a so-called crisis in which abdominal pain, boardlike rigidity of the abdomen and absence of breath sounds simulate conditions requiring surgical intervention. Symptoms are thought to be due to vascular obstruction by sickled cells. At the time of the crisis these cells are probably increased in number and their sequestration in local areas is responsible for additional sickling with further obstruction. Infarcts may occur in many areas including the spleen, bones, gastrointestinal tract, kidneys, lungs, heart and brain.

In other cases the first signs of the disease, which are pallor, jaundice and hepatosplenomegaly, are related to infections. In infants the disease may take the form of the "hand-foot" syndrome in which hands and/or feet swell and are tender. The metaphyses of the radius and ulna, metacarpals and phalanges develop radiolucencies indicative of bone infarction, and new bone is laid down under the rim (Fig. 28–6). Eventually the bone is restored to normal. In some infants the process is associated with systemic Salmonella infection, particularly in

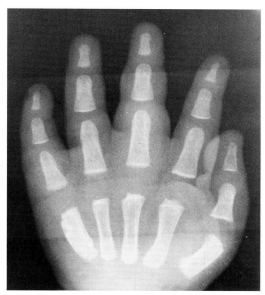

Fig. 28–6. – Sickle cell disease. Roentgenogram of the hand of a young infant with the hand-foot syndrome with swollen fingers and elevation of the periosteum of the fifth metacarpal. (Courtesy Dr. E. B. D. Neuhauser.)

the tropics, and the first symptoms may be fever and diarrhea. In many other cases careful investigation fails to reveal Salmonella (Hendrickse and Collard; Burko *et al.*). The condition has been recognized as early as 1 month of age (Ivy and Howard).

The character of the lesions accounts for the wide range of symptoms. A test for sickling should be included as part of the physical examination of all Negro patients.

Except during a crisis, the only symptoms are those indicative of a chronic hemolytic process and include pallor, anemia and mild jaundice. Mild indirect hyperbilirubinemia is common. Sickling may be present in ordinary blood smears during a crisis but at other times must be brought out by one of several laboratory procedures. The presence of S hemoglobin can be demonstrated by electrophoretic studies.

Crises tend to diminish with age but prognosis must always be guarded. The infant or young child has a less than average life expectancy, and only with careful treatment will he or she reach adult life.

Anatomic manifestations in fatal cases include generalized hemosiderosis and hyperplasia of erythroid elements of bone marrow. Bony abnormalities may resemble those of congenital spherocytosis. Arteriosclerosis may be prominent, especially in the lungs, and thrombosis of vessels of the

brain may be associated with local hemorrhage and necrosis. The spleen or other organs may be infarcted, and most of the erythrocytes may be sickled.

OTHER HEMOLYTIC ANEMIAS ASSOCIATED WITH ABNORMAL HEMOGLOBIN. – In addition to the well-recognized A hemoglobin of normal adult erythrocytes, F hemoglobin of the normal fetus and thalassemia and S hemoglobin of sickle cell anemia, many others have been discovered by electrophoresis. They may be produced by a heterozygous or homozygous state of the responsible gene. The heterozygous form is usually not accompanied by symptoms unless combined with another gene responsible for the presence of some other abnormal hemoglobin, as in thalassemia–hemoglobin S disease. When the gene is in the heterozygous form, the condition produced is known as a trait; when present in homozygous form it is known as a disease. Hemoglobins that have been recognized in addition to those mentioned above have been designated C, D, E, G, H, I, J and K, and others have remained unclassified. Combinations of abnormalities have included sickle cell anemia with hemoglobins C, D, E and G; thalassemia with hemoglobins S, C, E and G; spherocytosis and hemoglobin S; elliptocytosis and hemoglobin disease.

Symptoms due to the presence of abnormal hemoglobins vary, with the majority producing only moderate anemia even when the responsible gene is homozygous. The possibility of abnormal hemoglobin should be considered in every case of unexplained hemolytic anemia. Treatment is symptomatic. Pathologic changes have not been described.

CONGENITAL PORPHYRIA. – This congenital hereditary metabolic disorder is usually transmitted by a recessive gene, although one family with a dominant hereditary pattern was described by Smith. The basic difficulty is in the biosynthesis of heme in the red cell precursors. Failure of conversion of uroporphyrin to coproporphyrin leads to accumulation of the former in body fluids and tissues, with deposition in dentine, bone matrix and interstitium of the skin with resulting pigmentation of the teeth and bone and in light hypersensitivity of the skin. The skin response to light is one of erythema and blister formation.

The anemia associated with congenital porphyria is mild but is accompanied by punctate basophilia, polychromasia and erythroblastemia as well as the other common alterations of hemolytic processes. The urine and feces darken on exposure to sunlight. The nucleated red cells in the bone marrow have an intense red fluorescence, chiefly in their nuclei.

CONGENITAL METHEMOGLOBINEMIA. — Normally the amount of methemoglobin in the blood does not exceed 0.4% of total hemoglobin, but in rare instances a deficiency of the coenzyme factor that accelerates the reduction of methemoglobin to hemoglobin is responsible for an accumulation of 20–40%. Since methemoglobin does not carry oxygen, severe cyanosis that cannot be relieved by administration of oxygen is present at birth and persists thereafter. Polycythemia develops to compensate for the reduction in oxygen-carrying capacity of the cells and, except for cyanosis, symptoms of hypoxia are usually minimal. Freshly drawn blood is chocolate brown, and on spectroscopic examination a characteristic band is found at 630 millimicrons that disappears following the addition of potassium cyanide. Ascorbic acid and methylene blue reduce methemoglobin; since the proper administration of either substance causes diminution of the cyanosis, they may be used both diagnostically and therapeutically.

Methemoglobinemia, like most other abnormalities of hemoglobin, is inherited as a recessive character, producing symptoms only when homozygous (Dine).

CONGENITAL SULFHEMOGLOBINEMIA. — Few individuals who have this abnormality as a result of inheritance have been observed, although Miller reported a case that was definitely diagnosed soon after birth in a family with other similarly affected members. It is found more often following the ingestion of certain drugs or toxins. Possibly, some cases have been missed and described as methemoglobinemia since methemoglobin masks sulfhemoglobin. If methemoglobin is removed by the addition of potassium cyanide, the characteristic spectroscopic band at 618 millimicrons can be identified. Sulfhemoglobin is an inert pigment, useless for oxygen transport, and it is said that 0.5 gm% will produce cyanosis equal to that resulting from the presence of 5 gm% of reduced oxygen.

ANEMIA FROM EXCESSIVE CELL DESTRUCTION

Infections, especially those caused by hemolytic staphylococci or streptococci, may cause anemia through excessive cell destruction. Loss of blood from chronic bleeding decreases the stores of iron and results in anemia.

AUTO-IMMUNE HEMOLYTIC ANEMIA. — This develops when the body produces an antibody against an antigen introduced into the body (e.g., penicillin) and the antigen becomes attached to a receptor on the red cell surface, or when an antibody is formed against a haptene attached to the red cell surface (thus making a complete antigen), so that hemolysis occurs. Typical acute hemolytic anemia results.

There is no known genetic predisposition to this disorder, but when an auto-immune anemia is present in the mother, the antibodies may cross the placenta and attach to the infant's red cells, thus being responsible for a positive Coombs test on the infant's blood. Auto-immune processes that have their origin in the newborn are uncommon since the very young infant is a poor former of gamma globulin, but one such case has been recorded at 6 weeks of age (Smith).

Congenital Dysfunction of White Blood Cells

CHEDIAK-HIGASHI SYNDROME. — This lethal autosomal recessive disorder (Kritzler et al.) begins a few months after birth with the appearance of zones of decreased pigmentation, photophobia, horizontal nystagmus and hepatosplenomegaly. Recurrent infections, which are common, may result in early death from sepsis; skin infections are more common in older individuals.

Aplastic anemia is accompanied by leukopenia with decreased peripheral and marrow leukocytes and a paucity of leukocytes in bacterial abscesses. The polymorphoneutrophils and lymphoid cells contain characteristic large azurophilic cytoplasmic granules (Fig. 28–7). In the peripheral blood these granules contain a cerebroside (Kritzler et al.), although the ultrastructure has some of the characteristics of lysozymes (Lackman et al.). Splenomeg-

Fig. 28—7. — Chediak-Higashi syndrome. Smear of bone marrow showing inclusions in the cytoplasm of the polymorphonuclear cells. (Courtesy Dr. G. Vawter.)

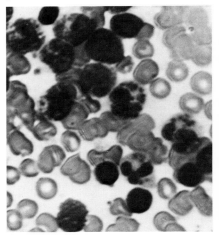

aly, when present, is accompanied by thrombocytopenia, probably secondary to hypersplenism.

At autopsy, histiocytes are found infiltrating lymph nodes, spleen, adventitia of the aorta, connective tissue of the liver, retroperitoneal fat and perivascular areas of the brain. In the latter areas the cells contain a large paranuclear lipid inclusion. Histiocytic infiltration of peripheral nerves may be associated with myelin degeneration.

FAMILIAL CHRONIC GRANULOMATOUS DISEASE.—In this inherited sex-linked recessive disorder the polymorphonuclear cells are capable of phagocytosis but incapable of digesting the engulfed bacteria. The abnormality appears to be related to disturbances in energy metabolism inasmuch as the increases in respiration and oxidation of glucose normally associated with phagocytosis and intracellular digestion do not occur (Holmes *et al.*). Because of this, infections cannot be overcome in the usual way and chronic lingering suppuration results.

In the usual case the symptoms begin in the first few months of life, although death does not occur for several years and one patient has been recorded who survived to adult life (Bridges *et al.*). The first symptom may be diarrhea, which is eventually followed by suppuration of superficial lymph nodes (Carson *et al.*). Dermatitis, acute and chronic pneumonitis and rhinitis are usually present; less common are osteomyelitis, empyema, peritonitis, meningitis and deep or superficial abscesses. Accompanying the inflammatory lesions are the usual systemic reactions to severe infection such as anemia, increased sedimentation rate, leukocytosis, hypergammaglobulinemia and hyperplasia of bone marrow.

The process acquires its name from the characteristic granulomatous nature of the terminal lesions in the lymph nodes, liver, lungs (Fig. 28–8) and spleen. Active abscesses are surrounded by broad zones of fibrous tissue with a granulomatous reaction and many multinucleated cells. In the lungs there is also a mild diffuse infiltration of mononuclear cells. Landing and Sharkey noted the presence in older children of pigmented histiocytes in the liver, spleen, adrenal glands, lymph nodes and bone marrow. In younger infants the process may be less characteristic histologically. Salmonella sepsis often occurs as a terminal event.

ALDRICH'S SYNDROME.—In this recessive hereditary syndrome, which affects males only, there is an increased susceptibility to infection, especially of the skin and respiratory system, in spite of a normal level of gamma globulin. Thrombocytopenia

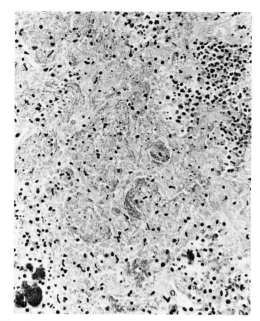

Fig. 28–8.—Familial chronic granulomatous disease. Lung showing zone of necrotic parenchyma with polymorphonuclear cells in upper right and masses of bacteria in the lower left.

is present at birth, and in a third of all cases death results from uncontrollable bleeding. There are no specific pathologic findings, and the defect in the immunologic apparatus has not been identified (Gordon).

CONGENITAL DEFICIENCY OF POLYMORPHONUCLEAR LEUKOCYTES.—A form of cellular deficiency in which granulocytes are absent from the peripheral blood and few are found in the bone marrow was first described by Fanconi. Skin infections occur commonly, and death often results from sepsis (Smith). No hereditary pattern has been established and no cases have been observed in siblings.

LEUKEMIA.—Leukemia is rare in young infants, but symptoms may be well advanced at birth or appear in the first few days of life. Pierce found 45 such cases reported by 1959, of which 37 were myelogenous, five lymphatic, two stem cell and one reticuloendothelial. The incidence of leukemia is three times greater among individuals with Down's syndrome than among those of the general population, and this is even greater in the newborn period. This association is of interest because myelogenous leukemia in the nonmongolian is accompanied by a partial deletion of chromosome 21, and in Down's syndrome it is this chromosome that is trip-

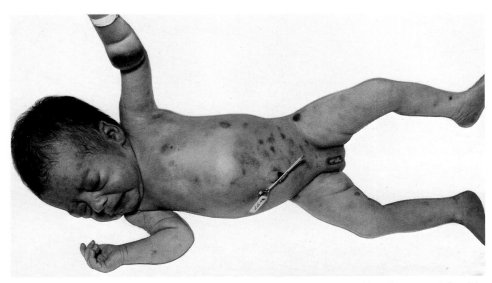

Fig. 28–9.—Myelogenous leukemia. Multiple flat and elevated areas of involvement of the skin. Largest area is in the left antecubital fossa. Death at 2 days.

Fig. 28–10 (left).—Myelogenous leukemia. Blood smear showing great numbers of promyelocytes. From infant shown in Fig. 28–9.

Fig. 28–11 (right).—Myelogenous leukemia. Elevated area in skin caused by dense infiltration by promyelocytes. From infant shown in Fig. 28–9.

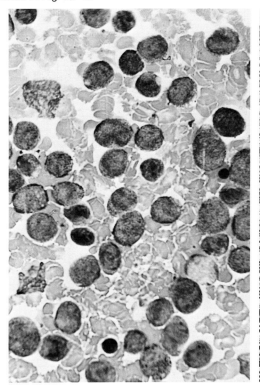

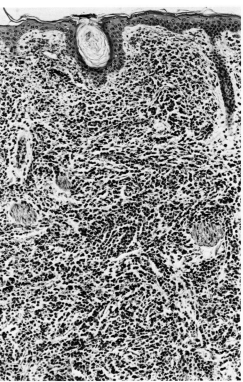

loid. In some cases of Down's syndrome with mye-logenous leukemia the leukemic process is transient. Engel *et al.* reported a number of such cases, and one mongolian infant with clinical myelogenous leukemia seen at the Boston Children's Hospital Medical Center had no evidence of leukemia at autopsy; the infant died of a cardiac malformation. Neonatal leukemia was reported in siblings by Campbell *et al.*

At the Chicago Lying-in Hospital three infants were studied, two of whom died at about 2 months and one at 2 days, all with severe manifestations of the disease. At birth the last infant had numerous indurated, flat, elevated skin lesions, some of which were hemorrhagic and some of normal skin color. They varied in diameter from a few millimeters to several centimeters and were most numerous over the trunk although they were also present on the face and extremities. The largest individual lesion was in the left antecubital fossa (Fig. 28–9). Immediately after birth the blood had a total count of 369,000 nucleated cells per cu mm. The majority were large immature mononuclear cells with basophilic cytoplasm. The chromatin of the nuclei was finely divided and evenly distributed. Nucleoli were occasionally present, and most cells contained a large number of fine azure granules. Peroxidase stain revealed granules in many cells that were interpreted as promyelocytes (Fig. 28–10). The infant did poorly from birth; when death occurred, the liver weighed 220 gm and the spleen 13.2 gm, but other viscera were of approximately normal weight. The external surface of the liver was covered by interlacing narrow white bands that histologically were composed of connective tissue densely infiltrated by promyelocytes (see Fig. 20–23). Histologic examination revealed an amazing number of cells similar to those in the blood in almost all of the tissues of the body. They were found in all connective tissue, and their presence between individual muscle cells caused a striking distortion of most muscles. They were present in the dermis of the entire body, with excessive infiltration being responsible for obliteration of all normal structures in the areas that were elevated above the body surface (Fig. 28–11). Lymphoid tissue was reduced. The thymus was small, weighing only 4.7 gm, and myeloid cells were absent except in the interlobular connective tissue. Wide zones of immature cells extended outward from the portal triads in the liver. The normal structures of the pancreas were almost obliterated by similar cells. None was found in the thyroid, adrenal glands or brain except in the blood vessels and the surrounding connective tissue. Malpighian corpuscles were not visible in the spleen, but immature myeloid cells were present in the pulp and sinuses.

Lymphomas

Lymphomas have not been described in the early months of life. Among 1,269 cases Rosenberg *et al.* found none with an onset earlier than 22 months of age.

Congenital Abnormalities of Bleeding and Clotting Time

THROMBOCYTOPENIC PURPURA. – This disease has been reported infrequently in the newborn period or later infancy, and clear-cut criteria for its diagnosis have not been established. Widespread "purpuric" hemorrhages in the skin, positive response to the tourniquet test and reduction in blood thrombocytes are generally given as the most outstanding characteristics. Melena is common, and major hemorrhage may occur in any part of the body. Bleeding time is ordinarily prolonged, and clotting time is normal although clot retraction is delayed and incomplete.

In the newborn the condition may be secondary to various causes such as destruction by placentally transmitted maternal antibodies, toxic substances derived from a dead twin or removal of platelets from the circulation, as in a giant hemangioma. It may be a primary failure of platelet formation or of unknown cause. In later infancy it may result from infections such as syphilis and cytomegalic inclusion disease, it may be associated with congenital aplastic anemia, leukemia or erythroblastosis, or it may result from sensitivity to certain drugs such as quinine.

A mother with thrombocytopenic purpura does not transmit this disease to her child, but about 60% of the infants of affected mothers have low platelet counts for 4 to 6 weeks as a result of placentally transmitted antibodies, and symptoms of purpura may be present during that time. This may be true even though the mother has had a splenectomy that has successfully controlled her own disease (Harrington *et al.*). Rarely, a mother may develop antibodies against the platelets of the fetus, and a few instances have been reported in which mother and fetus both developed antibodies against the cells of the other (Epstein *et al.*).

In some cases thrombocytopenia may be secondary to disseminated intravascular coagulation. In multiple pregnancies in which one twin dies and becomes macerated, on rare occasions disseminated intravascular coagulation is produced in the other twin by abnormal circulating substances arising from the dead conceptus. In the nonmacerated twin, renal and cerebral necroses as well as splenic infarcts have been seen at autopsy. In some cases advanced cerebral encephalomalacia has been found as an indication of an infarctive episode weeks or months before the termination of pregnancy (Moore *et al.*).

Disseminated intravascular thromboses without obvious cause have been found in various locations, including the cerebral sinuses, and have been responsible for infarcts of the lungs and adrenal glands (Leissring and Vorlicky). At the Boston Hospital for Women disseminated intravascular coagulation has been seen in some newborn infants with generalized viral infections such as herpes and rubella.

The term *purpura fulminans* has been applied to cases in which extensive thrombosis of small superficial blood vessels, usually of the extremities, is accompanied by necrosis of the skin. Such lesions are usually caused by infection or a hypersensitivity reaction (Morse *et al.*).

A few women observed at the Chicago Lying-in Hospital have had a diagnosis of thrombocytopenic purpura made either before or during pregnancy. Their infants have had cutaneous petechiae and low platelet counts for a few days following delivery, but all have been normal by 10 days of life. Children have also been seen with widespread petechiae whose mothers had no history of purpura. Platelet counts in these children have varied, a few being low, others normal. The hemorrhages have disappeared promptly without treatment, and no other symptoms have developed.

HEMORRHAGIC DISEASE.—Hemorrhagic disease at present is usually defined as a condition in which a prolongation of prothrombin time due to a lack of vitamin K is associated with evidence of gross bleeding, usually from the gastrointestinal tract, less often from other sites. The original definition of Townsend in 1894 was of spontaneous external or internal bleeding occurring in newborn infants, unrelated to trauma, accident or definite disease. Later the hemorrhage was found to be associated with prolongation of coagulation time, and it was thought that the intravascular injection of blood would decrease coagulation time and prevent bleeding. Arguments were numerous as to which cases should be included under this diagnosis and as to whether a prolongation of coagulation time was a necessary part of the disease.

Absent antihemophilic globulin, plasma thromboplastin component (PTC) or thrombocytopenia, either from maternal antibody activity acting on fetal platelets or congenital or acquired disease of the fetus, may cause hemorrhage, but the use of the term for such hemorrhage dilutes it to a symptomatic description.

It is now known that vitamin K deficiency causes not only low prothrombin levels but also a deficiency of other vitamin K–dependent factors such as factors VII, IX (plasma prothrombin component) and X (Stuart-Prower factor) (Ehling). Corrections of such factors by supply of vitamin K is not immediate, and often blood transfusions are required to stop bleeding until these substances can be manufactured in the body.

Other deficiencies of blood coagulation factors may accompany prothrombin deficiencies but are rarely the sole cause of hemorrhage in the newborn. Proconvertin levels follow prothrombin levels and may be as low as 3% of the normal adult level.

Since many infants with severe prolongation of prothrombin time have no evidence of hemorrhage, some inciting factor in addition to the change in prothrombin level seems to be necessary for the initiation of bleeding. Hemorrhage from intracranial vessels, liver, adrenal glands and lungs can usually be directly attributed to trauma or anoxia; although it is impossible to prove that the hemorrhage was not exaggerated by prolongation of prothrombin time, the latter cannot be considered the only cause of the bleeding, and such cases are eliminated on the basis of Townsend's original description.

The use of the diagnosis has come to be limited largely to infants with bloody emesis or melena. Occasionally, hemorrhage from the stump of the umbilical cord is included, but this can usually be attributed to local trauma. Any blood loss from the vagina is usually slight, hormonal in origin and not related to hemorrhagic disease. It has been shown that the amount of blood necessary to produce tarry stools is only about 2 ml (Potter), and melena may result from very slight blood loss.

The mortality appears to have dropped remarkably since the introduction of vitamin K therapy, although fatal cases are occasionally still reported despite treatment with this substance.

HEMOPHILIA.—Hemophilia is an hereditary hemorrhagic disease characterized by a delay in blood coagulation that is responsible for a tendency to bleed. Platelet count, clot retraction, fibrinogen and prothrombin concentrations, tourniquet test and bleeding time are normal. The clinical picture of severe hemorrhage from minor injury can be produced by a deficiency of any one of several clotting factors.

Hemophilia A, which is true or classic hemophilia, results from inability to produce adequate antihemophilic globulin (AHG). Inherited as a sex-linked recessive trait, it is found almost exclusively in males, the causative gene being transmitted through the female because of its position on the X chromosome. The tendency to bleed is present from birth and may be responsible for severe hemorrhage from circumcision. Hemorrhages in other locations are not common until after the child begins to walk, when minor trauma may cause bleeding in any tissue or organ.

Hemophilia B, or Christmas factor disease, is caused by deficiency of the plasma thromboplastin component (PTC). Like true hemophilia, it is inherited as a sex-linked recessive trait found only in males. It is responsible for about 15% of all hemophilia. The symptoms are identical to those of hemophilia A.

Hemophilia C is the result of a defect in synthesis of plasma thromboplastin antecedent (PTA). It is inherited as an autosomal dominant trait and affects both males and females. Although it may appear in the first hours of life, the tendency to hemorrhage is ordinarily not as great as in hemophilia A and B.

Von Willebrand's syndrome resembles hemophilia A in the tendency to bleed and the occurrence of hematomas in infancy. In this disease a vascular abnormality appears to be the main cause of deficient hemostasis, but in some instances a mild deficiency of antihemophilic globulin is associated. The suggestion has been made that the first be termed pseudohemophilia and the second autosomal vascular hemophilia. Both varieties are transmitted as autosomal dominant traits affecting both sexes.

Congenital Afibrinogenemia

Although this disease has rarely been diagnosed in the newborn, it must be suspected in any infant with evidence of hemorrhage. Older children with this diagnosis often have a history of prolonged bleeding from the umbilicus, great susceptibility to bruising and uncontrollable but usually mild hemorrhage from minor cuts or lacerations. The diagnosis is based on absent or unusually low values of fibrinogen in the blood, the normal in the newborn—according to Taylor—being 231 mg per 100 ml. The platelet count is variable, at times being abnormally low. Capillary resistance is usually diminished, the bleeding time prolonged and the blood incoagulable. The disease appears to be hereditary; it occurs in siblings, and a high degree of consanguinity has been reported in the parents. There is a strong likelihood that at least some of the cases of so-called hemorrhagic disease belong in this category. In afibrinogenemia the prognosis is poor, and death usually occurs in early childhood. With hypofibrinogenemia the life-span may not be shortened; it may accompany any severe disease of the hepatic parenchyma.

REFERENCES

Allen, F. H., Jr., and Diamond, L. K.: *Erythroblastosis Fetalis* (Boston: Little, Brown & Co., 1958).

Bartman, J., and Driscoll, S. G.: Fetal adrenal cortex in erythroblastosis fetalis, Arch. Pathol. 87:343, 1969.

Borum, A., Lloyd, H. O., and Talbot, T. R., Jr.: Possible fetal hemorrhage into maternal circulation, J.A.M.A. 164:1087, 1957.

Bridges, R. A., Berendes, H., and Good, R. A.: A fatal granulomatous disease of childhood, Am. J. Dis. Child. 97:387, 1954.

Burko, H., Watson, J., and Robinson, M.: Unusual bone changes in sickle cell disease in childhood, Pediatrics 80:957, 1957.

Burman, D.: Congenital spherocytosis in infancy, Arch. Dis. Child. 33:335, 1956.

Campbell, W. A. B., MacAfee, H. L., and Wade, W. G.: Familial neonatal leukemia, Arch. Dis. Child. 37:93, 1962.

Carson, M. J., et al.: Thirteen boys with progressive septic granulomatosis, Pediatrics 35:405, 1965.

Cook, C. D., Brodie, H. R., and Allen, D. W.: Measurement of fetal hemoglobin in newborn infant: Correlation with gestational age and intrauterine hypoxia, Pediatrics 20:272, 1957.

Cooper, M. D., Kincade, P. W., and Lawton, A. R., III: Thymic and Bursal Function, in Kagan, B. M., and Stiehm, E. R. (eds.): *Immunologic Incompetence* (Chicago: Year Book Medical Publishers, Inc., 1971), p. 81.

Corston, J. McC. D., et al.: Five years' experience with intrauterine transfusion, Can. Med. Assoc. J. 103:594, 1970.

Craddock, C. G., Longmire, R., and McMillan, R.: Lymphocytes and the immune response, N. Engl. J. Med. 285:324, 1971.

Dancis, J., Brenner, M. A., and Money, W. L.: Some factors affecting the permeability of the guinea pig placenta, Am. J. Obstet. Gynecol. 84:570, 1962.

Darrow, D. C., and Carry, M. K.: Serum albumen and globulin of newborn, premature and normal infants, J. Pediat: 3:573, 1933.

Diamond, L. K., Allen, D. M., and Magill, F. B.: Congenital (erythroid) hypoplastic anemia, Am. J. Dis. Child. 102:149, 1961.

Dignan, D. St. J., Mauer, A. M., and Frank, C.: Phocomelia with congenital hypoplastic thrombocytopenia, and myeloid leukemoid reactions, J. Pediatr. 70:561, 1967.

Dine, M. S.: Congenital methemoglobinemia in newborn period, Am. J. Dis. Child. 92:15, 1956.

Ehling, L. R.: Hemorrhagic disease of the newborn, Am. J. Dis. Child. 101:241, 1960.

Eng, L. L.: Alpha chain thalassemia and hydrops fetalis in Malaya—report of five cases, Blood 20:581, 1962.

Engel, R. R., et al.: Transient congenital leukemia in 7 infants with mongolism, J. Pediatr. 65:303, 1964.

Epstein, R. D., et al.: Congenital thrombocytopenic purpura: Purpura haemorrhagica in pregnancy and in the newborn, Am. J. Med. 9:44, 1950.

Fanconi, G.: Familiäre infantile pernizioaartige Anämie (perniziöses bluthild und Konstitution), in Jahrbuch der Kinderheilkunde, Vol. 117, p. 257, 1927.

Forrester, R. M., and Miller, J.: Dental changes associated with kernicterus, Arch. Dis. Child. 30:224, 1955.

Gairdner, D., Marks, J., and Roscoe, J. D.: Blood formation in infancy: IV. Early anemia of prematurity, Arch. Dis. Child. 30:203, 1955.

Gilmour, J. R.: Normal hematopoiesis in intrauterine and neonatal life, J. Pathol. Bacteriol. 52:25, 1941.

Gitlin, D.: Development and Metabolism of the Immune Globulins, in Kagan, B. M., and Stiehm, E. R. (eds.): Immunologic Incompetence (Chicago: Year Book Medical Publishers, Inc., 1971), p. 3.

Good, T. A., Carnazzo, S. F., and Good, R. A.: Thrombocytopenia and giant hemangioma in infants, Am. J. Dis. Child. 90:260, 1955.

Gordon, R. R.: Aldrich syndrome: Familial thrombocytopenia, eczema, infection, Arch. Dis. Child. 35:259, 1960.

Gudson, R. P., et al.: Amniotic fluid antibody titers and other prognostic parameters in erythroblastosis fetalis, Am. J. Obstet. Gynecol. 108:85, 1970.

Harrington, W. J., Minnick, V., and Arimura, G.: Autoimmune thrombocytopenias, Prog. Hematol. 1:166, 1956.

Henderson, J. L., Donaldson, G. M. M., and Scarborough, H.: Congenital afibrinogenaemia, Q. J. Med. 38:101, 1945.

Hendrickse, R. G., and Collard, P.: Salmonella osteitis in Nigerian children, Lancet 1:80, 1960.

Holmes, B., Page, G. R., and Good, R. A.: Studies of metabolic activity of erythrocytes from patients with a genetic abnormality of phagocytic function, J. Clin. Invest. 46:1472, 1967.

Hughes, D. W. O'G.: Hypoplastic anemia in infancy and childhood: Erythroid hypoplasia, Arch. Dis. Child. 26:349, 1961.

Ivy, R. E., and Howard, F. H.: Sickle cell anemia with unusual bone changes, J. Pediatr. 43:312, 1953.

Jaffe, E. R., and Heller, P.: Methemoglobinemia in Man, in Moore, C. V., and Brown, E. B. (eds.): Progress in Hematology (New York: Grune & Stratton, 1969), Vol. IV.

Johnstone, R. B., and McMurray, J. S.: Chronic familial granulomatous disease, N. Engl. J. Med. 277:899, 1967.

Katz, J.: Transplacental passage of fetal red cells in abortions; increased incidence after curettage and effect of oxytocic drugs, Br. Med. J. 4:84, 1969.

Kritzler, R. A., et al.: Chediak-Higashi syndrome, Am. J. Med. 36:583, 1964.

Lackman, L. A., Kennedy, W. R., and White, J. G.: The Chediak-Higashi syndrome: Electro-physiological and electron microscopic observations on the peripheral neuropathy, J. Pediatr. 70:742, 1967.

Landing, B. H., and Sharkey, H. S.: A syndrome of recurrent infection and infiltration of viscera by pigmented lipid histiocytes, Pediatrics 20:431, 1957.

Leissring, J. C., and Vorlicky, L. W.: Disseminated intravascular coagulation in a neonate, Am. J. Dis. Child. 115:100, 1968.

Matsumura, T., et al.: Quoted by Gitlin, D., in Development and Metabolism of the Immune Globulins, in Kogan, B. M., and Strehan, E. R. (eds.): Immunologic Incompetence (Chicago: Year Book Medical Publishers, Inc., 1971), p. 3.

Mattelaer, P. M., and Riley, H. D., Jr.: Leukemia in the neonatal period, Ann. Pediatr. 203:124, 1964.

Mauer, A. M.: Pediatric Hematology (New York: McGraw-Hill Book Co., 1969).

Mauer, A. M., DeVaux, W., and Lohey, M. E.: Neonatal and maternal thrombocytopenic purpura due to quinine, Pediatrics 19:84, 1957.

McLorey, D. C., and Fish, S. A.: Fetal erythrocytes in maternal circulation, Am. J. Obstet. Gynecol. 95:824, 1966.

Miller, A. A.: Congenital sulfhemoglobinemia, J. Pediatr. 51:233, 1957.

Minagi, H., and Steinboch, H. L.: Roentgen appearance of anomalies associated with hypoplastic anemias of childhood. Fanconi's anemia (erythrogenesis imperfecta), Am. J. Roentgenol. 97:100, 1966.

Mitchell, A. P. B., Anderson, G. S., and Russell, J. K.: Perinatal death from foetal exsanguination, Br. Med. J. 1: 611, 1957.

Mollison, P. L., and Cutbush, M.: Hemolytic disease of the newborn due to fetal maternal ABO incompatibility, Prog. Hematol. 2:153, 1959.

Moore, C. M., MacAdams, A. J., and Sutherland, J.: Intrauterine disseminated intravascular coagulation syndrome of multiple pregnancy with a dead twin fetus, J. Pediatr. 74:523, 1969.

Morse, T., Dorive, M. I., and Hartigan, M.: Purpura fulminans, Arch. Surg. 93:268, 1966.

Necheles, T. F., and Allen, D. F.: Heinz body anemias, N. Engl. J. Med. 280:203, 1969.

Page, A. R.: The Chediak-Higashi syndrome, Blood 20: 330, 1962.

Pearson, H. A., Shanklin, D. R., and Brodine, C. R.: Alpha-thalassemia as a cause of nonimmunologic hydrops, Am. J. Dis. Child. 109:168, 1965.

Pierce, M. I.: Leukemia in a newborn infant, J. Pediatr. 54:691, 1959.

Potter, E. L.: Present status of Rh factor, Am. J. Dis. Child. 68:32, 1944.

Potter, E. L.: Effect on infant mortality of vitamin K administered during labor, Am. J. Obstet. Gynecol. 50: 237, 1945.

Potter, E. L.: Diagnosis of erythroblastosis in the macerated fetus, Arch. Pathol. 41:233, 1946.

Potter, E. L.: The Rh factor, Med. Clin. North Am. 31:236, 1947.

Potter, E. L.: Rh: Its Relation to Erythroblastosis Fetalis and Intragroup Transfusion Reactions (Chicago: Year Book Medical Publishers, Inc., 1947).

Potter, E. L.: Reproductive histories of 322 mothers of infants with erythroblastosis, Pediatrics 2:369, 1948.

Potter, E. L.: Outlook for future pregnancies in women immunized to Rh, Am. J. Obstet. Gynecol. 75:348, 1958.

Potter, E. L.: Antenatal background of blood diseases of infancy, J. Pediatr. 54:552, 1959.

Potter, E. L., and Bernstein, H. E.: Hematologic studies on children of Rh-negative women compared to those of

Rh-positive women, J. Pediatr. 32:246, 1948.

Rosenberg, S. A., *et al.*: Lymphosarcoma—a review of 1269 cases, Medicine 40:31, 1961.

Schoen, E. J., King, A. L., and Duane, R. T.: Neonatal thrombocytopenic purpura, Pediatrics 17:72, 1956.

Shapiro, G. M., *et al.*: Hereditary spherocytosis in neonatal period: Diagnosis, incidence and treatment, J. Pediatr. 50:308, 1957.

Shiller, J. G.: Shock in the newborn caused by transplacental hemorrhage from fetus to mother, Pediatrics 20: 7, 1957.

Smith, C. A.: *Physiology of the Newborn Infant* (3d ed.; Springfield, Ill.: Charles C Thomas, 1959).

Smith, C. H.: *Blood Disease in Infancy and Childhood* (St. Louis: C. V. Mosby Co., 1966).

Spurling, C. L., Sacks, M. S., and Jiji, R. M.: Juvenile pernicious anemia, N. Engl. J. Med. 271:995, 1964.

Stern, K., Davidsohn, I., and Buznitsky, A.: Neonatal serologic diagnosis of hemolytic disease of newborn caused by ABO incompatibility, J. Lab. Clin. Med. 50: 550, 1957.

Taylor, P. M.: Concentration of fibrinogen in plasma of newborn infants, Pediatrics 19:233, 1957.

Valentine, W. N., and Tanaka, K. R.: Pyruvate Kinase and Other Hereditary Enzyme Deficiencies, in Stanbury, J. B., *et al.* (eds.): *Metabolic Basis of Inherited Disease* (3d ed.; Baltimore: Williams & Wilkins Co., 1972), p. 1338.

Walker, J., and Turnbull, E. P. N.: Haemoglobin and red cells in human foetus: III. Foetal and adult haemoglobin, Arch. Dis. Child. 30:111, 1955.

Watson, R. J., *et al.*: Hand-foot syndrome in sickle cell disease in young children, Pediatrics 31:975, 1963.

Zuelzer, W. W., Neel, J. V., and Robinson, A. R.: Abnormal hemoglobins, Prog. Hematol. 1:191, 1956.

Zuelzer, W. W., and Ogden, F. W.: Megaloblastic anemia in infancy: Common syndrome responding specifically to folic acid therapy, Am. J. Dis. Child. 71:211, 1946.

Index

AMNIOTIC FLUID IN -- 281-282